naon

Core Curriculum for Orthopaedic Nursing

4th Edition 2001

Delores C. Schoen, PhD, RN,C, FAAN
Editor
Adjunct Professor, School of Nursing
The Pennsylvania State University
University Park, Pennsylvania

Published for NAON by
Anthony J. Jannetti, Inc., East Holly Avenue Box 56, Pitman, New Jersey 08071-0056

CORPORATE SPONSORS

The Core Curriculum for Orthopaedic Nursing was funded in part through generous education grants from the following companies:

AMGEN® DePuy a Johnson & Johnson company PURDUE™

For more information about these corporate sponsors, see page 567.

NAON also thanks SYNTHES® *for its additional support of this publication.*

The National Association of Orthopaedic Nurses (NAON) is the professional specialty organization of nurses who provide musculoskeletal health care. NAON's mission is to advance the quality of musculoskeletal health care by promoting excellence in research, education, and nursing practice.

Contact NAON at:
East Holly Avenue, Box 56, Pitman, NJ 08071-0056
Phone: 800.289.NAON (6266)
Fax: 856.589.7463 or 856.256.2349
E-mail: naon@ajj.com
Web Site: naon.inurse.com or orthopaedicnurse.org

ISBN 1-892665-11-5

TABLE OF CONTENTS

TABLE OF CONTENTS

TABLE OF CONTENTS

TABLE OF CONTENTS

TABLE OF CONTENTS

TABLE OF CONTENTS

TABLE OF CONTENTS

PREFACE

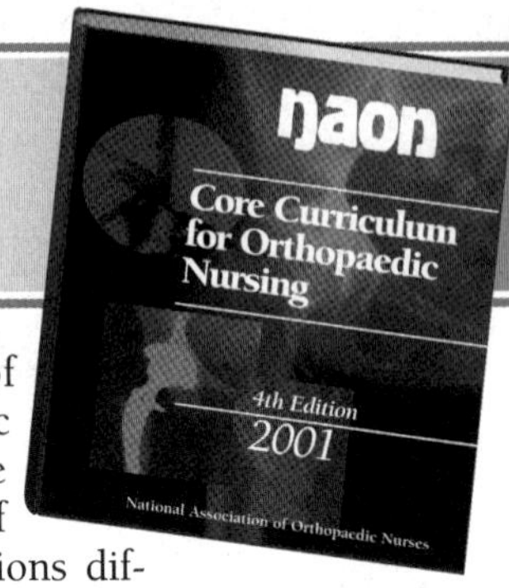

Nursing is a profession undergoing rapid change in the face of a global transformation in health care. Despite all the changes that have occurred in nursing and in the workplace, orthopaedics provides nurses opportunities for professional experiences in a wide variety of settings, with many types of pathologies, and with patients of all ages.

Whether the nursing care setting is acute care, subacute care, home care, case management, pediatrics, geriatrics, clinical/office practice, operating room nursing, advanced practice, education, or research, it is still orthopaedic nursing practice.

The mission of the National Association of Orthopaedic Nurses (NAON) is to advance the quality of musculoskeletal health care by promoting excellence in orthopaedic nursing research, education, and practice. NAON, as a dynamic specialty nursing organization, has been continually evolving to better meet the needs of its members and the patients they serve. As part of that effort, NAON strives to provide educational offerings and materials to meet the diverse needs of its members.

The content of the 4th edition of the *Core Curriculum for Orthopaedic Nursing* provides information to assist nurses in learning and/or reviewing the broad scope of orthopaedics and is relevant to all clinical settings. There were three major goals in the development of the 4th edition:

1. To explicate the critical nursing roles and responsibilities in the care of individuals with orthopaedic conditions.
2. To present new knowledge about the care of individuals at risk for or with an orthopaedic condition.
3. To incorporate NAON's revised *Scope and Standards of Orthopaedic Nursing Practice*.

NAON intends for this resource on orthopaedic nursing to serve the needs of a number of audiences. First, this is an ideal reference text for a senior level undergraduate or graduate level nursing course. For faculty teaching courses designed for associate degree, diploma, or baccalaureate students, the content greatly facilitates the preparation of lectures and presentations. Second, the text is an extremely useful resource for graduate nurses starting to work in the field of orthopaedics. Third, it is a great source of information for orthopaedic nurses changing their work setting from acute care to subacute, clinic, home care, or other settings. Fourth, the *Core Curriculum* is an excellent resource for a nurse returning to the work force in orthopaedics. Fifth, the text is an excellent resource for nurses to use in preparing for the orthopaedic nursing certification (ONC) examination. Sixth, it is a good resource for orthopaedic nurse researchers. Finally, the book is of value to both nurses and non-nurses as a general reference on orthopaedic nursing.

The content stresses those principles unique to orthopaedic nursing and addresses the critical nursing roles and knowledge required. Emphasis is placed on care for patients in the major clinical settings: office/clinic, acute hospital care, and rehabilitation/home care. Pediatric conditions are the focus of Chapter 11, and pediatric and/or geriatric aspects are identified in each chapter if the care for these populations differs from standard care for adults. Trauma is the subject of Chapter 14, and information on trauma and sports injuries is included throughout the book where appropriate.

Each chapter begins with a title page that includes the name of the author(s), their credentials, and a listing of the chapter's contents (with page numbers). The next page outlines the chapter's objectives and key points, with the text beginning on the third page. For each pathology/condition, the content is organized under broad headings as follows:

I. Overview (including definition, etiology, pathophysiology, incidence, considerations across the lifespan, and complications).
II. Assessment (including history, physical examination, and diagnostic tests).
III. Common therapeutic modalities.
IV. Nursing diagnoses, outcomes, and interventions.
V. Practice setting considerations.

Each chapter concludes with a bibliography and study questions.

The content presented in each chapter ranges from basic information to advanced practice in that area of orthopaedic nursing. Chapter 1 (Practice Settings for Orthopaedic Nursing) is a new chapter that describes the many different practice settings for orthopaedic nurses and outlines job qualifications. Chapters 2-15 and 17-18 present revised and updated materials on chapters that appeared in the 3rd edition of the core. Chapters 16 and 19-21 are new and present the nursing care of orthopaedic patients with conditions related to The Shoulder; The Hip, Femur, and Pelvis; The Knee; and The Foot and Ankle.

I would like to take this opportunity to thank the editors, authors, and reviewers of the previous Cores for their work. It was the foundation on which the present editor, authors, and reviewers were able develop the 4th edition. My thanks and appreciation also go to our sponsors AMGEN Inc.; Depuy, a Johnson and Johnson company; Purdue Pharma L.P.; and Synthes (USA) for their financial support; to Dr. Lorry Schoenly for her advice and support; to Janet D'Alesandro for her superb editorial work; to Maryanne Hatfield for her many roles from editing to communicating with authors and reviewers; to Jack Bryant and Darin Peters for the cover design and the addition of color; and to Dr. Robert Schoen for all of his love, support, understanding, and encouragement when things did not go as planned. My thanks also go to the NAON Executive Board and the Director of Education for allowing me the opportunity to edit the 4th edition of NAON's *Core Curriculum for Orthopaedic Nursing*.

Delores C. Schoen, PhD, RN,C, FAAN

Editor, NAON *Core Curriculum for Orthopaedic Nurses*, 4th Edition

Authors

Nancy Abbate, RN, CNOR, ONC
Nurse Clinician
Dr. David Altchek
New York, NY

Cindy Bagwell-Crum, MEd, BSN, RN, CNOR, CST
Chairman/Assistant Professor
University of Arkansas for Medical Sciences
Veteran Affairs Healthcare System
Little Rock, AR

Donna M. Barker, MS, RN, ONC
Staff Nurse
Personalized Family Care
Barrington, IL

Rebecca Jo Carpenter, BSN, RN, ONC
Nurse Manager Ortho/Neuro Unit
Proctor Hospital
Peoria, IL

Judith A. Chase, BS, MA, RN,C, ONC
Adult Nurse Practitioner
Carle Clinic
Urbana, IL

Sharon G. Childs MS, CRNP-CS, ONC
Assistant Professor
Johns Hopkins University
Nurse Practitioner
Department of Orthopaedic Surgery
Johns Hopkins Bayview Medical Center
Baltimore, MD

John P. Davis, BS, RN, ONC
Nurse Clinician/Quality Manger
Richard S. Laskin, MD
Hospital for Special Surgery
New York, NY

Kathleen A. Geier, MS, RN, ONC
Orthopaedic Clinical Nurse Specialist
Webster Orthopaedic Medical Group/Jackson Arthitis Center
Oakland, CA

Kimberly K. Haynes, MS, RN, CS, ONC
Clinical Nurse Specialist
Mid-America Sarcoma Institute
Overland Park, KS

Margaret Hickey, MS, RN, ONC
Clinical Nurse Specialist
Rush-Presbyterian St. Luke Medical Center
Chicago, IL

Victoria M. Hoshowsky, MSN, RN, CRNP, ONC
Family Nurse Practitioner
Rising Sun Family Practice Center
Philadelphia, PA
(Previously employed as Perioperative Clinical Nurse Specialist, Jeffferson University Hospital, Philadelphia, PA)

Marianne Genge Jagmin, PhD, RN, ONC
Assistant Professor - Per Diem Faculty
Rush University
Chicago, IL

Cathleen E. Kunkler, BSN, RN, CNA, ONC
Independent Nurse Consultant
Nichols, NY

Phyllis Lisanti, PhD, RN
Clinical Associate Professor
New York University - Division of Nursing
New York, NY

Ann Butler Maher, MS, RN, APNC, ONC
Family Nurse Practitioner
Sussex Family Practice
Sussex, NJ

Kimberly J. Mason, MSN, RN
Coordinator of Patient Care Systems and Standards
The Children's Hospital of Philadelphia
Philadelphia, PA

Nancy S. Morris, PhD, RN, CS
Assistant Professsor
University of Vermont
Adult Nurse Practitioner
Colchester Family Practice
Burlington, VT

Nina A. Rauscher, MS, RN,C, CRRN, ONC
Corporate Director - Performance Improvement and Quality
The North Shore Medical Center
Salem, MA

Dottie Roberts, MSN, MACI, RN,C, CNS, ONC
Medical-Surgical Clinical Nurse Specialist
Penrose-St. Francis Health Services
Colorado Springs, CO

Mary Faut Rodts, MS, MSA, RN, ONC
Assistant Professor
Rush University
Chicago, IL

Susan C. Ruda, MS, RN, ONC
Clinical Nurse Specialist
Parkview Musculoskeletal Institute
Palos Heights, IL

Maureen (Moe) Schmitt, MN, FNP, ONC
Nurse Practitioner - Orthopaedics
Crouse Hospital
Syracuse, NY

Karen A. Sikorski, MS, RN
Clinical Nurse Specialist/Pain
OSF Saint Anthony Medical Center
Rockford, IL

Luann M. Theis, BSN, RN, ONC
Director Ortho/Neuro & Rehab Units
Wausau Hospital
Wausau, WI

Janet S. Tompkins, MS, Ed, MSN, ARNP-C
Instructor/Nurse Practitioner
Department of Orthopaedics and Rehabilitation
University of Miami School of Medicine
Miami, FL

Karen E. Zorn, BSN, RN, ONC
Practice Coordinator
Resurgens Orthopaedics
Atlanta, GA

REVIEWERS

Elizabeth B. Abrahams, MSN, RN, ONC
Clinical Nurse Specialist, Materials Management
Inova Health System
Falls Church, VA

Shirley K. Bole, RN, ONC
Nurse Coordinator, Orthopaedic Oncology
Emory Clinic
Atlanta, GA

Toni Cawley, RN, ONC
Nurse Specialist II
University of Miami/Spine Institute
Miami, FL

Jo Anne Greene, MS, RN, CS, ONC
Clinical Nurse Practitioner
Wesley Glen
Columbus, OH

Jacqueline L. Harris, MNSc, RN, ONC
Assistant Professor of Nursing
Harding University
Searcy, AK

Katherine M. Hart, BSN, RN
Director, Orthopaedics
Children's Healthcare of Atlanta
Atlanta, GA

Kimberly K. Haynes, MS, RN, CS, ONC
Clinical Nurse Specialist
Mid-America Sarcoma Institute
Overland Park, KS

Amy Helmuth, MS, RN, ONC
Nurse Manager, Ortho/Neuro
Pinnacle Health Hospitals
Harrisburg, PA

Arleen L. Hodge, MS, RN, ACNP-C
Nurse Practitioner - Adult Orthopaedic Spine
Associate in Orthopaedics
Adjunct Faculty
Vanderbilt University Medical Center
Nashville, TN

Lori Huelskamp, MSN, RN, ONC
Case Manager
Wound Clinic
St. Luke's Northland Hospital
Kansas City, MO

Barbara A. Kahn, BS, RN, ONC
Orthopedic Nurse Clinician
The Hospital for Special Surgery
New York, NY

Dianne L. LaGow, RN, CNOR, RNFA, ONC
Nurse Manager, Sterile Processing Dept.
Holy Cross Hospital
Silver Spring, MD

Barbara L. Liscum, MSN, RN, ONC
Clinical Nurse Specialist - Orthopaedics
Touro Infirmary
New Orleans, LA

Miki M. Patterson, MS, RN, CS, NP, ONC
Orthopedic Trauma Coordinator
University of Massachusetts Memorial Medical Center
Worcester, MA

Kathleen Rourke, BSN, RN,C, ONC
Orthopedic Nurse Practitioner
Harvard Vanguard Medical Associates
Boston, MA

Lorry Schoenly, DNSc, RN,C
Director of Education
National Association of Orthopaedic Nurses
Pitman, NJ

Corinne M. Seidl, MS, RN,C, ANP, ONC
Nurse Practitioner
University Hospital SUNY; Department of Orthopaedics
Stonybrook, NY

Barbara L. Shoemaker, MSN, RN
Clinical Nurse Specialist Pediatric Orthopaedics
Shriners Hospitals for Children, Northern California
Sacramento, CA

Sidni Anna Smith, BSN, MS, FNP, ONC
Family Nurse Practitioner
Jacksonville CBOC Clinic and Urgent Care
Jacksonville, NC

Ann Marie Szoke-Halal, MSN, RN, CRNP, ANP-C, ONC
Nurse Practitioner, Geriatrics Institute
St. Luke's Hospital Health Services
Bethlehem, PA

Nancy Lynn Whitehead, MS, RN,C, CSN
Clinical Nurse Examiner
Midwestern Performance Assessment Center, Inc.
Madison, WI

Karen E. Zorn, BSN, RN, ONC
Practice Coordinator
Resurgens Orthopaedics
Atlanta, GA

NATIONAL OFFICE STAFF

Staff Executive
Cynthia R. Nowicki, EdD, RN,C

Director of Education
Lorry Schoenly, DNSc, RN,C

Managing Editor
Janet Perrella-D'Alesandro

Editorial Coordinator
Maryanne R. Hatfield

Art Director
Jack M. Bryant

Layout and Design
Darin Peters

Role and Value of the Orthopaedic Nurse

Role

The orthopaedic nurse diagnoses and treats human responses to actual and potential health problems related to musculoskeletal function. Orthopaedic nursing practice facilitates the promotion of wellness and self-care, the maintenance of health, and the prevention of injury and illness in the care of individuals of all ages with degenerative, traumatic, inflammatory, neuromuscular, congenital, metabolic, and oncologic disorders of the musculoskeletal system.

The professional orthopaedic nurse practices in all health care settings where individuals with musculoskeletal conditions receive care, including the home, ambulatory, inpatient, and extended care settings, and where the health education of patients, families, health care professionals and consumers takes place. The professional orthopaedic nurse works either independently or as a member of the interdisciplinary team. The professional orthopaedic nurse bases clinical judgement and decision making on the nursing process, nursing theory, and research, as well as specific orthopaedic knowledge. The professional orthopaedic nurse provides direct care or collaborates with other health care professionals to provide appropriate, effective, and efficient care and education by:

1. Performing a holistic assessment of an individual and/or family specifically assessing the impact of musculoskeletal conditions including self-care needs, environmental management, resources, and support systems;
2. Identifying and treating the following nursing diagnoses that frequently occur in the orthopaedic population: a) activity intolerance, b) disuse syndrome, risk for, c) adjustment, impaired, d) physical mobility, impaired, e) skin integrity, impaired, risk for, f) infection, risk for, g) pain, acute, h) pain, chronic, i) peripheral neurovascular dysfunction, risk for, j) post-trauma response, k) knowledge, deficient, l) self-care deficient, m) ineffective coping, risk for, and other nursing diagnoses as identified;
3. Developing and implementing a plan of care including mutually set goals that are unique to the individual and are evaluated on an ongoing basis;
4. Maintaining current orthopaedic knowledge through formal and informal education;
5. Participating in peer review to assure competent practice;
6. Designing and implementing systems to evaluate care based on identified criteria;
7. Serving as educator, mentor, and role model for nursing colleagues, students, and others;
8. Informing other health professionals and the community about the specialty of orthopaedic nursing;
9. Participating in professional nursing associations that promote educational and professional activities;
10. Applying research findings to clinical practice and contributing to nursing research;
11. Using appropriate resources to clarify and resolve ethical dilemmas; and
12. Being politically aware and proactive concerning health care issues.

The advanced orthopaedic nurse provides expertise in diagnosing and caring for individuals with musculoskeletal conditions as well as education and support to community groups interested in health promotion and illness/injury prevention. Advanced orthopaedic nursing practice requires substantial theoretical knowledge and clinical expertise in orthopaedic nursing and at least master's degree preparation. The advanced orthopaedic nurse may fulfill the roles of direct caregiver, consultant, educator, researcher, administrator, and/or primary health care provider.

Value

Specialized orthopaedic knowledge enhances the nurse's ability to serve as an advocate for the patient and the family in all aspects of care. As a vital link in the health care team, the orthopaedic nurse works with the patient and other health care providers to develop, interpret, implement, and evaluate the plan of care for patients. Their expertise equips orthopaedic nurses with knowledge and skills necessary to anticipate specific patient needs and potential problems throughout the course of a patient's care. Timely recognition of symptoms helps prevent complications and decrease length of stay. The increased knowledge and expertise of the orthopaedic nurse serves to decrease the cost of health care through timely and appropriate identification of patient needs, effective and efficient health care delivery, and timely and appropriate health education, maintenance, and prevention programs. Specialized orthopaedic nurses provide consistent delivery of care that ensures quality health care opportunities for all consumers. Advanced practice orthopaedic nurses, as primary health care providers, enhance the delivery of accessible and affordable health care for all consumers.

Maintaining a balance between technology, specialty knowledge, clinical expertise, research, political awareness, and caring, the role of the orthopaedic nurse is clearly that of patient advocate and, more importantly, as the gatekeeper in the delivery of orthopaedic patient care. The value of the orthopaedic nurse is significantly demonstrated through positive effects on access, cost, and quality for all consumers of musculoskeletal health care.

Catherine M. Smrcina, PhD, RN,C, ONC
NAON President, 1992-1993

Delores C. Schoen, PhD, RN,C, FAAN
NAON President, 1995-1996

Bibliography

American Nurses Association. (2001). *Code of ethics for nurses with interpretive statements.* Washington, DC. Author.

American Nurses Association. (1995). *Nursing's social policy statement.* Washington, DC: Author.

American Nurses Association. (1995). *Scope and standards of gerontological nursing practice.* Washington, DC: Author.

American Nurses Association. (1996). *Scope and standards of advanced practice registered nursing.* Washington, DC: Author.

American Nurses Association. (1996). *Statement on the scope and standards of pediatric clinical nursing practice.* Washington, DC: Author.

American Nurses Association. (1997). *Cultural diversity in nursing: Issues, strategies, and outcomes.* Washington, DC: Author.

American Nurses Association. (1998). *Standards of clinical nursing practice.* 2nd ed. Washington, DC: Author.

American Nurses Association. (1999). *Scope and standards of home health nursing practice.* Washington, DC: Author.

National Association of Orthopaedic Nurses. (1995) *Advanced practice resources: Graduate curriculum, job descriptions, preceptor guidelines.* Pitman, NJ: Author.

National Association of Orthopaedic Nurses. (1999) *Orthopaedic nursing core competencies: Adult acute care.* Pitman, NJ: Author.

National Association of Orthopaedic Nurses. (2001) *Scope and standards of orthopaedic nursing practice* (2nd ed.). Pitman, NJ: Author.

National Association of Orthopaedic Nurses. (2001) *Philosophy* [On-line]. Available: http://naon.inurse.com/About.

Chapter 1 *Practice Settings for Orthopaedic Nursing*

Susan C. Ruda, MS, RN, ONC

Contents

OBJECTIVES

At the completion of this chapter, the learner will be able to:

- Identify various practice settings for the orthopaedic nurse.
- Define the role of the orthopaedic nurse in multiple practice settings.
- Discuss the responsibilities of the orthopaedic nurse in various settings.
- Discuss the knowledge base required for the orthopaedic nurse in various settings.

KEY POINTS

- A nurse may practice in various settings in either the hospital or nonhospital setting and maintain a specialty in orthopaedics.
- Active participation in professional nursing organizations including but not limited to NAON is vital to a nurse's career progression and success.
- Orthopaedic nurses must take an active role in educating the public about health promotion and illness prevention in regards to the musculoskeletal system.
- Ongoing professional education is necessary regardless of employment position. This may be done on a formal basis (academic courses) and an informal basis (reading professional journals, attending hospital sponsored inservices, and attending orthopaedic conferences).
- Orthopaedic nurse certification (ONC) is a vital part of every career level.
- Nurses may begin a specialty in orthopaedics at any level in their career.

CHAPTER 1

PRACTICE SETTINGS FOR ORTHOPAEDIC NURSING

ORTHOPAEDIC NURSING IN ACUTE CARE OR EXTENDED CARE FACILITIES

I. STAFF NURSE

A. Acute care facility.

1. Role definition.
   a. Provide direct patient care.
   b. Serve as a liaison between the patient and physician.
2. Role responsibilities.
   a. Use the nursing process as a systematic way to organize patient care.
      (1) Assess and collect information relevant to the patient's health status.
         (a) Sources.
            i. Direct:
               - Interviews.
               - Observation.
               - Examination.
            ii. Other:
               - Available records.
               - Results of diagnostic tests
               - Information from family and significant others.
               - Information from other health care providers.
         (b) Classification of data.
            i. Subjective nonmeasurable data:
               - Observation.
               - Interview.
               - Information received indirectly from the patient.
            ii. Objective measurable data: observable and measurable by others.
      (2) Nursing diagnosis: assessment data are analyzed and interpreted and explicit statement is then made about the patient's health.
      (3) Goal formulation and plan:
         (a) Various nursing actions are considered
         (b) Plan is developed for promoting, maintaining, and restoring the patient's health.
         (c) Goals are set which describe the observable outcomes.
         (d) Priorities are set and specific plans are identified.
            i. What is to be done.
            ii. How is it to be done.
            iii. When it is to be done.
            iv. Where it is to be done.
            v. Who is to do it.
         (e) Plan prescribes the nursing actions.
      (4) Intervention: the action step where all therapeutic actions, identified in the plan, are implemented.
         (a) Nursing procedures.
         (b) Measures for patient comfort.
         (c) Teaching.
         (d) Counseling.
         (e) Purposeful socialization.
         (f) Coordinating and/or collaborating with other health care team members.
         (g) Whenever possible, encourage the patient, the patient's family and/or significant other to take an active part in the interventions.
      (5) Evaluation/Outcomes: compare the post-intervention status of the patient with observations relative to the desired outcomes.
   b. Serve as patient and family advocate.
   c. Administer therapies, treatments, and medications as prescribed by the physician.
   d. Collaborate with other disciplines such as physical and occupational therapy and dietary in caring for orthopaedic patients.
   e. Participate in developing and implementing clinical pathways.
   f. Evaluate and communicate outcomes of interventions to appropriate authority (supervisor, physician).
   g. Teach patient about home care.
   h. Participate in discharge plan.
   i. Serve on facility committees, as appropriate.
   j. Serve as role model for less experienced nurses.
   k. Join and participate in professional nursing organizations, especially the National Association of Orthopaedic Nurses (NAON).
3. Knowledge base.
   a. Basic anatomy and physiology with an emphasis on the musculoskeletal system.
   b. Good body mechanics.
   c. Good transfer techniques.
   d. Knowledge of common orthopaedic procedures and surgery.
   e. Knowledge of nursing diagnosis.
   d. Knowledge of clinical pathways.
   f. Basic physical assessment skills.
   g. Knowledge of preoperative, perioperative, and postoperative nursing care.
   h. Specific knowledge base for specialty areas including ICU, pediatrics, and surgical nursing.

4. Requirements.
    a. An absolute necessity is an up-to-date license for the registered nurse (RN), licensed practical nurse (LPN), or licensed vocational nurse (LVN) for the state in which the nurse is practicing, except federal employee nurses who need only an up-to-date license from any state.
    b. Minimal or no clinical experience is required.
    c. Initial employment positions involve a range of levels of experience from entry level to advanced.
    d. Orthopaedic nurse certification (ONC) is strongly recommended.
    e. Additional education and/or clinical experience are usually necessary to practice in specialty areas such as pediatrics or surgery.
    f. Ongoing inservice and workshop participation.
    g. Participation in the formal orientation for the care of the orthopaedic patient provided by the institution.
    h. Highly encouraged: join and participate in professional nursing organizations, especially NAON.
5. Areas of practice.
    a. Orthopaedic unit.
    b. Medical-surgical unit.
    c. Ambulatory or outpatient unit.
    d. Pediatric unit.
    e. Surgery.
    f. Same-day surgery.
    g. Post-anesthesia recovery.
    h. Operating room.
    i. Intensive care unit.
    j. Discharge planning.
    k. Rehabilitation unit.
    l. Home care

B. Extended care facility.

1. **Role definition.**
    a. Provide direct patient care.
    b. Serve as a liaison between the patient and physician.
2. Role responsibilities.
    a. Use the nursing process as a systematic way to organize patient care (see I. Role Responsibilities for Staff Nurse in an Acute Care Facility).
    b. Serve as patient and family advocate.
    c. Administer therapies, treatments, and medications as prescribed by the physician.
    d. Collaborate with other disciplines such as physical therapy and dietary in caring for orthopaedic patients.
    e. Supervise care administered by nursing aides, assistants, and family members as appropriate.
    f. Prepare discharge plan for patient.
    g. Consult with home health care nurse, as appropriate.
    h. Evaluate and communicate outcomes of interventions to appropriate authority (supervisor, physician).
    i. Serve as a role model for nurses with less education and experience, and unlicensed health care providers.
    j. Join and participate in professional nursing organizations, especially NAON.
3. Knowledge base.
    a. Basic anatomy and physiology with an emphasis on the musculoskeletal system.
    b. Good body mechanics.
    c. Good transfer techniques.
    d. Knowledge of common orthopaedic procedures and surgery.
    e. Broad base of knowledge about health problems and issues which affect the older adult.
    f. Knowledge of nursing diagnosis.
    g. Knowledge of clinical pathways.
    h. Knowledge of rehabilitation process/rehabilitation care.
    i. Knowledge of discharge planning.
    j. Basic physical assessment skills.
4. Requirements.
    a. An absolute is an up-to-date license for the RN, LPN, or LVN for the state in which the nurse is practicing.
    b. Acute care nursing experience may be required.
    c. Gerontological nursing experience may be highly recommended or even required, depending on the patient population of the unit.
    d. ONC is strongly recommended
    e. Rehabilitation and/or gerontological nursing certification are also strongly recommended.
    f. Ongoing inservice or workshop participation is required.
    g. Attend professional organization meetings, including those sponsored by NAON.
5. Areas of practice.
    a. Rehabilitation unit.
    b. Extended care facility.
    c. Long-term care facility.
    d. Skilled nursing facility.
    e. Nursing home.

II. HEAD NURSE/UNIT MANAGER/NURSING SUPERVISOR

A. Role definition.

1. Supervise, evaluate, and assist in the modification of the care provided by nursing and other health care providers.
2. Serve as liaison between the staff and administration.

B. Role responsibilities.

1. Interpret hospital policies and governmental laws for nursing personnel, patients, and family.
2. Provide direct communication with nursing personnel and administrative personnel.
3. Participate in evaluation of nursing personnel.
4. Participate in budget, scheduling, and staffing decisions.
5. Delegate tasks to appropriate personnel.
6. Promote an environment of professional growth

among the nursing staff.
7. Mentor newer and/or less experienced orthopaedic nurses.
8. Join and participate in professional nursing organizations, especially NAON.

C. Knowledge base.
1. Advanced knowledge of anatomy and physiology with an emphasis on the musculoskeletal system.
2. Advanced physical assessment skills.
3. Knowledge of staff development, interpersonal relations, and productivity.
4. Knowledge of labor relations.
5. Knowledge of nursing service standards and policies.
6. Knowledge of the budget process.

D. Requirements.
1. Supervisory experience.
2. Experience in health care budgeting is recommended.
3. Strong leadership skills.
4. Experience in caring for the orthopaedic patient.
5. Bachelor's degree or master's degree may be required, depending on the institution.
6. ONC is strongly recommended.
7. Up-to-date RN licensure from the state where the nurse is practicing is required.

III. CLINICAL NURSE SPECIALIST (CNS)

A. Role definition: the role of the clinical nurse specialist incorporates the primary components of expert orthopaedic clinical practice, consultation, education, and research, and in some institutions, administration.
1. Direct care component refers to actual interaction with selected clients, families, or groups.
2. Indirect care component refers to services, such as education and consultation, which enhance patient care.
3. CNS uses research findings in orthopaedic nursing practice and identifies researchable problems.

B. Role responsibilities.
1. Interpret literature and research findings for the nursing personnel.
2. Participate in clinical research.
3. Identify researchable problems.
4. Develop collaborative research projects.
5. Aid in the integration of appropriate research findings into practice.
6. Educate patients and their families on various orthopaedic subjects.
7. Provide education that will enhance patient care; educate providers who are actually involved with the patient.
8. Serve as consultant in care of the complex orthopaedic patient.
9. Provide patient care as negotiated between the institution and the CNS.
10. Serve as role model for other nursing colleagues.
11. Publish research-based and nonresearch-based articles on subjects related to orthopaedic nursing.
12. Give presentations on orthopaedic nursing at the local, state, or national levels.
13. Assist administration with the interpretation, implementation, and evaluation of institutional policies.
14. Educate community groups about musculoskeletal conditions with an emphasis on health promotion and illness/injury prevention.
15. Join and participate in professional nursing organizations, especially NAON and the American Nurses Association (ANA).

C. Knowledge base.
1. Advanced knowledge of anatomy and physiology with an emphasis on the musculoskeletal system.
2. Advanced physical assessment skills.
3. Advanced knowledge of pathophysiology.
4. Advanced knowledge of nursing diagnoses and clinical pathways.
5. Strong theoretical base in musculoskeletal nursing.
6. Knowledge of research design and statistical analysis.
7. Communication skills.
8. Problem solving skills.

D. Requirements.
1. Clinical expertise in orthopaedic nursing.
2. Strong leadership skills.
3. Physical assessment skills.
4. Speaking ability.
5. Writing ability.
6. Problem solving skills.
7. Excellent communication skills and ability to work efficiently with others.
8. Knowledge of the teaching/learning process.
9. Nursing research experience.
10. RN licensure for the appropriate state is required.
11. Masters degree in nursing is required.
12. ONC is strongly recommended.

ORTHOPAEDIC NURSING OUTSIDE THE HOSPITAL SETTING

I. OFFICE/CLINIC NURSE

A. Role definition.
1. Provide care of the orthopaedic patient in the office or clinic setting.
2. Work with other health care providers as appropriate.

B. Role responsibilities.
1. Assist in minor procedures within the office.
2. Provide treatment or therapies as prescribed by the physician.
3. Educate patients and families on proper administration of medication and side effects.
4. Educate patients and families on orthopaedic procedures, equipment, complications, and possible emergency situations.
5. Interpret diagnostic tests for patients and families.
6. Coordinate patient care within the office with other disciplines.
7. Identify possible emergent situations based on telephone conversation.
8. Delegate non-nursing tasks to appropriate personnel.
9. Join and participate in professional nursing organizations, especially NAON.

C. **Knowledge base.**
1. Advanced knowledge of anatomy and physiology with an emphasis on the musculoskeletal system.
2. Knowledge of outpatient nursing.
3. Advanced physical assessment skills.
4. Knowledge of pathophysiology.
5. Knowledge of pharmacology, side effects, and interactions of medications.
6. Knowledge of diagnostic tests.
7. Knowledge of the teaching/learning process

D. **Requirements.**
1. Strong background in orthopaedic nursing.
2. Depending on the practice, experience in adult, geriatric, or pediatric nursing.
3. Physical assessment skills.
4. Cast removal and application experience is beneficial.
5. Strong telephone triage skills.
6. Excellent communication skills.
7. Ability to handle multiple tasks at once is strongly recommended.
8. LPN or RN licensure for the appropriate state is required.
9. ONC is strongly recommended.
10. Coding experience is beneficial.
11. Experience dealing with insurance carriers is strongly recommended.
12. Management and leadership experience may not be required but is very useful.

E. **Areas of practice.**
1. Orthopaedic physician's office.
2. Podiatrist office.
2. Clinic.
3. HMO office.
4. Primary care physician's office.
5. Sports medicine clinic.
6. Nursing Center.

II. SCHOOL NURSE

A. **Role definition.**
1. Participate in the care of children within the school setting.
2. Role may include care of students with non-orthopaedic disorders.

B. **Role responsibilities.**
1. Administer first aid as needed.
2. Maintain school records of vaccinations, allergies, and medical history on each student.
3. Educate students and their families about a student's condition.
4. Educate students about health promotion and illness prevention.
5. Administer medication and therapies as prescribed by the student's physician.
6. Coordinate screening programs for scoliosis and various other disorders.
7. Be a student advocate between student, parents, and administration.
8. Join and participate in professional nursing organizations, especially ANA and NAON.

C. **Knowledge base.**
1. Advanced knowledge of anatomy and physiology with an emphasis on the musculoskeletal system of the child.
2. Advanced physical assessment skills for children.
3. Knowledge of growth and development.
4. Knowledge of pathophysiology of pediatric conditions.
5. Knowledge of pediatric pharmacology, side effects, proper dosing, and interactions of medications.
6. Knowledge of school policies and local, state, and national legislation.

D. **Requirements.**
1. Pediatric experience.
2. Knowledge of trauma and first aid care.
3. Pediatric and young adult physical assessment skills.
4. Knowledge of growth and development.
5. Ability to communicate with a wide variety of people including children, parents, teachers, and school administrators.
6. Successful completion of school nurse certificate program based upon individual state and school district requirements.
7. RN licensure for the appropriate state is required.
8. Bachelor's degree may be required, based upon individual state and school district requirements.
9. ONC is strongly recommended.

E. **Areas of practice.**
1. Elementary education up to college or university setting.
2. Camp nurse will have similar requirements.

III. HOME HEALTH NURSE

A. **Role definition: provide care for an individual with an orthopaedic disorder in the person's home that requires a different perspective from acute care.**
1. Assessment skills: complete, physical, social, psychological, economic, environmental assessment, and a determination of home safety and family issues.
2. Autonomy: 24-hour care plan for the patient.
3. Communication with the physician: assessment skills and concise communication in a timely manner regarding significant changes in patient's condition.
4. Determining frequency and duration of care: in collaboration with physician, Medicare coverage criteria, and patient's needs.
5. Direct care: improvise equipment for clients with limited resources and teach a variety of skills to clients and caregivers.
6. Documentation: documentation covers anticipatory guidance to prevent future problems, provision of direct treatments of current conditions, and client teaching.
7. Patient teaching: teaching is a skilled service that is Medicare reimbursable and is one of the main roles of the home care nurse.
8. Referral to community resources: knowledgeable, over time, of the community resources available

both locally and nationwide, and ensure that the patient and family are aware of what might be helpful.

9. Reimbursement: validates and discusses reimbursement issues with the client and family in the home and verifies the client's eligibility for home care services with the physician.
10. Safety: read a map, manage home visiting safety issues, and assess troublesome situations.
11. Work environment: always a guest in the home with the presence of family, the need to adjust to variations in a client's environment, and based on need collaboration with others via phone.

B. Role responsibilities.

1. Educate patient and family about patient's orthopaedic disorder and the recommended treatment.
2. Assess patient's symptoms and clinical findings.
3. Assess patient's home environment for safety hazards and adaptability needed to maximize his/her independence.
4. Educate patient and family about health promotion and illness prevention, and prescribed treatments, and allow them to make choices when possible.
5. Administer prescribed treatments.
6. Evaluate and communicate outcomes of interventions to appropriate authority (supervisor, physician).
7. Assist patient in obtaining necessary equipment and help arrange for any necessary home modifications.
8. Join and participate in professional nursing organizations, especially NAON.

C. Knowledge base.

1. Advanced knowledge of anatomy and physiology with an emphasis on the musculoskeletal system.
2. Advanced physical assessment skills.
3. Knowledge of pathophysiology.
4. Knowledge of pharmacology, side effects, proper dosing, and interactions of medications.
5. Knowledge of rehabilitation of the orthopaedic patient.
6. Knowledge of common health problems of the older adult.

D. Requirements.

1. Recent clinical experience in orthopaedics, medical-surgical, and gerontological nursing is beneficial.
2. Strong physical assessment skills.
3. Strong environmental assessment skills.
4. Creativity in developing plans of care to maximize patients' independence within their own environment.
5. Time management skills.
6. Knowledge of community resources.
7. RN licensure for the appropriate state is required.
8. Bachelor's degree may be required.
9. ONC is useful.

ORTHOPAEDIC NURSING PRACTICE INSIDE/OUTSIDE THE HOSPITAL AND NON-HOSPITAL SETTINGS

I. NURSE PRACTITIONER (NP)

A. Role definition.

1. Administer primary care to a patient with an orthopaedic disorder within the acute care or extended care setting, the clinic or office setting, or the home environment.
2. Perform procedures such as aspiration of a joint, closed reduction of a simple fracture, cast application, and suturing a wound.
3. Inherent in the NP role is accountability and responsibility for decisions made and actions rendered.

B. Role responsibilities.

1. Assess patient's condition.
2. Prescribe diagnostic tests, treatment, and medication within the regulations of each individual state's nurse practice act.
3. Perform interventions and treatments within the regulations of each individual state.
4. Educate patient and family on illness/injury prevention and health promotion.
5. Help educate nurses in other disciplines; educate other health care providers.
6. Collaborate with other health care and medical care providers.
7. Serve as a role model and mentor to nursing colleagues.
8. Join and participate in professional organizations, especially NAON, ANA, and the National Organization of Nurse Practitioners.

C. Knowledge base.

1. Advanced knowledge of anatomy and physiology with an emphasis on the musculoskeletal system across the lifespan.
2. Advanced physical assessment skills.
3. Advanced knowledge of pathophysiology.
4. Knowledge of pharmacology, side effects, proper dosing, and interactions of medications.
5. Advanced knowledge of diagnostic tests.
6. Excellent communication skills.
7. Knowledge of the teaching/learning process.

D. Requirements.

1. RN licensure for the appropriate state is required.
2. Completion of accredited nurse practitioner program such as:
    a. Adult nurse practitioner.
    b. Pediatric nurse practitioner.
    c. Family nurse practitioner.
    d. Gerontologic nurse practitioner.
3. Certification from appropriate certification body for nurse practitioners.
4. ONC is strongly recommended.
5. Strong clinical background and experience in orthopaedic nursing.
6. Strong physical assessment skills.
7. Excellent communication skills.

8. Malpractice insurance may be required based upon the state of practice.
9. Join and participate in professional organizations, especially ANA, NAON, and the National Organization of Nurse Practitioners.

E. Areas of practice.

1. Orthopaedic physician's office.
2. Primary care physician's office.
3. Podiatrist office.
4. Clinic.
5. HMO office.
6. Hospital.
7. Sports medicine clinic.
8. Nursing center.

II. CASE MANAGER

A. Role definition.

1. Coordinate care of specified group of patients.
2. Serve as liaison between patient and physician, insurance carrier, workman's compensation carrier, and other health care disciplines.

B. Role responsibilities.

1. Oversee care of specified group of patients.
2. Attend therapy and physician appointments as negotiated by patient, lawyer, and/or insurance company.
3. Negotiate services and equipment needs on patient's behalf.
4. Serve as patient advocate.
5. Join and participate in professional nursing organizations, including but not limited to NAON and ANA.

C. Knowledge base.

1. Advanced knowledge of anatomy and physiology with an emphasis on the musculoskeletal system.
2. Physical assessment skills.
3. Knowledge of pathophysiology.
4. Knowledge of pharmacology, side effects, and interactions of medications.

D. Requirements.

1. Strong background and experience in orthopaedic nursing.
2. Occupational health nursing experience is strongly recommended.
3. Rehabilitation nursing experience is strongly recommended.
4. Strong leadership skills.
5. Physical assessment skills.
6. Strong communication skills.
7. Ability to function in an autonomous role.
8. Knowledge and experience of the insurance industry.
9. ONC is strongly recommended.
10. Occupational health nursing certification is strongly recommended.
11. RN licensure for the appropriate state is required.
12. Bachelor's degree may be required.

III. ACADEMIC FACULTY

A. Role definition: provide education to all levels of nursing student (undergraduate and graduate).

1. Teaching:
   a. Teach students at all levels.
   b. Advise students regarding education, practice, and research.
   c. Evaluate students' class and clinical performance.
2. Research.
   a. Identify researchable topics.
   b. Evaluate research proposals.
   c. Analyze published research for applicability for clinical practice.
   d. Develop and implement research proposals.
   e. Publish results.
   f. Write grant proposals for funding of research.
3. Service.
   a. Departmental committees
   b. College committees.
   c. University committees.

B. Role responsibilities.

1. Provide classroom and clinical education to nursing students (undergraduate or graduate).
2. Participate in student evaluation and promotion.
3. Evaluate effectiveness of teaching techniques.
4. Perform research on subjects related to orthopaedic practice.
5. Publish on topics pertinent to education, practice, and research.
6. Mentor professional orthopaedic nurses in advancing their careers.
7. Join and participate in professional nursing organizations, especially NAON and ANA.

C. Knowledge base.

1. Advanced knowledge of anatomy and physiology with an emphasis on the musculoskeletal system.
2. Advanced physical assessment skills.
3. Advanced knowledge of pathophysiology.
4. Knowledge of pharmacology, side effects, and interactions of medications.
5. Knowledge of effective teaching techniques.
6. Knowledge of research design and analysis.
7. Expert clinician.

D. Requirements.

1. Master's degree is the minimum requirement. Doctoral degree required for most positions in colleges and universities.
2. Excellent teaching skills.
3. Excellent communication skills.
4. Strong clinical background in orthopaedics.
5. Strong research background.
6. Strong leadership skills.
7. RN licensure for the appropriate state.
8. ONC is not required but is strongly recommended.

E. Areas of practice.

1. Community college.
2. Diploma nursing programs.
3. Colleges and universities.
4. Medical centers.
5. Hospitals.

IV. NURSE RESEARCHER

A. Role definition: performs research on topics of significance for orthopaedic nursing practice.

B. Role responsibilities.

1. Perform scientific research on subjects related to orthopaedic practice.
2. Publish on topics pertinent to orthopaedic practice.
3. Present research findings at conferences.
4. Aid in the implementation of research findings.
5. Apply for research funding.
6. Join and participate in professional nursing organizations, especially NAON and ANA.

C. Knowledge base.

1. Advanced knowledge of anatomy and physiology with an emphasis on the musculoskeletal system.
2. Physical assessment skills.
3. Knowledge of pathophysiology.
4. Knowledge of the funding process.
5. Grant writing skills.
5. Advanced knowledge of research design and statistical analysis.
6. Clinical expert.

D. Requirements.

1. Master's degree is the minimum requirement. Doctoral degree is required for most positions.
2. Strong clinical background in orthopaedics.
3. Strong research background.
4. Knowledge of qualitative and quantitative research methods.
5. Statistical analysis experience.
6. Strong leadership skills.
7. RN licensure for the appropriate state.
8. ONC is not required but is useful.

E. Areas of practice.

1. University.
2. Governmental agency.
3. Pharmaceutical company.
4. Medical centers.

V. NURSE ENTREPRENEUR

A. Role definition: develop a unique service or product for the orthopaedic population (nurse, physician, patient, and/or family, or the general community).

B. Role responsibilities.

1. Perform needs assessment to determine the significance or need of the product or service.
2. Market service or product to the appropriate audience.
3. Oversee product or service delivery to ensure quality.
4. Evaluate effectiveness of service or product.
5. Modify service or product according to the changing needs of the target population.
6. Participate in relevant research involving service or product.
7. Educate others on the effectiveness of the service or product.
8. Join and participate in professional nursing organizations, including ANA and NAON.

C. Knowledge base.

1. Knowledge of anatomy and physiology with an emphasis on the musculoskeletal system.
2. Physical assessment skills.
3. Knowledge of pathophysiology.
4. Knowledge of pharmacology, side effects, and interactions of medications.
5. Advanced knowledge of service or product.
6. Knowledge of effective sales techniques.

D. Requirements.

1. Strong clinical background in orthopaedics.
2. Creativity.
3. Ability to function in an autonomous role.
4. Strong leadership skills.
5. Strong business, marketing, and administrative skills.
6. RN licensure for the appropriate state.
7. ONC is not required but is useful.

VI. REGISTERED NURSE FIRST ASSISTANT (RNFA)

A. Role definition: the RN first assistant-at-surgery.

1. Collaborates with the surgeon in performing a safe operation with optimal outcomes for the patient.
2. Practices perioperative nursing and does so with acquired specific knowledge, skills, and judgment.
3. Practices under the supervision of the surgeon during the intraoperative phase of the perioperative experience.
4. Does not concurrently function as a scrub nurse.

B. Role responsibilities.

1. The scope of practice of the nurse performing as first assistant is a part of perioperative nursing practice.
2. Performs first assistant responsibilities in accordance with the State Nurse Practice Act.
3. Activities of the first assistant are further refinements of perioperative nursing practice and may include:
   a. Preoperative assessment of the patient and the development of a nursing care plan based on the assessment.
   b. Assistance in the positioning, skin preparation, and draping of the patient.
   c. Performs the following activities during the surgical procedure:
      (1) Hemostasis.
      (2) Wound exposure.
      (3) Tissue handling so as to reduce potential for injury.
      (4) Skillful use of surgical instruments in ways consistent with their design and purpose
      (5) Suturing of tissue.
      (6) Application of dressings under the direction of the surgeon.
   d. Provides assistance in transporting the patient post-operatively.
   e. Communicates information to the postanesthesia care unit personnel.
   f. Communicates information to the family, as appropriate.

g. Evaluates the patient post-operatively and participates in discharge planning.
4. Functions under the direct supervision of the surgeon who is being assisted.
5. Employed by the Department of Perioperative Nursing (Hospital-Employed RNFA), Physician-Employed RNFA, or Self-Employed RNFA.

C. Knowledge base.

1. Knowledge of perioperative nursing (preoperative, perioperative, and postoperative nursing).
2. Basic anatomy and physiology with an emphasis on the musculoskeletal system.
3. Knowledge of common orthopaedic procedures and surgery.
4. Knowledge of surgical anatomy, physiology, and operative technique related to the operative procedures in which the RN assists.
5. Knowledge of principles of asepsis and infection control.
6. Documentation of proficiency in perioperative nursing practice as both a scrub and circulating nurse.
7. Good body mechanics and transfer techniques.
8. Excellent physical assessment skills.
9. Knowledge and application of the nursing process.
10. Knowledge of clinical pathways.
11. Specific knowledge base for specialty areas of pediatrics and geriatrics.
12. Performs effectively in stressful and emergency situations.
13. Knows safety hazards and is aware of appropriate preventive and corrective actions to be taken.
14. Performs effectively and harmoniously as a member of the operative team.
15. Knowledge and behaviors unique to the RN first assistant (as defined).

D. Requirements. should include, but are not be limited to:

1. Current RN licensure.
2. Minimum of 3 years of perioperative nursing experience in both a scrub and circulating role.
3. Certification in perioperative nursing (CNOR).
4. Has successfully completed an RNFA program that includes didactic and at least 120 hours of a clinical component.
4. Certification as an RNFA (CRNFA), highly recommended.
5. ONC is highly recommended
6. Documentation of proficiency in perioperative nursing practice as both a scrub and circulating nurse.
7. Ability to apply principles of asepsis and infection control.
8. Knowledge of surgical anatomy, physiology, and operative technique related to the operative procedures in which the RN assists.
9. Ability to perform basic cardiac life support (BCLS) required, advanced cardiac life support (ACLS), preferred.
10. Ability to perform effectively in stressful and emergency situations.
11. Ability to recognize safety hazards and initiate appropriate preventive and corrective action.
12. Ability to perform effectively and harmoniously as a member of the operative team.
13. Ability to demonstrate skill in behaviors unique to the RN first assistant (as defined).
14. Meets requirements of statutes, regulations, and institutional policies relevant to RN first assistants.

E. Areas of practice.

1. Physician-Employed RNFA.
   a. Physician is the employer and the RNFA is the employee.
   b. Both parties negotiate the terms of the agreement in their own best interest.
      (1) The starting point is to answer the question "How much am I worth?"
      (2) Determine how much of the third-party reimbursement the physician will receive for the RNFA services and how much is due and payable to the RNFA.
   c. RNFA must promote financial value to the physician and the office manager.
   d. Collaborate with the physician to develop a formal statement concerning the use of an RNFA as first assistant in surgery (to include permission to bill the patient's insurance company for RNFA services if the physician does not bill for the RNFA).
   e. Collaborate with the physician to develop a financial policy that includes RNFA charges.
   f. Collaborate with the physician to develop a standard letter for insurance claims processors that identifies the RNFA's credentials and emphasizes the cost-effectiveness and value of the RNFA services.
2. Self-Employed RNFA: requires that the RNFA become knowledgeable about the claims process to file claims for reimbursement.
   a. Health Care Financing Administration (HCFA) 1500 form (Secondary insurance with Medicare).
   b. Medicare.
      (1) Federally funded and pays for health care services to people ages 65 and older regardless of income or ability to pay (Part A covers hospital and Part B covers physician and outpatient services).
      (2) Medicare only recognizes the RNFA if he/she is certified as an advanced practice nurse or certified nurse midwife.
      (3) Patients may have one of two types of secondary insurance policies to cover costs that are not covered by Medicare and a possible source for RNFA billing.
         (a) Supplemental insurance, commonly referred to as Medigap insurance, will not pay RNFA.
         (b) Secondary insurance – there is a possibility they will pay.
         (c) All supplemental policies are secondary to Medicare, but not all secondary policies are supplemental to Medicare.

c. Medicaid.
   (1) Funded jointly by the federal and state governments, but administered solely by the state.
   (2) Most states do not recognize RNFA as surgical assistants, but will issue provider numbers and consider claims for preoperative and postoperative care.
   (3) Florida provides direct Medicaid reimbursement of RNFAs at same rate that is paid to a physician for the same service.
d. CHAMPUS: the Civilian Health and Medical Program for the Uniformed Services may reimburse the RNFA for providing preoperative and postoperative care services.
e. Workers' Compensation.
   (1) Workers' Compensation varies by state.
   (2) All states base payment on a set fee-for-service.
   (3) Provider is prohibited from billing patient for unpaid services.
f. Commercial Insurance Carriers: most understand cost saving through the use of RNFAs and reimburse for their services.
g. Self-Insured Plans: vary in that some will pay for RNFA service and others will not.
h. Blue Cross/Blue Shield (BCBS): varies state by state.

3. Hospital-Employed RNFA.
   a. Hospital billing for services performed by an RNFA employee varies.
   b. Decision of the financial department of the institution whether to seek reimbursement.
   c. Institutions that do bill are doing so by:
      (1) Incorporating the charge into the room charge.
      (2) Adding an additional staff member.
      (3) Using a line item charge for the first assistant fee.

Bibliography

Association of Operating Room Nurses. (1997). *RN first assistant guide to practice.* Denver: Association of Operating Room Nurses, Inc.

Barnum, B.S., & Kerfoot, K.M. (1995). *The nurse as executive (4th ed.).* Gaithersburg, MD: Aspen Publications.

Buppert, C. (1998). *Nurse practitioner's business practice and legal guide.* New York: Aspen.

Curtin, L. (1996). *Nursing into the 21st century.* Springhouse, PA: Springhouse.

Fenstermacher, K., & Hudson, B.T. (1997). *Practice guidelines for family nurse practitioners.* Philadelphia: WB Saunders.

Fitsimmons, L., Hadley, S.A., & Shively, M. (1999). The education of advanced practice nurses: A contemporary approach. *Critical Care Nursing Quarterly, 21*(4), 77-85.

Hawkins, J.W., & Thibodeau, J.A. (1993). *The advanced practitioner: Current practice issues (3rd ed.).* New York: The Tiresias Press, Inc.

Hamric, A.B., Spross, J.A., & Hanson, C.M. (Eds.). (1996). *Advanced nursing practice: An integrative approach.* Philadelphia: WB Saunders.

Henry, P.F. (1996). The legal aspects of sports medicine for the nurse practitioner. *Nurse Practitioner Forum, 7*(3), 102-103.

Hickey, J.V., Ouimette, R.M., & Venegoni, S.L. (Eds.) (1999). *Advanced practice nursing: Changing roles and clinical applications.* Philadelphia: Lippincott.

Humphrey, C.J., & Milone-Nuzzo, P. (1996). *Orientation to home care nursing.* Gaithersburg, MD: Aspen Publications.

Pastorino, C. (1998). Advanced practice nursing role: Nurse practitioner. *Orthopaedic Nursing, 17*(6), 65-69.

Poster, E.C., & Marcontel, M. (1999). School nursing role and competence. *Journal of School Nursing, 15*(2), 34-42.

Ross, S.K. (1999). The clinical nurse specialist's role in school health. *Clinical Nurse Specialist, 13*(1), 28-33.

Rothrock. J.C. (1993). *The RN first assistant: An expanded perioperative nursing role (2nd ed.).* Philadelphia: Lippincott-Raven.

Stone, K.R. (1996). The role of the nurse practitioner in the orthopaedic sports medicine surgical practice. *Nurse Practitioner Forum, 7*(3), 100-101.

STUDY QUESTIONS

1. What is the single requirement that all nurses must have to practice as an orthopaedic nurse in any clinical setting?
   a. Graduate from a nursing program.
   b. Nursing certification.
   c. Clinical practice experience.
   d. State license.

2. The role of a staff nurse on an orthopaedic unit would include which of the following:
   a. Prescribe diagnostic tests as indicated by the patient's condition.
   b. Market orthopaedic services or products to orthopaedic patients in need.
   c. Collaborate with other health care disciplines to provide care for the patient.
   d. Maintain school and health records of students with orthopaedic conditions.

3. Which orthopaedic nursing position requires that the nurse have at least one nursing certification?
   a. Clinical Nurse Specialist.
   b. RN First Assistant.
   c. Nurse Practitioner.
   d. Nurse Entrepreneur

4. Which of the following are required of all orthopaedic staff nurses?
   a. Use the *Orthopaedic Nursing* journal to keep their practice current.
   b. Attend orientation and staff inservices on the orthopaedic unit.
   c. Local and/or national nursing meetings for continuing education.
   d. Attend continuing education classes in orthopaedics to update their practice.

5. A school nurse would be expected to perform which of the following:
   a. Conduct scoliosis screening on both males and females.
   b. Prescribe medication for a child with juvenile rheumatoid arthritis.
   c. Conduct a community program on osteoarthritis for parents.
   d. Educate nursing students about perioperative care of the patient.

6. Which of the following would **not** be expected of a nurse in the role of case manager?
   a. Contact a patient's insurance company to verify coverage for a surgical procedure.
   b. Discuss a patient's anticipated return date with his employer after a hip arthroplasty.
   c. Discuss rehabilitation and plan of care with a patient, family, and significant others.
   d. Conduct a financial analysis to determine type and financing of home care services.

7. A staff nurse practicing on a rehabilitation unit would be expected to do which of the following:
   a. Help the patient and family prepare a discharge plan.
   b. Do a financial impact study of staff overtime expenses.
   c. Determine need and order a wound culture and sensitivity.
   d. Prescribe an antibiotic for a patient who has erythema at the incision.

8. A unit manager on an adult medical/surgical unit with orthopaedic patients requires a strong knowledge of all of the following except:
   a. Labor and union relations.
   b. Governmental laws as they relate to inpatient care.
   c. Budget process within a health care institution.
   d. Musculoskeletal growth and development.

9. Which of the following is an inappropriate mentor for an experienced staff nurse on an orthopaedic unit in a general hospital?
   a. A more experienced staff nurse.
   b. Head nurse on a medical/surgical unit.
   c. An academic orthopaedic instructor.
   d. An orthopaedic nurse entrepreneur.

10. A clinical nurse specialist would perform which of the following:
    a. Help develop a care plan for a multiple trauma patient pelvic and neck fractures.
    b. Promote an orthopaedic product designed by a corporate sponsor to reduce infections.
    c. Serve as a mediator for the staff nurses' union regarding patient care issues.
    d. Submit a balanced 5-year budget plan for the hospital.

Chapter 2 ANATOMY AND PHYSIOLOGY

Judith A. Chase, BS, MA, RN,C, ONC

Contents

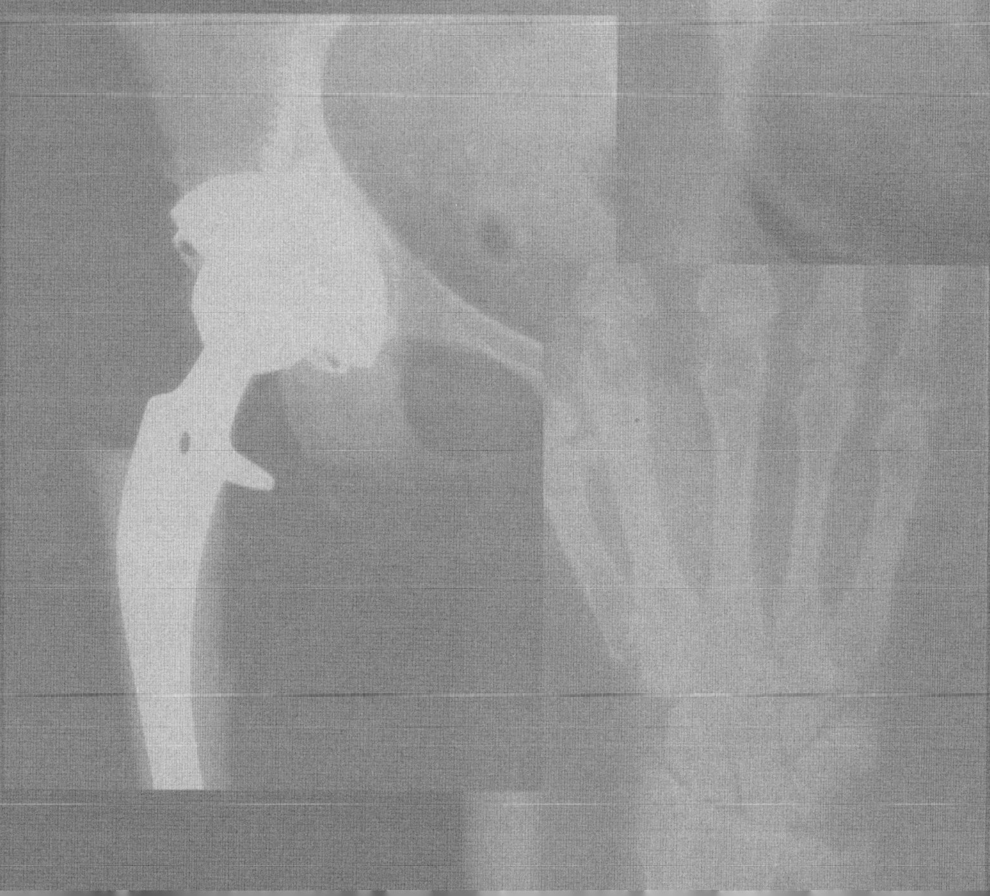

OBJECTIVES

At the completion of this chapter, the learner will be able to:

- Define anatomic position.
- Identify the nine terms of location.
- Describe the composition of bone.
- Describe bone development.
- Identify the characteristics of a muscle.
- Describe the functions of the musculoskeletal system.
- Identify the structures within the musculoskeletal system.
- Identify major muscle groups.
- Classify joints and describe specific motions.

CHAPTER 2

ANATOMY AND PHYSIOLOGY

I. ANATOMIC TERMINOLOGY

A. Anatomic position: legs and arms straight, feet together, legs together, palms forward.
1. Prone: lying face down.
2. Supine: lying face up.
3. Sagittal section: cut anterior to posterior, dividing the body into left and right sections.
4. Horizontal or transverse: cut producing upper and lower sections.
5. Coronal or frontal: cut separating anterior and posterior sections.
6. Oblique: a plane that is not coronal, sagittal, or transverse.

B. Terms of location.
1. Anterior or ventral: closer to the front.
2. Posterior or dorsal: closer to the back.
3. Superior, cranial, or cephalic: closer to the head.
4. Medial: closer to the midline.
5. Lateral: farther from the midline.
6. Superficial or external: nearer the surface.
7. Internal or deep: inside, opposite of superficial.
8. Proximal: closer to specified point of reference.
9. Distal: farther from specified point of reference.

II. BONE

A. Microscopic structure.
1. Haversian system.
   a. Contains blood vessels and lymphatics.
   b. Maintains and supplies nutrients to bone tissue.
2. Cell types.
   a. Osteoblast: forms new bone and bone matrix.
   b. Osteocyte: maintains bone.
   c. Osteoclast: resorbs bone.
3. Constituents.
   a. Organic.
      (1) 35% of bone.
      (2) Primarily collagen.
      (3) Gives bone elasticity.
   b. Inorganic.
      (1) 65% of bone.
      (2) Mineral.
      (3) Gives bone hardness.

B. Formation.
1. Embryonic development.
   a. Mesoderm-mesenchyme-bone, cartilage, ligaments, muscle, tendon, fascia.
   b. Chronologic development (during uterine life).
      (1) 5th week: mesenchyme limb buds develop.
      (2) 6th week: cartilaginous model of bone developing.
      (3) 7th week - 6th month: cartilage and bone development. Osteoblasts secrete collagen and mucopolysaccharide matrix and calcium deposition leads to immature bone.
      (4) 6th month: medullary cavity developed.
2. Endochondral ossification.
   a. Cartilage replaced by bone.
      (1) Embryo.
      (2) Fracture healing.
      (3) Some bone tumors.
   b. Responsible for longitudinal growth.
3. Intramembranous ossification.
   a. Transforms connective tissue to bone.
   b. Responsible for circumferential growth.
4. Center of ossification.
   a. Lies centrally in soft tissue and spreads centrifugally toward ends of bones.
   b. Appears between 6th - 10th week of intrauterine life.
   c. Primary center: appears near middle of long bones between 6th and 16th week in utero.
   d. Secondary center: appears at ends of bones just before birth to late teenage years.
5. Aging effects: osteopenia.
   a. Normally bones become thinner and weaker.
   b. Osteoblast activity starts to decrease, ages 30-40 years.
   c. After age 40, women lose 8% of bone mass every decade.
   d. After age 40, men lose 3% bone mass every decade.

C. Types of bone.
1. Cortical.
   a. Compact bone.
   b. Forms shaft of long bones.
   c. Hard outer layer of all bones.
   d. Poor blood supply.
2. Cancellous or trabecullar.
   a. Light, porous, spongy bone; absence of haversian system.
   b. Metaphysis and epiphysis of bone.
   c. Rich blood supply.

D. Functions.
1. Provides rigid framework and support for the body.
2. Serves as levers for skeletal muscles.
3. Protects vital organs.
4. Stores minerals, calcium and phosphate ions, lipids, and marrow elements.
5. Forms new red blood cells and other blood elements.

E. Shapes.
1. Long bones (bones in which length exceeds breadth and thickness).
   a. Structure.
      (1) Diaphysis.
         (a) Shaft.
         (b) Provides strength; resists bending forces.

(c) Compact bone with central cavity.

(2) Metaphysis.

(a) Flared portion between diaphysis and epiphysis.

(b) Growing portion.

(c) Area of greatest blood supply.

(3) Epiphysis.

(a) End.

(b) Primarily cancellous bone.

(c) Assists with bone development.

(4) Epiphyseal line/plate.

(a) Between metaphysis and epiphysis.

(b) Cartilage growth in length of diaphysis and metaphysis.

(c) Appositional growth increases girth of bone deposited by osteoblasts under periosteum.

(d) Ossification of plates fuses epiphyses with shaft.

i. Occurs earlier in girls.

ii. Usually complete by 18-21 years.

(5) Periosteum.

(a) Connective tissue covering bone.

(b) Continues at end of bone with joint capsule but does not cover articular cartilage.

(6) Perrochondrium: connective tissue covering cartilage.

b. Blood supply.

(1) Nutrient artery.

(a) Tunnel in diaphysis of long bone.

(b) Supplies bone with nutrients.

(2) Periosteal vessels supply compact bone of the diaphysis.

(3) Metaphyseal and epiphyseal vessels supply the spongy bone and marrow of the epiphysis.

2. Short bones.

a. Equal in main dimensions.

b. Found mainly in hands and feet.

c. Types.

(1) Accessory bones not normally present.

(2) Sesamoid.

(a) Embedded in tendons or joint capsulcs.

(b) May be mistaken for fractures on x-ray.

i. Have no callus.

ii. Edges are smooth.

iii. Are often bilateral.

3. Flat bones are primarily made up of cancellous bone tissue.

4. Irregular bones.

III. SKELETAL MUSCLE

A. Gross structure.

1. Bundles of muscle cells.

2. Fascia.

a. Sheet of connective tissue; contains numerous proprioceptive endings.

b. Covers muscles and provides origins and insertions for muscles.

c. Carries network of blood, nerves, and lymph vessels.

3. Tendon.

a. Extends beyond muscle fibers.

b. Attaches muscle to bone.

c. Properties of strength, extensibility, and flexibility.

4. Ligaments.

a. Bands of fibrous tissue.

b. Connect bones, primarily at the joint.

5. Aponeurosis.

a. Tendinous expansion.

b. Insertion for a muscle; connects muscle with the part it moves.

6. Bursae.

a. Sacs of connective tissue.

b. Filled with synovial fluid.

c. Function is to minimize friction.

d. Locations.

(1) Where tendons rub against bone, ligaments, or other tendons.

(2) Where skin moves over a bony prominence.

B. Characteristics.

1. Irritability.

2. Contractibility.

3. Extensibility.

4. Elasticity.

C. Main functions.

1. Produce movement.

a. Attachments

(1) Origin:

(a) More proximal and fixed.

(b) Closer to center of portion of body.

(2) Insertion: more moveable and distal.

b. Prime mover: directly brings about a desired motion. Example: the biceps brachii (prime mover) contracts to flex the elbow.

c. Antagonist (opponents): muscle that directly opposes the movement under consideration. Example: the biceps brachii flexes the elbow and the triceps (antagonist of the biceps) contracts to extend the elbow.

d. Fixation muscle:

(1) Essential: generally stabilizes a joint or part thereby maintaining position while prime mover acts. Example: in the pinch mechanism, the long thumb flexor and the long index flexor contract to form the pinch, while the radial wrist flexors and extensors simultaneously contract to stabilize the wrist.

(2) Postural: prevents the body being toppled by movements of heavy parts shifting center of gravity. Example: bending at the waist

e. Synergist: a muscle that contracts simultaneously with another muscle to produce the same or similar action. Example: the biceps brachii and brachialis contract simultaneously to flex the elbow.

f. Paradoxical actions: counter force of gravity. Example: biceps contract when elbow extended while lowering heavy weight.
2. Maintain posture and body position.
3. Support soft tissue.
4. Guard entrances and exits to digestive and urinary tracts.
5. Maintain body temperature.

D. Muscle action.

1. Controlled by central nervous system.
2. Functions are complex, variable, and often involuntary.
3. Contractions.
   a. Isometric: increase in tension without change in length.
   b. Isotonic: muscle shortens when weight is lifted.

E. Nerve supply.

1. Motor and sensory fibers derived from spinal nerves.
   a. Posterior primary rami: extensor muscles of spine.
   b. Anterior primary rami: all other muscles.
2. "Motor point" is entry point of nerve into muscle.

F. Blood supply from adjacent vessels.

G. Aging and muscular system.

1. Skeletal muscle fibers become smaller in diameter.
2. Skeletal muscles becomes smaller and less elastic.
3. Tolerance for exercise decreases.
4. The ability to recover from muscular injuries decreases.

IV. JOINTS

A. Gross structure.

1. Cartilage.
   a. Hyaline.
      (1) Covers ends of bone, articular surfaces.
      (2) Is avascular, nerveless, and relatively acellular.
      (3) Resilient and elastic.
      (4) Nonradiopaque.
      (5) Nourished by synovial fluid.
   b. White fibrocartilage.
      (1) Greater tensile strength than hyaline cartilage.
      (2) Found in wrist, knee joint, at ends of clavicle, in intervertebral discs, and in areas of insertion of tendon into bone.
   c. Consists of chondrocytes.
2. Synovial membrane.
   a. Encapsulates and lines the joint.
   b. Made of vascular connective tissue.
   c. Produces synovial fluid.
      (1) Lubricates.
      (2) Nourishes the articular cartilage.

B. Classifications.

1. Synarthrosis or fibrous.
   a. Immovable.
   b. Bones connected by fibrous tissue or cartilage.
2. Amphiarthrosis or cartilaginous: slightly moveable.
   a. Symphysis: connected by broad, flat disc of fibrocartilage.
   b. Syndesmosis: bony surfaces are united by an interosseous ligament.
   c. Suture: joints in the skull that allow accommodation for the growing brain.
3. Diarthrosis or synovial: freely moveable.
   a. Characteristics:
      (1) Articular surfaces covered with hyaline cartilage enclosed by joint capsule containing synovial fluid.
      (2) Intrinsic ligaments: thickening of capsule.
      (3) Accessory ligaments: limit movement of joint but separate from capsule.
   b. Types.
      (1) Gliding.
      (2) Hinge or ginglymus.
      (3) Condyloid.
      (4) Saddle or stellar.
      (5) Pivot or trochoid.
      (6) Ball and socket or spheroidal.

C. Motions.

1. Flexion: forward or anterior.
   a. Dorsiflexion: toe up motion of the ankle.
   b. Plantar flexion: toe down motion of the ankle.
2. Extension: backward or posterior.
3. Hyperextension: extension beyond 0 degrees.
4. Lateral flexion: trunk bent to either side.
5. Abduction: away from the midline.
6. Adduction: toward the midline.
7. Circumduction: combination of abduction, adduction, flexion, and extension.
8. Rotation.
   a. Medial or internal: toward the midline.
   b. Lateral or external: away from the midline.
9. Version:
   a. Eversion: sole of foot turned directed outwardly.
   b. Inversion: sole of foot turned directed medially
10. Pivot: rotation of head on neck.
11. Pronation: forearm so palm faces posteriorly or down
12. Supination: forearm turned so palm faces anteriorly or up.

IV. SKULL

A. Structures.

1. Cranial bones.
   a. Frontal.
   b. Parietal (pair).
   c. Occipital.
   d. Temporal (pair).
   e. Sphenoid.
   f. Ethmoid.
2. Facial bones.
   a. Zygomatic (pair).
   b. Maxillae (pair).
   c. Nasal (pair).
   d. Lacrimal (pair).
   e. Vomer.
   f. Palatine (pair).
   g. Inferior conchae (pair).
   h. Mandible.

Table 2.1
Muscles of the Upper Extremity

Muscle	Action	Origin	Insertion	Innervation
Rotator Cuff				
Supraspinatus	Abduction of humerus	Supraspinous fossa of scapula	Greater tuberosity of humerus	Suprascapular
Infraspinatus	Lateral rotation of humerus	Infraspinous fossa of scapula	Greater tuberosity of humerus	Suprascapular
Teres minor	Lateral rotation of humerus	Lateral margin of scapula	Greater tuberosity of humerus	Branch of axillary
Subscapularis	Medial rotation of humerus	Subscapular fossa of scapula	Lesser tuberosity of humerus	Subscapular
Scapular Stabilizers				
Trapezius	Scapular rotation	Occipital bone, spinous processes of seventh cervical and all thoracic vertebrae	Clavicle, acromion process, and spine of the scapula	Accessory and third and fourth cervical
Rhomboideus major	Retraction and elevation scapula	Spinous processes of second, third, fourth, and fifth thoracic vertebrae	Vertebral margin of the scapula	Dorsal scapula
Levator scapulae	Elevation of scapula	Transverse processes of first four cervical vertebrae	Vertebral border of the scapula	Anterior branches of third and fourth cervical nerve
Serratus anterior	Forward movement of scapula	First eight or nine ribs	Vertebral border of the scapula	Long thoracic
Pectoralis minor	Forward and downward displacement of shoulder	Third to fifth ribs	Coracoid process of the scapula	Medical pectoral

VI. SHOULDER GIRDLE

A. Structure.

1. Clavicle.
2. Scapula.
   a. Acromion.
   b. Coracoid process.
   c. Glenoid fossa or cavity.
   d. Spine.
   e. Inferior notch.
   f. Superior, medial, and lateral borders.
   g. Scapular notch.
   h. Supraspinous fossa.
   i. Infraspinous fossa.
3. Humeral head.

B. Muscles (see Table 2.1).

1. Rotator cuff.
   a. Supraspinatus.
   b. Infraspinatus.
   c. Teres minor.
   d. Subscapularis.
2. Scapular stabilizers.
   a. Trapezius.
   b. Rhomboideus major.
   c. Rhomboideus minor.
   d. Levator scapulae.
   e. Serratus anterior.
   f. Pectoralis minor.
3. Principal movers of shoulder (see Table 2.2).
   a. Deltoid.
   b. Pectoralis major.
   c. Latissimus dorsi.
   d. Teres major.
   e. Coracobrachialis.

C. Joints.

1. Acromioclavicular.
2. Sternoclavicular.
3. Glenohumeral.
4. Coracoclavicular.
5. Coracoacromial.
6. Coracohumeral.

D. Nerves: brachial plexus.

1. Median.
2. Ulnar.
3. Radial.
4. Musculocutaneous.
5. Axillary.

E. Major arteries.

1. Subclavian.
2. Axillary.
3. Brachial.

VII. UPPER EXTREMITY

A. Arm: humerus.

1. Largest bone in upper extremity.
2. Structure.
   a. Head.
   b. Greater and lesser tubercles.
   c. Tuberosities.
   d. Anatomic neck.
   e. Surgical neck.

Table 2.2
Principal Movers of Shoulder

Muscle	Action	Origin	Insertion	Innervation
Deltoid	Abduction of the arm	Clavicle, acromion, and the scapular spine	Deltoid tuberosity of humerus	Axillary
Pectoralis major	Flexion, adduction, and internal rotation of the arm	Sternum, clavicle, and cartilages of first to sixth ribs, aponeurosis of obliqus externus abdominus	Crest of bicipital groove of humerus	Medial and lateral pectoral, brachial plexus
Latissimus dorsi	Adduction, extension, and internal rotation of the humerus	Spines of thoracic and lumbar vertebrae, lumbodorsal fascia, iliac crest, lower ribs, and inferior angle of scapula	Bicipital groove of humerus	Thoracodorsal
Teres major	Adduction, extension, and internal rotation of the arm	Inferior angle of scapula	Bicipital groove of humerus	Subscapular
Coracobrachialis	Flexion and adduction of the arm	Coracoid process of scapula	Medial surface of humeral shaft	Musculocutaneous

f. Capitulum.
g. Trochlea.
h. Epicondyles.
(1) Medial.
(2) Lateral.
i. Bicipital groove.
j. Shaft.
k. Coronoid fossa.
l. Olecranon fossa.

B. Forearm: radius.
1. Smaller bone of the forearm.
2. Structure.
a. Head.
b. Tuberosity.
c. Styloid process.
d. Neck.
e. Ulnar notch.

C. Forearm: ulna.
1. Larger bone of the forearm.
2. Structure.
a. Olecranon process.
b. Coronoid process.
c. Trochlear notch.
d. Styloid process.
e. Tuberosity.
f. Radial notch.

D. Muscles acting on the forearm (see Table 2.3).
1. Flexors.
a. Biceps brachii.
b. Brachialis.
c. Brachioradialis.
d. Pronator teres.
2. Extensor: triceps brachii.
3. Supinators.
a. Supinator.
b. Biceps brachii.
4. Pronators.
a. Pronator teres.
b. Pronator quadratus.

E. Joints.
1. Elbow.
2. Humeroulnar.
3. Humeroradial.
4. Proximal radioulnar.
5. Distal radioulnar.
6. Interosseous.

F. Ligaments.
1. Collateral.
a. Ulnar.
b. Radial.
2. Orbicular.

G. Nerves.
1. Axillary.
2. Musculocutaneous.
3. Radial.
4. Median.
5. Ulnar.

H. Major arteries.
1. Axillary.
2. Brachial.
3. Radial.
4. Ulnar.

VIII. WRIST, HAND, AND FINGERS

A. Structure.
1. Carpals.
a. Proximal.
(1) Scaphoid.
(2) Lunate.
(3) Triquetrium.
(4) Pisiform.
b. Distal.
(1) Trapezium.
(2) Trapezoid.
(3) Capitate.
(4) Hamate.
2. Metacarpals.
a. Five long bones forming framework of palm.
b. Numbered 1-5 starting with thumb.
c. Structure.
(1) Head: articulates with phalanges.
(2) Shaft.
(3) Base: articulates with carpals.
3. Phalanges.
a. Each hand has 14.
b. Each finger has three except the thumb which has two.
c. Structure.
(1) Distal phalanx.
(2) Middle phalanx.
(3) Proximal phalanx.
4. Sesamoid.
5. Carpal tunnel.
a. Groove formed by carpal bones.
b. Deep part of flexor retinaculm.
c. Long digital flexor muscle tendons.
d. Median nerve.

B. Muscles (see Table 2.4).
1. Flexors.
a. Flexor carpi ulnaris.
b. Palmaris longus.
c. Flexor carpi radialis.
d. Flexor digitorum superficialis or sublimus.
e. Flexor digitorum profundus.
f. Flexor digiti minimi brevis manus.
2. Extensors.
a. Extensor carpi ulnaris.
b. Extensor digiti minimi.
c. Extensor indicis proprius.
d. Extensor carpi radialis longus.
e. Extensor carpi radialis brevis.
f. Extensor digitorum communis.
3. Other muscles acting on the hand and fingers.
a. Opponens digiti minimi.
b. Abductor digiti minimi manus.
c. Lumbricals.
d. Palmar interosseous.
e. Dorsal interosseous manus.
4. Muscles acting on the thumb.
a. Extensor pollicis longus.

Table 2.3
Movers Acting on the Forearm

Muscle	Action	Origin	Insertion	Innervation
Flexors				
Biceps brachii	Flexion and supination of the forearm	Short head from coracoid process and long head from upper border of glenoid fossa	Radial tuberosity and deep fascia of the forearm	Musculocutaneous
Brachialis	Flexion of the forearm	Anterior surface of humerus	Coronoid process of the ulna	Musculocutaneous and radial
Brachioradialis	Flexion of the forearm	Lateral supracondylar ridge of humerus	Distal radius	Radial
Pronator teres	Pronation and flexion of the forearm	Medial epicondyle of humerus and coronoid process	Lateral surface of the radius	Median
Extensor				
Triceps brachii	Extension of the forearm	• Long head: infraglenoid tubercle of scapula • Lateral head: posterior surface of humerus; lateral intermuscular septum • Medial head: posterior surface of humerus below radial groove, medial border of humerus, medial intermuscular septa	Olecranon process of the ulna	Radial
Supinators				
Supinator	Supination of the forearm	Lateral epicondyle of the humerus	Radius	Deep radial
Biceps brachii	Supination and flexion of the forearm	• Short head: apex of coracoid process • Long head: superior border of glenoid cavity	Radial tuberosity and deep fascia of the forearm	Musculocutaneous
Pronators				
Pronator teres	Pronation of the forearm	Medial epicondyle of humerus and coronoid process	Lateral surface of the radius	Median
Pronator quadratus	Pronation of the forearm	Anterior surface and border of distal third or fourth of the ulna	Distal fourth of the radius	Anterior interosseous

Table 2.4
Muscles of the Wrist, Hand, and Fingers

Muscle	Action	Origin	Insertion	Innervation
Flexors				
Flexor carpi ulnaris	Wrist flexion and adduction	Medial epicondyle of humerus, olecranon, and intermuscular septum	Pisiform and fifth metacarpal, hamulus of hamate	Ulnar
Palmaris longus	Wrist flexion	Medial epicondyle of humerus	Flexor retinaculum and palmar aponeurosis	Median
Flexor carpi radialis	Wrist flexion and abduction	Medial epicondyle of humerus	Base of second metacarpal	Median
Flexor digitorum superficialis or sublimus	Middle phalangeal flexion	Medial epicondyle of humerus, coronoid process of radius	Middle phalanges	Median
Flexor digitorum profundus	Distal phalangeal flexion	Shaft of ulna	Distal phalanges	Ulnar and anterior interosseous
Flexor digiti minimi	Little finger flexion	Hamulus of hamate and transverse carpal ligament	Medial proximal phalanx of little finger	Ulnar
Extensors				
Extensor carpi ulnaris	Wrist extension and adduction	Lateral humeral epicondyle and dorsal border of ulnar	Base of fifth metacarpal	Deep radial
Extensor digiti minimi	Little finger extension	Common extensor tendon, lateral epicondyle of humerus	Tendon of extensor digitorum to little finger	Radial
Extensor indicis proprius	Index finger extension	Dorsal surface of ulna and interosseous membrane	Common extensor tendon of index finger	Deep radial
Extensor carpi radialis longus	Wrist extension and abduction	Lateral supracondyle of humerus	Base of second metacarpal	Radial
Extensor carpi radialis brevis	Wrist extension and abduction	Lateral epicondyle of humerus	Base of third metacarpal	Radial
Extensor digitorum communis	Finger and wrist extension	Lateral epicondyle of humerus	Common extensor tendon each finger	Deep radial
Other Muscles Acting on the Hand and Fingers				
Opponens digiti minimi	Fifth metacarpal abduction and rotation	Transverse carpal ligament and hamulus of hamate	Medial aspect fifth metacarpal	Ulnar
Abductor digiti minimi manus	Little finger abduction	Pisiform and flexor carpi ulnaris	Medial proximal phalanx of little finger	Ulnar

Table 2.4 (continued)
Muscles of the Wrist, Hand, and Fingers

Muscle	Action	Origin	Insertion	Innervation
Other Muscles Acting on the Hand and Fingers (continued)				
Lumbricals	Flexion metacarpophalangeal joint and extension middle and distal phalanges	Flexor digitorum profundus	Extensor tendons of four lateral fingers	Ulnar and median
Palmar interosseous	Adduction and flexion proximal phalanx	Sides of second, fourth, and fifth metacarpals	Extensor tendons of second, fourth, and fifth fingers	Ulnar
Dorsal interosseous manus	Abduction and flexion proximal phalanx	By two heads from adjacent sides of metacarpals	Extensor tendons of second, fourth, and fifth fingers	Ulnar
Muscles Acting on the Thumb				
Extensor pollicis longus	Extension thumb	Dorsal surface of ulna and interosseous membrane	Posterior surface of the base of the distal phalanx of the thumb	Deep radial
Flexor pollicis longus	Thumb flexion	Anterior surface of the radius	Base of distal phalanx of the thumb	Anterior interosseous
Extensor pollicis brevis	Thumb extension	Dorsal surface of radius and interosseous membrane	Dorsal surface of proximal phalanx of the thumb	Deep radial
Flexor pollicis brevis	Thumb flexion and abduction	Transverse carpal ligament, ridge of trapezium	Base of proximal phalanx of the thumb	Median and ulnar
Abductor pollicis longus	Thumb abduction and extension	Posterior surfaces of radius and ulna	Radial side base of first metacarpal	Deep radialis
Abductor pollicis brevis	Thumb abduction and extension	Ridge of trapezium, transverse carpal ligament, and scaphoid	Lateral surface of base of proximal thumb	Median
Adductor pollicis	Thumb adduction	• Caput obliquum: sheath of flexor carpi radialis, anterior carpal ligament, capitate, and bases of second and third metacarpals • Caput transversum: distal two thirds of anterior surface of third metacarpal	Medial surface of base of proximal phalanx	Ulnar
Opponens pollicis	Thumb flexion and opposition	Ridge of trapezium and transverse carpal ligament	Radial side of first metacarpal	Sixth and seventh cervical through median

b. Flexor pollicis longus.
c. Extensor pollicis brevis.
d. Flexor pollicis brevis.
e. Abductor pollicis longus.
f. Abductor pollicis brevis.
g. Abductor pollicis.
h. Opponens pollicis.

C. Joints.
1. Radiocarpal.
2. Carpometacarpal.
3. Metacarpophalangeal.
4. Interphalangeal.

D. Ligaments.
1. Collateral: radial and ulnar.
2. Intercarpal, radiocarpal, ulnarcarpal: palmar, and dorsal.
3. Palmar and dorsal carpometacarpal.
4. Metacarpal: palmar and dorsal.
5. Transverse.
6. Palmar accessory.
7. Hamatometacarpal.
8. Pisohamate.
9. Pisometacarpal.

E. Arteries.
1. Common interosseous.
2. Anterior and posterior interosseous.

IX. THORACIC CAGE

A. Ribs: 12 pairs.
1. True.
2. False.
3. Floating.

B. Sternum.
1. Manubrium.
2. Body.
3. Xiphoid process.

X. SPINE: VERTEBRAL COLUMN

A. Vertebrae.
1. Cervical: 7 vertebrae between the skull and thorax.
   a. Atlas.
      (1) First cervical vertebra.
      (2) Skull rests on it.
   b. Axis.
      (1) Second cervical vertebra.
      (2) Site of the odontoid process or dens.
2. Thoracic: 12 vertebrae between cervical and lumbar vertebrae.
3. Lumbar: 5 vertebrae between thoracic and sacral.
4. Sacrum: 5 vertebrae, fused.
5. Coccyx: 4 vertebrae, usually fused.

B. Structure of a vertebra.
1. Body.
   a. Gives strength.
   b. Supports weight.
   c. Mostly spongy bone.
   d. Separated from other bodies by intervertebral disc.
2. Vertebral canal: passageway for the spinal cord and spinal nerves.
3. Lamina: right and left lamina from vertebral arch.
4. Spinous process: posterior spinal projections.
5. Transverse process: lateral spinal projections.
6. Articular process.
7. Pedicle.
8. Facet.
9. Vertebral foramen.
10. Zygopophyseal joints.

C. Structure of intervertebral disc.
1. Annulus fibrosus.
   a. Outer ring.
   b. Circular concentric layers of fibrocartilage
2. Nucleus propulsus.
   a. Inner portion.
   b. Collagen and reticular fibers composed of 75% water.

D. Sagittal curvatures of the adult vertebral column.
1. Cervical.
2. Thoracic; secondary.
3. Lumbar.
4. Sacral.

E. Abnormal curvatures of the spine.
1. Kyphosis: increased roundback, anterior concavity.
2. Lordosis: increased lumbar curvature, posterior concavity.
3. Scoliosis: lateral curvature.

F. Abnormalities of the spine.
1. Spina bifida: failure of posterior arch formation.
2. Spondylolysis: disruption of pars interarticularis.
3. Spondylolisthesis: slip forward of vertebral body.

G. Muscles of the neck and back (see Table 2.5).
1. Superficial.
   a. Trapezius.
   b. Latissimus dorsi.
   c. Levator scapulae.
   d. Rhomboidei: minor and major.
2. Intermediate.
   a. Serratus posterior superior.
   b. Serratus posterior inferior.
3. Deep.
   a. Splenius capitus.
   b. Splenius cervicis.
   c. Semispinalis thoracis, semispinalis cervicis, semispinalis capitis.
   d. Multifidi.
   e. Rotatores cervicis, rotatores thoracis, rotatores lumborum.

H. Ligamentous structures.
1. Anterior longitudinal ligament: anterior to vertebral bodies.
2. Posterior longitudinal ligament: posterior to vertebral bodies.
3. Annulus fibrosis: between vertebral bodies in area composing intervertebral disc space.
4. Ligamentum flavum: bounds intervertebral foramen posteriorly.
5. Interspinous ligament: anterior ligament.
6. Supraspinous ligament: posterior ligament.

I. Nerves.
1. Cervical: 8 pairs.

Table 2.5
Muscles of the Neck and Back

Muscle	Action	Origin	Insertion	Innervation
Superficial				
Trapezius	Elevation, rotation, and dorsal motion of scapula; elevates and lowers shoulders	Cervical spinous processes and spines of thoracic vertebrae	Lateral third of clavicle, acromion, and scapular spine	Spinal accessory third and fourth cranial nerves
Latissimus dorsi	Extension, abduction, and medial rotation of humerus	Six caudal thoracic, all lumbar spines, sacrum, and iliac crest	Intertubercular sulcus humerus	Thoracodorsal nerve of the brachial plexes C 6-7-8
Levator scapulae	Upward and medial pulling of the scapulae	Transverse processes C 1-4	Superior angle and base of spine of scapula	Cervical plexes and dorsal scapular
Rhomboidei: minor and major	Upward and medial pulling of the scapulae	Major: spines of T 2, 3, 4, 5; minor: C 7, T 1	Medial border scapula to spine of scapula	Dorsal scapula or nerve C 4, 5
Intermediate				
Serratus posterior superior	Elevation of first four ribs; assists in inspiration	Spinous processes C7 and T 1, 2, 3	Ribs 2-5 lateral to their angles	Intercostal
Serratus posterior inferior	Pulls last four ribs caudally, helps in expiration	From T 11 and 12 and L1 and 2 spinous processes	Inferior borders of last four ribs, lateral to their angles	Intercostal nerves
Deep				
Splenius capitus	Extension of the head and neck, rotation of head to the same side	Spinous processes C 3 to T 3 and upper thoracic spine	Lateral nuchal line and mastoid process of temporal bone	Posterior rami
Splenius cervicis	Extension of the head and neck, rotation of head to the same side	Spines of T 3-6	Transverse processes C 1-3	Posterior rami
Semispinalis thoracis Semispinalis cervicis Semispinalis capitis	Extension of the head and vertebral column; supports head	• Thoracis and cervicis: transverse processes of thoracic vertebrae • Capitis: transverse processes of 3 cervical and 6 thoracic vertebrae	• Thoracis and cervicis: spinous processes of 4 to 6 segments higher than their origin, including the spines of the axis • Capitis: between the superior and inferior nuchal line	Dorsal rami of cervical and thoracic nerves
Multifidi	Extension of the vertebral column; lateral motion and rotation of vertebrae	Dorsal surface of sacrum; transverse processes lumbar and thoracic vertebrae	Spinous processes lumbar, thoracic and cervical vertebrae	Dorsal rami of spinal nerves (cervical, thoracic, and lumbar)
Rotatores cervicis Rotatores thoracis Rotatores lumborum	Extension of the vertebral column; lateral motion and rotation of the vertebrae	• Cervicis: transverse processes of cervical vertebrae • Thoracis: transverse processes thoracic vertebrae • Lumborum: transverse processes lumbar vertebrae	Roots of the spinous processes of the adjacent or second vertebrae above	Dorsal rami of spinal nerves (cervical, thoracic, and lumbar)

2. Thoracic: 12 pairs.
3. Lumbar: 5 pairs.
4. Sacral: 5 pairs.
5. Coccygeal: 1 pair.
6. Cauda equina: mass of spinal nerves below spinal cord starting at L1.

J. **Major arteries.**
1. Common carotids.
    a. Internal.
    b. External.
2. Vertebral.

XI. PELVIC GIRDLE

A. **Structure.**
1. Sacrum.
2. Ox coxae.
    a. Ilium.
    b. Ischium.
    c. Pubis.
3. Acetabulum.
4. Iliac crest.
5. Greater sciatic notch.
6. Obturator foramen.
7. Rami.
    a. Superior pubis.
    b. Inferior pubis.
8. Ischial tuberosity.
9. Ramus of ischiium.
10. Male pelvis.
    a. Subpubic arch:
        (1) 70-75 degrees.
        (2) Canal long and tapered.
    b. Inlet triangular.
11. Female pelvis.
    a. Subpubic arch:
        (1) 90-100 degrees.
        (2) Canal shorter and parallel sides.
    b. Inlet larger and oval.

B. **Joints.**
1. Sacroiliac joints.
2. Symphysis pubis.

C. **Ligaments.**
1. Sacroiliac.
    a. Interosseous.
    b. Ventral.
    c. Dorsal.
2. Sacrotuberous.
3. Sacrospinous.

D. **Major nerves.**
1. Lumbar plexus.
    a. Femoral.
    b. Saphenous.
2. Sacral plexus.
    a. Posterior femoral cutaneous.
    b. Sciatic.
        (1) Tibial.
        (2) Common peroneal.

E. **Major arteries.**
1. Common iliac.
    a. Internal.
    b. External.
2. Obturator.
3. Femoral.

F. **Major veins.**
1. Femoral.
2. Greater saphenous.

XII. LOWER EXTREMITY

A. **Hip.**
1. Formed by the articulation of the acetabulum and femur.
2. Structures.
    a. Acetabulum.
        (1) Superior dome.
        (2) Fovea centralis.
        (3) Posterior lip.
        (4) Labrum.
    b. Femur.
        (1) Femoral head.
        (2) Femoral neck.
        (3) Trochanters.
            (a) Lesser.
            (b) Greater.
        (4) Intertrochanteric region.
        (5) Subtrochanteric region.
        (6) Gluteal tuberosity.
3. Muscles (see Table 2.6).
    a. Gluteus maximus.
    b. Gluteus medius.
    c. Gluteus minimus.
    d. Tensor fasciae latae.
    e. Piriformis.
    f. Obturator internus.
    g. Obturator externus.
    h. Quadratus femoris.
    i. Gemellus inferior.
    j. Gemellus superior.
4. Ligaments.
    a. Capsular.
    b. Iliofemoral.
    c. Teres.
    d. Transverse.
5. Nerves.
    a. Femoral.
    b. Obturator.
    c. Sciatic.
6. Major arteries.
    a. External iliac.
    b. Common femoral.
        (1) Superficial.
        (2) Deep.

B. **Femur.**
1. Structure.
    a. Femoral head.
    b. Femoral neck.
    c. Trochanters.
        (1) Lesser.
        (2) Greater.
    d. Shaft.
    e. Condyles.

Table 2.6
Muscles of the Lower Extremity

Muscle	Action	Origin	Insertion	Innervation
Gluteus maximus	Extension and external rotation of the thigh	Lateral surface of ilium, dorsal surface of sacrum and coccyx, sacrotuberous ligament	Iliotibial band of fascia lata, gluteal tuberosity of femur	Inferior gluteal
Gluteus medius	Abduction of the thigh	Lateral surface of ilium between anterior and posterior gluteal lines	Greater trochanter of femur	Superior gluteal
Gluteus minimus	Abduction and internal rotation of the thigh	Lateral surface of ilium between anterior and inferior gluteal lines	Greater trochanter of femur	Superior gluteal
Tensor fasciae latae	Extends knee	Iliac crest	Iliotibial band of fascia lata	Superior gluteal
Piriformis	External rotation of thigh	Ilium, second to fourth sacral vertebrae	Superior border of greater trochanter	First and second sacral
Obturator internus	External rotation of thigh	Pelvic surface of femur, margin of obturator	Greater trochanter of femur	First, second, and third sacral
Obturator externus	External rotation of thigh	Pubis, ischium, and superficial surface of obturator membrane	Trochanteric fossa of femur	Obturator
Obturator femoris	Abduction and external rotation of thigh	Superior ischial tuberosity	Quadrate tubercle of femur	Sacral plexus
Gemellus inferior	External rotation of thigh	Ischial tuberosity	Greater trochanter of femur	Sacral plexus
Gemellus superior	External rotation of thigh	Spine of ischium	Greater trochanter of femur	Sacral plexus

(1) Medial.
(2) Lateral.
f. Linea aspera.
2. Muscles of posterior thigh: hamstring muscles (see Table 2.7).
a. Semimembranosus.
b. Semitendinosus.
c. Biceps femoris.
3. Muscles of medial thigh: adductors.
a. Pectineus.
b. Adductor brevis.
c. Adductor longus.
d. Adductor magnus.
e. Gracilis.
4. Muscles of the anterior thigh (see Table 2.8).
a. Sartorius.
b. Quadriceps femoris: consists of rectus femoris, vastus lateralis, vastus intermedius, and vastus medialis.
c. Rectus femoris.
d. Vastus lateralis.
e. Vastus intermedius.
f. Vastus medialis.
g. Iliopsoas: iliacus and psoas major.
h. Iliacus.
i. Psoas major.
5. Nerves.
a. Saphenous.
b. Sciatic.
c. Femoral.
6. Major artery: femoral.
a. Deep.
b. Superficial.

C. Knee (genu).
1. Formed by the articulation of the distal femur with the proximal tibia.
2. Bony structures.
a. Patella.
b. Tibia.
(1) Tibial condyle.
(a) Medial.
(b) Lateral.
(2) Intercondylar eminence.
c. Tibial tubeosity.
d. Distal femur.
(1) Femoral epicondyle.
(a) Medial.
(b) Lateral.
(2) Femoral condyle.
(a) Medial.
(b) Lateral.
(3) Intercondylar fossa.
(4) Adductor tubercle.
(5) Patellar groove.
3. Other structures.
a. Suprapatellar pouch.
b. Prepatellar bursa.
c. Retropatellar fat pad.
4. Ligaments.
a. Collateral.
(1) Medial.
(2) Lateral.
b. Cruciate.
(1) Anterior.
(2) Posterior.
c. Menisci.
(1) Medial.
(2) Lateral.
d. Posterior capsule.
e. Patellar tendon.
f. Ligament of the fibular head.
5. Major nerve: peroneal.
6. Major artery: popliteal.

D. Tibia.
1. Larger bone in lower leg.
2. Structure.
a. Plateaus.
(1) Medial.
(2) Lateral.
b. Condyles.
(1) Medial.
(2) Lateral.
c. Tubercle.
d. Shaft.
e. Medial malleolus.

E. Fibula: smaller bone in lower leg.
1. Head.
2. Neck.
3. Shaft.
4. Lateral malleolus.

F. Muscles of the leg (see Table 2.9).
1. Anterior compartment: dorsiflexors.
a. Tibilalis anterior.
b. Extensor digitorum longus.
c. Extensor hallucis longus.
d. Peroneus tertius.
2. Lateral compartment: plantar flexion.
a. Peroneus longus.
b. Peroneus brevis.
3. Superficial posterior compartment.
a. Popliteus.
b. Triceps surae muscles:
(1) Plantaris.
(2) Soleus.
(3) Gastrocnemius.
4. Deep posterior compartment.
a. Tibialis posterior.
b. Flexor digitorum longus.
c. Flexor hallucis longus.
d. Popliteus.

G. Ligaments of the lower leg.
1. Tibiofibular.
2. Interosseous.

H. Nerves of the lower leg.
1. Peroneal.
a. Deep.
b. Common.
c. Superficial.
2. Nervus cutaneous patella.
3. Sural.

Table 2.7
Muscles of the Posterior and Medial Thigh

Muscle	Action	Origin	Insertion	Innervation
Posterior Thigh: Hamstring Muscles				
Semimembranosus	Knee flexion, thigh extension, and medial rotation	Ischial tuberosity	Medial tuberosity	Tibial
Semitendinosus	Thigh flexion, extension, and medial rotation	Ischial tuberosity	Superior and medial surface of tibia	Tibial portion sciatic
Biceps femoris	Thigh flexion and extension	Short head from linea aspera of femur, long head from ischial tuberosity	Head of fibula, lateral tibial condyle	Peroneal and tibial
Medial Thigh: Adductors				
Pectineus	Flexion and adduction of thigh	Superior ramus of pubis	Femur distal to lesser trochanter	Obturator and femoral
Adductor brevis	Flexion, adduction, and rotation of thigh	Lateral inferior pubic ramus	Superior to linea aspera of femur	Obturator
Adductor longus	Flexion, adduction, and rotation of thigh	Crest and symphysis of pubis	Linea aspera of femur	Obturator
Adductor magnus	Adduction and extension of thigh	Crest and symphysis of pubis, ramus of ischium, and ischial tuberosity	Linea aspera of femur and adductor tubercle of femur	Sciatic and obturator
Gracilis	Thigh adduction and knee flexion	Inferior ramus of pubis and ischium	Medial tibia	Obturator

Table 2.8
Muscles of the Anterior Thigh

Muscle	Action	Origin	Insertion	Innervation
Sartorius	Thigh flexion, abduction	Anterior superior iliac spine	Medial side of proximal tibia	Femoral
Rectus femoris	Leg extension and thigh flexion	Anterior inferior iliac spine, brim of acetabulum	Patella	Femoral
Vastus lateralis	Leg extension	Hip capsule, lateral femur	Common tendon of quadriceps femoris, patella	Femoral
Vastus intermedius	Leg extension	Anterior and lateral femur	Common tendon of quadriceps femoris, patella	Femoral
Vastus medius	Leg extension	Medial femur	Common tendon of quadriceps femoris, patella	Femoral
Iliacus	Thigh flexion	Iliac fossa and inferior sacrum	Lesser trochanter of femur	Femoral
Psoas major	Trunk flexion	Lumbar vertebrae and fascia	Lesser trochanter of femur	Second and third lumbar

4. Posterior tibial.

I. Major arteries of the lower leg.
1. Popliteal.
2. Anterior tibial.
3. Posterior tibial.
4. Peroneal.

J. Ankle and foot.
1. Ankle.
   a. Ankle: formed by the articulation of the distal fibula and tibia with the talus.
   b. Structure.
      (1) Medial malleolus.
      (2) Structure.
      (3) Lateral malleolus.
   c. Tendons.
      (1) Achilles.
      (2) Anterior tibial.
      (3) Posterior tibial.
2. Foot.
   a. Structures.
      (1) Tarsus.
         (a) Calcaneus.
            i. Tuberosity.
            ii. Sustenaculum tali.
         (b) Talus.
            i. Head.
            ii. Body.
            iii. Trochlea
         (c) Cuboid.
         (d) Scaphoid.
         (e) Cuneiforms.
         (f) Navicular.
      (2) Metatarsals.
         (a) Hallux (great toe)
         (b) Head.
         (c) Base.
      (3) Phalanges.
      (4) Sesamoids.
      (5) Plantar aponeurosis.
      (6) Plantar fascia.
      (7) Fat pad.
   b. Arches.
      (1) Medial longitudinal.
      (2) Lateral longitudinal.
      (3) Transverse.
   c. Flatfoot: Loss of height of medial longitudinal arch.
3. Muscles (see Table 2.10).
   a. Extensor digitorum brevis.
   b. Adductor hallucis.
   c. Flexor hallucis brevis.
   d. Flexor digiti minimi brevis pedis.
   e. Interosseous plantaris.
   f. Interosseous dorsalis pedis.
   g. Quadratus plantar.
   h. Abductor hallucis.
   i. Abductor digiti minimi pedis.
   j. Lumbricals pedis.
   k. Flexor digitorum brevis.

Table 2.9
Muscles of the Leg

Muscle	Action	Origin	Insertion	Innervation
Anterior Compartment: Dorsiflexors				
Tibialis anterior	Inversion and dorsiflexion of foot	Tibia, interosseous membrane	Medial cuneiform and first metatarsal	Deep peroneal
Extensor digitorum longus	Extension of toes	Anterior surface of fibula, lateral condyle of tibia, interosseous membrane	Common extensor tendon of four lateral toes	Deep peroneal
Extensor hallucis longus	Dorsiflexion of ankle joint and extension of great toe	Anterior tibia and interosseous membrane	Dorsal surface of base of distal phalanx of great toe	Deep peroneal
Peroneus tertius	Eversion and dorsiflexion of foot	Medial surface of fibula	Fifth metatarsal	Deep peroneal
Lateral Compartment: Plantar Flexion				
Peroneus longus	Plantar flexion, abduction, and eversion of foot	Lateral surface of fibula and lateral condyle of tibia	First metatarsal, medial cuneiform	Superficial peroneal
Superficial Posterior Compartment				
Popliteus	Flexion and lateral rotation of femur	Lateral condyle of femur	Posterior surface of tibia	Tibial
Plantaris	Plantar flexion of foot, knee flexion	Lateral condyle of femur	Posterior part of calcaneus	Tibial
Soleus	Plantar flexion of ankle	Fibula, tibia, and popliteal fascia	Calcaneous by tendocalcaneous (Achilles)	Tibial
Gastrocnemius	Plantar flexion of foot and knee flexion	Popliteal surface of femur, superior medial condyle and capsule of knee; lateral condyle	Aponeurosis unites with tendon soleus to form calcaneal tendon (Achilles)	Tibial
Deep Posterior Compartment				
Tibialis posterior	Inversion and plantar flexion of foot	Tibia, fibula, and interosseous membrane	Navicular tuberosity; bases of metatarsals and tarsals except talus	Tibial
Flexor digitorum longus	Flexion of toes and extension of foot	Posterior surface of tibial shaft	Distal phalanges of four lateral toes	Tibial
Flexor hallucis longus	Flexion of great toe	Posterior surface of fibula	Base of phalanx of great toe	Tibial

Table 2.10
Muscles of the Foot and Ankle

Muscle	Action	Origin	Insertion	Innervation
Extensor digitorum brevis	Toe extension	Dorsal surface of calcaneus	Extensor tendons of second, third, and fourth toes	Deep peroneal
Adductor hallucis	Flexes metatarsophalangeal joint of great toe	• Caput obliqum: bases of second, third, and fourth metatarsals and sheath of peroneus longus • Caput transversum: capsules of metarsophanlangeal joints of three lateral toes	Lateral side of base of proximal great toe	Lateral plantar
Flexor hallucis brevis	Great toe flexion	Under surface of cuboid and middle and lateral cuneiform	Base of proximal phalanx of great toe	Medial and lateral plantar
Flexor digiti minimi brevis pedis	Flexion of little toe	Base of fifth metatarsal, plantar fascia	Lateral surface of base of proximal phalanx of little toe	Lateral plantar
Interosseous plantaris	Adduction and flexion of toes	Medial surface third, fourth, and fifth metatarsals	Extensor tendons of third, fourth, and fifth toes	Lateral plantar
Interosseous dorsalis	Abduction and flexion of toes	Surfaces of adjacent metatarsals	Extensor tendons of second, third, and fourth toes	Lateral plantar
Quadratus plantae	Flexion of toes	Calcaneus and plantar fascia	Tendons of flexor digitorum longus	Lateral plantar
Abductor hallucis	Abduction and flexion of great toe	Medial tuberosity of calcaneus, plantar fascia	Medial surface of base of proximal phalanx of great toe	Medial plantar
Abductor digiti minimi pedis	Flexion and abduction of little toe	Medial and lateral tubercles of calcaneus, plantar fascia	Base of proximal phalanx of fifth toe	Lateral plantar
Lumbricals pedis	Extends toes at interphalangeal joints	Tendons of flexor digitorum longus	Extensor tendons of four lateral toes	Medial and lateral plantar
Flexor digitorum brevis	Flexion of toes	Medial tuberosity of calcaneus and plantar fascia	Middle phalanges of four lateral toes	Medial plantar

4. Major ligaments.
   a. Deltoid.
   b. Talofibular.
   c. Calcaneofibular.
   d. Tibiofibular.
   e. Collateral
5. Nerves.
   a. Plantar.
   b. Posterior tibial.
   c. Peroneal.
6. Arteries.
   a. Posterior tibial.
   b. Dorsalis pedis.

XIII. GAIT

A. Line of gravity:

1. Straight line going in front of atlanto-occipital joints.
2. Front of 11th thoracic vertebra.
3. Behind head of femur.
4. Through the patella.
5. To the arch of the foot.

B. Gait cycle.

1. Stance phase:
   a. 60% of cycle.
   b. Starts with heel strike to midstance and ends with toe off.
2. Swing phase:
   a. 40% of cycle.
   b. Starts with toe off to swing phase and ends with heel strike.

Bibliography

Alcamo, I.E. (1996). *Anatomy and physiology.* Hauppauge, NY: Barron's Educational Series, Inc.

Ellis, H. (1997). *Clinical anatomy: A revision and applied anatomy for clinical students* (9th ed.). Cambridge: Blackwell Scientific Publishers.

Martini, F., & Bartholomew, E. (1997). *Essentials of anatomy and physiology.* Upper Saddle River, NJ: Prentice Hall.

Scott-Conner, J.A., & Dawson, R.E. (1994). *Operative anatomy* (2nd ed.). Philadelphia: Lippincott-Raven.

Snell, R. (1996). *Clinical anatomy: An illustrated review with questions and explanations* (2nd ed). Philadelphia: Lippincott-Raven.

Snell, R. (2000). *Clinical anatomy for medical students.* Baltimore: Lippincott, Williams, & Wilkins.

Van de Graaff, K., & Rhees, R.W. (1997). *Theory and problems of human anatomy and physiology* (2nd ed.). New York: McGraw-Hill.

STUDY QUESTIONS

Don, a 17-year-old high school football player, sustained an injury to his posterior thigh during an exhibition game. He was evaluated on the sidelines and found to have point tenderness in the mid portion of the medial posterior thigh. (Questions 1-3)

1. Muscles of the posterior thigh (hamstring) are:
   a. Sartorius, quadriceps femoris, rectus femoris.
   b. Rectus femoris, vastus lateralis, vastus medialis.
   c. Semimembranosus, semitendinosus, and biceps femoris.
   d. Iliacus, psoas major, piriformis.

2. The primary functions of the hamstring are:
   a. Thigh extension and internal rotation.
   b. Thigh flexion and external rotation.
   c. Thigh extension and lateral rotation.
   d. Thigh flexion and medial rotation.

3. The muscle of the anterior thigh include:
   a. Gracilis, rectus femoris, and sartorius.
   b. Rectus femoris, quadriceps femoris, and sartorius.
   c. Gracilis, sartorius, psoas major.
   d. Rectus femoris, psoas major, and sartorius.

Ron, a 27-year-old softball pitcher, has been inactivated due to a torn rotator cuff in his pitching shoulder. (Questions 4-6)

4. The rotator cuff is comprised of:
   a. Trapezius, rhomboideus major, and pectoralis minor.
   b. Deltoid, teres major, and pectoralis major.
   c. Supraspinatus, infraspinatus, teres minor, and subscapularis.
   d. Coracoacromial, coracoclavicular, rhomboideus minor.

5. Which of the following is **not** a nerve innervating the brachial plexus?
   a. Suprascapular.
   b. Ulnar.
   c. Branch of the axillary.
   d. Radial.

6. Which movement is **not** performed by the rotator cuff?
   a. Abduction of the humerus.
   b. Adduction of the humerus.
   c. Lateral rotation of the humerus.
   d. Medial rotation of the humerus.

Ted was evaluated by an orthopaedic surgeon for pain and swelling in his left knee. After an initial radiograph was found to be within normal limits, the physician suggested further studies to more definitively diagnose his problem. (Questions 7-9)

7. In evaluating joint pain, it is important to be aware of which of the following?
   a. Hyaline cartilage covers articular surface, is avascular and nonradiopaque.
   b. Cartilage encapsulates and lines all joints in the body.
   c. Cartilage consists of vascular connective tissue that is radiopaque.
   d. Hyaline cartilage, connective tissue, and bone tissue all cause pain.

8. Tendons connect:
   a. Bone to muscle.
   b. Bone to bone.
   c. Ligaments to bone.
   d. Muscle to ligaments.

9. Fascia:
   a. Extends beyond muscle fibers to connect muscles.
   b. Acts as the insertion for a muscle to bone.
   c. Is a sac filled with synovial fluid that serves as a cushion.
   d. Covers and provides origins/insertions for muscles.

Susan is a 32-year-old auto accident victim who was a belted driver of a small sports car that veered off the road and hit a telephone pole. She was brought to the emergency department by ambulance and was found to be hypotensive and complaining of pain in her left low back and left leg. (Questions 10-12)

10. The nurses caring for Susan should be aware that one of the major arteries in the pelvis is the:
    a. Common superficial femoral artery.
    b. Vertebral artery.
    c. Common deep femoral artery.
    d. Common iliac arteries.

11. In consideration of the pelvic structures, it is important to note that the:
    a. Hip joint is part of the pelvis.
    b. Acetabulum is part of the pelvis.
    c. Symphysis articulates with the acetabulum.
    d. Greater sciatic notch comes through the acetabulum.

12. The sciatic nerve branches to these two more distal nerves:
    a. The tibial and common peroneal nerves.
    b. The peroneal and femoral nerves.
    c. The femoral and obturator nerves.
    d. The common peroneal and saphenous nerves.

Jim is a 47-year-old construction worker who enjoys biking on weekends and holidays. While biking on a path, he hit a hole and was thrown from the bike. He felt some discomfort in the calf of his right leg but was able to mount the bike and continue on the path. That night he noticed increased discomfort and swelling in the right calf. The following day he went to see his family physician for continued problems in the calf. (Questions 13-15)

13. The calf is divided into the following four compartments:
    a. Peroneal, tibial, fibular, and extensor.
    b. Anterior, lateral, superficial, and extensor.
    c. Posterior, medial, lateral, and intermediate.
    d. Tibial, fibular, medial, and lateral.

14. The calf muscles are responsible for motion of the:
    a. Hip, knee, and ankle.
    b. Hip and knee.
    c. Foot and ankle.
    d. Knee, foot, and ankle.

15. The nerve responsible for inversion and dorsiflexion of the foot is the:
    a. Superficial peroneal.
    b. Tibial.
    c. Deep peroneal.
    d. Posterior tibial.

Chapter 3 *Musculoskeletal Assessment*

Nina A. Rauscher, MS, RN,C, CRRN, ONC

Contents

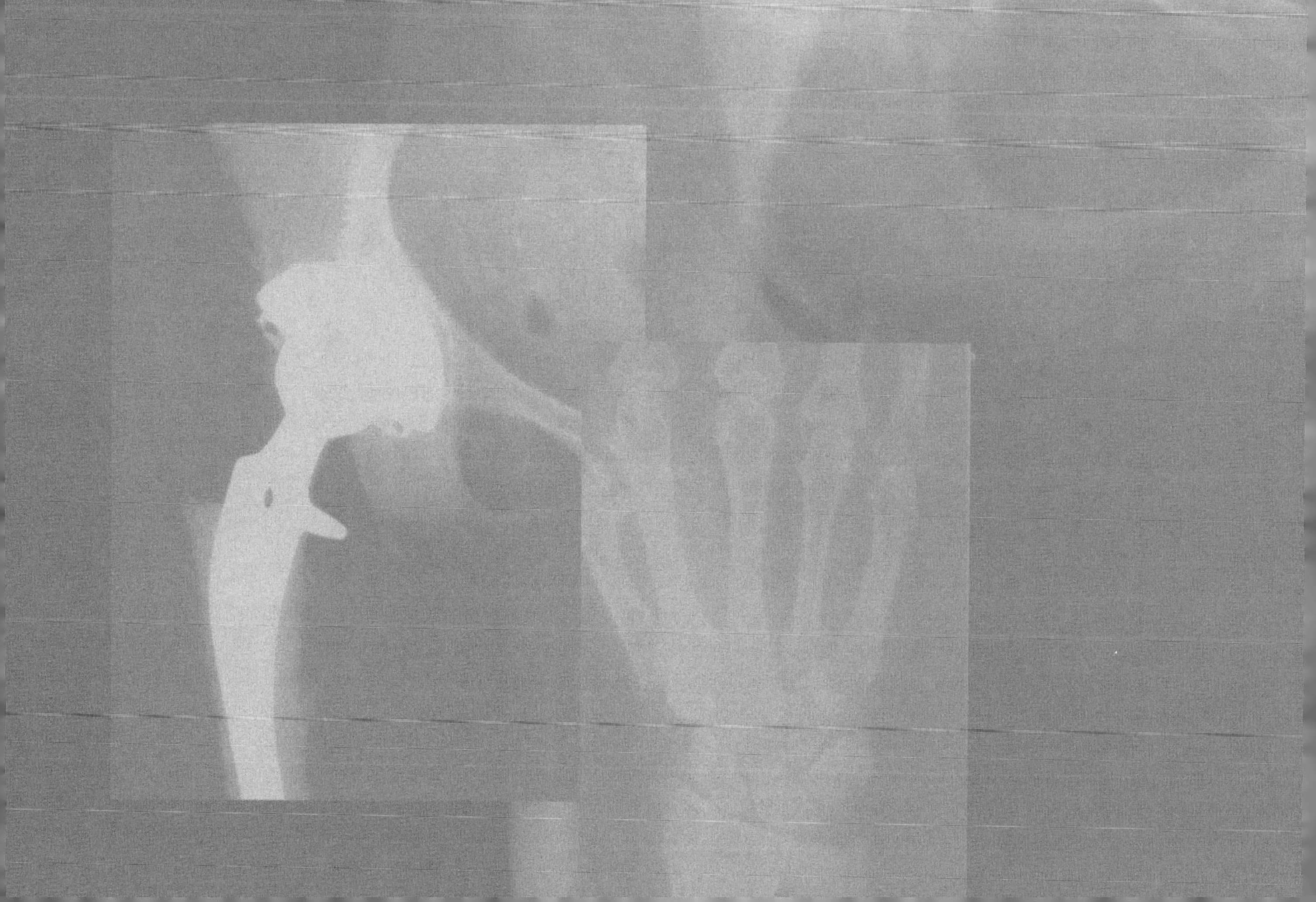

OBJECTIVES

At the completion of this chapter, the learner will be able to:

- Recognize terminology used in musculoskeletal assessment.
- Develop a list of data gathered during the history-taking process.
- Describe the steps in physical assessment, taking into consideration changes that occur throughout the lifespan.
- Recognize the tools needed for performing a musculoskeletal assessment.
- Describe abnormal symptoms found during physical assessment of the musculoskeletal system.
- Identify normal and abnormal gaits.
- Describe the steps in performing a neuromuscular evaluation.
- Identify specific tests performed to evaluate a musculoskeletal injury or compromise.
- List the steps in the assessment of sports injury.

KEY POINTS

- Many changes associated with aging result from normal physiologic change and gradual loss of function.
- The key to assessing the elderly is to ascertain their ability to perform activities of daily living.
- If a patient has experienced a traumatic injury to the cervical spine, do not move the neck or remove the cervical collar until radiographs confirm the absence of a fracture.
- Injuries due to sports or related activities occur frequently, and if left undiagnosed or untreated, can hamper or end further participation in sports.
- The key to assessing children is to use language they can understand.

CHAPTER 3

MUSCULOSKELETAL ASSESSMENT

I. OVERVIEW

A. Definition: musculoskeletal assessment is a comprehensive, organized collection of pertinent information from which the problems or physiologic needs of an individual with a musculoskeletal disorder can be identified and evaluated.

1. A plan of care can be developed and the individual returned to a state of improved health or pre-injury health.
2. The musculoskeletal physical assessment requires a thorough understanding of anatomic structures, physiologic function, and changes occurring throughout the lifespan that influence assessment.
3. Attaining a competence level in the art of history taking, using descriptive terminology, using specific tools for the collection of musculoskeletal data, and hands-on assessment techniques allow for the collection of pertinent data.
4. Table 3.1 defines musculoskeletal terminology.

II. THE HEALTH HISTORY

A. Data may be collected in a variety of ways.

1. Interviews with the individual, family, or significant others.
2. Review of past medical records, electronic lifetime clinical records, which include a previous episode(s) of care.
3. Consultation and collaboration with other health care professionals, and spiritual/cultural influences.
4. Physical examination.
5. Diagnostic studies.

B. The interview.

1. Introduce yourself/explain your professional role.
2. Assure the patient's level of comfort and privacy, clarifying with the patient who he or she would like present during the interview.
3. Encourage questions and validate patient's understanding of process.
4. In order to assess patient, holistic approach is needed.
   a. Cultural history.
   b. Social history.
   c. Psychological history.
   d. Spiritual history.
5. Consider influence of culture and spirituality upon patient's health care beliefs.
   a. Special traditions to maintain health.
   b. Use of non-traditional health care.
   c. Impact of religion or spirituality on quality of life.
6. Have patient use his or her own words to describe symptoms and pain.
7. Restate significant findings to the patient for confirmation.

C. Components of the health history.

1. Chief complaint (CC): ascertain in the patient's own words the reason for seeking medical attention.
2. History of present illness (HPI).
   a. Chronologically explore all symptoms and complaints leading up to the illness or hospitalization.
   b. Describe the patient's usual state of health.
      (1) Physical.
      (2) Social.
      (3) Psychological.
      (4) Spiritual.
   c. Include all traditional and nontraditional interventions used and whether effective.
3. Past medical history (PMH): information pertaining to previous episodes of illness, injuries (including violence), treatments, surgeries, hospitalizations, and immunizations, (when and why).
4. Current health status (CHS). Obtain data regarding:
   a. Smoking history: type of tobacco, how much, how long, last time used.
   b. Alcohol consumption: types, frequency, quantity, last time consumed.
   c. Medications: name/dosage/schedule/last time taken, prescription, vitamins, herbal, over-the-counter, and recreational usage.
   d. Allergies: environmental, drug, latex.
   e. Nutrition: 24-hour dietary recall and weight loss or gain?
   f. Exercise: types, frequency, duration, last time performed.
5. Family history (FH).
   a. Information about age/health of parents, siblings, grandparents, children.
   b. Pertinent information regarding the family unit, such as major health problems or genetic disorders.
6. Review of systems: an orderly review of subjective symptoms from each physiologic system (general, head, skin, nose, eyes, ears, throat, respiratory, cardiovascular, gastrointestinal, neurological, reproductive, musculoskeletal, endocrine, genitourinary).

D. Special considerations: examine in detail the signs of the current illness, such as the sequence of the development and distinct characteristics of each of the symptoms as well as any interaction between them.

1. Trauma.
   a. After life-threatening priorities have been assessed and treated, the nurse must do a rapid, yet thorough and systematic, physical assessment.
   b. Care must be taken so the dramatic injury does not cause a less obvious yet potentially more serious injury to be overlooked.
   c. If the trauma is violence related, be aware of the need for preserving evidence.

Table 3.1
Musculoskeletal Terminology

Abduction: motion in which a body part moves away from a defined line, for example, the midline of the body.

Adduction: motion in which a body part moves toward a defined line.

Ankylosis: abnormal fusion, immobility of a joint due to pathologic changes; may occur if a joint is surgically fused.

Atrophy: deterioration, wasting, or degeneration of tissue.

Causalgia: severe burning pain related to paraesthesia or partial injury of peripheral nerves.

Circumduction: swinging motion or movement, abduction, adduction, flexion, and extension totaling 360 degrees or a full circle of motion; this motion is seen in the shoulder, hip, and ankle.

Contracture: abnormal shortening or contraction of soft tissue and muscles often seen about a joint(s).

Coxa vara: deformity of hip associated with a decrease in the angle of the femoral neck.

Deformity: malformation or defect of any part of the body.

Leg-length discrepancy: inequality in the length of legs genetically or iatrogenically induced.

Dislocation: displacement of joint surfaces altering alignment, caused by traumatic injury, congenital defect, or pathology (disease, infection, or inflammation).

Dorsiflexion: movement of a body part up toward the dorsum as when the ankle moves to point the toes toward the head.

Dysplasia: abnormal development of tissue.

Eversion: turning outward of the foot and ankle.

Extension: motion involving an increase in the angle of a joint between two bones; pulling or extending.

External rotation: the rotating motion of a joint outward.

Flexion: motion involving a decrease in the angle of a joint between two bones; bending or contracting.

Gait: a definite pattern or style of achieving upright bipedal locomotion.

Goniometer: instrument used for measuring joint movement and angle.

Hallux valgus: lateral deviation of the great toe toward the second toe.

Hyperextension: excessive extension of a joint.

Internal rotation: rotating motion of a joint inward.

Inversion: turning inward of the foot and ankle.

Kyphosis (round back): excessive angulation, curvature, or convexity of the thoracic spine due to disease (osteoporosis, arthritis, rickets) or other pathologic conditions.

Lateral: the area toward the outer aspect of the body away from the midline.

Lordosis: concavity of the vertebral column; a normal curvature existing in cervical and lumbar areas, which may become pathologic if accentuated.

Medial: area nearest the midline of the body.

Palmar flexion: motion of the wrist moving the hand down.

Plantar flexion (equinus): motion of the ankle moving the foot downward.

Palsy: inability to move a part as in paralysis.

Planes:
- Cardinal frontal: the plane that divides the body into front and back segments.
- Cardinal horizontal: the plane that divides the body into top and bottom segments.
- Cardinal sagittal: the plane that divides the body into left and right sides.
- Midsagittal: divides the body in the cardinal sagittal plane.

Passive movement: any body movement that occurs without muscle contraction.

Pronation: motion of the forearm characterized by the palm down or movement toward the posterior of the body in the anatomic position.

Range of motion: the full motion a joint can move.

Recurvatum: hyperextension of the joint as in the knee or genu recurvatum.

Relaxation: stage during which the force of contraction is diminishing to inactivity.

Rotation: motion that involves turning on an axis in a circular movement.

Scoliosis: lateral curvature of the spine.

Subluxation: a sideways force causing slipping, shifting, displacement, with partial or incomplete dislocation of the joint surfaces.

Supination: the motion of the forearm characterized by the palm up or movement toward the anterior portion of the body in the anatomic position.

Tonus: the residual low level turgor or feeling of firmness found even in a relaxed muscle.

Tophi: deposits of urate crystals in the soft tissue in and about a joint with a resemblance to nodules.

Torque: twisting or rotation about a pivotal point.

Torsion: twisting or rotation about the axis of a structure.

Transverse: lying across or horizontally.

Valgus: deformity characterized by angulation away from the midline of the body distal to the anatomic part named as in valgus knee deformity, or knock-kneed.

Varus: a deformity characterized by angulation toward the midline of the body and distal to the anatomic part named as in varus knee, or bowleggedness.

(1) Photographs should be taken before removing or cutting clothing (cut along seams of clothing).
(2) Photographs may also need to be taken prior to some wound care.
(3) For rape victims, depending on the law in each state, law enforcement should be notified. (Any felonious assault must be reported.) Calls need to be made to a crisis center, rape care advocate, and/or a Sexual Assault Nurse Examiner. Support patient, inform patient of available support-system options, obtain appropriate patient consent, and notify appropriate parties.

d. Questions that should be asked:
(1) What was injured?
(2) How did it happen?
(3) Where did the injury occur?
(4) What was the specific mechanism of the injury?
(5) What was the force?
(6) What was the direction of the force?
(7) When did the injury occur?
(8) When was the onset of pain or disability?
(9) When did the swelling, redness, discoloration, numbness, or temperature change occur?
(10) What was done and by whom?
(11) If a motor vehicle accident, was the patient the driver?
(12) Was the steering wheel or windshield broken?
(13) Did a seat belt, car seat, child safety belt, or air bag restrain the injured person?
(14) Were splints, ice, heat, or any type of first aid administered, and what was the result?
(15) Were any analgesics used, and what was the effect?
(16) How was the patient transported to the health care facility?
(17) How do the current symptoms influence activities of daily living (ADL)?
(18) Last tetanus booster/immunization?

2. Chronic problem.
a. When did the symptoms begin?
b. How long have the symptoms been present?
c. Are the symptoms continuous or intermittent?
d. How did the symptoms begin?
e. Why does the patient believe the symptoms began?
f. What helps or irritates the condition?
g. What interventions have been used (both traditional and nontraditional) and their effect?
h. Response of condition to heat or cold?
i. Has the condition influenced ability to exercise?
j. What position causes pain?
k. Medications, herbs, over-the-counter products that have been used and what was the effect?
l. Complementary or alternative therapies that have been used such as therapeutic massage, acupuncture, aromatherapy, etc?
m. How has the condition affected patient's ability to work, attend school, sleep, and have sexual relations?

3. Congenital.
a. Was there any prenatal care?
b. Did anything occur of significance during the prenatal period or during the delivery?
c. What were the developmental milestones?
d. What is the family history?
e. How has the condition influenced the ability to attend school and have social relationships?
f. What is the influence on ADL?

III. CONSIDERATIONS ACROSS THE LIFESPAN

A. Children.

1. Height/weight.
2. School history including attendance and grades.
3. Home situation.
4. Consider abuse when frequent health care encounters for injuries are identified.
5. Previous illness, especially recent earaches or throat problems.
6. Age of menstruation.
7. Eating habits: anorexia or bulimia.
8. Nutritional intake: calcium, balanced diet.
9. Identify potential risky behavior patterns:
   a. Smoking.
   b. Drug use.
   c. Alcohol use.
   d. Unprotected sex.
   e. New driver.
   f. Lack of protective gear when engaging in sports.
10. Consider repetitive injury secondary to computer use.
11. Back injury may be related to carrying heavy backpacks.
12. Teens may not reveal changes in their body (scoliosis) to their parents.
13. Special needs of children:
   a. Size of child does not equate to maturity.
   b. Explain special needs using terminology children will understand.
   c. Permit children to feel equipment (as safety allows).
14. Older children may wish to be examined and interviewed alone, without the presence of parent.
15. Children need privacy whenever possible.

B. Elderly.

1. Mental status, as age does not equate to mental agility.
2. Ability to communicate: assess hearing, eyeglass use.
3. Many changes associated with aging result from subtle loss of function due to physiologic change.
4. Community ambulator or homebound.
5. Ability to perform ADL with or without assistive devices.
6. Support from family, friends, or outside agencies.
7. Impact on social and sexual relationships.

8. Assess home environment for access and safety.
   a. Single family versus multiple units in building.
   b. Elevator.
   c. Stairs: number and location.
   d. Lighting.
   e. Rugs.
   f. Gas/electric/oil heat.
   g. Air conditioning.
   h. Telephone.
9. Transportation available. Type.
10. Quality of life.
11. Impact on spirituality.

IV. GENERAL TECHNIQUES OF MUSCULOSKELETAL PHYSICAL EXAMINATION

A. Primary techniques used in musculoskeletal examination include inspection, palpation, and range-of-motion techniques.

1. Inspection of the musculoskeletal system includes:
   a. Visual scanning of the two sides of the body for symmetry, contour, and size.
   b. Observe for gross deformities, areas of swelling or inflammation, skin changes such as ecchymosis or other discoloration, and muscle atrophy.
2. Palpation is used to:
   a. Detect pain, tenderness, swelling, localized temperature changes.
   b. Marked changes in muscle shape, muscle tone, and resistance to pressure.
   c. Crepitus, abnormal bone development, bone or joint pathologies.
3. Range of motion of joints to:
   a. Determine the active and passive range of motion of joints.
   b. Evaluate muscle tone and muscle strength.
   c. Sensory and motor skills.

B. General guidelines for musculoskeletal assessment.

1. The examination should be performed after providing privacy to the patient.
2. Patient should be dressed in a way that allows full visualization of the body and facilitates examination without needlessly exposing him/her.
3. Wash hands before proceeding with examination.
4. The examination should proceed in an orderly fashion from head to toe, proximal to distal.
5. Compare one side of the body to the other, frequently alternating the assessment of one part of the body to the other side.
6. Examination should reflect the influence upon ADL, including impact on school and work.
7. Questions should be worded in a way that helps ascertain this information. For example:
   a. Are you able to get into and out of the bathtub?
   b. Can you stand at work?
   c. Can you comb your hair?
   d. Can you lift your backpack?

C. Equipment/tools used for musculoskeletal assessment.

1. Active listening skills.
2. Goniometer.
3. Reflex hammer.
4. Tape measure.
5. Flashlight.
6. Object to determine sharp/dull senses (Wartenberg pinwheel).
7. Cotton wisp.

D. Muscle function testing.

1. Muscle function testing is a method of examination that provides the following information:
   a. Strength of individual muscles or muscle groups that form a functional unit.
   b. Size, extent, and progress of peripheral nerve lesions.
   c. Nature of simple movement patterns.
   d. Conditions for physiotherapy and capability for physical work by body part being tested.
2. When performing a muscle function test properly, it is essential for the examiner to be knowledgeable about individual muscles and their movements.
3. Careful assessment is essential, especially in cases where there is decreased range of movement, contractures, or pain.
4. Technical rules: to perform muscle function tests properly, the following principles must be observed:
   a. Entire range of movement (not only the beginning or end of the range) must be tested.
   b. Movement must occur at an even, steady speed throughout.
   c. The limb being tested must be held by the examiner to assure stability.
   d. At the point where the limb is being held, neither the tendon nor the muscle must be under pressure.
   e. Resistance must be applied continuously and always against the direction of movement.
   f. Resistance must be applied with uniform strength throughout.
   g. Resistance must not be applied over two joints.
   h. The person being tested must start to perform movement as he/she is accustomed; only after recording the movement pattern is it corrected if necessary.
5. Test of muscle strength. Note that the tests are based on the fact that some muscle strength is always required to move a specific part of the body. The strength is adapted to the circumstances under which movement is carried out. Muscle test is scored as follows:
   a. Muscle can overcome a resistance directed against the movement.
   b. Muscle can overcome gravity.
   c. Muscle can work, but only when gravity is eliminated.
   d. Muscle can contract, but no movement results.

E. Muscle grading is the method of grading muscle function and has changed many times, although the principles have remained the same. The following is the simplest and most often used method.

1. Grade 5: N (normal):
   a. A normal, very strong muscle with full range of movement and ability to overcome considerable resistance.

   b. This does not imply that the muscle is normal in all circumstances (for example, when at the onset of fatigue or in a state of exhaustion).
2. Grade 4: G (good): a muscle with good strength, full range of movement, and ability to overcome moderate resistance.
3. Grade 3: F (fair): a muscle with complete range of movement against gravity only when resistance is not applied.
4. Grade 2: P (poor): a very weak muscle with complete range of movement only when careful positioning of the patient eliminates gravity.
5. Grade 1: T (trace): a muscle with evidence of slight contractility but no effective movement.
6. Grade 0: a muscle with no contractility.

F. Normal range of motion for joints (see Table 3.2).

G. Neurovascular assessment: evaluation of sensation, motion, and circulation of extremity: always compare one side of the body to the other.

1. Color: pink, pale, cyanotic, mottled, red, blue-tinged.
2. Temperature: hot, warm, cool, cold.
3. Capillary refill: rapid, sluggish, or absent (normal is 2 seconds).
4. Edema: absent, mild, moderate, pitting, dependent.
5. Pulses: bounding, strong, weak, not palpable or detected by Doppler®.
6. Sensation: normal, hyperesthetic (increased sensation, tingling, etc.), hypoesthetic (decreased sensation).
7. Pain: constant, intermittent, sharp, dull, burning, aching, with activity, at rest.

H. Reflex testing.

1. Reflex is a stereotypical involuntary motor response by the nervous system to a specific stimulus.
2. To test a reflex, the tendon must be partly stretched and lightly tapped (usually with the reflex hammer).
3. Always repeat several times and alternate with other limb, comparing response.
4. A nervous patient may react strongly or may stiffen giving a misleading response; therefore it may be necessary to repeat the reflex evaluation later in the examination.
5. The reflex consists of the following cycle: stimulus→travels along sensory nerve→synapses in spinal cord→travels back along motor nerve fiber→neuromuscular junction→stimulates muscle→jerk.
6. Using a straw man diagram of the body, mark reflex response next to area tested.
   a. Grade 4+: hyperactive, extremely brisk response.
   b. Grade 3+: response brisker than normal.
   c. Grade 2+: within normal limits.
   d. Grade 1+: response hypoactive, diminished.
   e. Grade 0: no response, flaccid.

I. Analysis of gait. Gait is a definite pattern or style of achieving upright bipedal locomotion.

1. Inspection begins while escorting the patient to the examination room.

Table 3.2
Normal Range of Motion for Joints

Joint	Range of Motion
Cervical spine	
Flexion	80-90 degrees
Extension	70 degrees
Lateral flexion	20-45 degrees
Rotation	70-90 degrees
Lumbar spine	
Flexion	40-60 degrees
Extension	20-35 degrees
Lateral flexion	15-20 degrees
Rotation	3-18 degrees
Shoulder	
Flexion	160-180 degrees
Extension	50-60 degrees
Abduction	170-180 degrees
Adduction	50-75 degrees
External rotation	80-90 degrees
Internal rotation	60-100 degrees
Circumduction	200 degrees
Elbow	
Flexion	140-160 degrees
Extension	0-10 degrees
Supination	90 degrees
Pronation	80-90 degrees
Wrist	
Flexion	80-90 degrees
Extension	70-90 degrees
Ulnar deviation	35-45 degrees
Radial deviation	15 degrees
Pronation	85-90 degrees
Supination	85-90 degrees
Hip	
Flexion	110-120 degrees
Extension	10-15 degrees
Abduction	30-50 degrees
Adduction	30 degrees
External rotation	40-60 degrees
Internal rotation	30-40 degrees
Knee	
Flexion	0-130 degrees
Extension	0-15 degrees
Medial rotation	20-30 degrees
Lateral rotation	30-40 degrees
Ankle	
Plantar flexion	50 degrees
Dorsiflexion	20 degrees
Inversion	30 degrees
Eversion	20 degrees
Subtalar inversion	5 degrees
Subtalar eversion	5 degrees
Forefoot adduction	20 degrees
Forefoot abduction	10 degrees
Great toe flexion	45 degrees
Great toe extension	70 degrees

2. Inspection: observe walking for 10-20 feet; note the phases of gait.
   a. Stance phase (weight bearing).
      (1) Heel strike.
      (2) Foot flat.
      (3) Midstance.
      (4) Push-off.
   b. Swing phase (nonweight bearing).
      (1) Acceleration.
      (2) Midswing.
      (3) Deceleration.
      (4) Note the body alignment while ambulating, position of head, shoulders, spine, pelvis (oscillates 2 inches vertically and shifts 1 inch laterally), knees, and feet.
      (5) Note rhythm of walk as pelvis rotates forward 40 degrees while arms swing in tandem.
      (6) Note the width of the gap (ankle to ankle) between the feet while walking (2-4 inches).
      (7) Note the length of the step (approximately 15 inches heel to heel).
      (8) Note that the body center of gravity is centered midline.
      (9) Note any muscle wasting or atrophy.
      (10) Note unstable gait due to leg length discrepancy, joint problems, lack of coordination, contractures.
      (11) Document use of assistive devices, splints, and special shoes.
      (12) Note the amount and location of wear on shoe soles.
3. Listen for:
   a. Foot slapping gait.
   b. Scraping of shoe at toe.
   c. Stomping gait.
   d. Unequal rhythm of steps.
   e. Abnormal gait that is caused by: (see Table 3.3 for causes and descriptives).
      (1) Pain.
      (2) Muscle weakness.
      (3) Structural deformity.
      (4) Instability.

V. ASSESSING SPORTS INJURIES

Injuries due to sports or related activities occur frequently and to people of all ages. Although many injuries of this type heal without medical intervention, some injuries if left undiagnosed and untreated can hamper or end further participation in sports.

A. Inherent to many sports are injuries varying from minor bumps and bruises to major muscle tears or broken bones. The following guidelines may be helpful in determining when to seek medical attention.
1. Pain: prolonged, or nonsubsiding, or continuing 2 weeks after episode.
2. Joints: any injury that occurs in or near a joint.
3. Function: any loss of function.
4. Healing:
   a. Any injury that does not heal in 3 weeks, or in which the structure is apparently abnormal.
   b. Any sign of infection on or under the skin, presence of pus, red streaks, swollen lymph nodes, or fever.
5. Alterations in sensation.

B. Assessing muscle injuries.
1. Site of muscle injury.
   a. Within the muscle body (occurs in 40% of all cases).
   b. At junction of muscle to tendon.
   c. Away from its bone origin.
   d. The tendon from the muscle.
2. The best way to assess any type of muscle injury is to gently palpate the whole muscle at its origin, body, and insertion.
3. There are three grades of muscle injury:
   a. Grade 1: the muscle is strained due to stretching of a few muscle fibers with minimal tearing of fibers; there is no defect palpated; less than 10% of muscle fibers are involved.
   b. Grade 2: there is a partial tear of muscle fibers; palpation reveals a defect in the muscle; 10%-50% of muscle fibers torn.
   c. Grade 3: there is an extensive tear or complete rupture: 50%-100% of muscle fibers torn to complete rupture of muscle.

C. Special considerations when assessing sports injuries.
1. In most sports, after a certain level of strength is achieved, the overall strength of the body is not essential for success.
2. Each sport has its unique movements, requiring specific neuromuscular coordination and strength in particular muscle groups.
3. Athletes who concentrate on one sport may overdevelop some muscles and not develop others.
   a. Runners may have weak underdeveloped upper bodies and abdominal muscles.
   b. Swimmers tend to have weak, underdeveloped hamstrings.
4. It is important to keep opposing muscle groups in balance.
   a. The quadriceps extends the leg at the knee and the hamstrings flex the leg.
   b. In the case of cyclists and sprinters, the quadriceps overdevelop in relation to the hamstrings, predisposing them to many sports-related injuries due to unbalanced muscle groups.
5. There are two key points to remember:
   a. The examiner should remember muscle balancing when performing an assessment of an athlete.
   b. It may be necessary to refer the patient for further testing.
6. The best way to evaluate muscle balance is to test the strength of opposing muscle groups with isometric measuring devices. These devices also are used for isokinetic exercise (exercise involving constant resistance through full range of movement).

Table 3.3
Abnormal Gaits

Gait	Cause	Descriptive
Antalgic	Multiple disorders	Pain or discomfort on weight bearing. Ambulates on affected extremity as little as possible. Shortened stride. Expresses pain verbally, by gesture, by expression on face, or by posture while walking.
Ataxic	Neurogenic (cerebellar)	Staggering, uncoordinated gait. Sway may be evident. Foot stomping, slapping, or double tap.
Festinating	Neurogenic (Parkinson Disease)	Body held rigidly. Trunk leans forward. Short, quick, shuffling steps. Delayed start.
Quadriceps	Neurogenic (muscle or nerve injury)	Hand on thigh to support gait. Decreased quadriceps function. Knee flexion contracture.
Short leg	Structural (degenerative joint disease, congenital dislocated hip, fracture)	Leg-length discrepancy of 1 inch or more. Vertical telescoping with dip on affected side.
Senile	Aging	En bloc turning, hesitant, short steps. May need to support self to get started. Once started, able to ambulate with no apparent associated gait problems.
Spastic	Neurogenic (Cerebral palsy, hemiplegia)	Jerky, uncoordinated movement. Short steps with dragging or scraping of foot. Crossed knee (scissors) gait. Severe spasticity.
Steppage	Neurogenic (peroneal nerve injury, tertiary syphilis, paralyzed dorsiflexor muscles)	Increased hip and knee flexion in order to clear the floor. Foot slaps or drags along ground. Drop foot evident.
Trendelenberg	Myogenic (coxa vara, congenital dislocated hip)	Known as the gluteus medial lurch. Typical gait associated with positive Trendelenburg test. Duck-like waddle or sailor's sway. Pelvic drops on unaffected side displaying that gluteus medius is not functioning.

7. The speed of motion is controlled through the entire exercise. This can also be accomplished by using exercise equipment or free weights.

D. Assessing ligament injuries.

1. A ligament is a strong band of connective tissue that joins bones to other bones or to a cartilage in the joint area.
2. Ligaments tend to be pliable but not elastic, permitting limited movement while holding attached bones in place.
3. All sprains are ligament injuries, usually caused by stretching the ligament beyond its limit.
4. As with muscle injuries, there are three grades of ligament injuries.
   a. Grade 1: the ligament is stretched with no tear to up to 20% torn.
   b. Grade 2: the ligament is torn 20%-75%.
   c. Grade 3: the ligament is torn 75% to complete disruption.

E. Assessing fractures.

1. A stress fracture exists when the bone is cracked but not displaced.
2. Stress fractures are more difficult to assess.
3. The following is evident when a stress fracture exists:
   a. Point tenderness of bone except in the case of the femur.
   b. Soft tissue swelling.
   c. Full and painless range of movement at the adjacent joints.
   d. Painless resisted active movement of the joint.
   e. In time, callus can be palpated at the fracture site.
   f. If the fracture is in the lower extremity, there will be an alteration in gait due to pain upon weight bearing.
   g. Muscular atrophy may occur, especially in the anterior tibial and gastrocnemius-soleus groups on the affected side.
4. An area with a fracture will swell immediately, there will be pain with movement, and deformity may be present (displaced fracture).

5. A stable fracture is a fracture that does not have motion at the fracture site.
6. If motion is present at the fracture site, the fracture is considered unstable and there is potential for severe trauma to adjacent structures.
7. Aside from stability, fractures are classified as to:
    a. Location (proximal, middle, distal thirds of long bones).
    b. Type (transverse, oblique, segmental, longitudinal, intra-articular, etc.).
    c. See fractures, Chapter 14, Trauma.

VI. THE MUSCULOSKELETAL PHYSICAL EXAMINATION FROM HEAD TO TOE

A. Temporomandibular joint. This joint has been associated with arthritis, headache, and neck problems. Examination of the joint is often overlooked; dental and neurologic evaluation should be performed to confirm diagnosis.

1. Inspection.
    a. Observe the mandible at rest and in motion.
        (1) At rest, note the posture of the chin, discoloration, atrophy of musculature, or scars.
        (2) In motion, palpate for crepitus or clicking mouth is opened and closed.
    b. Observe teeth for dentition, wear or cracks from grinding teeth.
    c. Observe movement, function, and grimaces or verbalization of pain.
2. Listen for crepitus, clicking, or popping during movement.
3. Palpate:
    a. Bone structures from over the mouth to the ear, noting any irregularities in bone or tumors.
    b. Soft tissue for tumors while evaluating skin temperature.
4. Range of motion.
    a. Active: instruct the patient to:
        (1) Open mouth.
        (2) Close mouth.
        (3) Move jaw from side to side.
        (4) Jut jaw forward.
        (5) Normally, three fingers can be inserted sideways into the open mouth and the jaw motion side to side is 1-2 cm in each direction
    b. Passive: if the patient is unable to actively move mouth, open and close the patient's mouth for him/her.
5. Muscle testing.
    a. Instruct the patient to close mouth tightly; try to pull mouth open while pulling downward on the chin.
    b. Instruct the patient to open mouth; try to close mouth while pressing upward under the chin.
6. Reflex testing: jaw reflex is triggered by tapping on the stretched tendon associated with the trigeminal nerve.
7. Special tests.
    a. Chvostek's sign: tapping the facial nerve (CN VII) against the bone just anterior to the ear produces ipsilateral contraction of facial muscles. A positive Chvostek's sign may indicate hypocalemia found in such conditions as abnormal calcium metabolism, parathyroid hypofunction, vitamin D deficiency, tetany, and alkalosis.
    b. Trousseau's sign: blood pressure cuff is inflated on the patient's arm (creating enough pressure to stop venous circulation) for 1-5 minutes. If contractions of the fingers and hands (collectively referred to as carcopedal spasms) develop, tetany is present.

B. Cervical spine.

1. If the patient has experienced a traumatic injury, the cervical spine is immobilized until the neck injury has been ruled out (see Chapter 14, Trauma; and Chapter 18, The Spine for assessment of cervical spine injury).
2. Inspection.
    a. Evaluation is done best with the patient sitting.
    b. Walk around the patient to get a 360 degree perspective.
    c. Note how the head and neck are postured.
    d. Note how the neck moves the head (smoothly or stiffly).
    e. Note any scars, obvious deformity, muscle atrophy, or asymmetrical musculature.
3. Palpation.
    a. With head held in neutral position, palpate bony structure around the neck.
    b. Anterior: palpate the hyoid bone, thyroid cartilage, carotid pulses (one side at a time) and note structure of the first cricoid ring.
    c. Posterior, palpate the occiput, inion ("bump of knowledge"), superior nuchal line, mastoid processes, spinous processes of cervical vertebrae, and facet joints.
    d. Soft tissue should be palpated with the head held in neutral position.
        (1) From the front, feel the long sternocleidomastoid muscle, lymph node chains, thyroid gland, parotid gland, and supraclavicular fossa.
        (2) Posterior, palpate trapezius muscle, lymph nodes, and superior nuchal ligament.
4. Range of motion: do not perform if neck trauma or instability is suspected.
    a. Active flexion and extension.
        (1) Have patient flex neck (shake head "yes").
        (2) Have patient extend neck (place chin on chest and then look up toward sky).
        (3) Note reports of pain, stiffness, or limited motion.
    b. Active rotation.
        (1) Have patient turn head to right and left; if normal, the chin should line up with each shoulder.
        (2) Note reports of stiffness and pain.

c. Active lateral bending.
   (1) Have patient touch each ear to shoulder; 45 degrees is normal.
   (2) Note compensatory shoulder shrug.

d. Passive: due to relaxation of cervical muscles, range of movement may be increased.

e. Passive flexion and extension.
   (1) Gently assist patient to flex and extend neck.
   (2) Place hand on back of head and push forward so chin moves toward chest.
   (3) Place hand on forehead and push posterior on head.
   (4) Note reports of pain or stiffness.

f. Passive rotation.
   (1) Gently help patient rotate head and neck (shake head "no"); chin should line up with each shoulder.
   (2) Note reports of pain and stiffness.

g. Passive lateral bending.
   (1) Gently guide patient's ear to the shoulder by pressing on head, to 45 degrees without shoulder shrug.
   (2) Note reports of pain or stiffness.

5. Muscle testing. The major muscle groups are: intrinsics, primary/secondary flexors, primary/secondary extensors, primary/secondary rotators, primary/secondary lateral benders. The patient should be seated and comfortable.
   a. Flexion.
      (1) While supporting patient at the sternum, apply increasing resistance and ask the patient to flex the neck.
      (2) Document the grade.
   b. Extension.
      (1) While supporting the patient's back, apply increasing resistance to the patient's occipital region and ask the patient to extend the neck.
      (2) Document the grade.
   c. Lateral rotation.
      (1) Place hand on the patient's shoulder and cup the opposite cheek while having the patient try to turn to the side against resistance.
      (2) Document the grade.
   d. Lateral bending.
      (1) While standing at patient's side, place one hand on the shoulder and place the other hand on the patient's head above the ear.
      (2) Ask patient to touch ear to shoulder against resistance.
      (3) Document the grade.

6. Sensory testing.
   a. Dermatomes are an area of the skin supplied by nerves originating from a single spinal nerve root.
   b. Test the distribution of dermatomes of C5 to T1 using a sharp object.
   c. C5 is the skin over the lateral arm and sensory distribution for the axillary nerve.
   d. C6 is the lateral forearm, thumb, index finger, and sensory distribution of musculocutaneous nerve.
   e. C7 is the middle finger.
   f. C8 is the ring and little finger, medial forearm, with sensory innervation by the medial antebrachial-cutaneous nerve from the posterior cord.
   g. T1 is the medial arm with sensory innervation by the medial brachial cutaneous nerve from the posterior cord.

7. Neurologic testing. Anatomically, eight nerves originate from seven cervical vertebrae (see Table 3.4 for the sensory distribution of C5-T1).

8. Major peripheral nerves (see Table 3.5).

9. Special tests: always evaluate adjacent structures, such as teeth, jaw, scalp, cardiac, or shoulder, for problems that may refer pain to cervical spine region.
   a. Distraction.
      (1) Used to determine if traction will help relieve symptoms.
      (2) Place one hand under chin and one hand on occiput, then gently pull up, increasing space between vertebrae.
   b. Compression.
      (1) Used to locate level of pathology by narrowing the foramen, increasing pressure on facet joints, and reproducing spasm.
      (2) May cause referred pain from neck to shoulder.
      (3) Place both hands on patient's head and gently push down, reproducing symptoms.
      (4) Document location and distribution.
   c. Valsalva maneuver.
      (1) Lesions such as tumor and herniated disc cause increased intrathecal pressure.
      (2) This test further increases the pressure, resulting in increased pain.
      (3) Ask the patient to hold his/her breath while bearing down as if to evacuate the bowel.
      (4) Have patient describe pain.
      (5) Patient may describe pain intensification with coughing or sneezing.
   d. Swallowing test.
      (1) Dysphagia or painful swallowing may occur when bony protrusions, osteophytes, or soft tissue involvement are present, secondary to tumor, infection, or hematoma in anterior cervical spine region.
      (2) Ask patient to swallow while fingers are gently pressed on either side of throat.
      (3) Document reports of painful swallowing.
   e. Adson test or maneuver.
      (1) Blood flow in subclavian artery may be compromised by presence of a cervical rib, tumor, hematoma, or infection that tightened the neck muscles.
      (2) While taking the radial pulse, abduct, extend, and externally rotate patient's arm.

Table 3.4
Sensory Distribution of Nerves of the Cervical Spine

Nerve	Motor	Reflex	Sensory
C5	Shoulder abduction/ deltoid/biceps	Biceps. Brachioradialis	Axillary nerve, lateral arm
C6	Wrist extension. Biceps	Biceps. Brachioradialis	Musculocutaneous nerve, lateral forearm, thumb, and index finger
C7	Wrist flexion/finger extension/triceps	Triceps	Middle finger
C8	Finger flexion/hand	Triceps	Medial antebrachial cutaneous nerve, medial forearm, and ulnar nerve, fourth finger, little finger on ulnar side
T1	Finger abduction	None	Medial brachial cutaneous nerve, upper half medial forearm and elbow

Table 3.5
Major Peripheral Nerves

Nerve	Motor	Sensory
Radial	Wrist, thumb extension	Dorsal web space between thumb and index
Ulnar	Abduction of all fingers. Ulnar deviation	Distal ulnar aspect of little finger (volar surface)
Median	Thumb pinch, opposition, abduction, and wrist flexion	Distal fat pad of index finger (volar surface)
Axillary	Deltoid	Lateral arm and deltoid patch on upper arm
Musculocutaneous	Biceps	Lateral forearm

(3) Have patient take a deep breath while turning head toward the arm being tested.
(4) If subclavian artery is compromised, the radial pulse will decrease or be obliterated.

C. **Shoulder.**
1. See Chapter 16, The Shoulder; and Chapter 14, Trauma.
2. Inspection.
   a. As patient enters the room, note the way the arms are held, swinging smoothly in tandem or if the shoulder is held protectively.
   b. Have patient disrobe from waist up.
   c. Female patients should remove bra or pull the straps down but remain draped.
   d. Have patient sit on a chair.
   e. Anterior, note shape of sternoclavicular joint, deformity of the clavicle, prominence of the acromioclavicular joint, bulging over clavicle (hematoma signifying fracture) or deltoid wasting.
   f. Laterally, note erythema, edema, or deformity.
   g. Posterior, note shape of scapula, winging, or deformity.
   h. While standing over patient, look down and note edema, deformity of the clavicle, and asymmetry of the supraclavicular fossa.
3. Palpation.
   a. Standing behind the seated patient, palpate the bony structure of the shoulder.
   b. Begin at the deltoid and move proximally toward the cervical spine.

c. Palpate the suprasternal notch, sternoclavicular joint, the length of the clavicle, and the coracoid process.
d. While patient rotates the arm, palpate the acromioclavicular articulation and note ease of movement.
e. Palpate the acromion, the greater tuberosity of the humerus, the bicipital groove, and the outer perimeter of the scapula, noting irregularities, tumors, or expressions of pain from the patient.
f. Palpate soft tissue about shoulder.
g. Note three components of the rotator cuff: the supraspinatus, the infra supraspinatus, and teres minor.
h. Note condition of the subacromial and subdeltoid bursa.
i. Palpate musculature of the shoulder girdle, sternocleidomastoid, pectoralis major, biceps, deltoid, trapezius, rhomboid minor/major, latissimus dorsi, and serratus anterior.
j. Palpate triangle-shaped axillary region and note presence of lymph nodes and presence of brachial pulse.

4. Range of motion.
   a. Apley "scratch" test (reaching behind head and touching the top of the opposite scapula) evaluates range of motion in the shoulder.
   b. Active adduction and internal rotation.
      (1) Have patient reach across front of body and touch opposite shoulder.
      (2) Have patient reach across back and touch opposite scapula.
      (3) Note reports of tenderness or stiffness.
   c. Passive.
      (1) Patient is assisted through the range of motion only if unable to do active range of motion.
      (2) Supporting the arm being tested by the elbow and anchoring the inferior angle of the shoulder, gently assist the patient through abduction, adduction, flexion, extension, and internal rotation.
5. Muscle testing.
   a. There are nine muscle groups for nine motions of the shoulder (see Chapter 2, Anatomy and Physiology).
      (1) Primary/secondary flexors.
      (2) Primary/secondary extensors.
      (3) Primary/secondary abductors.
      (4) Primary/secondary external rotators.
      (5) Primary/secondary adductors.
      (6) Primary/secondary internal rotators.
      (7) Primary/secondary elevators.
      (8) Primary/secondary retractors.
      (9) Primary/secondary protractors.
   b. Flexion.
      (1) Stand behind patient.
      (2) With the elbow flexed at 90 degrees, have the patient begin flexion of the elbow by moving forward as you provide maximum resistance by holding the area proximal to the elbow.
      (3) Stabilize patient by placing your hand on his/her back near the shoulder.
      (4) Document the grade.
   c. Extension.
      (1) Stand behind the patient.
      (2) Continue to stabilize shoulder; with elbow flexed at 90 degrees, have patient begin to push against your hand with his/her elbow, creating shoulder extension.
      (3) Document the grade.
   d. Abduction.
      (1) Stand at side of patient.
      (2) Stabilize shoulder by placing your hand on the lateral shoulder.
      (3) With elbow flexed at 90 degrees, have patient abduct against your hand for resistance.
      (4) Document the grade.
   e. Adduction.
      (1) Continue to stabilize the shoulder.
      (2) Have the patient try to pull own arm away from body while you apply resistance on the medial side.
      (3) Document the grade.
   f. External rotation.
      (1) Continue to stabilize the shoulder.
      (2) Hold patient by wrist and externally rotate the shoulder by having patient push out against resistance.
      (3) Document the grade.
   g. Internal rotation.
      (1) Continue to stabilize the shoulder.
      (2) Have patient try to pull in as you try to push out.
      (3) Document the grade.
   h. Scapular elevation.
      (1) Stand behind the patient.
      (2) With your hands on the patient's shoulders, ask the patient to shrug.
      (3) Document the grade.
   i. Scapular retraction.
      (1) Stand in front of patient.
      (2) Place your hands so your fingers are on the lateral aspects of the shoulder and your thumb on the posterior clavicle.
      (3) Ask patient to stand at attention with shoulders pulled back.
      (4) Document the grade.
   j. Scapular protraction.
      (1) Stand behind the patient.
      (2) Place your palm on the scapula while cupping the elbow, flexed at 90 degrees, with your other hand.
      (3) Ask patient to move his/her shoulder forward as if reaching for something while applying resistance.
      (4) Document the grade.
6. Reflex testing.

Table 3.6
Sensory Testing of the Shoulder

Nerve Root	Sensation
C5	Regimental patch area on lateral arm
T1	Medial arm
T2	Axilla
T3	Axilla to nipple
T4	Nipple

a. Lightly tap the elbow for the biceps and triceps tendon.
b. Document reaction.

7. Sensory testing.
   a. Using a sharp object, lightly prick the skin.
   b. Document patient's response (see Table 3.6).
8. Special tests: always evaluate adjacent structures, such as the lungs, abdomen, diaphragm, heart, cervical spine, spinous processes, ribs, or elbow, for problems that may refer pain to the shoulder.
   a. Yergason test/maneuver.
      (1) Determines biceps tendon stability in the bicipital groove.
      (2) Have patient flex elbow to 90 degrees while stabilizing the elbow by cupping and pulling downward.
      (3) Place other hand on the patient's wrist while externally rotating the arm as the patient attempts to resist.
      (4) If patient experiences sudden pain, the tendon may have popped out of the bicipital groove.
   b. Drop arm test.
      (1) Evaluate for tear of the rotator cuff.
      (2) Stand behind the patient.
      (3) Have patient abduct arms as high as possible.
      (4) Observe the muscles of the shoulder as each of the muscle groups transition to lower the arm.
      (5) If the arm suddenly drops, a tear in the rotator cuff is probable.
   c. Apprehension test.
      (1) In the shoulder, indicates shoulder laxity with history of dislocation/subluxation.
      (2) Standing behind the patient, place your hand on the acromion.
      (3) With your other hand, abduct and externally rotate patient's arm.
      (4) The patient will become noticeably "apprehensive" if the shoulder is about to sublux and will attempt to stop the examination.
9. Quick evaluation of shoulder.
   a. Pain: at rest, when lying on affected side at night, special motion (pitching).
   b. Hands behind head.
   c. Hands behind back.
   d. Hands across to other shoulder.

D. Elbow.

1. See Chapter 14, Trauma.
2. Inspection.
   a. As patient enters the examining room, observe posture and carrying angle of the elbow. The overall appearance of patient's gait should be smooth with arms moving in tandem.
      (1) Normal carrying angle: 5 degrees in males, greater than 15 degrees in females.
      (2) Cubitus valgus: greater than 5 degrees in males, less than 10 degrees in females.
      (3) Cubitus varus (gunstock deformity): less than 5 degrees in males, greater than 15 degrees in females.
   b. Observe the elbow for scars, deformity, and contusion.
   c. Note if hollows on either side of the elbow are present. If not, effusion may be present especially if the elbow is being held protectively in a semi-flexed position.
3. Palpation.
   a. Palpate bony structure of elbow beginning with epicondyles, medial supracondylar line of humerus, olecranon, ulnar border, olecranon fossa, lateral epicondylar line of humerus, and radial head for deformity, lesions, or tumors.
   b. Palpate soft tissue with elbow flexed to 90 degrees while extending and abducting the shoulder.
   c. Palpate ulnar styloid and flexor pronator muscles of the wrist.
   d. On the posterior aspect of the elbow, examine the olecranon bursa and the triceps muscle.
   e. On the lateral aspect, palpate the wrist extensors: brachioradialis, extensor carpi longus, and extensor carpi brevis muscles; lateral collateral ligament and annular ligament.
   f. On the anterior aspect, palpate the cubital fossa, the biceps tendon, and the brachial artery, checking the pulse.
4. Range of motion.
   a. Active flexion: have patient flex elbow and touch the same shoulder with hand.
   b. Active extension: ask patient to extend elbow.
   c. Active supination: have patient flex elbow to 90 degrees with arms held close to the body. Close the fist with palm down; ask patient to rotate wrist so palm points upward.
   d. Active pronation: position patient as for evaluating supination except the fist is closed with the palm up; ask the patient to rotate the wrist so the palm points downward.
   e. Passive range of motion: patient is assisted through range of motion only if unable to independently do active range of motion.

f. Passive flexion/extension: flex and extend patient's elbow while supporting at the wrist and cupping the elbow.
g. Passive supination/pronation: supinate and pronate by supporting the elbow and grasping in the "shake hands" position; gently rotate the wrist so the palm faces up and then the palm faces downward.

5. Muscle testing.
   a. Patient may sit or stand.
   b. There are four main muscle groups responsible for the four motions of the elbow (see Chapter 2, Anatomy and Physiology).
      (1) Primary/secondary flexors.
      (2) Primary/secondary extensors.
      (3) Primary/secondary supinators.
      (4) Primary/secondary pronators.
   c. Stabilize the elbow and use other hand to move the wrist.
   d. Active flexion: have patient flex elbow (pull up against resistance).
   e. Active extension: have patient extend arm (push down against resistance).
   f. Active supination: have patient externally rotate wrist, palm up.
   g. Active pronation: have patient internally rotate wrist, palm down.
6. Reflex testing.
   a. Lightly tap the biceps, brachioradialis, and triceps tendons to elicit a reflex.
   b. Document response.
7. Sensory testing.
   a. Using a sharp object, lightly prick the skin.
   b. Compare sensation of affected side to the sensation of the unaffected side.
   c. Document the patient's response (see Table 3.7).
8. Special tests: always evaluate adjacent structures for problems.
   a. Ligamentous laxity.
      (1) Determines stability of medial and lateral collateral ligaments of the elbow.
      (2) Cup elbow with your hand using the thumb and index fingers as a fulcrum; gently move forearm medially and laterally by holding the wrist.
      (3) Ligament laxity is present if any gapping is palpated.
   b. Tinel sign for neuroma.
      (1) Tap area between olecranon and medial condyle to elicit tenderness over a possible neuroma within the ulnar nerve.
      (2) If a neuroma is present, patient will experience a tingling sensation along the ulnar distribution to the hand.

E. Wrist and hand.

1. See Table 3.8; Chapter 14, Trauma; and Chapter 17, The Hand and Wrist.
2. Compare both hands throughout the examination.
3. Ascertain which is the dominant hand.
4. Note attitude or posture of the patient's hands as he/she enters the examination room.
5. Inspection.
   a. Have patient place both hands in lap with palms facing upward.
   b. Look for muscle wasting, webbing, ecchymosis, edema, and presence of sweat (absence of sweat could be indicative of nerve damage).
   c. Ask patient to place palms down.
   d. Look at general appearance of wrist and hand.
      (1) Note colors, presence of hair on fingers, muscle wasting, joint deformity, alignment, presence of edema, or shiny skin.
      (2) Note erythema.
   e. Look at fingernails.
      (1) Note color and condition of fingernails and presence of onychomycosis (fungus infection).
      (2) Note presence of:
         (a) Swan-neck deformity.
         (b) Boutonnière deformity.
         (c) Mallet fingers.
         (d) Herberden's nodes (bony growths).
         (e) Bouchard's nodes (swelling in the PIP joints).
         (f) Clubbing of fingers.
         (g) Presence of paronychia (abscess around the nail bed) or felon.
6. Palpation.

Table 3.7
Sensory Testing of the Elbow

Nerve Root	Sensation
C5	Lateral arm
C6	Lateral forearm
C7	Medial forearm
T1	Medial arm

Table 3.8
Key Assessment of Hand and Finger Injuries

1. Obtain a complete history, including the mechanism of the injury.
2. Perform meticulous physical examination: gently palpate all portions of hand and fingers.
3. Evaluate sensation in the hand and fingers with sharp object and cotton wisp.
4. Assess movement of affected part through range of motion: if unable to move, suspect tendon laceration.
5. Refer for an x-ray.
6. Consider treat with RICE (rest, ice compression, elevation).

Table 3.9
Sensory Testing of the Wrist and Hand

Nerve Root	Sensation
C6	Thumb, index, and half of the middle finger
C7	Middle finger
C 8 and T1	Ring and little finger

a. Note the temperature of the skin, dry areas, or callous formation.
b. Palpate the bony structures, such as the radial styloid, anatomic "snuff box," tubercle of the radius, ulnar styloid, metacarpals, metacarpophalangeal joints, and the phalanges.
c. Palpate each finger individually from metacarpal phalangeal (MCP), proximal interphalangeal (PIP), to distal interphalangeal (DIP) joints.
d. Palpate the soft tissue of the wrist, the radial styloid (the site of the de Quervain's tenosynovitis).
e. Palpate area of the tubercle of the radius, the ulnar styloid process, the pisiform, and the ulnar artery.
f. Palpate soft tissue of the hand, beginning with the thenar and hypothenar eminence.
g. With palm facing up, note presence of any trigger fingers or Dupuytren's flexion contracture, (an abnormal thickening of the fascia between the skin and tendons), thickened nodules on the ulnar side and proximal to the ring and little finger on the volar aspect.

7. Range of motion.
   a. Active wrist flexion and extension: ask patient to flex and extend wrist while stabilizing forearm with your hand.
   b. Active ulnar and radial deviation: ask patient to rotate the hand side to side while stabilizing forearm close to the wrist with your hand.
   c. Active supination and pronation: use same procedure as for the elbow.
   d. Active finger flexion and extension: ask patient to flex and extend fingers.
   e. Active abduction and adduction: ask patient to spread fingers as far apart as possible and then return to neutral position.
   f. Active thumb movement.
      (1) Have patient move thumb across the palm in order to touch pad at the base of the little finger.
      (2) Ask patient to spread thumb as far from hand as possible.
      (3) Ask patient to touch thumb to each of the fingertips to test opposition.
   g. Passive thumb movement.
      (1) Assist patient through range of motion only if unable to do active range of motion.
      (2) Gently move patient through range of motion, holding motionless the joint above the one being tested.
8. Muscle testing.
   a. Patient should be seated.
   b. The following are the muscle groups (see Chapter 2, Anatomy and Physiology).
      (1) Primary wrist extensors/flexors.
      (2) Primary finger extensors/flexors of the distal interphalangeal, proximal interphalangeal, and metacarpophalangeal joints.
      (3) Primary wrist abductors/adductors.
      (4) Primary thumb extensors/flexors of the metacarpophalangeal and interphalangeal joints.
      (5) Primary thumb abductors/adductors/opposers.
   c. Active wrist extension: stabilize the forearm while asking patient to cock-up the wrist against resistance.
   d. Active wrist flexion: with the hand in a fist, ask patient to flex against resistance.
   e. Active wrist supination and pronation are discussed in the section about elbow assessment.
   f. Active finger extension: stabilize the wrist in neutral position. Ask patient to extend the metacarpophalangeal joints while flexing the proximal interphalangeal joints. Place your hand on the dorsum of the proximal phalanges and try to force them into flexion.
   g. Active finger flexion: ask patient to flex fingers as you try to pull them out of flexion.
   h. Active finger abduction: ask patient to spread their fingers and not allow you to bring them together.
   i. Active finger adduction:
      (1) Place piece of paper between thumb and index finger.
      (2) Ask patient to squeeze the paper tightly as you attempt to pull it out.
      (3) Repeat for all fingers.
   j. Active thumb extension: have patient extend the thumb against resistance.
   k. Active thumb flexion: have patient touch the hypothenar eminence with his/her thumb as you hook your thumb around patient's and try to pull out of flexion.
   l. Active thumb abduction:
      (1) Ask patient to abduct the thumb while you stabilize the metacarpal joints.
      (2) Try to push patient's thumb back toward the palm.
   m. Active thumb adduction: ask patient to adduct the thumb against resistance as you stabilize the thumb and wrist.
   n. Pinch mechanism: ask patient to make an "O"

with thumb and index fingers and hold it while you try to break the circle.
o. Thumb/finger opposition: ask patient to touch thumb and little finger together while you try to pull apart the connection.

9. Sensory testing: using a sharp object, lightly prick the skin; document patient's response (see Table 3.10).
10. Special tests: always evaluate adjacent areas for all problems.
    a. Allen test.
        (1) Evaluate blood supply to the volar arch within the hand.
        (2) Have patient open and close the hand several times, pumping blood to the hand.
        (3) With hand closed in a fist, apply pressure to the radial and ulnar arteries, momentarily occluding the blood supply.
        (4) Have patient open hand as you release the pressure on the ulnar artery.
        (5) The hand should flush immediately. If it does not, the ulnar artery may be impaired.
    b. Finkelstein test.
        (1) Specific test for de Quervain's syndrome (tenosynovitis).
        (2) Ask patient to make a fist with the thumb inside while you stabilize the forearm.
        (3) Gently push the wrist to the ulnar side.
        (4) Sharp pain in the anatomic snuffbox indicates likelihood of stenosing tenosynovitis or de Quervain's disease.
    c. Phalen test.
        (1) Reproduces symptoms of carpal tunnel syndrome.
        (2) Ask patient to push the dorsa of the wrist together in front of them for at least 1 minute.
        (3) Tingling fingers indicate the probable presence of carpal tunnel syndrome.
    d. Tinel sign: gently tapping the volar surface of the wrist will produce a "tingling" sensation in the medial nerve distribution.

F. Spine.

1. Inspection.
    a. Observe patient as he/she enters the examination room, noting the gait and posture while standing, sitting, and supine.
    b. If possible, observe ability to undress and whether patient uses any strategies to make ADL easier.
    c. Note the normal curvatures of the spine, convex and concave.
    d. Note if the pelvis crests are level.
    e. Note if the shoulders are level.
    f. Observe the skin for redness, lipomata, hairy patches, café au lait spots, or birthmarks.
    g. Note any structural deformities, such as kyphosis, gibbus deformity, and scoliosis.
2. Palpation.
    a. Standing behind patient:
        (1) Palpate each spinous process.
        (2) Starting at the head and moving to the sacrum, and coccyx.
        (3) Note any tenderness or irregularities.
    b. Palpate each scapula for irregularities or point tenderness.
    c. Palpate the ischial tuberosities, greater trochanters, sciatic notches, iliac crests, and tubercles for irregularities or point tenderness.
    d. Standing in front of patient:
        (1) Palpate the structures of each rib.
        (2) Note any deformity or asymmetry.
    e. Standing behind patient:
        (1) Palpate soft tissue structures of the spine beginning with supraspinous and interspinous ligaments.
        (2) Note hard areas or tissue irregularities.
    f. Palpate for spasm in paraspinal muscles.
    g. Move down to the area of the iliac crests, noting the musculature of the gluteal muscles.
    h. Palpate distribution areas of the sciatic nerve for any irregularities and point tenderness.
        (1) Standing in front of patient.
        (2) Palpate the musculature of the abdomen.
        (3) Press gently in the inguinal areas.
3. Range of motion.
    a. There is more movement in the lumbar spine than in the thoracic spine.
    b. Active flexion.
        (1) Ask patient to touch toes while knees are kept straight.
        (2) If unable to touch toes, measure the distance from the fingertips to the floor to establish a baseline.
    c. Active extension.
        (1) Stand behind the patient as you support his/her lower back by placing your open palms on the iliac crests.
        (2) Ask the patient to bend back as far as he/she can.
        (3) Assure the patient that you are there to stabilize him/her.
    d. Active lateral bending.
        (1) While standing behind the patient with your hand placed on the iliac crests, ask patient to move laterally left and then right.
        (2) Note reports of stiffness or pain.
    e. Active rotation.
        (1) Detects only major restrictions in motion.
        (2) Even if patient has had a spinal fusion, there will be some motion.
        (3) While standing behind the patient, place your hand on his/her shoulder.
        (4) On the opposite side, place your hand on the iliac crest to stabilize the pelvis while asking the patient to twist torso.
    f. Passive: patient is assisted through range of motion only if unable to do active range of motion.
4. Sensory testing: using a sharp object, lightly prick patient's skin; document patient's response (see Table 3.10).

Table 3.10
Sensory Testing of the Spine

Nerve	Motor	Reflex	Sensory	Deficit/Compression
T12, L1	Iliopsoas	None	Anterior thigh between the inguinal ligament and knee	Dysfunctional bladder. Anal reflex is hyperactive. Paraplegics with pelvic stability can ambulate with braces.
L1, L2, L3	Iliopsoas	None	Anterior thigh between the inguinal ligament and knee	No voluntary control of bowel or bladder. No sensation of two-thirds of thigh distally. Decreased patellar reflex, absent Achilles reflex.
L2, L3, L4	Quadriceps, hip adductor	Patellar	Medial side of leg L2: anterior thigh L3: knee L4: medial calf	
L4 (overlap)	Tibialis anterior	Patellar	From the knee down, medial side of leg	
L5	Extensor halluces, gluteus medius, extensor digitorum longus, and brevis	None	Lateral leg and medial aspect of dorsum of foot	
S1	Peroneus longus and brevis, gastrocnemius soleus, gluteus maximus	Achilles	Lateral malleolus, lateral aspect of foot, and plantar surface of foot	
S2, S3, S4	Bladder muscles, intrinsic muscles of the foot	None	Three concentric rings around the anus: S2 outermost ring S3 middle ring S4 innermost ring Also S2 posterior thigh and knee	

5. Pathologic reflexes: if any of the following tests are abnormal, further tests may be indicated.
   a. Oppenheim test/sign.
      (1) With the flat handle of the reflex hammer, stroke distally on the medial tibia.
      (2) Normally there is no reaction; if the great toe extends dorsally, the test is positive.
   b. Babinski reflex/sign.
      (1) Run the handle of the reflex hammer or a key across the plantar surface of the foot from heel to toe, along the lateral border of the forefoot.
      (2) Normally the toes bunch up together; if the great toe extends while the other toes plantar flex and splay, the test is positive.
6. Special tests: always evaluate adjacent structures, such as the hip, lower gastrointestinal tract, pelvis, and genitourinary tract.
   a. Beevor's sign.
      (1) This sign is usually positive in patients with polio and meningomyocele.
      (2) Ask patient to do a quarter sit-up with arms held behind the head; observe the umbilicus for movement.
      (3) Normally no movement is apparent; if movement is present, the umbilicus moves toward the weak abdominal segment.
   b. Fabere (Patrick) test/sign.
      (1) If positive, may indicate sacroiliac joint involvement.
      (2) With patient supine, abduct the hip by placing the foot of the involved side on the opposite knee.
      (3) Externally rotate, flex, and abduct the hip. Pain may be caused by hip or sacroiliac joint involvement.
      (4) With patient in this position, press down on patient's flexed knee while stabilizing the opposite anterior iliac spine.
   c. Gaenslen test.
      (1) May indicate sacroiliac joint pathology.
      (2) With patient supine, ask him/her to flex both knees to chest.
      (3) Help patient move to the side of the table so the buttock extends over the edge of the examination table.
      (4) Allow unsupported leg to extend while keeping the other leg flexed.
      (5) Ask patient to report any pain in the sacroiliac joint.
   d. Hoover test.
      (1) May be helpful in determining if patient is malingering.
      (2) Instruct patient to raise leg; he/she will usually indicate inability to raise leg.
      (3) Cup one heel with your hand and again ask patient to try to straight-leg raise the other leg.
      (4) If patient is genuinely making an attempt, you will feel increased pressure from the heel to your hand.
   e. Kernig's sign.
      (1) If positive, may be a sign of meningeal irritation.
      (2) With patient supine, have him/her place hands under head in order to flex the head slightly forward.
      (3) Instruct the patient to express if he/she feels any pain along the spinal column.
   f. Brudzinski's sign: may indicate meningitis.
      (1) With patient supine, passive flexion of one leg results in a similar motion on the opposite side.
      (2) If the neck is passively flexed, flexion occurs in both legs.
   g. Milgrim test.
      (1) If positive, patient may have a herniated disc.
      (2) With patient supine, ask him/her to straight-leg raise both legs to about 2 inches off the examination table.
      (3) If patient can hold this position for 30 seconds, the test is negative.
   h. Naffziger test.
      (1) If positive, patient may be experiencing abnormal pressure on the spinal cord.
      (2) With patient supine, compress the jugular veins for 10 seconds; the face will become flushed.
      (3) Ask patient to cough or perform Valsalva maneuver.
      (4) The test is positive if the patient experiences pain.
   i. Pelvic rock test.
      (1) If positive, may indicate sacroiliac joint involvement.
      (2) Have patient lie supine while placing your fingertips on the iliac spines and palms on the iliac tubercles.
      (3) Push the pelvis toward the midline of the body.
      (4) Ask patient to report any pain in the sacroiliac joint area.
   j. Scoliosis test.
      (1) Scoliosis screening is done routinely in most schools (around 7th grade).
      (2) Patient is inspected posteriorly; note whether the spine is abnormally curved laterally.
      (3) Patient stands facing away from the seated examiner and then bends forward at the waist, keeping the knees straight.
      (4) The upper extremities are extended loosely in front of the body toward the floor with fingertips of each hand extended and touching (Diver's position).
      (5) This position enables the examiner to note subtle rotational differences in the thorax; normally the sides of the thorax are symmetrical.
      (6) Functional.
         (a) Due to a significant shortening of one leg.

(b) Will be present when patient is in an upright position but will disappear when patient bends forward.

(7) Structural: does not disappear when in the flexed position and may even be emphasized in comparison to when in the upright position.

k. Straight-leg test.
   (1) Reproduces back and leg pain, if positive.
   (2) With the patient supine, support the knee to keep it straight and lift leg slowly upward off examination table.
   (3) If there is pain in the posterior thigh, the hamstrings are tight.
   (4) Pain all the way down the leg could be indicative of sciatic nerve involvement.
   (5) This pain is usually exacerbated by dorsiflexing the foot while the leg is raised.
   (6) It should be documented how much of an angle of elevation causes severe pain.

l. Straight-leg uninvolved leg test.
   (1) With the patient supine, raise the uninvolved leg in the manner described above.
   (2) Positive if patient expresses pain in the lower back and sciatica pain on the opposite leg.

m. Valsalva maneuver.
   (1) If positive, patient may have bulging or ruptured intervertebral disc or spinal cord compromise.
   (2) With patient sitting, ask patient to bear down as if to move bowels.
   (3) If pain occurs down the legs or in the lower back or buttocks, the maneuver is positive.

G. Pelvis and hip.

1. Movement.
   a. Observe patient as he/she enters the examination room, noting gait and posture while standing, sitting, and supine.
   b. If possible, observe ability to undress and whether patient uses any strategies to make ADL easier.
   c. See Chapter 19, The Hip; and Chapter 14, Trauma.
2. Inspection.
   a. Observe patient from all sides.
   b. Note bruises, pressure spots, abnormal posture, or ecchymosis.
   c. Observe the shape of the patient's hips in proportion to rest of body.
   d. Note areas of muscle wasting, dimples, glottal folds, and the amount of lumbar lordosis.
   e. In the infant or young child, note any signs of congenital dislocated hip, such as asymmetry of the skinfolds, broadened buttocks, and widened perineum.
3. Palpation.
   a. Palpate:
      (1) The bony structures of the pelvis and hip.
      (2) The soft tissues around the hip and pelvis.
   b. With the patient supine:
      (1) Palpate the anterior superior iliac spines, the iliac crests, the iliac tubercles, greater trochanters, and symphysis pubis.
      (2) Abduct the hip and flex the knees so that the lower extremity crosses the opposite knee.
      (3) This should allow full visualization of the area known as the "femoral triangle."
      (4) There are three main structures in this area that should be palpated.
         (a) Inguinal ligament.
         (b) Sartorius muscle.
         (c) Adductor longus muscle.
      (5) Palpate patient's femoral pulse.
         (a) The femoral nerve and femoral vein are also present in this area.
         (b) These are not palpable.
   c. With the patient prone:
      (1) Feel the superior iliac spines, greater trochanters, ischial tuberosities, and the sacroiliac joint.
      (2) Palpate the soft tissues around the hip and pelvis.
   d. With the patient side lying, palpate the greater trochanter.
      (1) Note increased skin temperature, the presence of a trochanteric bursa, and the condition of the gluteus medius muscle.
      (2) Palpate the sciatic notch.
   e. Palpate the areas of the major hip and pelvic muscles.
      (1) The flexors found anteriorly include the:
         (a) Iliopsoas.
         (b) Sartorius.
         (c) Rectus femoris.
      (2) The adductors found medially include the:
         (a) Gracilis.
         (b) Pectineus.
         (c) Adductor brevis.
         (d) Adductor magnus.
      (3) The adductors found laterally include the gluteus medius.
      (4) The extensors found laterally include the gluteus maximus and hamstring.
4. Range of motion.
   a. Active abduction.
      (1) Ask patient to stand and spread legs as far apart as possible.
      (2) Be prepared to steady the patient.
   b. Active adduction: ask patient to cross one leg over the other while keeping the knee straight.
   c. Active flexion: ask patient to draw each knee up to the chest, while lying supine.
   d. Active extension: with the patient seated, ask patient to stand up without using hands.
   e. Active flexion and adduction: with the patient seated, ask patient to cross one leg over the other at the thigh.

f. Active flexion, abduction, and external rotation: with the patient seated, ask him/her to place the lateral side of foot on top of the opposite knee.
g. Active internal and external rotation: have patient, who is supine, roll legs so toes point in (internal) and then out (external).
h. Passive: assist patient through range of motion only if unable to do active range of motion.
i. Passive flexion: with patient supine on examination table, bring each knee to chest.
j. Passive extension.
   (1) With the patient lying prone, stabilize the pelvis by reaching over the patient with your arm so your hand is on the opposite hip.
   (2) With your other arm, support the leg under the thigh and smoothly lift off the examination table.
   (3) Be alert to limited extension due to contractures that may be present.
k. Passive adduction.
   (1) With the patient supine, stabilize the pelvis by reaching over the patient with your arm so your hand is on the opposite hip.
   (2) Gently move each leg so that it crosses over the opposite leg.
l. Passive abduction.
   (1) With the patient supine, stabilize the pelvis by reaching over the patient with your arm so your hand is on the opposite hip.
   (2) Gently move each leg away from the midline.
m. Passive internal rotation and external rotation. (Do not perform if patient has had a total hip arthroplasty or hip prosthesis.)
   (1) With the patient supine and legs extended, stand at the foot of the examination table.
   (2) Gently grasp the feet above the ankle and roll the leg inward (internal) and outward (external).
   (3) Note the position of the patella as the movement is carried out.

5. Muscle testing.
   a. Patient should be positioned according to test.
   b. The following muscle groups are tested (see Chapter 2, Anatomy and Physiology).
      (1) Primary/secondary flexors.
      (2) Primary/secondary extensors.
      (3) Primary/secondary abductors.
      (4) Primary/secondary adductors.
   c. Flexors: with patient sitting at the edge of the examination table, have patient lift each thigh off the table against resistance.
   d. Extensors.
      (1) With the patient lying prone, flex the knees while stabilizing the pelvis.
      (2) Ask patient to raise thigh off the table against resistance.
   e. Abductors.
      (1) With the patient side lying, place your hands on the lateral side of the hip and knee on top.
      (2) Ask patient to abduct against resistance.
   f. Adductors.
      (1) With the patient side lying, place your hands on the medial side of top hip and knee.
      (2) Ask patient to adduct against resistance.
   g. Abduction and adduction: with the patient lying supine, have patient try to swing legs out and back to neutral against resistance.
6. Sensory testing.
   a. Using a sharp object, lightly prick the patient's skin.
   b. Document patient's response (see Table 3.11).
7. Special tests: always evaluate adjacent structures, such as the lumbar spine, knee, lower gastrointestinal, and reproductive tract, for problems.
   a. Congenital dislocated hip.
      (1) All newborns are screened for dislocated hip.
      (2) Congenital dislocated hip has two characteristics: abduction is limited on the involved side and telescoping occurs when traction is applied to the knee.
      (3) Adduction.
         (a) With the infant or child supine, flex the hips to 90 degrees, then abduct them.
         (b) 90 degrees is normal; limited abduction of 20 degrees is an indication of abduction contracture.
      (4) Ortolani test.
         (a) Used to determine hip reducibility in the infant.
         (b) Known as the "click" test.
         (c) With the infant or child supine, abduct and lift to reduce the hip.
         (d) An audible "click" will be heard and a "clunk" palpated when you abduct and lift as the femoral head slides over the acetabular rim, causing hip reduction.
         (e) Done in conjunction with Barlow's maneuver.
      (5) Barlow's maneuver.
         (a) Used to determine the potential for the hip to dislocate in an infant.
         (b) Flex the femur and gently bring to midline.
         (c) Adduct 10-20 degrees.
         (d) As hip is adducted, a gentle posterior force is applied to see if the head will slide posterior within the acetabulum (sublux) or actually dislocate over the acetabular rim.
         (e) The hip is moved to abduction with gentle traction to relocate the femoral head.
         (f) The sequence is gently repeated 1-2 times to establish the degree of laxity.

Table 3.11
Sensory Testing of the Pelvis and Hip

Nerve Root	Sensation
T10	Transverse, slightly oblique band at the level of the umbilicus
T11	Transverse, slightly oblique band at the level between T10 and T12
T12	Transverse, slightly oblique band at the level above the inguinal ligament
L1	Lies below the inguinal ligament, parallel to the upper anterior portion of the thigh
L2	Lies below L1 area and most of the anterior thigh
L3	Knee including above and below the patella
Cluneal (L1, L2, L3)	Over the iliac crest between the posterior, suprailiac spine, the iliac tubercle, and the gluteus maximus

(Do not repeat too often as this may cause damage or dislocate the femoral head.)

(6) Galleazi's sign.
  (a) Used to determine femoral shortening in the older child.
  (b) Flex the hips to 90 degrees in neutral rotation and also in abduction and adduction.
  (c) The legs are kept parallel to the examination table while the hip is flexed.
  (d) The knees should be at the same level. Uneven knee height indicates a positive Galleazi sign.

(7) Allis sign.
  (a) Used to determine femoral shortening in the older child.
  (b) Flex the hips to 90 degrees in neutral rotation.
  (c) The child's feet are placed on the examination table.
  (d) The knees should be at the same level. Uneven knee height indicates a positive Allis.

(8) Telescoping.
  (a) With the infant or child supine, place your hand over the greater trochanter.
  (b) With the other hand, gently pull down the child's leg in order to apply traction to the leg at the knee.
  (c) This will cause the hip to move in and out of the acetabulum (telescoping).

b. Leg-length discrepancy test.
  (1) Determines if one leg is shorter than the other. Normal should be within 1 cm of each other.
  (2) Assess whether the shortness is occurring above or below the knee.
  (3) True leg length: with the patient lying supine, use a tape measure to measure from the anterior iliac spine to the medial malleolus.
  (4) Apparent leg length.
    (a) Determines if there is pelvic obliquity, adduction, or flexion deformity of the hip.
    (b) Done after the test for true leg length.
    (c) With the patient supine, measure from the umbilicus to the medial malleolus.
    (d) This method uses a nonfixed point (umbilicus) to a bony fixed landmark (medial malleolus).
    (e) If the measurement of true leg length is equal and the apparent leg length is unequal, further testing may be needed to determine source of shortening.
  (5) Tibial or femoral test.
    (a) Done at same time of true leg length test.
    (b) With the patient supine, have the knees flexed so the malleoli are level with feet flat on the examination table.
    (c) Note the level of the patellae.
    (d) If one knee projects further anteriorly than the other, the femur is the site of the discrepancy.
    (e) If one knee is higher than the other is, the tibia is the site of the discrepancy.

c. Ober test.
  (1) Indicates a contracture of the tensor fascia lata.
  (2) With the patient side lying with the involved leg up, abduct the leg as far as possible.
  (3) Flex the knee to 90 degrees, keeping the hip in neutral.
  (4) Release the abducted leg.
  (5) Normally the leg should drop into an adducted position.
  (6) If the leg remains abducted, the test is positive for a contracture of the iliotibial band or tensor fascia lata.

d. Thomas test.
  (1) Indicates when flexion contracture is present in the hip.
  (2) With the patient supine, stabilize the pelvis.
  (3) Ask the patient to flex the uninvolved hip to the chest (may need assistance in order to obtain this position).
  (4) Observe opposite leg.
  (5) If opposite leg lifts off the examination table, a flexion contracture is present.
  (6) Determine the amount of flexion contrac-

ture by measuring the angle between the posterior thigh and the table with a goniometer.
- e. Trendelenberg test.
  - (1) Evaluates strength of the gluteus medius muscle.
  - (2) Standing behind patient, observe the dimples over the posterior iliac spines.
  - (3) The level of those dimples should be equal if patient's weight is evenly distributed.
  - (4) When standing erect, the gluteus medius muscle should contract as the foot leaves the floor.
  - (5) When the pelvis is elevated on the unsupported side, the test is negative.
  - (6) If the pelvis on the unsupported side remains in position or descends and the gluteal folds drop, the muscle is not functioning, therefore indicating a positive test.
- f. Assessment for fractured hip.
  - (1) With patient lying on examination table or stretcher, gently palpate iliac crests.
  - (2) The iliac crests should be as level as possible level.
  - (3) Note if affected leg is internally rotated and shorter indicating a fracture of the hip.
  - (4) See Chapter 19, The Hip.

H. Knee.

1. Movement.
   - a. Observe the patient as he/she enters the examination room, noting gait and posture while standing, sitting, and lying down.
   - b. If possible, observe ability to undress and whether the patient uses any strategies to make ADL easier.
   - c. See Chapter 20, The Knee; and Chapter 14, Trauma.
2. Inspection.
   - a. Observe patient from all sides.
   - b. Inspect knees for edema, muscle wasting, overall general appearance, effusion, and scars.
   - c. Note the appearance of the skin, presence of blotches, dimpling, and the alignment of the knees while standing and seated.
   - d. Note any vascular changes, such as discoloration or varicosity.
   - e. Observe the presence of valgus (knock-knee), varus (bowlegs), or recurvatum (pushed-back) deformities.
   - f. Note the position of the patella.
3. Palpation.
   - a. Palpate the bony structures of the knee: (see Chapter 2, Anatomy and Physiology).
   - b. On the medial side, palpate the:
     - (1) Medial tibial plateau.
     - (2) Tibial tubercle.
     - (3) Medial femoral condyle.
     - (4) Adductor tubercle.
   - c. On the lateral side, palpate the:
     - (1) Lateral tibial plateau.
     - (2) Tibial tubercle.
     - (3) Lateral femoral condyle.
     - (4) Lateral femoral epicondyle.
   - d. Palpate the:
     - (1) Head of the fibula.
     - (2) Trochlear groove.
     - (3) Mobility of patellae.
   - e. With the leg extended and relaxed, place your fingers on the patella and gently move in all directions.
   - f. Patellae should have pain-free mobility.
   - g. Palpate the soft tissue of knee from the front. With patient seated, leg extended, note the:
     - (1) Quadriceps.
     - (2) Infrapatellar tendon.
     - (3) Patella bursa.
     - (4) Superficial Infrapatellar area.
     - (5) Prepatella area.
     - (6) Preanserine bursa.
   - h. Palpate the medial aspect of the knee for the:
     - (1) Medial joint space over meniscus.
     - (2) Medial collateral ligament.
     - (3) Sartorius muscle.
     - (4) Gracilis muscle.
     - (5) Semitendinosus muscles.
   - i. Examine the lateral structures of the knee.
     - (1) Lateral joint space over meniscus.
     - (2) Lateral collateral ligament.
     - (3) Anterior superior tibiofibular ligament.
   - j. Palpate the biceps femoris tendon, iliotibial tract, and fibular head.
   - k. Have patient lie prone to facilitate palpation of the posterior structures.
   - l. Palpate the popliteal fossa, noting the presence of bulging or swelling
   - m. Palpate the areas of the posterior tibial nerve, gastrocnemius muscle, popliteal vein and artery.
   - n. Evaluate skin temperature, noting the guidelines mentioned concerning RICE in sports-related injuries (see Chapter 14, Trauma).
4. Range of motion.
   - a. Active flexion.
     - (1) With patient standing, ask patient to perform a deep knee bend.
     - (2) Be prepared to steady the patient.
   - b. Active extension.
     - (1) With patient sitting at the edge of the examination table, ask the patient to fully extend legs.
     - (2) To fully extend the legs, the tibia will externally rotate.
   - c. Active internal and external rotation: with patient seated on examination table, ask the patient to internally rotate foot, then externally rotate foot.
   - d. Passive: patient is assisted through range of motion only if unable to do active range of motion.
   - e. Passive flexion.
     - (1) With patient seated at edge of the exami-

Table 3.12
Sensory Testing of the Knee

Nerve Root	Reflex	Sensation
L2		Lies below L1 area
L3		Lies above and below the patella
L4	Patellar or quadriceps	Anterior and posterior portion of medial knee, down the leg medially. The infrapatella branch of the saphenous nerve is the only sensory branch of the femoral nerve that continues in the leg. Often cut during surgical removal of the medial meniscus.
S2	None	A strip down the midline of the posterior thigh, covering the popliteal bursa and supplied by the posterior femoral cutaneous nerve.

nation table, place one hand on the ankle and the other supporting the knees.
 (2) Gently flex the knee as far as possible.
 (3) In children, the amount of flexion will be increased with foot flexing to make contact with the buttocks.

f. Passive extension.
 (1) With patient seated on examination table, place one hand on the thigh above the knee to stabilize the leg.
 (2) Gently pull the leg out with your other hand at the ankle to fully extend the patient's leg.

g. Passive internal and external rotation.
 (1) With patient seated, place your hand on patient's thigh just above the knee to stabilize the femur.
 (2) Grasp patient's ankle and gently rotate the tibia inward and outward.

5. Muscle testing.
 a. Patient should be positioned appropriately to elicit the test response.
 b. The following muscle groups are tested: (see Chapter 2, Anatomy and Physiology).
  (1) Primary flexors.
  (2) Primary extensors.
  (3) Primary rotators.
 c. Flexion.
  (1) With patient lying prone on the examination table, place your hand on the patient's thigh to stabilize it.
  (2) Apply gentle resistance to the hamstrings and at the ankle joint.
  (3) Ask patient to flex the knee as if to try to lift leg off the table.
 d. Internal and external rotation: these muscles cannot be separated for individual testing.

6. Sensory testing.
 a. Using a sharp object, lightly prick the skin of the patient
 b. Document the patient's response (see Table 3.12).

7. Special tests: always evaluate adjacent structures such as the lumbar spine, hip, and foot.
 a. Anterior drawer test.
  (1) Determines if anterior cruciate ligament (ACL) is compromised.
  (2) With patient lying on examination table, the hip is flexed to 45 degrees and the knees are flexed to between 60 and 90 degrees.
  (3) In order to prevent the patient's feet from forward movement; block that motion by leaning your body on top of the feet.
  (4) Cup the knee with your hands, placing the thumbs on the medial and lateral joint lines as the rest of your fingers grasp the posterior aspect of the knee.
  (5) Gently pull the tibia forward.
  (6) If you are able to feel and observe excessive forward movement of the tibia, the ACL may be compromised.
 b. Apprehension test.
  (1) Indicates if the patella has potential for dislocation.
  (2) With patient lying on examination table with legs extended and the quadriceps muscle relaxed, press the patella along the medial edge with your thumb.
  (3) Observe patient's face as you push the patella laterally.
  (4) If patient anticipates that patella will dislocate, they will become visibly apprehensive and try to stop further examination.
 c. "Bounce home" test.
  (1) Indicates probable cause of limited extension.
  (2) With patient lying supine, cup the heel in your hand, while supporting the knee with your other hand.
  (3) Ask patient to flex the knee into full flexion, and then passively move the knee into extension.
  (4) The knee movement will end with a bouncing motion into full extension.
  (5) If the knee cannot be fully extended, a loose body (torn meniscus, osteochondral fragment) may be the cause.
 d. Compression test.
  (1) Also known as the "grinding" test.
  (2) Indicates meniscus tears or tags.
  (3) With patient lying prone, lean on patient's thigh to stabilize the joint while asking patient to flex the leg to 90 degrees.

(4) Press upward on the heel of the affected leg in order to compress the medial and lateral menisci while rotating the tibia internally and externally.
(5) Ask the patient to indicate the location of any pain.
(6) Audible clicking of torn meniscus may be detected.

e. Distraction test.
(1) Indicates compromise to the ligament or meniscus.
(2) With patient lying prone, lean on patient's thigh to stabilize the joint while asking patient to flex the knee to 90 degrees.
(3) Apply traction to the leg while rotating the tibia internally and externally.
(4) Ask patient to indicate the location of any pain.

f. Posterior drawer test.
(1) Indicates posterior cruciate ligament (PCL) compromise.
(2) With patient lying on examination table, the hip flexed to 45 degrees, and the knees flexed between 60 and 90 degrees.
(3) In order to prevent patient's feet from forward movement, block motion by leaning your body on top of the patient's feet.
(4) Cup the knee with your hands, placing the thumbs on the medial and lateral joint lines as the rest of your fingers grasp the posterior knee.
(5) Gently push the tibia backward onto the femur.
(6) If you are able to feel and observe any backward movement of the tibia, the PCL may be compromised.
(7) Loss of dimpling on the medial aspect of the knee may indicate a PCL tear.
(8) Lift the affected leg in extension, if knee sags into a "back knee," a PCL tear is suspected.

g. Knee joint effusion.
(1) Determine if effusion is present in the joint.
(2) If effusion is the result of a sports-related injury, remember the protocol of "RICE" and how it may influence your assessment.
(3) Minimal effusion evaluation.
(a) With patient lying on examination table, place your hand above the suprapatellar pouch and gently milk the pouch downward and medially.
(b) When the fluid has been collected in the medial side of the pouch, gently tap, moving the fluid to the lateral side.
(4) Gross effusion evaluation (ballottement).
(a) With patient lying on examination table, have patient extend knee as much as possible.
(b) Inform patient that the examination may be uncomfortable.
(c) Encourage patient to relax quadriceps muscles and to take a deep breath.
(d) Gently push the patella into the trochlear groove and release it.
(e) The fluid collected in the joint surrounds the patella and then resumes its previous shape.
(f) The action of floating the patella and causing it to rebound is known as "ballottement."
(5) Aspiration for joint fluid analysis may indicate blood-tinged fluid. Blood in synovial fluid usually indicates torn ligament or intra-articular fracture.

h. Joint stability.
(1) Determines if collateral ligaments are compromised.
(2) With patient lying on examination table, envelop lower leg with your arm just below the knee joint.
(3) Use your other hand as a fulcrum on the thigh.
(4) Gently apply valgus and varus stress.
(5) If collateral ligaments are compromised, you will be able to palpate and observe opening of the joint laterally and/or medially.

i. Lachman test.
(1) Determines if ACL is compromised.
(2) With patient lying on examination table, the knees are flexed from full extension to 30 degrees.
(3) In order to prevent patient's feet from forward movement; block that motion by leaning your body onto the table.
(4) Grasp the thigh with one hand.
(5) Gently pull the tibia forward with the other hand.
(6) If you are able to feel and observe forward movement of the tibia, the ACL may be torn.

j. McMurray maneuver.
(1) Indicates possible medial meniscus tear.
(2) With patient lying on examination table, cup the heel in your hand and flex the involved leg fully.
(3) Place other hand around the knee joint with your fingers on the medial joint line and the thumb and thenar eminence on the lateral joint line.
(4) Rotate leg internally and externally to relax the knee joint.
(5) Push on the lateral side to apply valgus stress to the medial side of the joint while at the same time rotating the leg externally.
(6) Maintain the valgus stress and external rotation while extending the leg slowly as you continue to palpate the medial joint line.
(7) If you palpate or hear a "click" within the joint, there is a probable tear in the medial meniscus.

k. Patella femoral grinding.
(1) Indicates condition of the posterior patella

surface or the trochlear groove in the femur.
   (2) With patient lying supine, use your finger to push the patella distally.
   (3) Ask the patient to tighten quadriceps muscle as you apply gentle resistance as it moves proximally.
   (4) Movement of the patella should be smooth and glide easily without feeling of crepitus or geit.
   (5) If pain is present, degenerative changes or chondromalacia may be present.
   (6) Chondromalacia causes severe knee pain when descending stairs.
l. Reduction click.
   (1) The goal of this maneuver is to return a torn meniscus back into place by unlocking a locked knee.
   (2) With patient lying on the examination table, cup the heel in your hand and flex the involved leg.
   (3) Place other hand around the knee, with your fingers on the medial joint line and thumb and thenar eminence on the lateral joint line.
   (4) Flex knee while rotating leg internally and externally.
   (5) Rotate and extend leg repeatedly until you hear and palpate a "click" which indicates that the meniscus has slipped back into alignment.

I. Ankle and foot.

1. Movement.
   a. Observe patient as he/she enters the examination room, noting gait and posture while standing, sitting, and supine.
   b. If possible, observe ability to remove shoes and socks and whether the patient uses any strategies to make ADL easier.
   c. See Chapter 21, Foot and Ankle; and Chapter 14, Trauma.
2. Inspection.
   a. Observe condition of patient's shoes soles, noting areas of excessive wear or special accommodation such as a wedge.
   b. Observe patient standing, noting the arch and general condition of skin and toes.
   c. Ask patient to sit in a chair or on the edge of the examination table.
      (1) Note the nonweight-bearing foot, arch, color of skin with feet both dependent and elevated.
      (2) Note any callus formation, corns, or vascular compromise.
      (3) Observe any deformities, edema of ankle and foot.
      (4) Examine toes and note presence of hair on the dorsal side.
      (5) Observe each toe individually, noting shape and color of nails.
3. Palpation.
   a. Palpate bony structures of the ankle and foot.
   b. On the medial aspect, (see Chapter 2, Anatomy and Physiology) palpate the:
      (1) First metatarsocuneiform.
      (2) Navicular tubercle.
      (3) Head of the talus.
      (4) Medial malleolus.
      (5) Head of the first metatarsal and metatarsophalangeal joint.
   c. Palpate the sustentaculum tali and medial tubercle of the talus.
   d. On the lateral aspect, palpate the:
      (1) Fifth metatarsal bone.
      (2) Metatarsophalangeal joint.
      (3) Calcaneus.
      (4) Peroneal tubercle.
      (5) Lateral malleolus.
   e. In the sinus tarsi arc, palpate the inferior tibiofibular joint area.
   f. In area of the hindfoot, palpate the calcaneus and the medial tubercle.
   g. On plantar surface, note the metatarsal heads.
   h. Palpate soft tissue in area of the first metatarsal bone, looking for tophi, hallux valgus, or hallux rigidus.
   i. In area of the medial malleolus, palpate the deltoid ligament that commonly tears in a severe ankle sprain.
   j. Palpate tendons, including the:
      (1) Tibialis posterior.
      (2) Flexor digitorum longus.
      (3) Flexor hallucis longus.
   k. Assess the pulse of the posterior tibial artery.
   l. Note area of the long saphenous vein and the tibia nerve.
   m. Palpate dorsum of the foot between the malleoli for the:
      (1) Tibialis anterior.
      (2) Extensor hallucis longus.
      (3) Extensor digitorum longus tendons.
   n. Assess the dorsalis pedis pulse.
   o. In the area of the lateral malleolus, palpate the:
      (1) Anterior talofibula.
      (2) Calcaneofibula.
      (3) Posterior talofibular ligaments.
   p. Palpate:
      (1) The peroneus longus and brevis tendons.
      (2) Structures of the sinus tarsi, anterior to the lateral malleolus where the extensor digitorum brevis muscle is a common site for sprain.
   q. The head of the fifth metatarsal is the site of a Tailor's bunion or inflamed bursa.
   r. In area of the calcaneus, palpate length of the Achilles tendon, located at the distal one-third of the calf and attached to the calcaneus.
      (1) This area is a common site of inflamed bursa, including the retrocalcaneal and the calcaneal.
      (2) This area is also a common site for blistering from overuse.

s. Palpate:
   (1) The plantar surface of the foot for spurs.
   (2) The plantar fascia.
   (3) Each toe, beginning proximally and moving distally.
   (4) Note if any deformity is present, such as claw toes or hammertoes.
   (5) Note presence of corns or callouses.
   (6) Note condition of toenails, looking for fungal infections, ingrown toenails, breaks in skin, ulcers.

3. Range of motion.
   a. Be prepared to steady the patient.
   b. Active dorsiflexion: ask patient to walk on heels.
   c. Active plantar flexion: ask patient to walk on toes.
   d. Active inversion: ask patient to walk on the lateral sides of feet.
   e. Active eversion: ask patient to walk on medial sides of feet.
   f. Active forefoot adduction and abduction: unable to isolate these motions but are presumed normal if all other range of movement is possible.
   g. Active toe flexion: ask patient to flex the tips of toes downward.
   h. Active toe extension: ask patient to extend toes upward.
   i. Passive.
      (1) Patient is assisted through range of motion only if unable to do active range of motion.
      (2) Passive ankle dorsiflexion and plantar flexion.
         (a) While stabilizing the subtalar joint by holding the calcaneus firmly, grip whole forefoot.
         (b) Pull foot up into dorsiflexion 30 degrees and push down into plantar flexion about 50 degrees.
      (3) Passive subtalar inversion.
         (a) While stabilizing patient's tibia distally, hold patient's heel.
         (b) Invert than evert the heel.
      (4) Passive forefoot adduction and abduction.
         (a) While holding patient's heel, grip forefoot.
         (b) Move forefoot to the medial side then the lateral side.
      (5) Passive great toe flexion and extension.
         (a) Movement of the great toe is crucial to normal locomotion as it provides stability and balance.
         (b) While stabilizing the foot, flex and extend the great toe.

4. Muscle testing.
   a. The following muscle groups are tested (see Chapter 2, Anatomy and Physiology).
      (1) Dorsiflexion.
         (a) Primary dorsiflexors lie in the anterior tibial compartment and are innervated by the deep peroneal nerve.
         (b) Footdrop will occur if the deep peroneal nerve has been injured.
         (c) Heel walking is the primary means of assessing this group of muscles.
      (2) Flexion.
         (a) Ask patient to walk on medial borders of feet, than walk on toes.
         (b) Observe the gait.

5. Sensory testing: using a sharp object, lightly prick the patient's the skin; document patient's response (see Table 3.13).

6. Special tests: always evaluate adjacent areas, such as the lumbar spine, hip, and knee, for problems.
   a. Anterior drawer test.
      (1) Similar to test for the knee.
      (2) Indicates if anterior talofibular ligament is intact.
      (3) With patient seated on edge of examination table, cup heel and gently grasp the distal tibia.
      (4) Push forward at heel, while pushing backward on tibia.
      (5) Any motion indicates that the ligament is compromised.
   b. Flat feet test.
      (1) Ask barefooted standing or seated patient to flatten the foot.
      (2) In "rigid flat feet" the arch is not present when standing on the toes and is absent when standing flat on the floor.
         (a) Not passively correctable.
         (b) Heel frequently everted.
         (c) Forefoot may be abducted.
      (3) In "supple flat feet" the arch is present when standing on the toes but is absent when standing flat on the floor.
         (a) Nonweight-bearing foot looks normal.
         (b) Weight-bearing heels everted, forefoot pronated and abducted; loss of normal longitudinal arch.
   c. Homans' sign.
      (1) Indicates possible deep vein thrombosis in the calf.
      (2) With patient lying supine, grasp toes while dorsiflexing the ankle.
      (3) If pain is elicited in calf of extended leg, further testing for deep vein thrombosis indicated.
   d. Thompson squeeze test.
      (1) To assess the Achilles tendon.
      (2) Have patient lie prone.
      (3) Squeeze both sides of the calf muscle on the affected leg.
      (4) If the foot moves into plantar flexion, the Achilles is intact.
   e. Tibial torsion.
      (1) Indicates excessive internal rotation of the

Table 3.13
Sensory Testing of the Ankle and Foot

Nerve Root	Reflex	Sensation
L4		Medial aspect of calf and ankle
L5		Dorsum of the medial aspect of foot and lateral side of the leg
S1	Achilles	Lateral side of foot

tibia, also known as "toeing in."

(2) Measure distance from tibial tubercle to each malleoli.

(3) Drop a perpendicular line from the tubercle to a point on the line between the malleoli. Measure the angles of interception: 15 degrees of torsion is considered normal.

VII. THE QUICK ASSESSMENT

Step 1

- Examine cervical spine and upper extremities with patient seated.
- Examine lower extremities with patient supine and the torso with patient standing.

Step 2

- Observe gait and (if possible) the manner of undressing, noting any strategies used to perform ADL.

Step 3

- Obtain a patient history.

Step 4

- Inspect for asymmetry, swelling, deformity, and abnormal limb size.

Step 5

- Palpate for: muscle spasm; painful areas; joint effusion, tenderness, instability, credits, and warmth; bone shapes; check for patent pulses and limb temperature.

Step 6

- Measure range of motion.

Step 7

- Grade muscle strength.

Step 8

- Grade reflexes.

Step 9

- Test cervical spine.
  - ♦ Look over each shoulder.
  - ♦ Touch each ear to the shoulder without compensatory shrug.
  - ♦ Ask patient to touch chin to chest.
  - ♦ Put head as far back as possible.

Step 10

- Test shoulders.
  - ♦ Arms out to side and then rise upward as far as possible.
  - ♦ Arms behind back as if to touch opposite buttock.
  - ♦ Arms placed in front, swing to the side and swing behind.
  - ♦ Elbows at side, rotate arm outward and then place forearm over abdomen.

Step 11

- Test elbow.
  - ♦ Arms in front and then flex the elbow as far as possible.
  - ♦ Elbows at side, supinate, and then pronate.

Step 12

- Test wrist.
  - ♦ Flex and extend wrists as far as possible.
  - ♦ Dorsiflex then volarflex the wrist.

Step 13

- Test hand.
  - ♦ Flex fingers into fist.
  - ♦ Extend fingers and then abduct them.

Step 14

- Test back.
  - ♦ Stabilize hips and ask patient to twist right and left.
  - ♦ Stabilize pelvis and ask patient to bend to each side so fingertips move toward the floor.
  - ♦ With the examiner seated, ask patient to bend forward, stand up and bend backward.

Step 15

- Measure leg length.
  - ♦ Measure each leg from anterior iliac spine to medial malleolus.

Step 16

- Test hamstrings.
  - ♦ Stabilize pelvis with your arm; raise leg slowly keeping the knee straight.

Step 17

- Test hip.
  - ♦ Bend knee, then flex hip.
  - ♦ Stabilize pelvis with your arm, abduct then adduct the leg.
  - ♦ Flex hip and knee; internally and externally rotate the leg at the hip.

Step 18

- Test knee.
  - ♦ Flex knee as far as possible, then extend.
  - ♦ Place hand on lateral aspect of thigh and the other on the medial aspect of the patient's ankle.
  - ♦ Apply lateral and medial stress to knee.
  - ♦ Secure patient's foot under your thigh; apply stress to knee by pulling calf forward, then by pushing the tibia backward.

Step 19

- Test foot.
  - ♦ Plantarflex then dorsiflex the foot.
  - ♦ Stabilize the ankle, invert and evert forefoot.

VIII. CHANGES WITH AGE

A. Infants

1. Congenital dislocated hip.
2. Hip dysplasia.
3. Foot deformities such as clubfoot.
4. Fractured clavicle is a common birth trauma.
5. Fractures heal quickly.

6. Bones are mostly cartilage (soft).
7. Primitive reflexes.
8. Developmental milestones.

B. Toddlers.
1. Bruises/contusions secondary to accidents.
2. Head injury.
3. Physical abuse accounts for 10.6% of all blunt trauma in ages newborn to 4 years.
4. Developmental milestones continue.
5. Foot malalignments.

C. Children.
1. Sports injuries.
2. Bruises/contusions secondary to accidents.
3. Head injury.
4. Developmental milestones continue.
5. Tibial torsion
6. Genu varum (bowlegs)
7. Child with limp.

D. Adolescence.
1. Changes in:
   a. Size.
   b. Proportion.
   c. Strength.
2. Growth spurt.
   a. Boys: between ages of 12.5 and 15 years.
      (1) Gain an average of 8 inches in height.
      (2) 40 lbs in weight.
   b. Girls.
      (1) Growth spurt occurs about 2 years earlier.
      (2) Smaller in magnitude.
3. Bodily proportions change in regular sequence.
   a. Legs lengthen.
   b. Hips and chest widen.
   c. Shoulders broaden.
   d. Trunk lengthens and broadens.
   e. Chest lengthens.
   f. In boys, shoulders broaden; in girls, pelvis widens.
4. Muscles increase in size and strength especially in boys.
5. Growing pains.

E. Elderly. Musculoskeletal changes continue through adult years.
1. After maturity, height slowly decreases, especially in individuals with osteoporosis.
2. Significant shortening in old age.
   a. Most height loss occurs in the trunk.
   b. Intervertebral bodies become less spongy and thin.
   c. Vertebral discs shorten or collapse because of osteoporosis.
   d. Increased flexion at knees and hips may contribute to shortened stature.
3. Kyphosis, barreling of anterior chest increased thoracic diameter (especially in women).
4. Skeletal muscles decrease in muscle mass, bulk, and power.
5. Ligaments may lose tensile strength.
6. Range of motion may diminish.
7. Pain is not a given as one ages.

Bibliography

Bates, B. (1995). *A guide to physical examination and history taking* (6th ed.). Philadelphia: J.B. Lippincott.

DiScala, C., Sege, R., Li, G., & Reece, R. (2000). Child abuse and unintentional injuries: A 10-year retrospective. *Archives Pediatric Adolescent Medicine, 154*(1), 16-22.

Fernbach, S. (1998). Common orthopedic problems of the newborn. *Nursing Clinics of North America, 33*(4), 583-594.

Hoffinger, S. (1996). Evaluation and management of pediatric foot deformities. *Pediatric Clinics of North America, 43*(5), 1091-1111.

Hoppenfeld, S. (1976). *Physical examination of the spine and extremities.* New York: Appleton-Century-Crofts.

Maher, A.B. (1998). Assessment of the musculoskeletal system. In A.B. Maher, S.W. Salmond, & T.A. Pellino (Eds.), *Orthopaedic nursing* (2nd ed., pp.168-189). Philadelphia: W.B. Saunders.

Mercier, L., Pettid, F., Tamisiea, D., & Heiech, J. (2000). The physical examination. In L. Mercier, F. Pettid, D. Tamisiea, & J. Heiech (Eds.), *Practical orthopedics* (5th ed., pp. 1-4). St. Louis: Mosby.

Rodts, M. (1983). An orthopaedic assessment you can do in 15 minutes. *Nursing 83',* 65-73.

Schoen, D.C. (2000). Assessment of the orthopaedic patient. In D.C. Schoen, *Adult orthopaedic nursing* (pp. 11-42). Philadelphia: Lippincott.

Snider, R.K. (1997). General orthopedics. In R.K. Snider (Ed.), *Essentials of musculoskeletal care* (pp. 1-69). Rosemont, IL: American Academy of Orthopaedic Surgeons.

Seidel, H.N., Ball, J.W., Dains, J.E., & Benedict, G.W. (1998). *Mosby's guide to physical examination* (3rd ed.). St. Louis: Mosby Year Book.

Sims, L.K., S'Amico, D., Stiesmeyer, J.K., & Webster, J.A. (1995). *Health assessment in nursing.* Redwood, CA: Addison-Wesley.

STUDY QUESTIONS

Bob, a 27-year-old male, is admitted after falling off a mountain bike. He comes to the emergency room with a swollen left ankle. There is a possibility that it may be fractured. (Questions 1-3)

1. To assess the neurovascular status of the extremity the nurse should:
   a. Apply the principles of "RICE."
   b. Stretch the tendon and tap lightly.
   c. Score the reaction to touch in grades.
   d. Evaluate CMST and capillary refill.

2. There is a possibility of stress fracture. Which of the following is true of stress fractures?
   a. It is very easy to diagnose and plan treatment for stress fractures.
   b. There is usually very little soft tissue swelling with a stress fracture.
   c. A stress fracture may not be evident on an x-ray until a callus begins to form.
   d. There is excruciating joint pain upon movement with stress fractures.

3. The patient demonstrates an antalgic gait upon ambulation. Which of the following best describes an antalgic gait?
   a. Staggering or uncoordinated gait.
   b. Pain or discomfort on ambulation.
   c. Vertical telescoping of the hip.
   d. Foot slaps or drags along the ground.

Anna, a 56-year-old female, is seen in the orthopedic physician's office. She reports having increasing left knee pain. (Questions 4-6)

4. As Anna is escorted to the examination room, the nurse should:
   a. Evaluate her gait as she talks with her.
   b. Talk about the medications she takes for pain.
   c. Say nothing to assure confidentiality and review the medical record.
   d. Discuss the weather to put her at ease.

5. The nurse positions the patient for an anterior drawer test of the right knee. Which of the following statements is correct regarding the anterior drawer test?
   a. Another name for this test is the "bounce home" test.
   b. This test evaluates anterior stability provided by the anterior cruciate ligament.
   c. The anterior drawer is not a test to assess knee function.
   d. This test requires the examiner to sit on the examination table and push the tibia back.

6. Which of the following tests, when positive, indicates a possible tear of the medial meniscus?
   a. Trendelenburg test.
   b. Lachman test.
   c. McMurray test.
   d. Apprehension test.

Gabrielle, a 16-year-old high school volleyball player, is evaluated by the school nurse for "popping" and "cracking" in the left knee. (Questions 7-9)

7. One of the most common conditions that causes a crackling sound with flexion and extension of the knee is:
   a. Leg-length discrepancy.
   b. A dislocated hip.
   c. Chondromalacia of the patella.
   d. A positive Ortolani test.

8. If the knee is severely swollen and aspiration of the joint reveals blood-tinged synovial fluid, it is expected that:
   a. Evacuating the fluid from the knee will help it to heal faster.
   b. An internal structure may be torn or there may be an intra-articular fracture.
   c. There is always an infection in the joint.
   d. The cruciate ligaments are intact.

9. The patient with chondromalacia of the patella usually has the most severe pain when:
   a. Bearing weight on the affected leg.
   b. Performing straight leg lifts.
   c. Walking down stairs.
   d. Swimming.

10. Which of the following statements is true about the patient with "footdrop?"
   a. This patient has had an injury to the deep peroneal nerve.
   b. This patient will be able to walk on his/her heels.
   c. This patient will not be able to toe walk.
   d. This patient will not be able to compensate for the injury and will walk with a limp.

Mrs. Jones is a 72-year-old female with severe degenerative joint disease of the right hip. (Questions 11-14)

11. The characteristic gait that the nurse would expect Mrs. Jones to have is:
   a. A quadriceps gait.
   b. A spastic gait.
   c. A Trendelenburg gait.
   d. A steppage gait.

12. When evaluating the right leg, which of the following would you **not** expect to find:
   a. A decreased range of motion of the right hip.
   b. A flexion contracture of the right hip.
   c. Pain with motion of the right hip.
   d. Decreased circulation to the hip and leg.

13. Performance of the Valsalva maneuver may cause pain with which of the following conditions?
   a. Degenerative joint disease.
   b. Extruded lumbar disc.
   c. Torn meniscus in the knee.
   d. Subacromial bursitis.

14. The Thompson test evaluates the:
   a. Hip for arthritic changes.
   b. Knee for a torn cruciate ligament.
   c. Achilles tendon for function.
   d. Calf for thrombophlebitis.

Chapter 4 DIAGNOSTIC STUDIES

Rebecca Jo Carpenter, BSN, RN, ONC

Contents

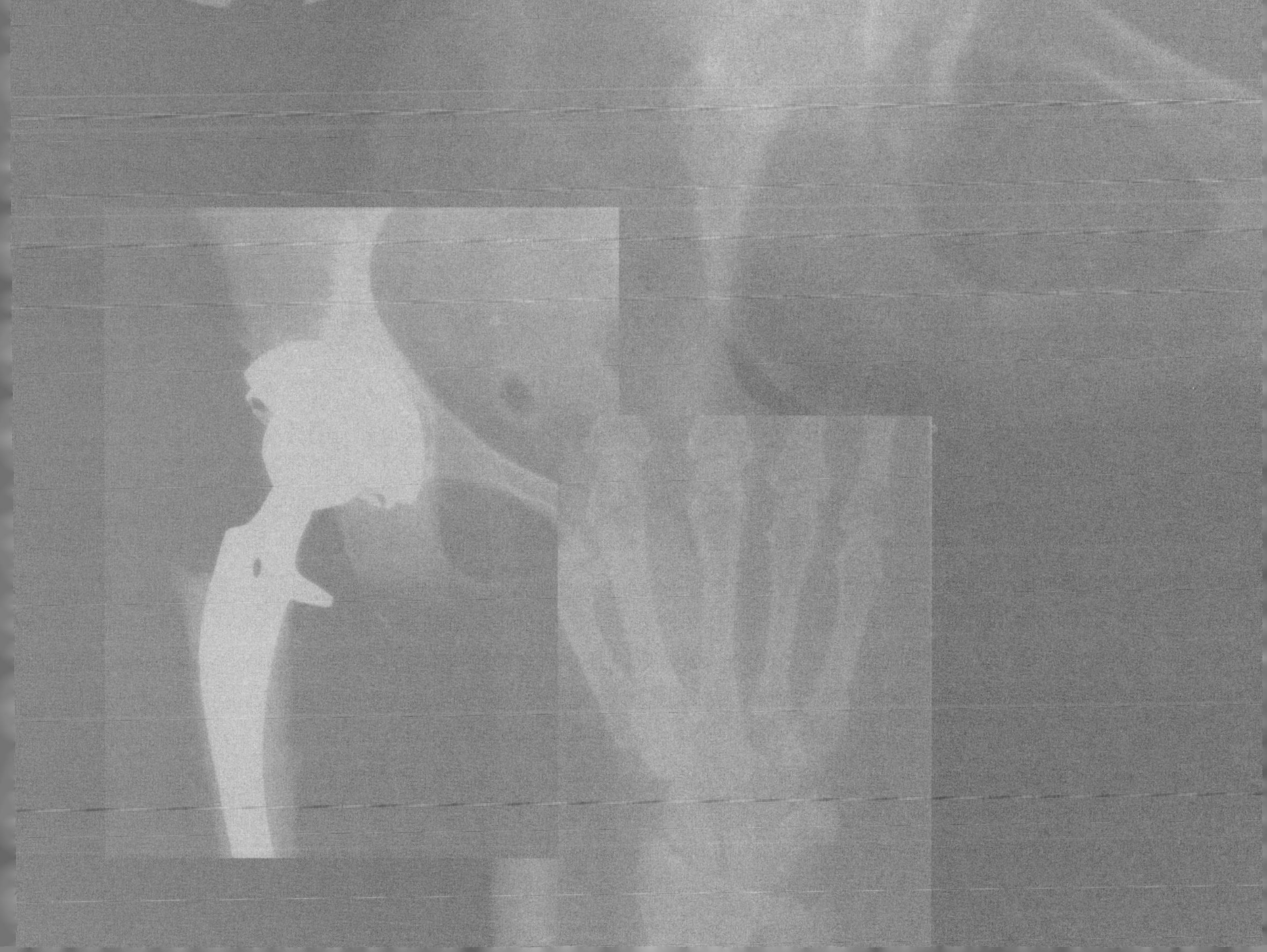

OBJECTIVES

At the completion of this chapter, the learner will be able to:

- Explain each diagnostic study including definition, purpose, and parameters of findings.
- Describe the indications for each diagnostic study.
- Synthesize the objective data for diagnostic therapeutic purposes.
- Describe patient preparation for each diagnostic procedure.
- Identify complications associated with each diagnostic procedure.
- Identify nursing implications for each diagnostic procedure.
- Describe the special diagnostic tests including procedures, purposes, complications, patient preparation, and diagnostic capabilities.

CHAPTER 4

DIAGNOSTIC STUDIES

LABORATORY STUDIES

I. BLOOD

A. Acid phosphatase (ACP).

1. Definition:
   a. Acid phosphatase is an enzyme found in erythrocytes, platelets, prostatic tissue, bone, liver, spleen, and kidney.
   b. The biologic role of this enzyme is not clearly understood.
   c. A large proportion of acid phosphatase is found in the prostate gland where acid phosphatase is 100 times higher than in other tissue.
2. Purpose: used in detecting prostatic carcinoma that has metastasized, Paget's disease and hyperparathyroidism with skeletal involvement, and with invasion of the bones by a variety of malignant neoplasms such as carcinoma of the breast.
3. Normal values.
   a. 1.0-4.0 King Armstron (mu)/dl.
   b. 0.5-2.0 Bodansky (mu)/dl.
4. Elevated serum levels of acid phosphatase are shown in patients with prostatic carcinoma, multiple myeloma, Paget's disease, hyperparathyroidism, hepatitis, obstructive jaundice, acute renal impairment, sickle cell crisis and any cancer that has metastasized to the bone. If the acid phosphatase is elevated; it can be further fractionated to differentiate the tissue of origin (prostate vs. other tissue).
5. Lower serum levels, an inborn error of metabolism, transmitted as an autosomal recessive trait, caused by a deficiency of lysosomal ACP. The deficiency presents in the neonatal period and is rapidly fatal. It can be detected by prenatal analysis of amniotic fluid.

B. Aldolase (ALD).

1. Definition: aldolase is a glycolytic enzyme, which catalyzes the cleavage of fructose 1.6-diphosphate into glyceraldehyde phosphate and dihydrosyaceton phosphate.
2. Purpose: this enzyme is most useful in monitoring diseases affecting muscle.
3. Normal values: 1.0-7.5 U/100 ml.
4. Elevated aldolase levels are shown in muscular dystrophy, dermatomycosis, trichinosis, skeletal muscle necrosis, myocardial infarction, granulocytic leukemia, hepatic necrosis, and carcinomatosis. Adrenocorticotropic hormone (ACTH) and cortisone produce levels as much as five times normal.

C. Alkaline phosphatase (ALP).

1. Definition.
   a. Alkaline phosphatase is an enzyme originating mainly in bones, liver, placenta, kidney, and intestinal lining.
   b. It is particularly sensitive to mild biliary obstruction and hepatic lesions.
   c. However, since both skeletal and hepatic diseases can raise alkaline phosphatase levels, its most specific clinical application is in the diagnosis of metabolic bone disease.
2. Purpose: used chiefly as an index of liver and bone diseases when correlated with other clinical findings.
3. Normal values.
   a. Males: 90-239 U/liter.
   b. Females under 45 years old: 76-196 U/liter.
   c. Females over 45 years old: 87-250 U/liter.
   d. Children: will be elevated due to bone growth.
4. Elevated levels of alkaline phosphatase are shown in bone diseases characterized by increased osteoblastic activity: osteitis deformans, rickets, osteomalacia, hyperparathyroidism, healing fractures, osteoblastic bone tumors, pregnancy, normal growth, biliary obstruction, cirrhosis, tuberculosis, sarcoidosis, and amyloidosis. Alkaline phosphatase can be further fractionated to determine the tissue of origin.
5. Lower than normal levels of alkaline phosphatase are shown in hypophosphatasia, an inborn error of metabolism, and in malnourished patients.

D. Antinuclear antibody (ANA).

1. Definition.
   a. Antinuclear antibodies are gamma globulins that react to specific antigens when mixed in the laboratory.
   b. Such antibodies (anti-DNA, extractable antibody) are produced in response to the nuclear part of white blood cells.
   c. ANA forms antigen-antibody complexes that cause tissue damage.
2. Purpose: used to detect the presence of anti-nucleoprotein factor associated with certain autoimmune diseases.
3. Normal values:
   a. Negative is a titer of 1:32 or below.
   b. Positive is a titer of 1:32 or above.
4. Positive titer tests in ANA are associated with systemic lupus erythematosus, rheumatoid arthritis, rheumatic fever, mixed connective tissue disease, scleroderma, polyarteritis nodosa, chronic hepatitis, dermatomyositis, atypical pneumonia, Sjogren's syndrome, tuberculosis, anaplastic carcinomas, and Raynaud's disease.
5. False positives can occur. The test is highly nonspecific and ANA occurs in some liver diseases as well as in some healthy individuals.

E. Antistreptolysin O titer (ASO).

1. Definition: ASO test measures the relative serum concentrations of the antibody steptolysin-O; an oxygen-labile enzyme produced by group *β-hemolytic streptococci*.

2. Purpose: primarily used in the differential diagnosis of post-streptococcal diseases such as glomerulonephritis, rheumatic fever, bacterial endocarditis, and scarlet fever.
3. Normal values (less than or equal).
   a. Adults: < 166 Todd units/ml.
   b. Children.
      (1) Newborn: similar to mother's value.
      (2) Preschoolers: 85 Todd units/ml.
      (3) School-age children: 170 Todd units/ml.
4. Highly elevated titers are seen in post–streptococcal diseases, rheumatic fever, rheumatic arthritis, glomerulonephritis, and ASO titers also may be elevated in uncomplicated streptococcal diseases.

F. Calcium (Ca).

1. Definition.
   a. Calcium helps regulate and promote neuromuscular contraction, cardiac function, and transmission of nerve impulses and blood coagulation.
   b. Calcium levels vary inversely with phosphorus.
   c. The bulk of the body calcium (over 98%) is stored in the skeleton and teeth.
2. Purpose: used as a measure of parathyroid function and calcium metabolism.
3. Normal values.
   a. Adult: (total) 9.0-10.5 mg/100 ml.
   b. Children: 6.0-12 mg/100 ml.
4. Increased calcium levels may occur in hyperparathyroidism, parathyroid tumors, Paget's disease, multiple myeloma, metastatic cancers, multiple fractures, prolonged immobilization, sarcoidosis, Addison's disease, and renal disease.
5. Decreased calcium levels may occur in hypoparathyroidism, Cushing's syndrome, osteomalacia, rickets, renal failure, acute pancreatitis, and peritonitis.

G. Chymofast blood test.

1. Definition.
   a. Chymopapain is an enzyme used to treat herniated discs.
   b. The enzyme, when injected into the herniated disc, causes the herniated material to break down.
   c. Chymopapain can be highly allergenic.
2. Purpose: used to determine sensitivity to chymopapain.
3. Values.
   a. 0.00-0.03, minimal sensitivity.
   b. 0.04-0.05, potential sensitivity.
   c. 0.06 and greater, strong possibility of anaphylactic shock if chymopapain administered.

H. Creatine phosphokinase (CPK).

1. Definition: creatine phosphokinase is an enzyme that catalyzes the creatine-creatinine metabolic pathway in the heart and skeletal muscle and in much smaller concentrations in the brain tissue.
2. Purpose.
   a. Important in the diagnosis of myocardial infarction and as a reliable measure of skeletal muscle disease such as muscular dystrophy.
   b. Skeletal muscle contains two types of muscle fibers
      (1) Type I fibers, which contain only CPK-MM.
      (2) Type II fibers, which contain CPK-MB and compose 40% of the fibers in such muscles as the quadriceps.
      (3) In Duchenne's muscular dystrophy, especially in the early stages, the amount of CPK-MB may be increased, presumably due to skeletal muscle type II involvement, with CPK-MM increased to a much greater degree.
      (4) CPK-MB begins to rise in 2-4 hours, peaks in 12-24 hours in myocardial infarction.
3. Normal values.
   a. CPK-MM: 5-70 IU/liter.
   b. CPK-MB: undetectable to 7 IU/liter.
4. Elevations of CPK-MB and CPK-MM levels are associated with muscular dystrophy, polymyositis, myoglobinuria, and muscle damage from trauma such as surgery and IM injections, and myocardial damage.

I. C-reactive protein (CRP).

1. Definition.
   a. CRP is a somatic polysaccharide of the pneumococcus, thought to be synthesized mainly in the liver.
   b. Presence of CRP in the blood serum can be detected 1-24 hours after the onset of tissue damage.
   c. Has roughly the same usefulness as the erythrocyte sedimentation rate.
2. Purpose.
   a. Used to diagnose and evaluate inflammatory diseases, particularly rheumatoid arthritis, myocardial infarction, active widespread malignant diseases.
   b. Often used to monitor the status of orthopaedic infections following total joint replacement.
3. Normal values: trace amounts.
4. Elevated levels in rheumatoid arthritis, rheumatic fever, lupus erythematosus, myocardial infarction, active widespread malignancy, pneumonia, and bacterial and viral infections.

J. Creatinine.

1. Definition.
   a. Creatinine is a metabolic product of creatine-phosphate dephosphorylation in muscle.
   b. Daily production of creatine, and subsequently creatinine, depends on muscle mass; unlike creatine, the kidney with minimal reabsorption easily excretes it.
2. Purpose: used to diagnose impaired renal function.
3. Normal values:
   a. Males: 0.8-1.2 mg/100 ml.
   b. Females: 0.06-0.09 mg/100 ml.
4. Increased levels occur in glomerulonephritis, pyelonephritis, acute tubular necrosis, urinary obstruction, gigantism, and acromegaly.
5. Decreased levels occur in muscular dystrophy.

K. **Enzyme-linked immunosorbent assay test (ELISA).**

1. Definition.
   a. The blood or serum is exposed to surface antigens of killed HIV virus: if antibodies are present, a positive reaction occurs.
   b. The test is simple to perform and is sensitive to the point of 99.8% accuracy.
2. Purpose: used to screen donated blood and blood products for the human immunodeficiency virus (HIV) protein; also used to detect the presence of Lyme disease.
3. Results:
   a. If the first ELISA test is positive, a second test is run; if this test is positive, a Western Blot test is used for confirmation.
   b. A positive test does not diagnose acquired immunodeficiency syndrome (AIDS); it merely indicates exposure to the HIV virus at some time.
   c. A false negative does exist, as the person's exposure may be recent and the disease could still be in the acute stage - also called nonreactive.
   d. When used to detect the presence of Lyme disease, the test may reveal a false negative when only erythema migrans is present but will convert to positive late in the disease.
   e. A false positive may result in the presence of other spirochetal illnesses (syphilis); however, these patients also will have a positive treponema reagin test and Lyme disease patients will not.
4. Other comments: home testing kits are now available, as are oral tests.

L. **Erthyrocytes (red blood cells [RBCs]).**

1. Definition.
   a. Main function of erythrocytes is to carry hemoglobin, which in turn carries oxygen to the body tissues and carbon dioxide from the tissue to the lungs.
   b. This process is achieved by means of the hemo globin in the red cells, which combines easily with oxygen and carbon dioxide.
   c. The combination of hemoglobin and oxygen gives arterial blood a bright red appearance, and also has a function in acid-base balance.
2. Purpose: used to evaluate anemia or polycythemia, and measures the total number of erythrocytes.
3. Normal values.
   a. Males: 4.2-5.4 million/mm^3.
   b. Females: 3.6-5.0 million/mm^3.
4. Increased erythrocyte levels are associated with polycythemia vera, severe diarrhea, dehydration, acute poisoning, pulmonary fibrosis (during and immediately following hemorrhage), hypernephroma, cirrhosis of liver, scurvy, splenomegaly, hyperthyroidism, and cardiac decompensation.
5. Decreased erythrocyte levels are associated with aplastic anemia, sphereocytosis, hemolytic anemia, Fanconi's syndrome, chronic renal disease, Addisons' disease, hyperthyroidism, intoxication with chemical agents (arsenic), malignant lymphoma, chronic lymphocytic leukemia, lupus erythematosus, infectious mononucleosis, most viral infection, multiple myeloma, rheumatic fever, and subacute endocarditis.

M. **Erythrocyte sedimentation rate (ESR).**

1. Definition:
   a. Tests the rate at which erythrocytes settle out of unclotted blood within 1 hour, with an increased rate of settling indicating the presence of inflammation and necrotic processes.
   b. The test has three main limitations:
      (1) Is sensitive but not specific.
      (2) May present normal results in the presence of active disease.
      (3) Results may be considerably influenced by technical factors.
2. Purpose: test for inflammation and necrosis since these processes cause an alteration in blood proteins, resulting in an aggregation of red cells which make them heavier and more likely to fall rapidly when placed in a special vertical test tube.
3. Normal values.
   a. Wintrobe.
      (1) Males: 0-5 mm/hr.
      (2) Females 0-15 mm/hr.
   b. Westergren.
      (1) Males: 0-15 mm/hr.
      (2) Females: 0-20 mm/hr.
4. Increased values are shown in acute and chronic infections, all of the collagen diseases, tissue necrosis, infarction, inflammatory diseases, carcinoma, acute heavy metallic poisoning, toxemia, Lyme disease, and certain physiologic stress situations such as pregnancy.
5. Decreased values are shown in polycythemia vera, sickle cell anemia, congestive heart failure, phyofibrinogenemia due to any cause, hyperviscosity, or low protein level.

N. **Erythropoietin.**

1. Definition.
   a. Measures the level of erythropoietin in the peripheral circulation.
   b. The hormone erythropoietin controls the production of (RBCs) in the bone marrow.
   c. It is very sensitive to changes in tissue oxygen levels.
   d. Tissue hypoxia stimulates production of erythropoietin therefore decreasing the production of RBCs.
2. Purpose: used to differentiate between primary and secondary polycythemia.
3. Normal values: 4-20 U/L.
4. Increased level in secondary polycythemia caused by renal cysts, hepatic carcinoma, hypernephroma, chronic obstructive pulmonary disease (COPD), and cyanotic congenital heart disease.
5. Decreased level in polycythemia vera, as excess RBCs suppress production of erythropoietin.

O. Ferritin level.

1. Definition.
   a. Ferritin is the iron storage protein.
   b. Found in all tissues but primarily in reticuloendothelial cells and liver.
2. Purpose.
   a. Measures the intracellular iron stores.
   b. Used to differentiate iron deficiency anemia from other types of anemia.
   c. Used to monitor iron levels in chronic renal failure.
   d. Used to monitor patient with iron deficiency, or diagnose (along with total iron binding capacity [TIBC] and serum iron) iron deficiency.
3. Normal values.
   a. Male mean: 123 ng/ml.
   b. Female mean: 56 ng/ml.
   c. Iron depletion at less than 30 ng/ml.
   d. Absent iron stores at less than 10 ng/ml.
4. False positive in patients with active liver disease.
5. Decreased level in iron deficiency anemia.

P. Fluorescent treponemal antibody absorption test (FTA-ABS).

1. Definition: the fluorescent treponemal antibody absorption test uses indirect immunofluorescence to detect antibodies that cause syphilis, the spirochete Treponema pallidum in serum.
2. Purpose.
   a. Differentiates biologic false positives from true syphilis positives.
   b. Diagnoses syphilis when definite clinical signs of syphilis are present but other tests are negative.
3. Normal values: negative.

Q. Hematocrit.

1. Definition.
   a. Whole blood is made up essentially of RBCs and plasma.
   b. After centrifugation, the percentage of packed RBCs gives an indirect estimate of the number of RBC/100 ml of whole blood.
   c. The measure is recorded in terms of the volume of cells found in 100 ml of blood.
2. Purpose: measures the percentage of RBC mass to original blood volume.
3. Normal values.
   a. Males: 40-54/100 ml.
   b. Females 37-47/100 ml.
4. Increased volume is found in erythrocytosis, polycythemia vera, severe dehydration, and shock (when the hemoconcentration rises).
5. Decreased volume is found in anemia, leukemia, hyperthyroidism, cirrhosis, acute massive blood loss, and hemodilution.

R. Hemoglobin.

1. Definition.
   a. Hemoglobin is the main component of RBCs.
   b. Serves as the vehicle for the transportation of oxygen and carbon dioxide, and hydrogen.
   c. Is composed of amino acids that form a single protein called "globin," a compound called "heme," which contains iron atoms, and the red pigment porphyrin.
   d. Each erythrocyte contains about 200-300 million molecules of hemoglobin.
   e. Hemoglobin has an important role in determining acid-base balance.
2. Purpose.
   a. Used as an index of the oxygen-carrying capacity of the blood.
   b. Often used to determine need for blood transfusion.
3. Normal values:
   a. Males: 14-16.5 gm/100 ml.
   b. Females: 12-15 gm/100 ml.
4. Increased hemoglobin levels are associated with COPD, congestive heart disease, polycythemia vera, severe burns, and dehydration.
5. Decreased hemoglobin levels are associated with iron deficiency anemia, sideroblastic anemia, Coolery's anemia, hyperparathyroidism, liver, cirrhosis, severe hemorrhage, incompatible blood transfusion, chemical reactions such as lead or copper intoxication, drug reactions, severe burns, Hodgkin's disease, leukemia, lymphoma, systemic lupus erythematosus, carcinomatosis, renal cortical necrosis, and sarcoidosis.

S. Human leukocyte antigen B-27 (HLA B-27).

1. Definition.
   a. The HL-A system is a complex antigen group of white blood cells (WBCs) and is found in nucleated cells of tissues other than WBCs.
   b. The HL-A system has been closely identified with tissue transplant compatibility to such a degree that some refer to HL-A as histo-compatability leukocyte-A; it has been found to have a relationship with various diseases.
   c. HLA-B is one of the four major subgroups of HL-A and has been identified to have eight antigens, HLA B-27 being one of the eight.
2. Purpose.
   a. Used to diagnose ankylosing spondylitis and variants of rheumatoid arthritis.
   b. Also of prime importance for skin and organ transplantation and for platelet and leukocyte transfusions in matching donor and recipient.
3. Normal values: negative reaction.
4. Positive reactions occur in ankylosing spondylitis, juvenile rheumatoid arthritis in over 50% of patients, arthritis associated with Reiter's syndrome, arthritis associated with psoriasis, and enteropathic arthritis associated with ulcerative colitis, Crohn's disease, or Yersinia enterocolitica.

T. Indirect immunofluorescence assay (IFA).

1. Definition: uses immunofluorescence to detect abnormal immune complexes caused by the spirochete *B. burgdorferi*, the causative organism of Lyme disease.
2. Purpose: used to detect Lyme disease.
3. Normal values: negative reaction.

4. False positive may occur with other spirochetal illnesses such as syphilis; however, these patients will have a positive FTA-ABS in addition to the IFA.

U. Iron (serum iron concentration).

1. Definition: serum iron concentration combined with TIBC can differentiate iron deficiency anemia and chronic illness or disorders.
2. Purpose: used in differentiation of hypochromic anemia when blood loss cannot be documented.
3. Normal values.
   a. Adult: 65-175 ug/dl.
   b. Newborn: 100-200 ug/dl.
   c. 4 months to 2 years: 40-100 ug/dl.
   d. 2 years to adult 85-150 ug/dl.
4. Increased levels in hemoglobin breakdown as in sickle cell anemia, patients taking estrogen, oral contraceptives, or chloramphenicol, or patients having high dietary intake.
5. Decreased levels in iron deficiency anemia, periods of rapid growth, chronic blood loss, and patients receiving ACTH drugs, infection, repeated pregnancies, decreased dietary intake, and physiologic diurnal variation (normally lower in the evening).

V. Leukocytes (white blood cells [WBCs]).

1. Definition: the main function of leukocytes is to fight infection and defend against invading microorganisms by phagocytosis. The types of WBCs are:
   a. Neutrophils.
      (1) Most numerous and most important type of WBC in the body's reaction to inflammation.
      (2) Constitute a primary defense against microbial invasion through the process of phagocytosis.
   b. Eosinophils.
      (1) Exact function is unknown, but it is believed that eosonophils may play a role in the breakdown of protein material and a specialized role in phagocytizing antigen-antibody complexes.
      (2) It is known, however, that allergens, foreign proteins, and products of protein breakdown produce the eosinophils' response and that they are inflammatory exudates.
   c. Basophils: function is not clearly understood, but basophils are considered to be phagocytic and to contain heparin and histamines.
   d. Lymphoctyes: are subgrouped as B cells and T cells, and are closely involved in the immune response and antibody formation of the body.
   e. Monocytes.
      (1) May be converted into large macrophages in tissue with increased phagocytic and digestive capacity.
      (2) Interact with antigen-antibody complement complexes to promote phagocytosis.
2. Normal values.
   a. Leukocytes: 5,000-10,000/cc. mm.
   b. Neutrophils: 60%-70%.
   c. Eosinophils: 14%.
   d. Basophils: 0.5%-1%.
   e. Lymphocytes: 20%-40%.
   f. Monocytes: 2%-6%.
3. Increased:
   a. Neutrophils: an increased percentage is associated with bacterial infections, granulocytic leukemia, myeloproliferative disorders, physical and emotional stress, and drugs such as catecholamines, corticosteroids, ACTH, and sulfonamides.
   b. Eosinophils: an increased percentage is associated with allergies, parasitic diseases, myelogenous leukemia, Hodgkin's disease, polyarteritis nodosa, and subacute infection.
   c. Basophils: an increased percentage is associated with myeloproliferative diseases, chronic inflammation, polycythemia vera, and the healing phase of inflammation. Increased percentage also results following radiation.
   d. Lymphocytes: an increased percentage is associated with pertussis, syphilis, tuberculoses, mumps, infectious mononucleosis, German measles, ulcerative colitis, and chronic infectious states.
   e. Monocytes: an increased percentage is associated with viral infections such as mononucleosis, chicken pox and mumps, certain protozoa and ricketsial diseases such as malaria, Rocky Mountain spotted fever, and typhus; bacterial infections such as brucellosis, subacute bacterial endocarditis, collagen diseases, multiple myeloma, myelocytic leukemia, and lymphomas.
4. Decreased:
   a. Neutrophils: a decreased percentage is associated with acute viral infections, blood disorders such as aplastic and pernicious anemia, agranulocytosis, acute lymphoblastic leukemia, toxic agents, and hormonal diseases such as Addison's disease, thyrotoxicosis, and acromegaly.
   b. Eosinophils: a decreased percentage is associated with infectious mononucleosis, aplastic and pernicious anemia, hypersplenism, congestive heart failure, Cushing's syndrome, and use of certain drugs such as epinephrine and thyroxin.
   c. Basophils: a decreased percentage is associated with anaphylactic reaction, hyperthyroidism, stress reactions, pregnancy, aging, and ovulation. A decreased percentage also results following prolonged steroid therapy.
   d. Lymphocytes: a decreased percentage is associated with high levels of adrenal corticosteroids, renal failure, and immunosuppressive drugs.

W. Lupus erythematosus cell preparation (LE cell prep).

1. Definition.
   a. LE cells are neutrophils that contain in their cytoplasm large masses of depolymerized DNA from the nuclei of polymorphonuclear leukocytes.

b. LE factors are present in the gamma globulin fraction of the serum protein and have the characteristics of an antinuclear antibody.
c. Certain drugs interfere with the test result.

2. Purpose: used in the diagnosis of systemic lupus erythematosus.
3. Normal values: negative
4. Positive results are associated with LE, chronic active hepatitis, rheumatoid arthritis, scleroderma, and blood sensitivity reaction.

X. Phosphorus (P).

1. Definition.
   a. Phosphorus is necessary for mineralization of bones and teeth, energy metabolism, and fatty acid transport.
   b. Phosphorus levels are determined by calcium metabolism, parathormone, and to a lesser degree by intestinal absorption.
   c. Because an inverse relationship exists between calcium and phosphorus, a decrease in one mineral results in an increase in the other.
   d. Various drugs cause increased and decreased values in phosphorus levels.
2. Purpose: used to measure phosphorous levels in blood.
3. Normal values.
   a. Adults: 2.5-4.5 mg/100 ml.
   b. Children: 3.5-5.8 mg/100 ml
4. Increased levels are found in chronic renal failure, hypoparathyroidism increased dietary or intravenous intake, pseudohypoparathyroidism as well as tetany of the newborn when this is caused by excessive phosphorus retention.
5. Decreased levels are found in rickets associated with malabsorption syndrome, renal tubular dystrophies, and inadequate dietary ingestion of phosphorus, chronic antacid ingestion, hyperparathyroidism, and hypercalcemia.

Y. Rheumatoid factor (RA factor).

1. Definition.
   a. In rheumatoid arthritis, "renegade" IgG antibodies, produced by lymphocytes in the synovial joints, react with other IgG or IgM to produce immune complexes.
   b. These immune complexes can migrate from the synovial fluid to other areas of the body causing vasculitis, subcutaneous nodules, or lymphadenopathy.
   c. The IgG or IgM molecules that react with altered IgG are called rheumatoid factors.
   d. Two agglutination tests can detect rheumatoid factor.
      (1) Sheep cell agglutination test: in the sheep cell test, rabbit IgG absorbed onto sheep RBCs is mixed with the patient's serum in serial dilutions.
      (2) Latex fixation test:
         (a) In the latex fixation test, latex particles are coated with denatured IgG.
         (b) The serum from the patient is heated and then added to the suspension of coated latex particles.
         (c) If the serum contains the rheumatoid factor, the rheumatoid factor will react with the IgG and cause the latex particles to agglutinate.
2. Purpose: is the most useful serum measurement of the IgM immunoglobulin present in the patient with rheumatoid arthritis.
3. Normal values: titers above 1:80 are usually considered diagnostic for rheumatoid arthritis.
4. The rheumatoid factor is present in a significant number of other conditions in addition to rheumatoid arthritis such as aging, systemic lupus erythematosus, scleroderma, polymyositis, infectious mononucleosis, sarcoidosis, and syphilis.

Z. Serum glutamic-oxalacetic transaminase (SGOT).

1. Definition.
   a. SGOT is an enzyme that catalyzes the conversion of the nitrogenous portion of an amino acid to an amino acid residue. It is found in the cytoplasm and mitochondria of many cells, primarily in the liver, heart, skeletal muscles, kidneys, pancreas, and to a lesser extent in RBCs.
   b. In cases of acute cellular destruction, this enzyme is released into the blood stream from damaged cells.
      (1) Elevated values usually appear 8 hours after injury.
      (2) Serum levels reach a peak in 24-36 hours and then fall to normal (usually in 4-6 days).
2. Purpose: evaluate liver, heart, and to a larger extent skeletal muscle injury/disease.
3. Normal values: 8-20 U/liter
4. Elevations appear with acute viral hepatitis, skeletal muscle trauma, myocardial infarction, muscular dystrophy, dermatomyositis, hemolytic anemia, pancreatitis, and Lyme disease.

AA. Serum osteocalcin (bone Gla protein).

1. Definition: osteocalcin, a protein, attaches itself to the osteoblasts; as the osteoblastic activity increases there is a higher level of osteocalcin in the blood.
2. Purpose: osteocalcin is the biochemical indicator of osteoblastic activity, which is indicative of the rate of bone turnover.
3. Normal values.
   a. Males: 4.7-10.1 mg/ml.
   b. Females: 1.8-10.1 mg/ml.

BB. Total iron binding capacity (TIBC).

1. Definition: a test that measures the capacity of the blood globulin transferrin to combine with and transport iron.
2. Purpose.
   a. Used to differentiate iron deficiency anemia from other anemias.
   b. Used to monitor therapy for patient with either an iron deficiency or overload.
   c. Also used in conjunction with serum iron.
3. Normal values.
   a. Adults: 250-450 ug/dl.
   b. Newborn: 60-400 ug/dl.

c. 4 months to 2 years: 100-400 ug/dl.
d. 2 years to adult: 350-450 ug/dl.

4. Generally, conditions that decrease serum iron levels increase TIBC because the less iron available the more sites for iron to bind.

CC. Total protein albumin/globulin ratio (A/G Ratio).

1. Definition.
   a. Albumin/globulin ratio is the ratio of albumin and globulin concentrations in serum, usually determined by protein electrophoresis.
   b. Albumin, which comprises more than 50% of the total serum proteins, maintains oncotic pressure. Its osmotic influence is about four times that of globulin. Albumin transports substances that are insoluble in water alone, such as bilirubin, fatty acids, hormones, and drugs.
   c. Globulin seems to have more varied assignments and forms the main transport system for many substances as well as playing an active role in certain immunologic mechanisms.
   d. Serum electrophoresis is the most current method for measuring serum proteins.
   e. Although somewhat outdated, determinations of total protein and A/G ratio are still being performed.
2. Purpose: used to determine the total protein and the albumin/globulin in the serum.
3. Normal values.
   a. Total serum protein: 6.0-7.9 gm/100 ml.
   b. Albumin: 3.2-4.5 gm/100 ml.
   c. Globulin: 2.3-3.5 gm/100 ml.
4. Increased:
   a. Protein levels, by electrophoresis, appear in multiple myeloma, rheumatoid arthritis, osteomyelitis, chronic infections, monocytic leukemia, and early stage Laennec's cirrhosis.
   b. Globulin levels, by electrophoresis, appear in chronic syphilis, tuberculosis, multiple myeloma, collagen diseases, systemic lupus erythematosus, and rheumatoid arthritis.
5. Decreased:
   a. Albumin levels are evident in collagen diseases, systemic lupus erythematosus, rheumatoid arthritis, ricketsial diseases, liver diseases, and poor nutritional states.
   b. Globulin levels are evident in variable neoplastic and renal diseases, hepatic dysfunction, and blood dyscrasias.
   c. A low AG ratio may occur in cirrhosis, hepatitis, and other liver diseases, reflecting a diminished capacity of the liver to synthesize albumin and also, but not invariably, an increase in the albumin-globulin fraction.

DD. Uric acid.

1. Definition:
   a. Is an end product of the metabolism of a class of compounds known as purine bodies.
   b. Large amounts of purines are present in nucleic acids that are derived from dietary and endogenous sources.
   c. Uric acid clears the body by glomerular filtration and tubular secretion.
2. Purpose: used primarily to detect gout.
3. Normal values.
   a. Males: 2.1-7.8 mg/dl.
   b. Females: 2.0-6.4 mg/dl.
4. Increased levels are associated with gout or chronic impaired renal function, congestive heart failure with decreased creatinine clearance; glycogen storage diseases such as Lesch-Nyhan syndrome and Gierke's disease; starvation; lymphoma, and myeloproliferative diseases such as acute and chronic leukocytic and granulocytic leukemia, multiple myeloma; excessive ethyl alcohol intake, hypoparathyroidism, neoplasms, polycythemia; arthritis associated with psoriasis, sarcoidosis; and following therapy with thiazide diuretics, chemotherapy, and radiation therapy.
5. Decreased levels are associated with defective tubular absorption such as Fanconi's syndrome and Wilson's disease.

EE. Western blot test.

1. Definition.
   a. Uses electrophoresis to separate the killed virus on a special gel.
   b. The separated antigens are put on an electrophoretic sheet using a blotting technique; the serum is incubated and compared with two control specimens.
2. Purpose.
   a. Used as an alternative to the ELISA in screening blood confirmed for the HIV protein.
   b. Or as a confirmatory test to the ELISA.
3. Positive response confirms a positive ELISA test.
4. Negative response with a positive ELISA does not rule out the possibility of the presence of HIV.

II. URINE

A. Bence-Jones protein.

1. Definition: electrophoresis of urine used to identify Bence Jones protein, a specific low molecular weight protein in the urine.
2. Purpose: used to identify the presence of the Bence Jones protein in the urine.
3. Normal value: negative
4. Positive: found in 40% of multiple myeloma cases, tumor metastasis to the bone, chronic lymphocytic leukemia, amyloidosis, and macroglobulinemia.

B. Urinalysis.

1. Definition.
   a. The performance of clinical laboratory tests on urine specimens.
   b. Urine is a fluid that contains water and metabolic products. It is secreted by the kidneys, stored in the bladder, and discharged by way of the urethra.
   c. The largest component of urine by weight is water and the second largest is urea, followed by sodium chloride, phosphate, sulfate, and uric acid.
   d. Other normal components include potassium,

calcium, magnesium, and various organic compounds.

e. Routine analysis typically consists of:
   (1) Observing for any unusual color.
   (2) Noting any unusual odor.
   (3) Determining specific gravity: a determination of the weight of urine compared to the weight of an equal volume of distilled water.
   (4) Performing qualitative or semi-quantitative chemical screening tests for:
      (a) pH.
      (b) Protein: an important evaluation of glomerular function.
      (c) Glucose.
      (d) Ketones bodies: the products of incomplete fat metabolism in conditions when the body is using fatty acids as a principal source of metabolic energy or insufficient intracellular carbohydrate metabolism.
      (e) Occult blood.
      (f) Bilirubin, urobilinogen, and nitrite.
   (5) Screening for bacteriuria.
   (6) Examining centrifuged sediment microscopoically for:
      (a) Cells: typical cells include erythrocytes, leukocytes, renal tubular epithelial, transitional epithelial, or squamous epithelial cells and other cells of the genitourinary tract.
      (b) Casts: casts are an aggregate composed of material deposited in renal tubules and are classified according to the materials trapped in their matrices.
      (c) Crystals: crystals may include urate, oxalaate, cystine, tyrosine, and crystals of certain drugs. The importance of crystal formation in the urine is questionable, but crystals can contain clues to calculus formation or certain metabolic diseases.

2. Purpose.
   a. Used to reveal pathology anywhere in the urinary tract.
   b. In addition, systemic diseases may be revealed by quantitative or qualitative alterations of urine constituents or by the presence of abnormal substances, apart from their direct effects on the kidneys.
3. Normal values.
   a. Pale yellow to amber color.
   b. Slight acid reaction.
   c. Distinctive odor.
   d. Specific gravity: 1.003-1.035 (usually between 1.010-1.025).
   e. Protein: negative.
   f. Glucose: negative.
   g. Crystals: negative.
4. Increased:
   a. Specific gravity of urine with diarrhea, vomiting, excessive sweating, hypernatremia, uncontrolled diabetes mellitus, nephrotic syndrome, heart failure, and shock.
   b. Presence of protein in the urine occurs in severe muscular exertion, orthostatic proteinuria, multiple myeloma, hypertension, nephrotic syndrome, and post-collagen disease.
   c. Crystals that appear in acidic urine include calcium oxalate, uric acid, and urate. Crystals in alkaline urine are phosphate and carbonate.
5. Decreased: Specific gravity of urine with hyperthyroidism, diabetes insipidus, pyelonephritis, occasionally in sickle cell anemia, renal failure, and urine containing large amounts of urea.

C. Urine calcium.

1. Definition: test to determine the level of calcium in the urine.
2. Purpose.
   a. To help evaluate calcium metabolism and excretion and monitor deficiency.
   b. Procedure.
      (1) All excreted urine is collected for 24 hours.
      (2) Concurrent administration of medications should be noted.
      (3) Patient should avoid contaminating urine with stool or tissue.
3. Normal values: may vary with dietary intake.
   a. Males: 275 mg calcium per 24 hours.
   b. Females: 250 mg calcium per 24 hours.
4. Increased calcium excretion may occur in hyperparathyroidism, vitamin D intoxication, metastasis, and multiple myeloma.
5. Decreased calcium excretion may occur in hypoparathyroidism, nephrosis, nephritis, renal insufficiency, and osteomalacia.

D. Urine creatinine clearance.

1. Definition.
   a. Creatinine is formed and excreted in a continuous manner by an irreversible reaction.
   b. It is an end product of creatine and proportional to total muscle mass.
   c. The test determines how efficiently the kidneys are clearing creatinine from the blood.
   d. The rate of clearance is expressed in the amount of blood that can be cleared of creatinine in 1 minute.
   e. Approximately half the nephrons must be damaged before creatinine levels become abnormal.
2. Purpose.
   a. The test helps assess renal function.
   b. Procedure.
      (1) Urine specimens are collected at timed intervals over a 24-hour period, usually at 2, 6, 12, and 24-hour periods
      (2) Urine is stored in a container with a preservative to prevent breakdown of creatinine.
      (3) Urine should be kept cool (on ice or in refrigerator) during the collection period.

(4) A blood sample is obtained during the collection period to determine plasma creatinine concentration.
3. Normal values.
   a. Males: 90 ml/minute.
   b. Females: 84 ml/minute.
4. A low creatinine clearance may result from reduced blood flow to the kidney, nephritis, renal lesions, congestive heart failure, or severe dehydration.
5. A high creatinine clearance may result from a high cardiac output, pregnancy, burns, or carbon monoxide poisoning.

RADIOGRAPHIC STUDIES

I. ANGIOGRAPHY

A. Definition.

1. Study of vascular structures using x-ray: radiopaque contrast medium used (fluoroscopy may be used for selective catheter placement into vessel).
2. Serial x-ray films taken of selected vascular area.
3. Types.
   a. Arteriography: examination of arterial system.
   b. Venography.
      (1) Examination of venous system.
      (2) Used primarily to identify deep vein thrombosis or suitable veins for arterial bypass grafting.
   c. Digital subtraction angiography (or transverse digital subtraction).
      (1) Examination of arterial system using venous catheterization.
      (2) Computer-based imaging method.
      (3) Advantages over regular arteriography.
         (a) No arterial puncture necessary.
         (b) Reduced risk of trauma and emboli.
         (c) Outpatient procedure.
         (d) Lower cost.

B. Purpose.

1. Assessment of peripheral vascular perfusion: determination of amputation level.
2. Confirmation of vascular integrity in:
   a. Traumatic lesions.
   b. Bone tumors.
   c. Orthopaedic surgery.
   d. Chemotherapy.
   e. Free muscle transfers.

C. Procedure.

1. Regular angiography.
   a. Patient placed supine on x-ray table.
   b. Local anesthetic injected at site of catheter injection.
      (1) Catheter with a guidewire introduced.
      (2) Fluoroscopy may be used for direction to site under examination.
   c. Perform a sterile prep at the site.
   d. Injection of dye followed by serial x-ray films.
   e. Catheter removed and pressure dressing applied to site.
   f. Time 1-2 hours.
2. Digital subtraction angiography (DSA).
   a. Right antecubital or femoral area used.
   b. Local anesthetic injected.
      (1) Catheter advanced over guide wire to superior vena cava.
      (2) Dye injected at selected time intervals via power injector in selected amounts.
   c. Pictures taken and stored on magnetic tape or videodiscs.
   d. Catheter removed, site bandaged.
   e. Time: 30-45 minutes.

D. Nursing implications.

1. Before procedure.
   a. Consent forms necessary.
   b. Explain purpose, procedure, and patient's role.
      (1) Procedure not painful but may cause some discomfort
      (2) Explain that a warm, flushed feeling may accompany dye injection.
      (3) Explain necessity to remain still during procedure.
      (4) Encourage any questions.
   c. Ascertain if allergic to iodine, contrast media, or shellfish.
   d. NPO 8-12 hours.
   e. Cleansing enema if ordered.
   f. Start IV infusion.
   g. Administer glucagon if ordered for DSA study.
   h. Anticoagulant therapy should be discontinued several hours to days before the procedure.
   i. Shave injection site and prep as ordered.
   j. Record vital signs.
   k. Remove jewelry or metallic objects.
   l. Pre-medicate with a sedative or narcotic analgesic 1-hour before the procedure or as ordered.
   m. Have patient void.
   n. Have patient remove dentures.
2. After the procedure.
   a. Regular angiography (via arterial approach).
      (1) Pressure maintained on insertion site 5-10 minutes.
      (2) Pressure dressing or sandbag applied to site.
      (3) If pressure device used, reduce and remove pressure as ordered.
      (4) Bed rest maintained 12-24 hours.
      (5) Restricted activities next 24 hours.
      (6) Leg or arm kept straight for 6-8 hours.
      (7) Check site and vital signs frequently.
         (a) Every 15 minutes for 1 hour.
         (b) Every 30 minutes for 2 hours.
         (c) Every hour for 4 hours.
      (8) Check temperature every 4 hours for 24-48 hours.
      (9) Report site swelling, bleeding, hematoma formation.
      (10) Assess peripheral pulses distal to injection site: use doppler if necessary.

(11) Note temperature and color of extremity distal to injection site.
(12) Observe for delayed allergic reactions.
(a) Tachycardia.
(b) Dyspnea.
(c) Skin rash.
(d) Hypotension.
(e) Decreased urine output.
(13) Encourage fluid intake unless contraindicated.

b. Digital subtraction angiography.
(1) Check vitals signs.
(2) Observe injection site for bleeding, hematoma formation.
(3) Observe for signs of allergic reactions.
(a) Tachycardia.
(b) Dyspnea.
(c) Skin rash, urticaria.
(d) Hypotension.
(e) Decreased urine output.
(4) Encourage fluid intake unless contraindicated.

E. Complications.
1. Allergic reactions to contrast media: range from mild rash to anaphylaxis.
2. Hemorrhage at site of arterial injection.

II. ARTHROGRAPHY

A. Definition.
1. A roentgenologic examination of a joint following injection of radiopaque dye and/or air.
2. Double-contrast arthrograms use both dye and air.
3. Outlines soft tissue structures and contour of joint not normally seen on routine x-ray films.

B. Purpose.
1. Diagnosis of joint damage or disease.
2. Persistent unexplained joint discomfort or pain.
3. Identification of acute or chronic tears of joint capsule or supporting ligaments of knee, shoulder, ankle, hips, or wrists.
a. Tears in the menisci.
b. Internal joint derangements.
c. Synovial cysts.
4. Abnormal filling of structures of encapsulated joint is seen in arthritis, dislocation, ligament tear, rupture of rotator cuff, and synovial abnormality.

C. Procedure.
1. Patient placed on back on an examining table.
2. Skin over joint cleansed with sterile technique.
3. Local anesthetic injected around puncture site.
4. Any joint effusion is aspirated.
5. Contrast agent injected into joint.
6. A x-ray examination made of soft tissue and encapsulated joint.
a. Tomographic examination may be included.
b. Also called body section radiography, planigraphy, laminography, or stratigraphy.
c. Allows more detail to be visualized: images structures lying in a pre-determined tissue plane.
7. Joint may be put through its range of motion under fluoroscopy while x-ray series is made.

D. Nursing implications.
1. Before procedure.
a. No physical preparation necessary.
b. Consent forms necessary.
c. Explain purpose, procedure, and patient's role.
d. Determine patient allergy to contrast media.
2. After procedure.
a. Joint rest for 12 hours.
b. Application of compression dressing for 12 hours.
c. Mild analgesia for pain if ordered.
d. Ice application for swelling and pain.
e. Patient education.
(1) Normally, clicking or cracking noises may be heard in joint for 1-2 days as dye and air are absorbed.
(2) If persistent, notify physician.

E. Complications: persistent joint crepitus.

F. Precautions: observe for evidence of allergic reaction to dye.

III. BONE SCAN (SCINTIGRAPHY)

A. Definition.
1. A radionuclide study.
a. Radioactive material administered intravenously.
b. Technitium tagged to phosphate (99 mTc).
c. Bone-seeking radioisotope.
d. Uptake related to bone metabolism.
2. Skeletal system imaged.

B. Purpose.
1. Confirm, evaluate, and diagnose disease or disorders, including unexplained bone pain and increased alkaline phosphate levels.
2. Indicates very early bone disease and healing.
a. A concentration of radioisotope at a higher rate than normal bone noted in the areas of increased metabolic activity.
b. Detects but does not differentiate.
(1) Bone tumors: benign and malignant.
(2) Arthritis.
(3) Fractures.
(4) Osteomyelitis.

C. Procedure.
1. Radioactive material injected intravenously.
2. 2-3 hour waiting period with no physical restrictions.
3. Patient instructed to drink at least 1 quart of liquid during waiting period.
4. Before scan begins, patient voids (full bladder masks pelvic bones).
5. Patient placed supine on a x-ray type table.
a. Patient must remain still for 30-60 minutes during scan.
b. A sedative may be given if necessary to maintain stillness during procedure.

D. Nursing implications.
1. Before procedure.
a. Consent form may be necessary.
b. Explain purpose, procedure, and patient's role.
(1) 2-3 hour waiting period after radioisotope injection.

(2) Need to drink 4-6 glasses of water during waiting period.
(3) Dose of radiation is harmless to patient and those with whom contact is made.
(a) Radiation involved is less than a chest x-ray.
(b) Radioactive isotope is excreted from the body in 6-12 hours.
(4) Painless.
(5) Lasts 30-60 minutes.

c. Obtain a health history.
(1) Recent exposure to radionuclides.
(2) Allergies.
(3) Current pregnancy.
(4) Current infant breastfeeding.

d. Have patient remove jewelry or metal objects.

e. Have patient void before scan.

f. Answer any questions patient or family may have.

g. Report undue anxiety to physician.

2. After procedure.
a. No physical restrictions.
b. Encourage fluid intake.
c. Observe for allergic reaction to radionuclides.
d. Advise patient not to schedule any other radionuclide tests for 24-48 hours.

E. Complications.

1. Allergy to radionuclide.
2. Factors affecting results.
a. Antihypertensives.
b. Two radionuclide tests given in one day.
c. Movement during scan.
d. Distended bladder.

IV. COMPUTER TOMOGRAPHY(CT)/ COMPUTED AXIAL TOMOGRAPHY(CAT) SCAN

A. Definition.

1. Use of narrow beam of x-ray to scan area in successive layers.
a. Multiple intersecting x-ray beams used.
b. X-ray beam used in conjunction with a computer, with mathematical reconstruction of values obtained.
c. Cross-sectional views provided to produce a three-dimensional picture.
d. Differentiates similar x-ray densities: absorption coefficient calculated by computer.
e. Anatomic details are shown: screen display of digital data.
2. Routine study, noninvasive.
3. Contrast study.
a. Frequently done to increase diagnostic accuracy.
b. Characterizes certain lesions.
(1) Enhances detection of small lesions.
(2) Clarifies margins of larger lesions.
c. Uses iodine-based dye injected intravenously or barium-like substance administered by mouth or by nasogastric or gastrostomy tube.

B. Purpose.

1. Head scans.
a. Evaluate disease, disorders, and trauma to brain, facial bones, and sinuses.
b. Differentiate normal and abnormal structures.
c. Evaluate headaches, loss of consciousness, and neurologic deficits.
2. Spine CT.
a. Diagnosis of spinal cord and peripheral nerve pathology.
b. Evaluation of disease progression.
c. Evaluate post-fusion complications.
(1) Pseudoarthrosis.
(2) Stenosis of central cord.
(3) Lateral recess of neural foramen.
3. Body CT.
a. Abdomen, chest, pelvis, joints.
b. Identification of soft tissue and/or bone tumors.
(1) CT scan is good choice for visualization of bone cortex.
(2) MRI may be better choice for soft tissue lesions and marrow changes.
c. Identification of injuries to ligaments and tendons.
d. Diagnosis of fractures in areas difficult to access due to overlying and/or surrounding structures.
4. CT guided biopsy.

C. Procedure.

1. General information.
a. X-ray beams projected horizontally.
b. Data displayed on a screen, photographed, or stored on magnetic tapes or discs.
c. Procedure takes 45-90 minutes: new light speed technology cuts scanning time dramatically.
d. If a contrast study is done, IV contrast medium is injected over a 2-minute period.
(1) Patient may feel flushed and warm and may report a metallic or salty taste.
(2) Patient may experience nausea and/or vomiting.
2. Specific information.
a. Head.
(1) Patient placed on a motorized table with head immobilized in a cradle.
(2) A clicking noise may be heard as scanner revolves around the patient's head.
b. Spine.
(1) Patient positioned supine on a table with hips and knees supported.
(2) IV or intrathecal contrast.
(a) Not routinely used for lumbar spine studies.
(b) Used for intradural process, arachnoiditis, or postoperative fibrosis evaluation.
c. Body.
(1) Patient in supine position on table with appropriate body part in scanner.
(2) Patient may be asked to hold breath occasionally.

(3) Patient may hear clicking noise.
(4) If contrast study is done, IV medium is injected over a 2-minute period.

D. Nursing implications.

1. Before procedure.
   a. Ascertain pregnancy: procedure is contraindicated in pregnancy.
   b. Consent form necessary.
   c. Explain purpose, procedure, and patient's role.
      (1) Some patients experience claustrophobic fears of being in machine, show a picture of scanner.
      (2) Explain need to be still during procedure, which can last from 20-90 minutes.
      (3) Noninvasive (unless contrast used).
      (4) Painless, any discomfort comes from disease, existing trauma, or lying still.
      (5) Scanner rotates about the body part.
   d. Contrast study.
      (1) Determine allergy to iodine, seafood, or other contrast media.
         (a) If allergy history, patient may be put on steroids for 3 days or antihistamines before test.
         (b) Additionally, diphenhydramine may be given orally or IV before test.
      (2) Teach that a warm, flushed, possibly nauseated sensation may accompany dye injection.
   e. NPO for 3-12 hours before the test, if ordered.
   f. Enema, if ordered.
   g. Remove jewelry or metal objects.
   h. Offer emotional support to patient and family. Inform that radiation received will be no more than from a series of regular x-rays.
   i. Retained barium can obscure images.
2. During procedure.
   a. Contrast study.
      (1) Have emergency drugs and equipment available for severe allergic reactions.
      (2) Observe for nausea and vomiting.
   b. Observe for allergic reactions.
   c. Offer verbal reassurance to patient.
3. After procedure.
   a. If contrast study, observe for delayed allergic reactions.
      (1) Urticaria, skin rashes, nausea, vomiting, headache, and swelling of parotid glands (iodism).
      (2) Administer oral antihistamines if symptoms persist.
   b. If contrast study, encourage fluids to assist excretion of dye.

E. Complications: if contrast study, allergic reaction.

F. Precautions.

1. Contraindicated in pregnancy.
2. Contrast study.
   a. Obtain allergy history.
   b. Administer pre-procedure drugs as ordered.
   c. Have emergency drugs and equipment available during procedure.
3. Studies using barium should be scheduled after CT scans.

V. DUAL ENERGY ABSORPTIOMETRY (DEXA)

A. Definition.

1. Method of measuring bone mineral density (BMD) using x-ray absorptiometry to test the hip and spine.
2. Laser x-ray scanner and computer technology record images and measure fracture risk.
3. A noninvasive and accurate measurement based on the fact that mineralized bone absorbs x-rays at different rates than soft tissue.
4. DEXA is the "gold standard" for BMD testing for hip and spine. Other ultrasound machines are available for fingers, wrists, and heels.

B. Purpose.

1. Determine bone mineral density and thus be able to diagnose low bone mass and osteoporosis.
2. Assess patient's response to treatment method for low bone mass and osteoporosis.
3. Predict potential fractures.

C. Procedure: patient position depends on body part imaged.

1. Foam block placed under knees for spine.
2. Brace is used for leg immobilization during femur scan.
3. Brace is used for arm during forearm scan.
4. Scan can take from 20-55 minutes.

D. BMD values.

1. World Health Organization (WHO) defines osteoporosis in terms of BMD.
2. Scores are based on a population of Caucasian women and are not necessarily applicable to all ages.
   a. Normal bone density is a T-score between +1 and -1.
   b. Osteopenia is defined as a T-score between -1 and 12.5.
   c. Osteoporosis is considered present when the T-score is below (more negative than) -2.5; is considered severe if the patient already has had a fracture.

E. Nursing implications.

1. Explain purpose, procedure, and patient's role.
2. Have patient remove metal objects (jewelry, braces, or prosthetic devices) from area to be scanned.
3. Obtain surgical history focused on any metal implants.
4. Inform patient that he/she will need to be still for at least 20 minutes.
5. Ascertain pregnancy.

E. Complications: none.

F. Precautions.

1. Remove any external metal objects to prevent interference with scan.
2. Implanted metal objects may interfere with scan.
3. Nuclear medicine studies with 72 hours may interfere with exam.

4. Barium studies done within last 7-10 days may interfere with exam.

VI. INDIUM-WBC SCAN

A. Definition/purpose.

1. A method of detecting infections or abscesses in deep body cavities; can locate infected site and determine if it is localized, walled off, and suitable for draining.
2. Replaces use of gallium scan in patients with neoplastic lesions or non-infected healing wounds as gallium gives false positive for these conditions.
3. Indium In 111 pentetic acid (also called indium-111-DTPA) is the agent of choice for radionuclide cisternography because its half-life of 2.8 days is suitable for 24-48 hour delayed scans.

B. Procedure.

1. Patient's blood sample is obtained; granulocytes are isolated and labeled with In-111 or Tc-99 m isotopes.
2. Cells are then re-injected intravenously.
3. Whole body scanning is done anywhere from 4-48 hours later for suspected infections.
4. Results can be confirmed with CT or ultrasound.

C. Nursing implications.

1. Explain purpose, procedure, and patient's role.
2. Preparation of tagged WBCs takes from 1-2 hours.
3. Patient's white count should be at least 4.0. Note: this is so there is enough volume of WBCs for the radionuclids to attach to.
4. Imaging takes approximately 1 hour.

D. Complications: none identified.

E. Precautions: verify correct patient when injecting tagged WBCs.

VII. MAGNETIC RESONANCE IMAGING (MRI)/NULCEAR MAGNETIC RESONANCE (NMR).

A. Definition.

1. Imaging modality that examines interaction between magnetic field, radio waves, and tissue cells. Image produced is dependent upon density of cells stimulated and magnetic interaction that differs in fat, muscle, bone, and blood.
2. Cross-sectional imaging device that can obtain images in sagittal, coronal, and transverse planes.
3. Tissue differentiation is more apparent in MRI than CT.

B. Purpose: used for visualizing marrow; soft tissue tumors; primary and metastatic bone tumors. Also anatomic delineation of muscles, ligaments, fat, nerves, blood vessels, and bones.

C. Procedure.

1. Patient completes questionnaire regarding any metal implants.
2. Patient removes all external metal objects and credit cards with magnetic strips.
3. Patient lies on table that moves into magnet.
4. Magnetic force is applied.
5. Cell nuclei respond to the force by resonating.
6. Magnetic force is stopped.
7. Nuclei release energy absorbed in the form of radio waves.
8. Antenna in MRI unit receives radio waves.
9. Computer amplifies and processes radio waves to produce image.
10. Contrast media (gadolinium, iron, or magnesium complexes) may be used.

D. Nursing implications.

1. Before procedure.
   a. Consent form may be necessary.
   b. Take detailed history.
   c. Contraindicated if patient has any metal implants.
   d. Explain purpose, procedure, and patient's role:
      (1) Patient may become claustrophobic in machine; show pictures of device and discuss need for complete cooperation.
      (2) Patient must lie still during entire procedure.
      (3) Non-invasive, painless.
      (4) Remove all external metal objects.
2. After procedure: patient may resume normal activity and diet.

E. Complications: metal aneurysm clips have been bent and pulled from cerebral vessels during test.

F. Precautions.

1. Magnet may attract metal objects including tools such as stethoscope, scissors, etc.
2. Patients with pacemakers, prostheses, metal braces, or any other metal implant may be restricted from having this procedure.

VIII. MYELOGRAPHY

A. Definition: an x-ray following injection of contrast medium or air into subarachnoid space of lumbar spine through a spinal puncture.

1. Fluoroscopic and x-ray examination done.
2. Spinal subarachnoid space outlined.
3. Distortion of spinal cord or spinal dural sac visualized.

B. Purpose.

1. Done to determine tumor sites, herniated intervertebral discs, cysts, or other lesions blocking subarachnoid space.
2. Usually requested before surgical treatment of ruptured vertebral disc.
3. Presence of unexplained back or leg pain.
4. Suspected intraspinal pathology.

C. Procedure.

1. Done in x-ray department.
2. Position as for lumbar puncture initially.
   a. Patient positioned prone and secured to table with straps.
   b. Shoulder and foot braces may be used.
3. Lumbar area shaved and prepped.
4. Area injected with local anesthetic: puncture level lower in children.
5. Lumbar puncture is done: introduction of hollow needle into lumbar subarachnoid space at L4-5.
6. Contrast medium or air is injected into subarach-

noid space of lumbar spine.

a. Air or oxygen.
   (1) Used for patients allergic to contrast media.
   (2) May be used for differential diagnosis of cervical cord lesions.
   (3) Tomography essential to improve visualization.
   (4) Difficulty controlling gas after introduction.
b. Metrizamide.
   (1) Water soluble contrast medium: 5-15 milliliters used.
   (2) Absorbed by body, excreted by kidneys.
   (3) Does not require removal from spinal canal.
   (4) Side effects due to central nervous system (CNS) irritation from drug.
      (a) Headache.
      (b) Seizures.
   (5) Advantages.
      (a) Better nerve root and nerve sleeve visualization.
      (b) Use of a smaller puncture needle possible.
      (c) Immediate removal of needle.
c. Iophendylate.
   (1) Oil-based iodine compound contrast medium: 5-15 ml used.
   (2) Removed by syringe and needle aspiration after procedure.
   (3) Irritation of tissues and poor absorption of oil by subarachnoid space may occur.

7. Head of examining table tilted downward: course of contrast medium observed fluoroscopically and films made serially.
8. Puncture site cleaned and covered with a sterile dressing.

D. Nursing implications.

1. Before procedure.
   a. Consent forms necessary.
   b. Check for allergy to iodine or contrast material.
   c. If metrizamide to be used ascertain absence of drugs that lower the seizure threshold (phenothiazides, tricyclic antidepressants, CNS stimulants, amphetamines).
   d. Instruct patient to force fluids the night before procedure.
   e. NPO is maintained 4-8 hours before the procedure.
   f. Cleansing enema may be ordered.
   g. Pre-medication with a sedative or narcotic analgesic and atropine, if ordered.
   h. Explain purpose, procedure, and patient's role.
      (1) Possible transient burning sensation and/or flushed/warm feeling as dye is injected.
      (2) Tilting of table will necessitate strapping.
      (3) Procedure will take approximately 1 hour.
   i. Have patient void before procedure.
2. After procedure.
   a. Metrizamide (water based).
      (1) Head elevated 15-40 degrees for 8 hours.
      (2) Progress to flat bed rest with bathroom privileges for 16 hours.
      (3) Do not give phenothiazines.
      (4) Avoid drugs that lower the seizure threshold (tricyclic antidepressants, phenothiazides, CNS stimulants, amphetamines) for 24 hours.
   b. Iophendylate (oil based).
      (1) Patient flat in bed 12-24 hours.
      (2) May turn side to side.
   c. Force fluids.
   d. Assess for bladder distention, ability to void.
   e. Maintain intake and output record.
   f. Frequent neurologic assessments and vital signs.
   g. Administer pain medications for headache or discomfort.
   h. Observe for complications as listed below.

E. Complications.

1. Bleeding or leakage at injection site.
2. Nausea and vomiting.
3. Headache.
4. Fever.
5. Seizure activity: most likely to occur 4-8 hours after myelogram.
6. Paralysis.
7. Arachnoiditis: inflammation of coverings of spinal cord.
8. Neck stiffness.
9. Sterile meningitis reaction.
   a. Severe headache.
   b. Slow EEG patterns.
10. Brain stem compression.
11. Brain stem herniation.

F. Precautions.

1. Procedure contraindicated in patients with multiple sclerosis in the acute stage as the edema of myelinated areas may resemble a lesion; in later stages there are areas of demylinated (unprotected) white matter which would be chemically traumatized by the dye.
2. Seizures possible with incorrect post-procedure positioning and care.
   a. Be certain to determine type of contrast media used.
   b. Metrizamide irritates the meninges.
      (1) Patient must be positioned first with head elevated to allow dye to be resorbed in spinal canal.
      (2) The head is then lowered to allow an adequate amount of fluid to re-enter and bathe cerebral meninges.
3. Gas or fecal material in gastrointestinal tract affect results.
4. Acute exacerbation of symptoms may be caused by manipulation of cerebrospinal fluid (CSF) pressure: immediate surgical intervention might be required.

IX. THERMOGRAPHY

A. Definition.

1. Measurement of the degree of heat radiating from

skin surface.
    a. Noninvasive.
    b. Pictorial representation of infrared radiation from area examined.
2. Skin temperature elevations or depressions localized.
    a. Can indicate inflammatory or malignant lesions.
    b. Hypothermic areas may indicate levels of spinal cord lesion.
    c. Objective documentation of subjective symptomatology.
    d. Premyelography screening.

B. Purpose.
1. Investigate inflamed, infectious, traumatic, and neoplastic diseases of spine and extremities.
2. Object method for documentation of remissions or relapses of certain conditions.
3. Method of diagnosing peripheral neuropathies.
4. Assessing and monitoring of treatment results, anti-inflammatory medications.
5. Utilized as a way to augment or complement other diagnostic studies.

C. Procedure.
1. Patient taken to a draft-free, air-conditioned room.
2. An instant camera records thermograms.
3. Techniques.
    a. Contact thermography, an inflated "air pillow" is used.
    b. Liquid crystal thermography.
        (1) Cholesterol derivatives that selectively reflect polarized light used.
        (2) Advantages over contact method.
            (a) Contact with patient's body unnecessary.
            (b) Adaptable to any part of body.
            (c) Larger body areas can be encompassed on each view.
            (d) Simplicity of apparatus.
            (e) High color contrast achievable.
4. If abnormal image seen, photography repeated at least three times in succession for confirmation.

D. Nursing implications.
1. Explain purpose, procedure, and patient's role.
    a. Noninvasive, painless.
    b. No radiation involved.
    c. Time approximately 5-10 minutes.
2. No smoking allowed the day of procedure.
3. Assure even temperatures in procedure room.
4. Area to be examined may require cooling with a water sponge bath for 10 minutes before procedure.

E. Precaution: no precautions necessary.

X. X-RAY (RADIOGRAPHS, ROENTGENOGRAMS)

A. Definition: a study using beams of radiation to produce images of various body tissues based on densities.
1. Densities in human body.
    a. Air: has less density, produces dark or black images.
    b. Water.
    c. Fat.
    d. Bone.
        (1) Has high density, produces light or white images.
        (2) Calcium in bone increases density and therefore, lightness.
2. Images produced are recorded on photographic film, as digital images, or imaged on video screen.

B. Purpose.
1. Bone films determine integrity, density, texture, erosion, and changes in relationship to other bones and tissue.
2. Bone cortex films reveal widening, narrowing, and irregularity.
3. Joint films detect fluid presence, spur formation, narrowing, irregularity, or changes in structure.
4. Help to define and intervene regarding trauma, surgery, pain, tumor, or disease conditions.

C. X-ray views.
1. Anteroposterior (AP): x-ray passes from front to back.
2. Apical lordotic: x-ray of chest with apices of the lungs as well as clavicle viewed.
3. Bruerton: x-ray of hand specifically to view early joint changes.
4. Carter Rowe: x-ray of hip from a 45-degree oblique angle.
5. Hughston: x-ray of knee in 60 degrees of flexion at a 55-degree angle.
6. Lateral: x-ray beam passes from side to side (left to right or right to left).
7. Mortise: x-ray of ankle rotated with lateral and medial malleoli parallel to the film.
8. Oblique: x-ray beam passes at an angle.
9. Posteroanterior (PA): x-ray beam passes from back to front.
10. Scanography: x-ray of hips, knees, and ankles using a ruler to determine leg lengths.
11. Sunset or tangential: x-ray of patella with knee flexed and a profile view of the knee.
12. Tunnel: x-ray of tibia, fibula, and femur with patella deflected and PA view of knee.
13. Von Rosen: x-ray of hips in abduction and internal rotation.
14. Routine orthopaedic areas.
    a. Thorax: chest, clavicle, ribs (anterior and posterior), scapula, shoulder, and sternum.
    b. Limbs:
        (1) Upper: shoulder, humerus, elbow, forearm, wrist, hands, and fingers.
        (2) Lower: hip, femur, knee, patella, tibia and fibula, ankle, foot, calcaneus, and toes.
    c. Spine and spinal area: cervical, thoracic, and lumbar spine, coccyx, pelvis, sacroiliac joints, and sacrum.

D. Precautions.
1. Patients in reproductive years should have genital areas protected during procedures.
2. Women in first trimester of pregnancy are at risk for

developing fetal abnormalities.

a. Only emergency films are taken.
b. Lead apron is used to shield abdominal and pelvic areas during radiation exposure.
c. Films for obstetric reasons are not to be repeated.

3. Genetic: mutation of reproductive cells might occur with exposure of genital organs to radiation.
4. Somatic: changes might occur in tissue in other parts of body following excessive or repeated exposure to radiation.
5. Effects of radiation exposure may be cumulative:
   a. Personnel and physicians should wear lead apron, gloves, and goggles in radiology laboratory.
   b. Patient's medical records should be reviewed closely to determine frequency and dosage of radiologic studies.

E. Advantages.

1. Rapidly and readily available in most institutions.
2. Ability to survey or screen a large anatomic area.
3. Useful as a screening procedure for decision-making regarding further diagnostic tests.

F. Procedure.

1. Position dependent upon x-ray view ordered. Patient may be standing, sitting, prone, supine, or side lying.
2. Patient instructed not to move during exposure.
3. Personnel and parts of patient's body should be protected from exposure to x-ray beams by lead aprons or lead screens
4. Time dependent upon views ordered; usually 5-10 minutes for routine procedure.

G. Nursing implications.

1. Before procedure.
   a. Explain purpose, procedure, and patient's role and assess patient's understanding.
   b. Inform patient that procedure usually takes 5-10 minutes.
      (1) Several pictures may be taken.
      (2) Patient may be asked to wait following exposure to be certain films are readable.
   c. Determine if female patients are pregnant.
   d. Determine elderly, traumatized, deformed, or debilitated patient's ability to assume required positions over periods necessary for procedure.
      (1) Schedule with this information in mind.
         (a) Allow rest time between procedures.
         (b) Administer analgesic medication before procedure if indicated.
      (2) Inform radiology department of patient's physical restrictions.
   e. If ordered, withhold food and drink.
   f. Encourage questions, expressions of fear or anxiety. Reassure patient and family members that x-ray equipment does not expose them to excessive radiation.
   g. Administer analgesics if ordered and indicated.
2. After procedure: analgesics or local heat or ice applications may be necessary for pain relief following lengthy procedures and/or painful positioning.

H. Complications: interfering conditions.

1. Obesity and ascites might interfere with clarity of some views.
2. Improper positioning of patient.
3. Patient movement during exposure.

SPECIAL DIAGNOSTIC STUDIES

I. ARTHROMETER

A. Definition: a method of measuring and documenting cruciate ligament laxity of the knee both actively and passively.

B. Purpose.

1. Diagnose anterior and/or posterior cruciate ligament (ACL and PCL) tears.
   a. Tears may be acute or chronic.
   b. ACL trauma usually caused by twisting or cutting motion.
   c. PCL trauma usually caused by blow to back of the knee.
   d. Additional diagnostic tool following physical examination of the knee including Lachman and pivot shift test.
2. Evaluate ACL and/or PCL stability intra-operatively.
3. Confirm ACL and/or PCL stability during and after a rehabilitation program.

C. Procedure.

1. Usually performed in the orthopaedist's office.
2. May be performed in operating room immediately pre-operatively, intra-operatively, or immediately postoperatively.
3. Patient is placed in a supine position on table.
4. Arthrometer is placed on non-injured leg
   a. Operating instructions for specific brand of arthrometer are followed.
   b. Measurements are made using distraction forces on the knee passively, actively, and manually.
5. Arthrometer is then placed on injured leg and measurements are taken.
6. Positioning parameters and arthrometer measurements are documented in patient's record.

D. Nursing implications.

1. Explain purpose, procedure, and patient's role.
   a. Patient must completely relax quadriceps and hamstrings during test.
   b. Test is not painful.
2. Test should be performed after physician examination, x-rays, and arthrocentisis (if necessary).
3. Patient may return to pre-test activities immediately.

E. Complications.

1. Disruption of fracture near and/or involving proximal tibia and fibula, distal femur, or patella.
2. Disruption of ACL graft if done with too much force early in rehabilitation phase.
3. Locked and swollen knee can abnormally restrict knee motion and result in a false negative test result.

F. Precautions.

1. Ensure that patient can attain full extension of

injured knee comfortably before test.
2. Check to see that x-rays have been evaluated before test.
3. Document date and method of reconstruction or injury on request form.

II. ARTHROSCOPY

A. Definition: surgical procedure enabling physician to directly visualize the inside of a joint.

B. Purpose: differential diagnosis and treatment of synovial, ligatmentous, meniscal, capsular, and articular cartilage tears, defects, and/or disease processes.

1. Musculoskeletal trauma.
   a. Fractures involving articular cartilage and joint integrity.
   b. Ligament, cartilage, and capsular tears.
   c. Ligament release, repair, or reconstruction.
   d. Foreign body within joint.
   e. Joint subluxation.
2. Inflammatory process.
   a. Differential diagnosis of rheumatic disease.
   b. Synovial biopsy.
   c. Therapeutic synovectomy.
   d. Impingement syndrome.
3. Osteochondritis dissecans.
4. Joint mice/loose bodies composed of osteochondral or meniscal tissue.
5. Adhesions within joint that limit joint function

C. Procedure.

1. Performed in operating room under local, regional, or general anesthesia.
2. Patient positioned to facilitate physician's access to affected joint.
3. Operative site prepared and draped in a sterile fashion.
4. Portals made for arthroscope and arthroscopic instrumentation.
5. Arthroscope inserted into joint.
6. Joint visually and dynamically examined with arthroscope and probe.
7. Abnormal pathology addressed when applicable.
   a. Synovial biopsy or removal.
   b. Meniscal repair or removal.
   c. Articular cartilage repair or reconstruction.
   c. Fracture reduction or fixation.
   d. Scar tissue debridement.
   e. Foreign body and loose body removal.
8. Sterile compression dressing applied.
9. Brace or cast may be used following some procedures.

D. Nursing implications.

1. Before procedure.
   a. Consent forms necessary.
   b. Explain purpose, procedure, and patient's role: patients with local or regional anesthesia may experience tightness if a tourniquet is used.
   c. NPO for 8-12 hours for general anesthesia.
   d. Shave and prep the operative area as ordered.
   e. Determine drug and anesthesia allergies.
   f. Record vital signs and pertinent medical history.
   g. Remove jewelry, contact lenses, glasses, etc.
   h. Pre-medicate if ordered.
2. After the procedure.
   a. May go to recovery room.
   b. Check operative site for bleeding.
   c. Monitor circulation and sensation distal to operative site.
   d. Resume diet and medications as tolerated.
   e. Resume activity/begin rehabilitation as ordered.
   f. Usually performed on an outpatient basis.

E. Complications.

1. Hemorrhage.
2. Infection.
3. Thrombophlebitis.
4. Neurovascular compromise.
5. Compartment syndrome.
6. Ligament/tendon rupture.
7. Bone fracture.

III. BONE MARROW ASPIRATION AND BIOPSY

A. Definition: removal of bone marrow (soft tissue contained in medial canals of the long bones and in interstices of cancellous bone) by aspiration, needle biopsy, or drilled core.

B. Purpose: used to determine cause of infection, type of tumor, anemia, osteoporosis, response to treatment, and effectiveness of chemotherapy.

C. Procedure.

1. May be performed under local or general anesthetic in patient's room, special procedure room, radiology, or operating room.
2. Common sites usually chosen are posterior superior iliac spines, midsternum, spinous process of vertebral body, body of vertebra, and proximal tibia.
3. Aspiration.
   a. Skin prepped and draped.
   b. Local anesthetic administered.
   c. Aspiration needle inserted into bone cortex.
   d. Stylet removed and syringe attached.
   e. 0.1-3.0 ml of bone marrow fluid aspirated.
   f. Needle may have to be repositioned if no specimen obtained.
   g. Sterile compression dressing applied.
4. Biopsy.
   a. As above for aspiration.
   b. Biopsy needle or drill inserted into bone at biopsy site.
   c. Sterile compression dressing applied.

D. Nursing implications.

1. Before procedure.
   a. May be NPO.
   b. Consent forms necessary.
   c. Determine sensitivity to local anesthetic/latex.
   d. Explain purpose, procedure, and patient's role.
2. During procedure: patient will feel pressure on insertion and pulling sensation on removal of marrow.
3. After procedure.
   a. Properly label specimens.
   b. May go to recovery room if general anesthesia used.

c. Check biopsy site for bleeding and hemorrhage.
d. Monitor vital signs closely following procedure.
e. Resume diet, routine medications, and activity as tolerated.
f. Teach patient or significant other to check site for infection.

E. Complications.
1. Hematoma.
2. Bleeding.
3. Hemorrhage.
4. Infection.
5. Sternal fractures if sternum is used.

F. Precautions.
1. Contraindicated in patients with severe bleeding disorders.
2. Send tissue specimen to lab immediately.

IV. DISKOGRAM (DISCOGRAM)

A. Definition.
1. Injection of radiopaque dye into intervertebral lumbar disc.
2. Performed under sterile conditions using fluoroscopy.

B. Purpose: identify internal derangement of disc.

C. Procedure.
1. Performed by radiologist or surgeon in radiology or surgical department using local anesthetic.
2. Skin prepped and draped in sterile fashion.
3. Local anesthetic infiltrated.
4. Long needle inserted in a posterolateral approach to the center of selected vertebral disc under fluoroscopy.
5. Radiopaque dye injected. If patient is allergic to dye, an "air acceptance test" is done.
6. Air injected and resistance determined: intact disc will exert more resistance than herniated disc.
7. Appropriate x-rays taken.

D. Implications.
1. Diskogram evaluated by configuration of dye pattern.
2. Leakage of dye can indicate herniated disc.
3. Normal disc will accept 1 ml of dye with strong residual pressure; abnormal disc will accept a greater amount of dye with minimal residual pressure.

E. Nursing implications.
1. Before procedure.
   a. Usually NPO a few hours before procedure.
   b. Explain purpose, procedure, and patient's role.
   c. Consent forms necessary.
   d. Determine allergy to local anesthetic, seafood, iodine, and radiopaque dye.
   e. Analgesic may be required.
2. During procedure.
   a. Observe patient for signs of anaphylaxis.
   b. Observe patient's pain response and report of radicular pain.
3. After procedure.
   a. Conduct neurologic assessments regularly until stable.
   b. Observe for anaphylaxis or allergy.

F. Complications.
1. Nerve root damage.
2. Injection in inappropriate space.
3. Dural tear.
4. Infection.

G. Precautions: in the past, was done before chymopapain injection (chemonucleolysis), but the current belief is that this may increase complications following chemonucleolysis.

V. JOINT ASPIRATION

A. Definition: diagnostic procedure carried out by inserting needle into synovial capsule of joint in order to withdraw fluid for examination.

B. Purpose: performed for pain relief when joint swelling and effusion are present.

C. Procedure.
1. Performed by physician using aseptic technique in office or hospital setting under local anesthesia.
2. Most common joint aspirated is knee.
3. Site cleansed with antiseptic solution.
4. Local anesthetic infiltrated, aspiration site indicated.
5. Sterile needle chosen that is long enough and gauge large enough to withdraw fluid. (Large sterile syringe used.)
6. Needle inserted into joint capsule and fluid withdrawn.
7. Fluid prepared for microscopic evaluation.
8. Puncture site cleansed and pressure dressing applied.

D. Implications.
1. Symptomatic indication of joint pathology is increased joint fluid.
2. Normal characteristics of synovial fluid.
   a. Straw colored and clear.
   b. Cell count less than 200.
   c. Glucose equivalent to two-thirds of blood.
   d. No crystals.
   e. Negative cultures.

E. Nursing implications.
1. Before procedure: explain purpose, procedure, and patient's role.
2. During procedure: support patient.
3. After procedure.
   a. Apply pressure to puncture sire.
   b. Patient may resume previous activity.

F. Complications: infection.

G. Precautions: procedure may have to be repeated as indicated.

VI. LUMBAR EPIDURAL VENOGRAM

A. Definition: procedure involving opacification of lumbar epidural venous plexus by catheterization and injection of contrast material into ascending and internal iliac veins.

B. Purpose: the visualization of vertebral veins to try and localize abnormalities.

C. Procedure.
1. Performed in radiology.
2. Local anesthetic injected into catheterization site.
3. Catheterization performed into ascending lumbar, internal iliac, or presacral veins and 35-50 ml of contrast material injected.

4. Repeated radiographs taken during injection.

D. Implications: anterior and inferior vertebral veins by relationship to vertebrae and discs and therefore localized asymmetry may represent abnormality.

E. Nursing implications.

1. Before procedure.
   a. No physical preparation necessary except NPO.
   b. Consent forms necessary.
   c. Explain purpose, procedure, and patient's role,
   d. Determine possible sensitivity to local anesthetic, radiopaque dye.
2. After procedure.
   a. Observe for complications, including anaphylactic shock, hematoma, hemorrhage, and infection.
   b. Monitor vital signs regularly every 15 minutes for 1 hour, then every 30 minutes for 2 hours, then every hour until stable.
   c. Check pulse and dorsalis pedis, popliteal arteries for volume, intensity, and rate.
   d. Support patient.
   e. Patient education, encourage rest first 24 hours, resume medications and diet as tolerated.

F. Complications: bleeding, hematoma, hemorrhage, emboli, anaphylactic shock, and infection.

G. Precautions.

1. Contraindicated in patients with severe bleeding disorders.
2. Observe patients on anticoagulants closely for bleeding.

VII. NERVE CONDUCTION STUDIES/ ELECTROMYOGRAPHY (EMG)

A. Definition.

1. Nerve conduction studies/electromyography measures electrical activity across muscle membranes by means of needle electrodes.
2. EMG is a recording of electrical activity of selected skeletal muscle groups at rest and during contraction.
3. Nerve conduction study measures time between stimulation of nerve and detected response of implanted electrodes where response is displayed on oscilloscope.

B. Purpose.

1. Procedure yields information on the condition of nerve impulses to muscles, as well as the response of those muscles to the nerve impulses.
2. Differentiate primary muscle disorders.
3. Determine disc disease characterized by central nerve degeneration.
4. Aid diagnosis of neuromuscular and peripheral nerve disorders.
5. Can differentiate between myopathy and neuropathy.

C. Procedure.

1. Patient sits or lies quietly.
2. Extremity positioned at rest.
3. Needle electrode inserted into select muscles and lead strap applied to ankle or wrist for grounding.
4. Stimulation of muscles results in electrical signal which is recorded during rest and contraction and viewed on an oscilloscope or recorded on graphs and often audio amplified.
5. Nerve conduction time measured simultaneously by knowing time between stimulation of nerve and detected response.
6. The speed is then determined by dividing distance between point of stimulation and recording electrode by time between stimulation and response.
7. Procedure can last from 30 minutes to 2 hours. With today's powerful computers the results can be interpreted immediately.

D. Nursing implications.

1. Before procedure.
   a. Explain tests, purpose, procedure, who will be performing test (usually a neurologist), and patient's role.
   b. No danger of electrical shock.
   c. Usually no restrictions for food and fluids.
   d. There may be a 2-3 hour restriction on nicotine and/or caffeine products before procedure.
   e. Alert patient to discomfort of electrode placement and muscle stimulation similar to shock from static electricity.
   f. Consent forms necessary.
   g. Review medical history for medications (muscle relaxants, anticholinergics, and cholinergics) that may interfere with results.
2. After procedure.
   a. Apply warm compresses if residual pain remains.
   b. Resume previous medications and activity.

E. Complications: extremely rare.

F. Precautions: contraindicated in patient with bleeding disorders.

VIII. PULMONARY FUNCTION TESTS

A. Definition: tests for lung volume and capacity.

B. Purpose.

1. Identifies obstructive and/or restrictive defects in respiratory system.
2. Used in prevention of postoperative respiratory complications.
3. Is preoperative evaluation tool for patients undergoing scoliosis corrective surgical procedures.
4. Used to evaluate patients with known obstructive respiratory disease (asthma, emphysema, COPD), or smoking history.
5. Used to evaluate patients with known restrictive respiratory disease (scoliosis, obesity, muscular dystrophy).
6. Used for postoperative evaluation of respiratory function.

C. Procedure.

1. Usually performed in pulmonary function lab.
2. Patient positioned for comfort, usually sitting.
3. Technique demonstrated to patient by technician; patient must breathe through mouth only.
4. Patient breathes as directed for each phase of test into a spirometer.
5. Most common levels evaluated.

a. Vital capacity (VC).
    (1) The maximum amount of air expired after normal inspiration.
    (2) Used to evaluate restrictive defects.
b. Forced vital capacity (FVC).
    (1) Vital capacity with a forced expiration.
    (2) Used to evaluate restrictive defects.
c. Forced expiratory volume (FEV).
    (1) The percent of vital capacity expressed in 1-3 seconds.
    (2) Used to evaluate severity of obstruction and effectiveness of bronchodilators.
d. Volume exhaled (VE).
    (1) Volume of air exhaled at rest in 1 minute.
    (2) Used to evaluate obstructive defects.
e. Maximum voluntary ventilation (MVV) or maximum breathing capacity (MBC).
    (1) The volume of air exhaled in 1 minute after patient breathes as deeply and rapidly as possible.
    (2) Used to evaluate obstructive defects.
f. Forced expiratory flows (FEF).
    (1) The speed with which a patient can exhale a specific volume of air.
    (2) Used to evaluate obstructive defects.

D. Nursing implications.
1. Explain purpose, procedure, and patient's role.
2. Patient should rest before the test so the respiratory system can function at its full capacity.
3. Bronchodilators and narcotics should not be administered before the test as they effect the true functional capacity of the respiratory system.
4. Patient may return to pretest activities immediately.

E. Precautions: no precautions necessary.

IX. SOMATOSENSORY EVOKED POTENTIALS (SSEP)

A. Definition.
1. Measures time in meters per second from the stimulation of a peripheral nerve through the response.
2. Measures conduction along nerve pathways not accessible with EMGs.
3. Documents axonal continuity when sensory nerve potential cannot be measured due to nerve trauma.

B. Purpose.
1. Evaluation of radiculopathies and peripheral nerve function.
2. Diagnostic of Charcot-Marie-Tooth disease, diabetic neuropathy, and Freidreich's ataxia.
3. Preoperative evaluation and intra-operative monitoring of spinal nerves during spinal instrumentation/stabilization.

C. Procedure.
1. Patient sits in a recliner or lies quietly.
2. Transcutaneous or percutaneous electrodes are applied to the skin; usually along median or peroneal nerve distributions.
3. The stimulus is applied to electrodes. Intervals calculated by the monitoring device.

D. Nursing implications.
1. Explain purpose, procedure, and patient's role.
2. Alert patient to mild discomfort, which may accompany electrode placement and stimulation.
3. No restrictions for food or fluids before testing.

E. Precautions: use transcutaneous electrodes for patients with bleeding tendencies.

Bibliography

Academy of Infrared Thermography. (1999). *Learn about thermography* [Online]. Available: www. infraredtraining.net/thermographer.htm

El-Khoury, G.Y. (1994). Imaging of the musculoskeletal system. In S.L. Weinstein & J.A. Buckwalter (Eds.), *Turek's orthopaedics: Principles and their application* (pp. 69-124). Philadelphia: J.B. Lippincott.

Fischbach, F. (2000). *A manual of laboratory diagnostic tests* (6th ed.). Philadelphia: Lippincott.

Lum, E., & Gross, T. (1998). *Interpretation of pulmonary function tests: spirometry. Virtual Hospital* [Online]. Available: www.vh.org/Providers/Simulations/Spirometry/SpirometryHome.html

MedicineNet.com Medical References. (2000). *Joint aspiration: Arthrocentesis* [Online]. Available: www.MedicineNet.com

Moye, C.E. (1998). Diagnostic modalities for orthopaedic disorders. In A.B. Maher, S.W. Salmond, & T.A. Pellino (Eds.), *Orthopaedic nursing* (pp. 190-211). Philadelphia: W.B. Saunders.

Schoen, D.C. (2000). Assessment of the orthopaedic patient. In D.C. Schoen, *Adult orthopaedic nursing* (pp. 11-42). Philadelphia: Lippincott.

STUDY QUESTIONS

1. Hyperpigmentation of the sacrum, buttocks, and lower extremities is indicative of fibrous dysplasia. The only laboratory finding confirming the diagnosis of fibrous dysplasia is an abnormal:
   a. Acid phosphatase.
   b. Alkaline phosphatase.
   c. Creatinine phosphokinase.
   d. C-reactive protein.

2. Mr. Atencio is a 36-year-old male who is unable to bear weight on his left foot. Examination reveals a swollen, tender, and inflamed great toe with an ingrown toenail. Medical management includes the use of allopurinol and indomethacin. What laboratory study should be ordered for a patient suspected to have gout/arthritis?
   a. Erythrocyte sedimentation rate/uric acid.
   b. Erythropoietin and urine creatinine.
   c. Enzyme assay test and urinalysis.
   d. Rheumatoid factor and antinuclear antibody.

3. Jean is a 70-year-old female who is concerned that she has ruptured a disc. For a week, she has been aware of dysesthesia and dysfunction in the left arm and lower extremity. She has a drop foot on the left and her short toe extensor is weak. The Achilles reflex is slightly diminished. The Babinski is questionable positive. The right lower extremity is normal. A neurologic evaluation is indicated. The preliminary study useful in determining a CVA is:
   a. Computed axial tomography.
   b. Magnetic resonance imaging.
   c. Thermography of the head.
   d. Bone scan.

4. Allyson, age 13, is seen in the physician's office for wrist pain. She complains of pain and tenderness on the flexor surface beneath the radial pulse at the insertion of the flexor carpi radialis. Pronation, supination, range of motion, and tests for carpal instability are negative. Neurologic physical examination of bilateral upper extremities is negative. X-rays of the right wrist (anteroposterior, lateral, and oblique) appear to be normal. The impression is overuse syndrome. The diagnostic study that should be used is:
   a. Bone scan.
   b. Bone marrow aspiration.
   c. Electromyography.
   d. Bone biopsy.

June is a 73-year-old homemaker with chronic obstructive pulmonary disease. She has experienced episodes of paroxysmal atrial fibrillation and has arteriosclerotic heart disease; she is oxygen dependent and has been taking corticosteroids for years. On presentation in the emergency room, June complained of left hip pain and loss of leg control. She has a varus deformity. (Questions 5-6)

5. Radiographic views to rule out a left hip fracture include:
   a. Anteroposterior/lateral.
   b. Von Rosen/oblique.
   c. Posteroanterior/tunnel.
   d. Carter Rowe/mortise.

6. The nurse's role in preparing the patient for x-ray procedures is to:
   a. Encourage the patient to find a comfortable position.
   b. Inform the patient that analgesic medication is unnecessary.
   c. Encourage the patient to ask questions and provide reassurance.
   d. Inform the patient that fears of radiation overdose are unfounded.

7. A laboratory test that is important in the diagnosis of myocardial infarction is:
   a. Antistreptolysin O titer (ASO).
   b. Erythrocyte sedimentation rate.
   c. Indirect immunofluorescence assay (IFA).
   d. Creatinine phosphokinase (CPK).

8. An increase of specific gravity from a routine analysis can be helpful in diagnosing:
   a. Sickle cell anemia.
   b. Pyelonephritis.
   c. Heart failure.
   d. Diabetes insipidus.

9. Jackie is a 64-year-old female with a complicated history of left knee pain. On examination, she has palpable swelling, extension is restricted by 15 degrees, and flexion is good. She has difficulty walking and pain in the anteromedial aspect of the knee. Radiographic studies indicate a genu valgus. The MRI was insignificant and a bone scan was negative. A differential diagnosis of suspected disease process within the knee joint is confirmed by:
   a. Bone biopsy.
   b. Tomography.
   c. Arthroscopy.
   d. Arthrometry.

10. Teresa is a 35-year-old female with pain in the anterior groin and anterior thigh. A systems review is negative. She does not drink or smoke. On examination, internal and external rotation are good. Tests for hip disease are negative. She describes tenderness in the distribution of the lateral femoral cutaneous nerve. Several radiolucent spots in the neck of the femur superiorly with remodeling of the femoral neck suggest neoplastic bone disease as seen in metastasis. Confirmation of metastasis not visible on routine x-rays can be made with a(n):
    a. Arthrogram.
    b. Bone scan.
    c. Thermogram.
    d. CAT scan.

Chapter 5 Perioperative Patient Care

Victoria M. Hoshowsky, MSN, RN, CRNP, ONC

Contents

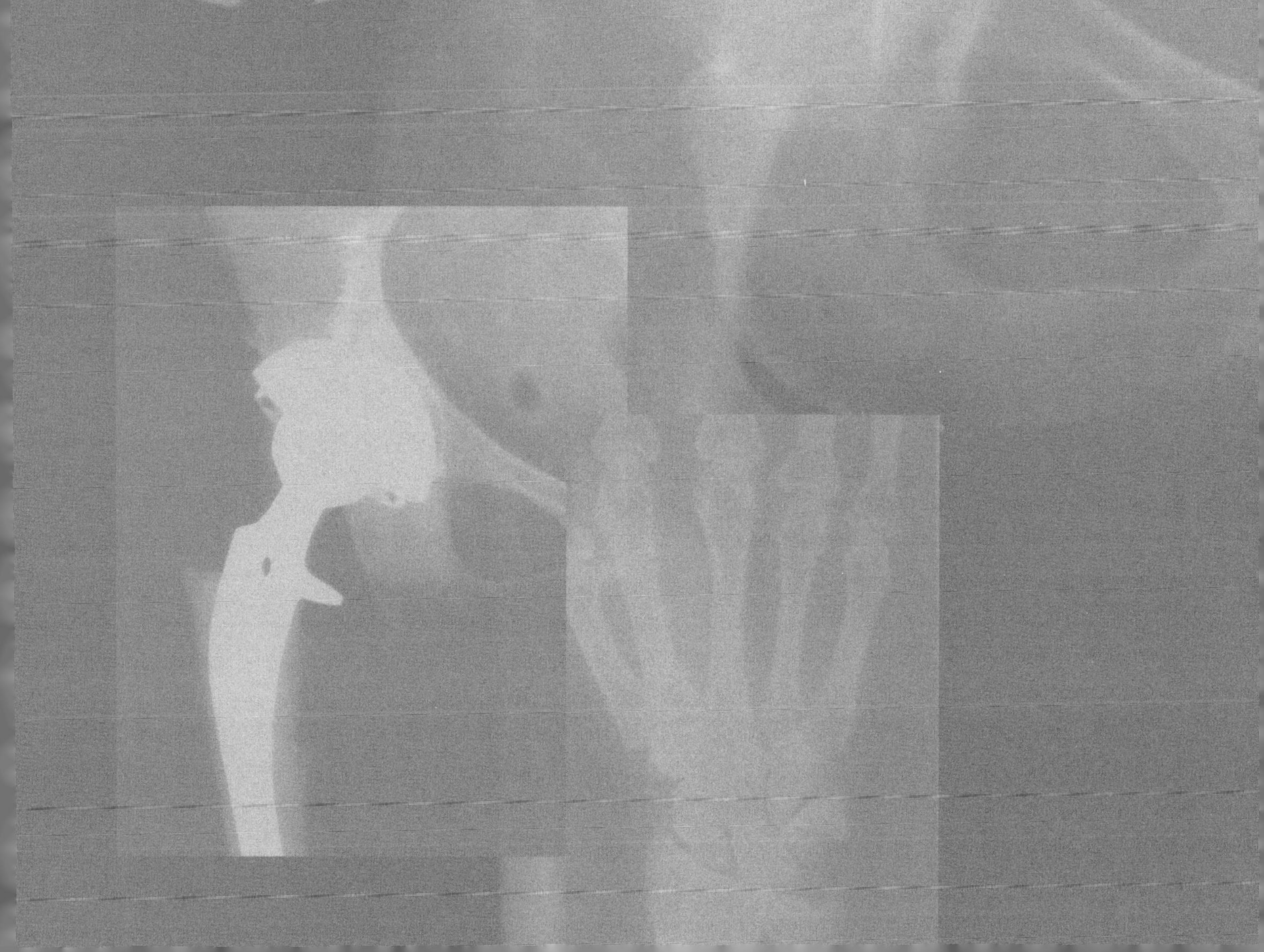

OBJECTIVES

At the completion of this chapter, the learner will be able to:

- Identify nursing care measures during the preoperative, intraoperative, and postoperative periods.
- Identify nursing implications for the different types of anesthesia used for the orthopaedic patient.

KEY POINTS

- Preoperative assessment is essential to identify patients at risk for developing intraoperative and postoperative complications and to intervene to prevent those potential complications.
- Nurses play a key role in assessment and intervention to protect the patient's safety during surgery.
- Postoperative nursing care is focused on interventions to help patients return to their optimal level of functioning.

CHAPTER 5

PERIOPERATIVE PATIENT CARE

PREOPERATIVE PATIENT CARE

I. OVERVIEW

A. The preoperative period begins with the patient's decision to have surgery and ends when he or she enters the operating room (OR). The preoperative period has two phases.

1. Phase 1 occurs from the decision to have surgery to admission to the same day surgery unit or hospital inpatient unit.
2. Phase 2 occurs from the patient's arrival in the holding area of the OR through admission to the OR.

B. The major goals of this period include:

1. Assessment of the patient's physical and psychological condition.
2. Education and preparation of the patient for surgery.

II. ASSESSMENT AND PREPARATION

A. History.

1. A complete history with emphasis on pre-existing medical conditions (coronary artery disease [CAD], hypertension [HTN], kidney or liver disease); previous surgical and anesthetic experiences and their complications.
2. An allergy history to food, medications, and latex are important as they may alter preparation of the patient's operating room.
3. A complete medication history (these may interact with anesthetic agents).
4. A family history (some anesthetic complications are inherited, such as malignant hyperthermia [MH] pseudocholinesterase deficiency).
5. A social history that includes an evaluation of the patient's home situation and availability of individuals to assist in caring for the patient upon discharge. This information should be used during discharge planning.

B. Physical examination.

1. Height and weight are essential for computing medication dosages and for proper positioning on the OR table.
2. Airway assessment is usually performed by anesthesia personnel and includes condition of the teeth, ability to open mouth, degree of neck flexion and extension, and history of sleep apnea. Patients with a temporomandibular joint (TMJ) disorder, facial deformity, immobility of the cervical spine, and patients with a short stocky neck or who are obese can pose a challenge to the anesthesiologist.
3. Complete a review of systems with the patient.

C. Assignment of anesthesia class.

1. Performed by the anesthesia provider when the history and physical are completed.
2. Anesthesia classes:
   a. Class I: normal, healthy patient. No organic physiologic, biochemical, or psychiatric disturbance.
   b. Class II: mild to moderate systemic disease usually well controlled (for example, HTN).
   c. Class III: severe systemic disease that limits activity but is not incapacitating (such as previous myocardial infarction [MI]).
   d. Class IV: severe systemic disease that is life threatening (cardiac failure).
   e. Class V: moribund patient not expected to survive 24 hours without surgery (ruptured aneurysm).
   f. Class E: emergency surgery.

D. Laboratory studies.

1. Confined to limited studies to promote cost-effectiveness.
2. Hemoglobin and hematocrit recommended for all patients.
3. Blood type and screen if blood loss is anticipated.
   a. Maximum Surgical Blood Order Schedule (MSBOS) determines the amount of blood necessary for surgery based on the type of procedure to be performed.
   b. Guideline is based on national averages of blood usage to curtail unnecessary blood sequestering and waste.
4. Additional diagnostic tests such as electrolytes, urinalysis, chest x-ray, and electrocardiogram are performed as determined by:
   a. The patient's age and physical condition.
   b. Surgical procedure to be performed.
   c. Physician and institutional policies and procedures.

E. Blood donation.

1. If blood loss and replacement is anticipated, blood may be obtained in any of the following three ways.
   a. Autologous donation: blood given by the patient several weeks before surgery.
      (1) Criteria for autologous donation.
         (a) Follow the American Association of Blood Banks criteria.
         (b) No history of cardiovascular or severe respiratory disease.
         (c) No history of seizures since infancy.
         (d) Must be between the ages of 12 and 75.
         (e) Adequate red blood cell count (hemoglobin 11 gms/deciliter or hematocrit of 34%).
         (f) Weight greater than 110 lbs. Donors less than 110 lbs may donate amounts determined by body weight.

(2) Procedure for predeposit autologous donation.
   (a) One unit of blood drawn every 4-7 days.
   (b) Maximum number of units drawn is usually 5 in either 31 or 39 days.
   (c) Last unit must be drawn no later than 72 hours before surgery.
   (d) Blood can be stored without freezing for 35-42 days.
   (e) Blood can be frozen as plasma or RBCs for up to 1 year.

b. Directed donor blood donation: family and friends with compatible blood type donate blood for a specific patient.

c. Bank blood.

F. Mental status: assess attitude, affect, mood, speech, thought processes, sensorium and reasoning, potential for danger.

G. Ability to communicate: assess the patient's verbal skills, language spoken, hearing ability, and comprehension.

H. Knowledge of procedure, pre and postoperative care.

1. Informed consent:
   a. Must be obtained for the surgical procedure and anesthesia.
   b. Explanations of the procedure and anesthesia type must be disclosed to patients in terms they can understand.
   c. The nature of the problem, treatment type, risks and benefits, consequences, alternatives to treatment, and expected outcome if procedure is not performed must be disclosed to the patient.
   d. Patients must have an opportunity to ask questions.
   e. No force or coercion can be used, consent is voluntary.
   f. If a patient changes his or her mind or if mental status changes, the nurse must notify the physician as soon as possible, rendering the consent invalid.
2. NPO status.
   a. Patients are NPO according to institutional policy and type of oral intake to avoid complications such as aspiration.
   b. Current practice guidelines from the American Society of Anesthesiologists state that the minimum fasting period differs for the types of food and liquids ingested.
      (1) Clear liquids require a fasting time of at least 2 hours.
      (2) Breast milk requires a fasting time of at least 4 hours.
      (3) Infant formula, nonhuman milk, light meal (toast and clear liquids) require a fasting time of at least 6 hours.
      (4) All other types of foods may require a fasting time longer than 6 hours.
   c. Patients should not eat, drink, smoke, chew gum, or suck on candy or cough drops as these stimulate the secretion of gastric acid in the stomach.
3. Preoperative education.
   a. Purpose: to decrease anxiety and increase patient compliance.
   b. Details of the pre, intra, and postoperative phases are disclosed.
   c. Escort: confirm availability of an escort home for the ambulatory surgery patient. If no escort is available, the surgery will be canceled.
   d. Discharge teaching: use of ambulation devices such as crutches should be taught and return demonstrated preoperatively.
4. Preoperative medications provide:
   a. Anxiety relief.
   b. Sedation.
   c. Amnesia.
   d. Analgesia.
   e. Drying of airway secretions.
   d. Reduction of gastric fluid volume.
   e. Increased pH of GI secretions.
   f. A reduction in anesthetic requirement.
   g. The facilitation of induction of anesthesia.
   h. Antiemetic effect.
   i. Prophylaxis against allergic reactions.
5. Phase 1: ends as the patient is escorted from the unit or preoperative area of the surgical center into the holding area of the operating room.
6. Phase 2: in this phase the following activities occur:
   a. Patient is interviewed and the chart is checked for completeness.
   b. IV access is established.
   c. Blood and blood byproduct availability is confirmed.
   d. The surgical consent is obtained or checked for accuracy and completeness.
   e. Anesthesia personnel visit the patient and discuss or confirm the anesthesia type to be used.
   f. Once all necessary activities are completed and in order, Phase 2 ends with escort of the patient into the operating room.

III. NURSING DIAGNOSES, OUTCOMES, AND INTERVENTIONS

A. Fear.
Anxiety.

1. Outcomes.
   a. Patient reports reduced anxiety and appears relaxed.
   b. Patient demonstrates knowledge of procedure by verbalizing understanding of surgical procedure and anesthesia prior to preoperative medication administration.
2. Nursing interventions.
   a. Reduce patient anxiety.
      (1) Assess anxiety by interviewing the patient and reviewing history.
      (2) Identify patient's perception of surgery by

allowing patient to verbalize fears related to the procedure and anesthesia.

(3) Provide adequate information regarding surgical intervention and anesthesia as requested by the patient.

b. Provide patient teaching.

(1) Provide explanations of preoperative, intraoperative, and postoperative preparation to patient and family.

(2) Instruct regarding coughing, deep breathing, turning, pain, drains and tubes, IV, and possible ventilator.

(3) Instruct regarding NPO, preoperative medications, IV line, shave, antiseptic scrub, length of surgery, family waiting area, etc.

c. Minimize anxiety related to powerlessness.

(1) Keep patient and family informed.

(2) Allow for flexible visiting hours if possible.

(3) Inform patient of scheduled times and changes that may occur.

B. Nutrition, imbalanced: less than body requirements. Nutrition, imbalanced: more than body requirements. Fluid volume, deficient.

1. Outcomes.

a. Patient maintains adequate nutritional balance.

b. Patient maintains adequate fluid and electrolytes.

2. Nursing interventions.

a. Maintain nutritional balance.

(1) Perform nutritional assessment.

(2) Nutritional supplement given prior to surgical intervention if nutritionally deficient.

(3) Monitor food and fluid intake. If patient is NPO for over 7-10 days, nutritional support is required, even if there is no previous deficit.

(4) Provide for additional nutritional support for catabolic/hypermetabolic conditions (trauma, multiple bone fractures, chemotherapy, or radiation therapy).

(5) Review lab results: BUN, electrolytes, CBC, protein.

b. Assess and maintain adequate intake and output of fluids.

(1) Assess for signs of dehydration or fluid overload.

(2) Provide fluids as needed.

(3) Monitor vital signs.

(4) Review lab results.

(5) Maintain and monitor intake and output.

C. Infection, risk for.

1. Outcome: patient remains free of infection.

2. Nursing interventions:

a. Use good hand washing technique and universal precautions when performing patient care activities.

b. Check for redness, tenderness, discoloration, and broken skin areas.

c. Monitor temperature.

d. Maintain aseptic technique when inserting invasive lines.

f. Administer preoperative medications as ordered.

D. Breathing patterns, ineffective.

1. Outcome: patient is free of respiratory complications.

2. Nursing interventions:

a. Evaluate results of pulmonary function studies in high-risk patients (scoliosis, chronic obstructive pulmonary disease [COPD]).

b. Assess respiratory status by auscultating breath sounds.

c. Instruct patient in deep breathing.

d. Instruct patient in respiratory treatments (intermittent positive pressure breathing [IPPB], incentive spirometer).

e. Monitor vital signs.

f. Discourage smoking.

g. Administer oxygen, as indicated.

INTRAOPERATIVE PATIENT CARE

I. OVERVIEW

The intraoperative period begins with the patient's transfer to the operating room bed and ends when the patient is admitted to the postanesthesia care unit (PACU).

II. ASSESSMENT

A. Assess patient and refer to documentation in patient record.

1. Ability to communicate.

a. Appropriate verbally.

b. Language spoken.

c. Hearing.

d. Sight.

2. Level of consciousness.

a. Alert.

b. Confused.

c. Drowsy.

d. Nonresponsive.

e. Premedicated.

3. Height and weight.
4. Vital signs.
5. Neurovascular status.
6. Skin integrity.
7. Circulatory status.
8. Respiratory status, including presence of endotracheal tube, tracheotomy, mechanical ventilation, etc.
9. Physical/musculoskeletal limitations.
10. Emotional status, anxiety, and fear.
11. Therapeutic devices, casts, external fixation.
12. History.

a. Allergies.

b. Previous surgical procedures.

c. Medications.

d. Prostheses (internal and external).

e. Substance abuse.

f. Infectious diseases, hepatitis, and HIV

13. Routine and specific diagnostic tests.

14. Danger potential (complications, risks).
15. Type of anesthesia used: local, regional, or general.

III. COMMON THERAPEUTIC MODALITIES

A. Maintain airway.

B. Provide anesthesia.

1. General.
2. Regional.
3. Local.

C. Assist with surgical positioning.

D. Prevent patient injury.

E. Create and maintain a sterile field.

F. Perform surgical counts.

G. Perform surgical procedure.

H. Prevent wound infection.

I. Manage fluids and electrolytes.

J. Assess vital signs and/or hemodynamic monitors.

K. Choose/apply type of implant, external fixation, traction, and/or cast, etc., as ordered by the surgeon.

IV. ANESTHESIA

A. Agents and techniques (see Tables 5.1 and 5.2).

B. Complications.

1. Pulmonary: aspiration occurs when the gag reflex is abolished and the patient is unconscious.
   a. May cause respiratory obstruction.
   b. Treatment involves airway suctioning and oxygenation.
2. Cardiovascular.
   a. Hypovolemia.
      (1) Related to decreased circulating volume due to hemorrhage and NPO status.
      (2) Treatment involves replacement with fluid and electrolyte solutions, and/or blood and plasma expanders, along with control of the source of the bleeding.
   b. Cardiac arrhythmias.
      (1) Ischemia or MI may result from a cardiac arrhythmia.
      (2) Treatment is directed at minimizing the oxygen demands of the tissue and optimizing myocardial oxygen consumption.
      (3) Administration of 100% oxygen, narcotics, and inhalation anesthetic agents is necessary.
3. Hypothermia.
   a. Defined: core body temperature less than 35°C (95°F).
   b. Patients at increased risk for hypothermia include:
      (1) Infants, children, elderly.
      (2) Patients undergoing general anesthesia.
      (3) Patients having surgery in which a major body cavity or the skull will be opened.
      (4) Patients undergoing surgery lasting greater than 1 hour.
   c. Adverse effects of hypothermia include:
      (1) Bradycardia, cardiac arrhythmias (atrial fibrillation), hypotension.
      (2) Peripheral vasoconstriction.
      (3) Increased oxygen consumption.
      (4) Increased bleeding due to platelets being sequestered in the spleen.
   d. Nursing actions to prevent hypothermia.
      (1) Increased ambient room air temperature to 70°F for adults and 75°F for children.
      (2) Limit body exposure.
      (3) Apply hot air warming blanket to patient's entire body preoperatively, then to exposed areas of the body intraoperatively.
      (4) If hot air warmer is not available, use plastic bags or reflective drapes to cover exposed areas of the body.
      (5) Warm inspired air, irrigation solutions, IV fluids, and blood and blood byproducts prior to entering the patient.
      (6) Monitor temperature intraoperatively.
4. Malignant hyperthermia (MH).
   a. Defined: an inherited hypermetabolic syndrome that is triggered by the neuromuscular blocking agent, succinylcholine chloride, and selected anesthetic inhalation agents (halothane, isoflurane, enflurane).
   b. Patient assessment: susceptible patients include:
      (1) Individuals with a family history of MH or any anesthetic complication.
      (2) A personal history of muscle disorders such as muscular dystrophy or central core disease.
      (3) Cola-colored urine following anesthesia.
      (4) Unexplained high fever or muscle rigidity during surgery.
   c. Signs of MH:
      (1) Apparent after anesthesia induction or during emergence.
      (2) Unexplained tachycardia, cardiac arrhythmias, and hypertension.
      (3) Rigidity of the masseter muscles, rapidly rising CO_2 level, tachypnea respiratory acidosis with hypoxemia.
      (4) Rapid rise in body temperature.
   d. Treatment.
      (1) Surgery is canceled, close patient as quickly as possible.
      (2) Discontinue inhalation agents and change to a clean anesthesia machine.
      (3) Hyperventilate patient with 100% oxygen.
      (4) Reconstitute and administer IV dantrolene.
      (5) Initiate cooling measures immediately.
      (6) Manage arrhythmias, correct fluid/electrolyte and acid/base imbalances.
      (7) Monitor patient for 12-24 hours for reemergence of MH, disseminated intravascular coagulation (DIC), or myoglobinuric renal failure.
5. Pseudocholinesterase deficiency.
   a. Defined: prolonged neuromuscular blockade following a normal dose of succinylcholine chloride.
   b. Treatment: maintenance of patient on ventilator until effects of succinylcholine chloride have disappeared.

Table 5.1
Anesthesia and Nursing Implications

Type of Anesthesia*	Nursing Implications
I. General Anesthesia • Reversible state of unconsciousness with amnesia, analgesia, reflex suppression, and muscle relaxation. • Components include induction, maintenance, and emergence. • Wide variety of agents and techniques used.	• Induction and emergence are critical times. • During induction the circulating nurse may need to apply cricoid pressure to displace the cricoid cartilage and close the esophagus when passing the endotracheal tube to decrease the risk of aspiration. Assess patient for bilateral breath sounds after passage of endotracheal tube. Warm blankets are applied before and during surgery to attenuate shivering and warm the patient. • Emergence assessments include airway patency, return of reflexes and muscle strength, and ability to follow commands. • Postoperative assessments include level of consciousness, airway patency, cardiovascular status, temperature, fluid balance, and return of neuromuscular function. Assess for nausea and vomiting. Determine need for postoperative analgesia based on patient comfort. Operative site assessments as appropriate.
II. Regional Anesthesia • Local anesthetics act on cell membrane, interrupting sensory pathways between surgical site and the brain. • All local anesthetics have the potential to produce side effects (influenced by maximal safe dose, vascularity, absorption, and other patient variables) and allergic reactions (rare). • Toxic reactions usually seen intraoperatively. • Duration of block depends on potency of drug, its duration of action, dose, technique, and patient variables. • Lidocaine hydrochloride (Xylocaine®) acts for 1-3 hours and is commonly used for infiltration, regional IV anesthesia, peripheral nerve block, epidurals, and spinals. • Bupivacaine (Marcaine®) acts for 3-10 hours and may be used for the same techniques as above. The addition of epinephrine to either of the local anesthetics may prolong the anesthetic action of the medications and cause vasoconstriction, which decreases bleeding at the infiltration site.	• Following administration, monitor for signs and symptoms of allergic reaction. • Signs and symptoms of toxicity primarily affect the central nervous system first and then the cardiovascular systems. Check for drowsiness, numbness of tongue, blurred vision, tinnitus, dizziness, restlessness, slurred speech, and muscular twitching, followed by convulsions. Hypotension, bradycardia, heart block, and arrest can occur as well. • Management includes stopping administration of local anesthetic, and resuscitation as appropriate with epinephrine, oxygen, intravenous fluids, aminophylline, and hydrocortisone. • Good for postoperative pain control.
A. Infiltration Techniques • Local Infiltration: subcutaneous injection at operative site. Provides sensory blockade of the skin and subcutaneous tissue of the operative area. • Intravascular infiltration, or Bier block, used for surgeries below elbow or knee. Double bladder tourniquet applied to operative extremity and inflated. Then local anesthetic injected into distal peripheral vein to provide anesthesia in operative extremity.	• Assess need for postoperative analgesia as sensation returns. Helpful to get oral or intramuscular analgesia on board *before* block wears off. • Tourniquet time crucial. Cannot be less than 30 minutes (inadequate for sufficient metabolism before release into systemic circulation) or greater than 90 minutes in upper extremity or 2 hours in lower extremity because of ischemia. Tourniquet must be deflated slowly and intermittently to avoid systemic bolus. Assessment of circulatory status critical postoperatively: monitor for return of normal sensation, color, and capillary refill.

B. Peripheral Nerve Blockade
• Local anesthetic injected around major nerve trunk supplying surgical site, producing both sensory and motor blockade.
  ◦ Brachial plexus block: used for procedures involving the upper extremity. Accomplished via axillary, interscalene, or supraclavicular approach. Interscalene, or supraclavicular approach useful for procedures of the shoulder; however, a more extensive block and pneumothorax are possible complications. Axillary technique often used for hand surgery.
  ◦ Femoral block: used for procedures involving the knee.
  ◦ Ankle block: used for procedures on the foot and toes.
	• Assess for sensory and motor blockade before incision.
	• Postoperatively, assess for return of sensory and motor function. Important to differentiate between paresthesias related to dissipation of anesthesia versus neurovascular compromise.
	• Proper positioning and support of extremity (sling or shoulder immobilizer) essential to protect from injury.
	• If able to ambulate, support lower extremity until recovery is complete. Use assistive devices for ambulation.

*Type of anesthesia depends on type and length of surgery, surgeon's and anesthesiologist's preference, and patient's condition and preference.

Table 5.1 (continued)
Anesthesia and Nursing Implications

Type of Anesthesia*	Nursing Implications

C. Central Nerve Blockade
• Local anesthetic injected into spinal canal with resultant sensory, motor, and autonomic blockade.
  • Spinal: injection made into subarachnoid space (dura is punctured).
  • Epidural: injection into epidural space. Indwelling catheter may be left in place for postoperative pain management.
	• Intraoperatively, assess patient's level of sensory and motor blockade using dermatomal landmarks. Common dermatomal landmarks include L_{1-2} (groin), T_{10} (umbilicus), and T_4 (nippleline). Assess for high spinal (anesthetic may travel as high as C_4) with breath sounds: equal bilaterally.
	• Postoperatively, monitor for return of sensory and motor function. Return of sensation can vary, with one leg regaining sensation before the other.
	• Return of sensation to both extremities and the rectal area (which represents the lower sacral segments) is a good indication that recovery is complete.
	• Assess motor functioning by having patient wiggle toes, dorsiflex ankles, and raise and flex legs as allowed by surgery.
	• Check for hypotension due to residual autonomic blockade. Management includes elevation of legs, intravenous fluids, oxygen, and pharmacologic intervention as necessary.
	• Check for urinary retention, as nerves supplying bladder are affected.
	• Check for complaints of spinal headache on second postoperative day (due to dural puncture with cerebrospinal fluid leak). Incidence decreased with 25-gauge needle for spinal injection and adequate hydration. Early ambulation does not affect incidence of headache. Symptoms include severe frontal or occipital pain that worsens in the upright position and possibly nausea, vomiting, double vision, tinnitus, and dizziness. Conservative treatment: bed rest, hydration, and analgesics. No response to conservative therapy, then an epidural blood patch can be done: 10 ml of the patient's own venous blood is injected using sterile technique into the spinal puncture site to seal the leak. Relief is usually instantaneous.
	• Other possible but rare complications include symptoms of meningeal irritation and cord compromise. Report complaints of fever, pain, tenderness, weakness, or paralysis to appropriate physician immediately for prompt investigation and treatment to avoid permanent neurologic impairment.

III. Intravenous Conscious Sedation to Accompany Local Anesthetics for Regional Techniques **A. Benzodiazepines** • Diazepam (Valium®) • Midazolam (Versed®)	• Intravenous conscious sedation is used to produce a depressed level of consciousness but allows the patient to maintain a patent airway and respond appropriately to verbal instruction or physical stimuli. The goals of conscious sedation are relaxation, sedation, amnesia, and analgesia, usually achieved with a balance of the two classes of medications. Intraoperative monitoring with pulse oximeter and frequent vital sign checks as per institution policy essential. Assess level of consciousness and emotional comfort. • Antianxiety agents: not for control of pain. • Often given with local anesthetics for relaxation and amnesia. Effects reversible with flumazenil (Romazicon®). Written discharge instructions essential in ambulatory setting.
B. Narcotics • Meperidine (Demerol®) • Morphine • Fentanyl (Sublimaze®)	• Analgesics control pain. • Assess for changes in level of consciousness, vital signs, and respiratory status. Effects reversible with naloxone (Narcan®). • Frequently cause nausea and vomiting and urinary retention as side effects.

*Type of anesthesia depends on type and length of surgery, surgeon's and anesthesiologist's preference, and patient's condition and preference.

Adapted from Mattocks-Whisman, F. (1996). Perioperative patient care. In S.W. Salmond, N.E. Mooney, & L.A. Verdisco (Eds.), *NAON: Core curriculum for orthopaedic nursing* (3rd ed., pp. 174-175). Pitman, NJ: NAON.

V. NURSING DIAGNOSES, OUTCOMES, AND INTERVENTIONS

A. Infection, risk for: intraoperative.

1. Outcome: patient will be free of infection.
2. Interventions:
   a. Universal precautions and operating room sanitation.
      (1) All patients are viewed as potentially contaminated. Personal protective attire (gowns, gloves, goggles, surgical attire) worn is the same for each patient and/or room cleaning.
      (2) The same precautions are maintained for each patient, no contaminated case technique exists.
      (3) Room sanitation is completed after each surgical case. Sanitation of OR tables, bed, and room surfaces is performed using a high level disinfectant moving from the cleanest to the most soiled area.
      (4) Terminal cleaning of the OR suite including walls, ceilings, floors, and all furniture is performed at the end of the daily OR schedule.
   b. Wound classification.
      (1) Purpose: to categorize surgical wounds to predict the patient's risk of acquiring an infection.
      (2) Class I: Clean – any surgery where the respiratory, gastrointestinal, or genitourinary tracts are not entered. Surgical wound is primarily closed, closed wound drainage system may be present, no evidence of infection. Risk of infection – 1%-5%.
      (3) Class II: Clean-Contaminated – any surgery where the respiratory, gastrointestinal, or genitourinary tracts are entered under controlled conditions. No breaks in aseptic technique, no evidence of infection. Risk of infection – 3%-11%.
      (4) Class III: Contaminated – any surgery involving an open, fresh, or traumatic wound, or where a major break in aseptic technique has occurred. Incisional infection is present. Risk of infection – 10%-17%.
      (5) Class IV: Dirty – any surgery where retained devitalized tissue is present or existing clinical infection is present. Risk of infection – >27%.
   c. Airflow and filtration.
      (1) Standard ORs have 25 air exchanges per hour, 5 of which should be fresh air.
         (a) Air is filtered via high efficiency particulate air (HEPA) filters.
         (b) Air enters at the ceiling and exits at the floor.
         (c) Slightly less air is exhausted from the room than is introduced into the room to create a positive pressure within the room.
         (d) This prevents potentially contaminated air from entering the room when the door is opened.
      (2) Laminar airflow: a specialized high-flow unidirectional air handling system that may circulate air under the hood up to 400 times per hour.
         (a) Provides a clean air environment by filtering the air at a rapid rate through HEPA filters to rid it of bacteria and particulate matter.
         (b) Air is delivered in a pattern that minimizes turbulence.
         (c) Care must be taken by the surgical team not to interfere with airflow and cause unwanted turbulence by positioning of the OR lights or personnel within the field.
         (d) Turbulence may increase the risk of infection. Laminar flow is used exclusively for total joint arthroplasty cases.
      (3) Body exhaust suits: consist of a helmet and an air filtering system that is worn by the surgical team scrubbed at the field.
         (a) Provides fresh air for the wearer to breathe.
         (b) System complements laminar flow, and provides a sterile barrier between the patient and the surgical team.
         (c) Protects the surgical team from the patient's blood and body fluids, and the patient's wound from respiratory secretions of the team members.
         (d) Type of system may be battery operated or connected to the laminar flow system. In either case, filter maintenance is imperative for effectiveness.
   d. Germicidal ultraviolet light.
      (1) Ultraviolet (UV) light has bacteriocidal qualities.
      (2) Mercury vapor tubes mounted in the OR suite supply UV light which kills 95% of the pathogenic microorganisms within 3 minutes, but it takes 20 minutes to destroy spores and fungi.
      (3) This type of disinfection is rarely used due to complications related to prolonged UV light exposure (skin erythema and burns, and conjunctivitis).
   e. Surgical attire: provides a barrier for infectious matter passing between personnel and patients.
      (1) Good hygiene is the cornerstone in controlling the type and amount of bacteria introduced into the OR. Individuals shed bacteria from skin surfaces, hair, and mucous membranes.
      (2) Wearing surgical attire, which includes a pantsuit and hair covering, decreases bacterial shedding.
      (3) Masks protect against respiratory secre-

Table 5-2
Anesthetic Agents and Adjuncts*

Agent+	Selected Comments
Induction Agents Thiopental sodium (Pentothal®) Methohexital sodium (Brevital®) Propofol (Diprivan®) Midazolam (Versed®) Etomidate	• Hypnotic agents, given intravenously to render the patient unconscious for induction. • Propofol (Diprivan®) and midazolam (Versed®) may also be used for maintenance of anesthesia. • Propofol is dissolved in lecithin, so it is used cautiously in patients with egg white allergy. • Midazolam can be reversed by Romazicon®. • Propofol and etomidate can cause burning sensation on injection. • Some studies show that patients emerge more quickly with propofol than with inhalation anesthesia.
Inhalation Agents Halothane (Fluothane®) Isoflurane (Forane®) Enflurane (Ethrane®) Desflurane (Suprane®) Sevoflurane Nitrous Oxide (N_2O)	• Potent respiratory depressant agents absorbed and eliminated primarily through the lungs. • May trigger malignant hyperthermia (MH) except N_2O. • Halothane decreases heart rate and blood pressure and can sensitize the heart to catecholamine-precipitating arrhythmias. Shivering is common on emergence. • Forane® provides effective muscle relaxation, causes less myocardial depression, but has a higher incidence of bronchospasm and laryngospasm during induction. • Ethrane® has marked central nervous system action. Should not be used in patients with a history of seizures. • Suprane® offers rapid induction and emergence, with less myocardial depression. • Sevoflurane is nonirritating to the respiratory tract and does not predispose the heart to arrhythmias or depress kidney or liver function. Cautious use in patients with increased intracranial pressure. • Nitrous oxide causes depression of the myocardium and decreased blood pressure. Usually given in combination with oxygen, narcotics, and muscle relaxants for balanced anesthesia. • All potent inhalation agents can cause transient elevation in liver enzymes.
Neuromuscular Blockers (Paralyzing Agents) ***Depolarizing Agent*** Succinylcholine chloride (Anectine®)	• All drugs in this category render the patient apneic. They should be used only by anesthesia providers who are experts in airway management.
Nondepolarizing Agents Mivacurium (Mivacron®) Atracurium (Tracrium®) Vecuronium (Norcuron®) Tubocurarine chloride (curare) Metocurine iodide (Metubine Iodide®) Pancuronium bromide (Pavulon®) Pipercuronium bromide (Arduan®) Doxacurium chloride (Nuromax®)	• All medication in this category interfere with the action of acetylcholine at the neuromuscular junction; they do not affect the central nervous system. Therefore, these drugs should be used only in conjunction with sedatives and narcotics to prevent patient awareness and distress. • Succinylcholine chloride has been identified as the primary triggering agent for MH. All others in this class can be used in patients with a history of MH. Effects of the nondepolarizing agents can be reversed with anticholinesterase inhibitors.
Reversal Agents ***Anticholinesterase Inhibitors*** Neostigmine methylsulfate (Prostigmin®) Pyridostimine Bromide (Mestinon®, Regonal®)	• Reverses effects of nondepolarizing neuromuscular blocking agents. Inhibits the action of acetylcholinesterase, allowing more acetylcholine to be available to compete with the neuromuscular blockers for the receptor sites. • May cause parasympathetic nervous system side effects (i.e., increased secretions, bronchospasm, bradycardia); should be given with atropine sulfate or glycopyrrolate (Robinul®).
Narcotic Inhibitors Naloxone (Narcan®)	• Effective in reversing depressant effects of narcotics only. • Patients must be observed carefully for renarcotization, as the action of the narcotic may last longer than the action of Narcan®. Careful titration when delivering medication IV push is important to avoid abolishing all analgesia and producing tachycardia, sweating, nausea, and vomiting.

**See references for additional information.*

+The anesthetic agents listed here are examples, and this list should not be considered exhaustive.

Table 5.2 (continued)
Anesthetic Agents and Adjuncts*

Agent+	Selected Comments
Benzodiazepine Inhibitor Flumazenil (Romazicon®)	• Reverses benzodiazepines only. Effect of flumazenil may be shorter than the sedation effect of midazolam; patient may appear awake and oriented for periods of 15-30 minutes, with the eventual return of a sedation state. • Use cautiously with narcotics. If rebound sedation occurs at same time narcotic is administered, respiratory depression and worsening of sedation are possible. If respiratory depression occurs, assisted ventilation is the first step in treatment. • Correlation exists between flumazenil and a mild increase in the incidence of postoperative nausea and vomiting. • Patients routinely taking benzodiazepines have an increased risk of seizure activity when they are reversed with flumazenil.
Anticholinergics Atropine sulfate	• Given to dry oral secretions, decrease gastric acidity, and possibly prevent peri-induction vagally mediated bradycardia. May cause tachycardia. Do not use in patients with narrow angle glaucoma.
Glycopyrrolate (Robinul®)	• Similar action to atropine; however, it is longer acting and causes less tachycardia. Affects the gastric contents by decreasing volume and increasing pH.
Narcotics Fentanyl citrate (Sublimaze®) Sufentanil citrate (Sufenta®) Alfentanil hydrochloride (Alfenta®) Morphine sulfate Meperidine hydrochloride (Demerol®) Hydromorphone (Dilaudid®)	• Used to provide analgesia intraoperatively and postoperatively. Varying potencies and durations of action (alfentanil is very short-acting, fentanyl is intermediate-acting, and morphine is long-acting.) • Effects are reversible with naloxone.
Narcotic Agonist-Antagonists Pentazocine (Talwin®) Butorphanol (Stadol®) Nalbuphine (Nubain®) Dezocine (Dalgan®)	• Opiate agonist antagonists. Actions range from potent analgesia to sedative effects. They exhibit varying degrees of respiratory and cardiac depressive effects. Patients displaying physical dependency on narcotics can precipitate withdrawal symptoms while taking these medications.
Antiemetics Prochlorperazine (Compazine®) Trimethobenzamide (Tigan®) Metoclopramide (Reglan®) Promethazine (Phenergan®) Ondansetron (Zofran®) Droperidol (Inapsine®)	• All of these medications decrease the side effects of nausea and vomiting. Zofran® is quite expensive. • Patients with allergy to Tigan® may have a similar reaction to local anesthetics. Avoid using atropine-like drugs with Tigan®. • Reglan® in combination with narcotics will decrease Reglan®'s effectiveness, whereas Reglan® combined with succinylcholine chloride will increase the effectiveness of the neuromuscular blocking agent. • Droperidol should be used with care, as it causes hypotension and tachycardia. When used with fentanyl, it may increase the patient's blood pressure and cause respiratory depression.
Miscellaneous Adjuncts Ketamine hydrochloride (Ketalar®, Ketaject®)	• Useful nonopioid intravenous anesthetic agent related chemically to PCP and LSD and has been associated with vivid dreams and hallucinations with accompanying wild behavior in early postoperative period. Strategies to prevent these side effects include maintaining a calm, quiet environment and reassuring and reorienting as needed. Incidence of hallucinations decreased with concomitant use of benzodiazepines. • Stimulates sympathetic nervous system, good for patient experiencing hypotension or bronchospasm. • Can be used alone as effective analgesic for short procedures because respiratory function and airway reflexes remain intact. Patients receiving ketamine in this fashion become dissociated from environment; they appear unconcerned with pain and amnesic for the event.
Ketorolac tromethamine (Toradol®)	• Nonsteroidal antiinflammatory drug. Injection during case can help with postoperative analgesia. • Also used on regular schedule for short-term postoperative pain control. • No side effect of respiratory depression.

LSD - lysergic acid diethylamide; PCP - phencyclidine hydrochloride.

**See references for additional information.*

+The anesthetic agents listed here are examples, and this list should not be considered exhaustive.

Reprinted with permission from Hoshowsky, V.M., & Reining, K.M. (1998). Perioperative considerations for the orthopaedic patient. In A.B. Maher, S.W. Salmond, & T.A. Pelligrino (Eds.), *Orthopaedic nursing* (2nd ed., pp. 273-275). Philadelphia: W.B. Saunders Co.

tions for different lengths of time, so the manufacturer must be contacted for specific product information.

(4) Protective eye wear, gloves, impervious aprons, and shoe coverings protect against splashing of hazardous fluids.

(5) Jewelry and acrylic nails harbor bacteria and should not be worn in the OR.

(6) Laundry of scrub suits should be performed by the institution, not by personnel in their homes.

(7) Institutional policies and procedures should be followed when wearing attire in the OR.

f. Traffic patterns:

(1) Purpose: control the movement of patients, personnel, and supplies throughout the OR suite.

(2) Consists of three distinct areas:

(a) Unrestricted: street clothes are worn here.

(b) Semi-restricted: consists of support areas of the surgical suite.

i. Supplies are stored here.

ii. Personnel wear surgical attire and hair coverings.

iii. Patients wear gowns and hair coverings.

(c) Restricted:

i. Surgery is performed.

ii. Sterilization of unwrapped items occurs.

iii. Surgical attire, hair coverings, and masks are required.

(3) Movement of soiled equipment is separate from the movement of clean and sterile supplies to prevent contamination.

(4) Doors to ORs remain closed so that proper airflow can occur.

g. Aseptic technique.

(1) Involves development of a "Surgical Conscience" by personnel which means that personnel act out the statement that all items of doubtful sterility are considered contaminated no matter the situation.

(2) Principles of aseptic technique according to the Association of Operating Room Nurses (AORN):

(a) Sterile personnel wear sterile gowns and gloves.

(b) Sterile drapes are used to establish a sterile field.

(c) Items used within a sterile field are sterile.

(d) All items introduced onto the sterile field are opened, dispensed, and transferred by methods that maintain sterility and integrity.

(e) Sterile fields should be constantly monitored and maintained.

(f) All persons moving within the sterile field should do so in a manner that maintains the integrity of the field.

h. Sterilization and packaging.

(1) Defined: the process of rendering instruments and equipment free of microorganisms including spores.

(2) Bioburden is the amount of microbial contamination present on the item after decontamination but before sterilization.

(3) Sterilization relies on decontamination, so for an item to be truly sterile, it must first be clean.

(4) Decontamination of items may be completed by using an approved decontamination agent with manual cleaning, ultrasonic washing, or both.

(5) Once the items are clean, they are assembled into sets placed into perforated container systems, wrapped, or peel packaged.

(6) Chemical and/or biological indicators are placed inside and outside the package so that sterility may be checked by the surgical team.

(7) Types of sterilization.

(a) Steam:

i. Used the majority of the time to sterilize metal instruments, linens, and paper.

ii. Flash steam sterilization is used only when an item is needed emergently.

(b) Ethylene oxide: used to sterilize fiberoptic or delicate instrumentation; not environmentally safe.

(c) Peracetic acid: used to sterilize fiberoptic instrumentation rapidly.

(d) Gas plasma: used to sterilize metal and plastic instrumentation, not useful for paper and linen; environmentally safe.

(e) Gamma irradiation: used by manufacturers only to sterilize all types of instruments, equipment, and supplies.

(8) Implant sterilization.

(a) According to manufacturer instructions.

(b) Biological indicators always included in trays.

(c) Implants may be sequestered until results of biological indicator known.

(d) Should never be flash sterilized.

i. Surgical skin preparation.

(1) Surgical hand scrub.

(a) Necessary for proper asepsis.

(b) Performed by all personnel scrubbed in at the field.

(c) Antimicrobial soap and mechanical friction remove gross dirt, oil, and transient bacteria. Residential microbial count on skin is decreased.

(2) Surgical skin prep.
  (a) Purpose: to decrease the patient's risk of acquiring a wound infection.
  (b) Preoperatively, patients may bathe or scrub themselves with an antimicrobial soap as directed by the surgeon.
  (c) Hair removal.
    i. Only removed if it interferes with surgery.
    ii. May be clipped, shaved, or removed with depilatory cream.
    iii. Preferred methods are clipping or depilatory as they interfere less with the patient's skin integrity and are associated with lower infection rates.
    iv. If shaving is to be used, it should be performed as close to the time of incision as possible. Increased lengths of time between shaving and incision are associated with increased infection rates.
    v. Use the wet shave method as opposed to dry shaving the patient to help to avoid skin nicks.
  (d) Skin cleansing.
    i. Use antimicrobial scrub and/or solution (iodophor chlorhexidine gluconate) depending upon the area to be cleaned and tissue type.
    ii. Begin at the cleanest part and move outward in a circular fashion.
    iii. Avoid pooling of solutions under patient and/or tourniquet cuff to prevent chemical burns of the skin.
    iv. If the area to be prepped is dirty or infected, begin at the cleanest part (periphery) and proceed inward to the most soiled part (center).

j. Implants and explants.
  (1) May be metallic, plastic, ceramic, chemical, or biological.
  (2) Avoid scratching any metallic, plastic, or ceramic implant as this may cause device failure secondary to a stress fracture.
  (3) Never alter an implant; always use the correct size and configuration.
  (4) Document:
    (a) Manufacturer name.
    (b) Type of implant.
    (c) Size of implant.
    (d) Amount of implant.
    (e) Catalog, model, lot and/or serial numbers of implant.
    (f) Sterilization load control number if the implant was sterilized inside the institution.
    (g) FDA tracking number if available.
    (h) Anatomic location of implanted item.
  (5) The above information will be used if the implant is ever recalled by the manufacturer or if the physician needs to remove the implant or place the same type in the contralateral side of the patient.
  (6) Document all items removed from the patient as explants, according to institution policies and procedures.
  (7) Chemical implant: polymethyl methacrylate (PMMA)/bone cement
    (a) Grouting material.
    (b) Used to secure implants to bone.
    (c) Comes as a monomer (liquid) and a polymer (powder).
    (d) May be hand mixed, vacuumed, or centrifuged to remove excess air.
    (e) A warm environment will decrease setting time of the cement. Setting time may be extended by cooling the monomer.
    (f) Monomer is very flammable and care should be taken not to spill the liquid or break the ampule.
    (g) When mixing cement, apply a fume evacuator to remove harmful fumes from the air.
    (h) Avoid contact with skin, mucous membranes, eyes, and contact lenses.
    (i) Pregnant personnel should not be present in the room during cementing
    (j) Notify anesthesia personnel prior to injecting cement into a canal, as this may cause hypotension.
    (k) The cementing process is an exothermic one. When cementing, surround patient tissues with cool sponges and avoid allowing cement to contact tissues.
  (8) Biologic implants (allograft tissue and bone).
    (a) Types:
      i. Fresh frozen.
      ii. Freeze-dried.
      iii. Decalcified.
      iv. Frozen cryopreserved.
    (b) Purchase from a company which adheres to the American Association of Tissue Banks (AATB) guidelines to minimize the risk of the patient acquiring a blood-borne disease.
    (c) Tissue should be handled, thawed, and reconstituted according the manufacturer directions. Usually bone is thawed or reconstituted in sterile Ringer's lactate or normal saline prior to cutting, contouring, or implanting bone.
    (d) Use of allograft tissue must be includ-

ed on the surgical consent form.
(e) Document:
i. Type of allograft tissue.
ii. Name of tissue bank from which it was purchased.
iii. Implanting surgeon name.
iv. Identification or access number of graft.
v. Location of implant.

B. Skin integrity, impaired.
Injury, risk for.

1. Outcome: patient will be free from injuries related to positioning and intraoperative care.
2. Intervention:
   a. Goals:
      (1) Optimal exposure of surgical site.
      (2) Access to airway, IV lines, monitoring devices.
      (3) Prevention of compromise of physiologic functions.
      (4) Protection of all body systems.
      (5) Protect patient dignity.
   b. Careful assessment and meticulous attention to detail will avoid postoperative complications for the patient.
   c. Anesthetic agents and surgical positioning affect body systems.
      (1) General anesthesia causes decreased peripheral venous blood flow causing vasodilitation and hypotension.
      (2) Depression of the central nervous system decreases the patient's ability to communicate and perform normal defense mechanisms.
      (3) Pain and pressure receptors surrounding joints are decreased leading to muscle relaxation.
      (4) Injuries occur from stretching, twisting, and compression of nerves, tendons, ligaments, and muscles.
   d. Complications of positioning.
      (1) Pressure ulcers.
         (a) Prevention is accomplished through identifying patients at risk and intervening appropriately.
         (b) Factors predictive of pressure sore formation:
            i. Age > 40 years.
            ii. Weight.
            iii. Anesthesia type.
            iv. Length of surgery.
            v. Time on the OR table > 2.5 hours.
            vi. Thermal blanket use.
            vii. Extracorporeal circulation use.
            viii. Presence of vascular disease.
         (c) OR table surface affects patient's risk of developing pressure sores. Viscoelastic overlays have been shown to be more effective than a standard mattress at preventing pressure sore formation.
      (2) Thrombus formation.
         (a) Inferior vena caval (IVC) pressure affects circulation when patients are in the prone position.
         (b) This causes decreased cardiac output and circulating blood volume, and hypotension.
         (c) Placement of a pillow under the patient's pelvis helps to relieve IVC pressure and prevents thrombus formation.
         (d) Use of antiembolic stockings and/or compression devices also prevent this complication regardless of surgical position used.
      (3) Impaired respiration.
         (a) Respiration is affected in the lateral and prone positions.
         (b) Surgical positions cause decreased lung expansion, chest wall, diaphragm movement, and vital capacity.
         (c) Anesthesia personnel ensure adequate oxygenation and prevent respiratory problems by:
            i. Monitoring oxygen saturation.
            ii. Supplying oxygen via nasal cannula or face mask.
            iii. Carbon dioxide monitoring.
            iv. Applying positive pressure as necessary.
      (4) Neuromuscular impairment.
         (a) Neurologic and musculoskeletal systems most vulnerable to injury.
         (b) Upper extremity: brachial plexus injury.
            i. Occurs when the arm is abducted > 90° or when pressure is applied to the axilla, clavicle, or elbow.
            ii. Patient experiences numbness, paresthesias, paralysis of arm, shoulder, or trunk.
            iii. Prevention: never abduct arm past 90°. Palms of hands face upward when arms are out on arm boards, and inward when arms are tucked at sides. When tucking arms, cover the entire elbow region with the drawsheet.
         (c) Lower extremity: sciatic, saphenous, peroneal, tibial, and sural nerve injuries.
            i. Sciatic nerve.
               - Uncommon, causes low back and leg pain, weakness, and numbness.
               - Occurs from severe abduction or flexion of the leg at the hip.

- Occurs when the nerve is stretched.
- Prevented by lifting the leg carefully and not exceeding the normal leg and hip range of motion.

ii. Saphenous nerve.
- Runs superficially at the medial thigh area.
- Injury is from direct compression of the nerve via the tourniquet or arthroscopic leg holder.
- Prevent this injury by applying ample padding under the tourniquet or leg holder.

iii. Peroneal nerve.
- Injury is due to compression of the nerve as it runs superficially at the lateral aspect of the fibular head.
- Causes foot drop.
- Prevent by applying adequate padding over the area of the fibular head.

iv. Tibial nerve.
- Occurs from compression as it splits at the popliteal fossa and travels down the back of the leg to the medial aspect of the ankle.
- Produces a sensory and/or motor loss to the calf and sole of the foot.
- Prevent by ensuring that the patient's legs are not crossed and that any pillow placed behind the knees is not too large.

v. Sural nerve.
- Found laterally at the ankle and foot.
- Injury causes sensation loss to the lateral aspect of the foot.
- Prevent by ensuring that the patient's feet are not crossed and by providing extra padding over this area.

(d) Pudendal and femoral nerve injuries:
i. Caused by traction on the legs and pressure on the perineum from positioning the patient on the fracture table.
ii. Prevent these injuries by providing extra padding to the perineal post and monitoring the amount of traction applied to the patient's legs.

e. Nursing interventions related to positioning.
(1) Assess patient's skin prior to and after surgery.
(2) Assess patient's neurovascular function prior to and after surgery.
(3) Document.
(a) Type of position.
(b) Positioning devices used.
(c) Location of positioning devices.
(d) Names of personnel who performed the positioning (anesthesia, surgeon, nurses).

f. Surgical positions.
(1) Supine.
(a) Used for anesthesia induction.
(b) Position for most extremity procedures; anterior cervical spine procedures; closed reduction and nailing of femur and tibial fractures; open reduction internal fixation (ORIF) of hip; and some total hip arthroplasty procedures.
(c) How to position:
i. Have patient move to the OR table.
ii. Provide a headrest to relax the neck muscles.
iii. Apply safety strap 2 inches above knees.
iv. Place arms out on arm boards or tucked at sides.
v. Assure legs are uncrossed and no part of the body is touching metal.
vi. Place small lumbar roll or pillow under knees to alleviate back pains.

(2) Modified supine.
(a) Beach chair or Semi-Fowlers position:
i. Used for shoulder procedures
ii. Position patient on OR table that has the back up and knee section of bed flexed.
iii. Secure the patient's head to a headrest being careful to protect the patient's neck and skin.
iv. Apply a side brace to the bed to keep the patient's torso in place while the operative shoulder is brought as far over to the edge of the bed as possible.
v. Operative arm is draped free on the field.
vi. Patient's legs are uncrossed.
(b) Lowered foot of the OR table:
i. Used for knee arthroscopy.
ii. Patient is supine with the knees at the lower table break.
iii. An arthroscopy leg holder is placed around the patient's upper thigh on the operative leg.
iv. The foot of the table is lowered.
v. The operative leg is draped free

on the field.
vi. The nonoperative leg is held in a padded Allen stirrup.
(c) Application of cervical traction/tongs:
i. Used for cervical spine procedures.
ii. The head section of the OR table is removed and replaced with a neurosurgical headrest.
iii. A cervical head halter or tongs are applied to the patient.
iv. Traction cording and weight are added.
(d) Application of finger traps:
i. Used for pins and plaster of the wrist and wrist arthroscopy.
ii. Apply finger traps to patient's fingers by compressing the netting, insert the digit, and then pull down to close.
iii. The set of finger traps may be hung from an IV pole and weight is applied to the upper arm via a felt sling for wrist distraction.
iv. Commercial distraction devices are best used for wrist arthroscopy.
(3) Lateral.
(a) Used for hip, femur, some elbow, and shoulder arthroscopy, and some anterior spine procedures.
(b) How to position:
i. Anesthetize patient supine.
ii. Turn patient's hips and shoulders simultaneously.
iii. Lower shoulder is brought forward slightly and pillows are placed between arms and legs.
iv. An axillary roll is placed under the down arm to relieve brachial plexus pressure.
v. Lower leg is flexed at the hip and knee and the upper leg is straight.
vi. Padding is placed at ankle and knee to protect bony prominences.
vii. Lateral position may be maintained with Vac Pac® or hip positioning frame (McGuire, etc.).
viii. Shoulder arthroscopy requires a shoulder holder device to position patient.
(4) Prone.
(a) Used for posterior thoracic and lumbar spine, some elbow, posterior cervical spine, and lower extremity procedures.
(b) How to position:
i. Anesthetize patient supine on stretcher.
ii. Logroll patient into prone position.
iii. Always have stretcher immediately available in case of emergency.
iv. Patient is maintained in prone position by either:
- Four poster frame (Relton-Hall, CHOP).
- Convex frame (Wilson, Kambin).
- Knee-chest frame (Andrews).
- Chest rolls.
v. All positioning devices require that the patient's genitals, abdomen, and breasts hang free, arms are brought through their normal range of motion and placed on arm boards palm side down and elbows flexed, the head is turned to one side without pressure on nose, eyes, or ears.

3. Electrical safety.
a. Electrosurgery is the cutting and coagulation of body tissues using high radio frequency current. This may be monopolar or bipolar type.
b. Monopolar.
(1) Requires an active electrode (pencil), generator, and dispersive pad.
(2) Current flows from the generator to the pencil, through the patient, and back into the generator through the dispersive pad.
(3) Dispersive pad site selection:
(a) A smooth fleshy area close to the operative site that is without hair or scars.
(b) Not over a bony prominence or a metallic implant.
(c) Never cut the dispersive pad.
(4) Ensure that no portion of the patient's body is touching metal.
(5) Ensure that EKG pads are not placed between the operative site and the dispersive pad.
(6) Ensure that no irrigation or prep solution contacts the pad.
(7) Ensure that the generator alarm is working and able to be heard during surgery.
(8) Scrub person should keep the pencil in the holster when not in use to avoid inadvertent activation.
(9) Once surgery is complete, slowly remove the dispersive pad and note any skin irritations.
(10) If skin problems are noted, they should be documented.
(a) Save the pencil, dispersive pad, and packaging material.
(b) Remove the generator from service and send to biomedical engineering to be checked.
c. Bipolar.
(1) Forceps are used to deliver the current to the tissues.

(a) Current flows from the generator to the forcep tip, through tissue, and back into the generator.
(b) No dispersive pad is necessary.
(2) Used for cauterization of delicate tissues.
d. Precautions.
(1) Pacemaker:
(a) Never position pencil and pad so that current flow is through the patient's heart.
(b) Ensure that there is a short distance between the pencil and pad and that this is as far from the pacer as possible.
(c) Monitor EKG throughout procedure, and have the defibrillator immediately available during the case.
(2) Automatic internal cardiac defibrillator (AICD): must be deactivated before using the electrosurgical unit (ESU).
(3) Monitor EKG throughout the case.
4. Radiographic safety.
a. X-rays may be used during any phase of the surgical experience.
b. Intraoperatively, it is important to protect both the patient and personnel from harmful radiation exposure.
c. The golden rule in minimizing radiation exposure includes time, distance, and shielding.
d. Personnel should wear x-ray badges according to institutional policy and procedures, usually on the outside of their lead garment, and maintain a distance of 6 feet from the radiation source.
e. Never turn your back on the source of radiation unless wearing a lead skirt or standing behind a full-length lead screen.
d. Patients should also be shielded with a lead garment whenever possible, but shielding should not interfere with the sterility of the operative site.
5. Surgical counts.
a. Critical to the delivery of safe intraoperative care.
b. Purpose: to prevent retention of a foreign body.
c. Based on the legal principle "res ipsa loquitor," or the evidence stands for itself.
d. All sponges, sharps, instruments, and accessory items must be accounted for before and after surgery.
e. Surgical counts occur between scrub and circulating nurses.
f. Counted items should not leave the OR.
g. Broken items must be accounted for in their entirety.
h. Count timing:
(1) Initial count occurs prior to the incision.
(2) Counts of items added to the field occur at the time of dispensing.
(3) Counts occur when personnel are relieved from their assignment in the room.
(4) Closing counts occur when the body cavity (peritoneum, pleura, fascia) is being closed and again when skin is being closed.
i. Document:
(1) Personnel performing the count.
(2) Results of the count.
(3) Actions taken if the count was incorrect.
(4) Rationale if a count was not performed.
j. Count discrepancy - if a count error occurs:
(1) Inform the surgeon.
(2) Recount.
(3) Search the operative field and wound for the missing item.
(4) Search the OR room (trash, linens, floor).
(5) If the item is not found after a complete search is completed.
(6) Then x-ray the patient.
6. Medications.
a. Antibiotics.
(1) Broad spectrum used.
(2) Usually, Ancef®, Bacitracin®, Polymixin B Sulfate®, Tobramycin®, or Vancomycin®.
(3) May be given IV or mixed into irrigation solution.
(4) Irrigation solutions commonly used include normal saline, lactated Ringer's, and Ringer's solutions.
(5) Irrigation may be delivered via bulb syringe or pulse lavage.
b. Vasoactive medications (antispasmodics): used topically to control vessel spasm in microsurgical cases.
c. Steroids: mixed with local anesthetics and injected intra-articularly when procedure is completed to decrease inflammation and joint effusion.
d. Local anesthetics: injected subcutaneously to anesthetize the skin and underlying tissues. Epinephrine may be added to the local anesthetic to control bleeding.
e. Hemostatic agents:
(1) Thrombin: catalyzes the conversion of fibrinogen to fibrin for clot formation.
(2) Avitene Hemostat®: a microfibrillar collagen agent used to aggregate platelets during conversion of prothrombin to thrombin.
(3) Gelfoam®: an absorbable gelatin sponge, which absorbs up to 45 times its weight in blood and fluid.
(4) Surgicel®: an oxidized cellulose product, which absorbs up to 10 times its weight in blood and fluids.
(5) Bone wax: processed beeswax; applied directly to the ends of cut bone to seal the interstices.
7. Tourniquets.
a. A compressive device applied circumferentially to the extremity.
b. Used during extremity surgery.
c. Prevents venous oozing without complete arterial occlusion.

d. Provides a bloodless operative field and prevents excess blood loss.
e. Contraindicated in patients with vascular insufficiency and neurologic impairment.
f. Prior to use:
   (1) Calibrate tourniquet gauge if needed.
   (2) Select cuff size to allow for a 3 inch overlap.
   (3) Apply high on the operative limb over a layer of cotton cast padding.
g. Settings:
   (1) Surgeon chosen.
   (2) Upper extremity: 135-255 mm Hg or 50-75 mm Hg above the patient's systolic blood pressure.
   (3) Lower extremity: 250-450 mm Hg or 100-150 mm Hg above the patient's systolic blood pressure.
h. Prior to inflation, the limb is exsanguinated using an Esmarch bandage, elastic wrap, or by gravity. The tourniquet is always inflated with the limb elevated.
i. Monitoring
   (1) The surgeon should be notified of the tourniquet time at 1 hour and every 15 minutes thereafter.
   (2) After 90-120 minutes have passed, the tourniquet is deflated for 10 minutes to allow for tissue perfusion.
   (3) Documentation: tourniquet site, pressure, tourniquet time, I.D. number of the tourniquet box, and skin integrity under the tourniquet cuff.

C. Fluid volume, deficient: electrolyte imbalance. Fluid volume, excess: electrolyte imbalance.

1. Intraoperative management.
   a. Estimated blood loss (EBL) is calculated by the circulating nurse.
   b. EBL = sponges (weighed) + suction (amount of fluid in suction canisters) – irrigation used.
   c. Prior to blood administration, hemodynamic stability may be maintained by administering volume expanders (Hespan®, albumin) and IV fluids.
   d. If blood must be administered, the following order applies:
      (1) Autologous blood first.
      (2) Donor-directed blood second.
      (3) Bank blood last.
   e. Intraoperative blood salvage - cell saver:
      (1) Blood is suctioned from the wound and collected in a canister combined with a heparin solution.
      (2) When the canister is full, the blood is spun down and may now be reinfused to the patient.
      (3) Contraindications include:
         (a) Presence of infection.
         (b) Presence of malignancy.
         (c) Presence of bowel contents.
2. Postoperative blood management: blood may be collected from the wound via a specialized closed wound drainage system (Solcotrans®). Once the unit is full, the blood may be reinfused to the patient.

INPATIENT POSTOPERATIVE CARE

I. OVERVIEW

A. Definition: the postoperative period begins with admission to the Post Anesthesia Care Unit (PACU) and ends with termination of treatment.

B. Postoperative phases.

1. Phase 1: encompasses the acute phase of recovery in the PACU.
2. Phase 2: this is the surveillance phase; occurs when the patient is admitted to the inpatient unit or when the patient is transferred to the ambulatory surgery discharge lounge.

II. ASSESSMENT AND INTERVENTION

A. Phase 1.

1. The patient is brought to the PACU by the anesthesia provider.
2. Patients are transported with oxygen and monitoring devices as needed.
3. Anesthesia gives report on the patient to include:
   a. Patient history and surgical procedure performed.
   b. Type of anesthesia and medications given.
   c. Intraoperative course and events.
   d. EBL and fluids given (intake) and urinary output.
4. Patient assessment in the PACU includes:
   a. Patency of airway.
   b. Vital sign stability.
   c. Fluid status.
   d. Level of consciousness.
   e. Neuromuscular status (sensory and motor function).
   f. Patency of lines.
   g. Operative site evaluation.
   h. Positioning.
   i. Skin color.
   j. Comfort level.
5. Complications.
   a. Airway.
      (1) Most common.
      (2) Pulse oximeter used to measure oxygen level of blood.
      (3) Oxygen applied during recovery.
      (4) Assess for hypoxia and hypoventilation.
      (5) Types of airway complications.
         (a) Upper airway obstruction.
            i. Tongue is cause.
            ii. Signs and symptoms include snoring or no sound at all, use of accessory muscles, hypoxia (confusion, agitation, cardiac arrhythmias are markers).
            iii. Use oral or nasopharyngeal artificial airway to prevent and treat

this complication.

(b) Respiratory depression/arrest.

i. Anesthesia and medications (narcotics) are cause.

ii. If narcotic induced, may be reversed with Narcan®. Assess for renarcotization 20-30 minutes after Narcan® use.

iii. Treatment:

- Encourage deep breathing.
- Incentive spirometry.
- Chest physiotherapy.
- Pain control.
- Manual ventilation if arrested.

(c) Airway spasm.

i. Bronchospasm:

- Contraction of the lower airways exemplified by wheezing.
- Treatment focuses on administration of bronchodilators and oxygen.

ii. Laryngospasm:

- Sudden vocal cord closure occurs.
- May be due to pain or secretions.
- Patient exhibits stridor or no sound at all, but they look panic stricken.
- Treat with positive pressure, oxygen, succinylcholine chloride to break the spasm, and suctioning as needed.
- Corticosteroids and bronchodilators may also be used.

(d) Aspiration:

i. Acidic vomitus is inhaled.

ii. May be caused by pulmonary edema and adult respiratory distress syndrome.

b. Hypothermia.

(1) Postoperative shivering is present in patients with hypothermia and due to anesthetic agents.

(2) Important to decrease shivering as it increases myocardial oxygen demand fourfold, inhibits release of oxygen from tissues, and makes the patient uncomfortable.

(3) Treat shivering with Demerol®.

(4) Monitor patient temperature.

(5) Apply hot air warmer as needed.

c. Fluid and electrolyte imbalance: direct treatment at cause of imbalance as indicated by the patient's diagnosis and laboratory values.

d. Urinary retention.

(1) Multiple causes:

(a) Medications such as narcotics.

(b) Large volumes of fluids.

(c) Pain.

(d) Anxiety.

(2) Patients at risk are:

(a) Orthopaedic patients who had surgery involving pelvic structures and total joint arthroplasty.

(b) Men, due to an enlarged prostate and inability to stand to void.

(c) Elderly individuals, due to decreased bladder capacity and sensory/motor function.

(3) Treatment is aimed at rapid assessment of the problem and insertion of a catheter.

e. Nausea and vomiting.

(1) Most common problem.

(2) Anesthesia agents and narcotics are cause.

(3) Treat intraoperatively and postoperatively with Doperidol® or Zofran®.

(a) If on the postoperative unit, may use Compazine®, Tigan®, Reglan®, or Phenergan®.

(b) Use nursing measures such as deep breathing, application of cool wash cloth to head, and minimizing rapid position changes.

(4) If patient is vomiting, position patient on side or allow to sit up to avoid aspiration.

f. Pain.

(1) Multiple methods of pain control are available (see Chapter 7, Pain).

(2) Alleviation or control of postoperative pain will decrease other complications.

g. Alteration in hemodynamic stability.

(1) Alteration of vital signs due to many causes such as:

(a) Anesthesia.

(b) Blood loss.

(c) Fluid overload.

(d) Hypothermia.

(2) Treatment is directed at the cause.

h. Neurovascular compromise.

(1) Assessment of neurovascular status is critical in the orthopaedic patient.

(a) Color.

(b) Capillary refill.

(c) Movement.

(d) Sensation.

(e) Pulses.

(f) Temperature.

(2) Treatment is aimed at correction of the problem (cast or splint removal, resolution of edema, or emergency fasciotomy).

6. PACU discharge criteria.

a. Recovered from anesthesia and hemodynamically stable.

b. Use of scoring system such as Aldrete to objectively rate the patient's condition and readiness for discharge is common.

(1) Scores are assigned to assessment findings.

(2) Includes categories of activity, respiration, circulation (BP), level of consciousness, and color.

(3) A score of 10 plus stable vital signs indicates readiness for discharge.
(4) Anesthesia personnel must see patient and sign them out of the PACU.
(5) Upon discharge to the unit or Phase 2, a full report is given.

B. Phase 2 - assessment upon admission to the inpatient unit includes:

1. Airway, respiration, adequate breath sounds.
2. Vital signs.
3. Level of consciousness.
4. Presence of nausea, vomiting, adequate bowel sounds.
5. Presence of urinary bladder distention, functioning of foley catheter if applicable.
6. Neurovascular status of extremities.
7. Status of incision, dressings, and drains.
8. Status of tubes, IVS, invasive and noninvasive monitoring devices, and appliances.
9. Skin turgor and integrity.
10. Comfort level.
11. Positioning, body alignment in the bed.
12. Intake and output.

III. COMMON THERAPEUTIC MODALITIES

A. Dependent on type of anesthesia used.

1. General.
2. Regional.
3. Local.

B. Fluid and electrolyte balance maintenance.

C. Nutritional support.

D. Antibiotics to prevent wound infection.

E. Pain control measures.

F. Measures for bowel and bladder control.

G. Laboratory tests.

H. Radiographic studies.

I. Care of cast, traction, external fixation, brace, and dressing.

J. Prevention of dislocation and/or disruption.

K. Discuss lifestyle alteration.

L. Discharge planning, including support services.

IV. NURSING DIAGNOSES, OUTCOMES, AND INTERVENTIONS

A. Peripheral neurovascular dysfunction, risk for.

1. Outcome: neurovascular status intact.
2. Nursing interventions:
   a. Implement a thorough assessment of neurovascular status with documentation.
   b. Observe pain as an indicator of complication.
   c. Elevate affected part above heart level.
   d. Reposition frequently.
   e. Use of ice as indicated and/or ordered.
   f. If necessary, alter cast or appliance.

B. Pain, acute.

1. Outcome: patient is comfortable.
2. Nursing interventions: (see Chapter 7, Pain).
   a. Assess pain for pathophysiologic cause.
   b. Reposition affected part and/or the whole body.
   c. Administer analgesics per provider order.
   d. Evaluate effectiveness of medications.
   e. Check appliances for fit and adjust in consultation with physician, orthotist, occupational/physical therapist.
   f. Organize nursing interventions to allow for uninterrupted periods of rest if possible.
   g. Observe for nonverbal cues: how patient holds body, sits; facial expressions; or cool fingers and/or toes.

C. Urinary elimination, altered pattern.

1. Outcome: patient reestablishes normal urinary elimination pattern.
2. Nursing interventions:
   a. Check voiding and monitor output.
   b. Assess for retention or incontinence.
   c. Report and document frequency, burning, pain, retention, color, and odor of urine.
   d. Perineal care to decrease the chance of infection and/or skin breakdown.
   e. Review lab values for renal function changes and infection.
   f. Adhere to regular bladder emptying schedule.
   g. Position urinary indwelling catheter for tube drainage to prevent reflux.
   h. Remove catheter as soon as possible.

D. Bowel elimination, altered pattern.

1. Outcome: patient reestablishes normal bowel elimination pattern.
2. Nursing interventions:
   a. Check baseline data regarding patient's normal bowel habits prior to admission.
   b. Assess bowel sounds.
   c. Palpate for distention.
   d. Encourage adequate fluid intake.
   e. Encourage adequate dietary intake of bulk, fiber, and roughage.
   f. Monitor bowel movements.
   g. Encourage individual exercise program.
   h. Give stool softeners, as indicated.

D. Infection, risk for.

1. Outcome: patient remains free of infection.
2. Nursing interventions:
   a. Maintain good handwashing technique prior to working with patient.
   b. Maintain dressing integrity including:
      (1) Use sterile dressing technique, when indicated.
      (2) Change or reinforce dressing, as ordered.
      (3) Assess if dressing is constricting circulation.
   c. Check for drainage, odor, increased pain, redness, and swelling.
   d. Maintain patency and integrity of drainage systems when present.
   e. Provide adequate nutrition to promote wound healing and supply needed calories if infection is present.
   f. Provide isolation, as indicated; monitor medication regimen.

g. Maintain sterile technique during all procedures.
h. Teach patient about signs and symptoms of infection.

F. Gas exchange, impaired.

1. Outcome: patient will maintain normal gas exchange.
2. Nursing interventions:
   a. Assess respiratory status (including breath sounds).
   b. Instruct patient to deep breathe and cough frequently to promote adequate gas exchange.
   c. Assist patient with respiratory treatments (IPPB, blow bottles, incentive spirometer).
   d. Discourage smoking.
   e. Encourage activity.
   f. Monitor vital signs.
   g. Administer oxygen as indicated.
   h. Observe for signs of pulmonary emboli.
   i. Observe for signs of fat emboli.

G. Physical mobility, impaired.

1. Outcome: patient resumes preoperative activity level.
2. Nursing interventions:
   a. Check for correct alignment of affected part and monitor the neurovascular status.
   b. Promote optimum positioning and comfort during transfer by use of adequate personnel.
   c. Support affected body parts/joints using pillows, foot supports, etc.
   d. Teach patient proper body mechanics, activity and movement restrictions, use of appliances, ambulatory devices, etc.
   e. Assess characteristics of pain.
   f. Assess degree of decreased motor agility.
   g. Instruct or reinforce adequate exercise program.
   h. Refer to physical/occupational therapy.
   i. Refer to home health agency, as indicated.

V. HOME CARE CONSIDERATIONS FOLLOWING ORTHOPAEDIC SURGERY

A. Home assessment: exterior.

1. Steps and sidewalks in good repair.
2. Handrails on stairs.
3. Nonskid treads on outside steps.

B. Home assessment: interior.

1. Lighting.
2. Rooms, hallways uncluttered for mobility.
3. Electrical/telephone cords removed from traffic path.
4. Area rugs removed or anchored.
5. Stairway railings.
6. Doors wide enough: adequate turnaround space.
7. Store commonly used supplies (kitchen, bathroom, bedroom) in cabinets or drawers to avoid excessive bending or reaching.
8. Toilet adequate height/elevated seat available.
9. Grab bars by toilet or bathtub if indicated.
10. Safety strips or rubber mat in bath/shower.
11. Tub seat/bench of appropriate height and secured.
12. Hand-held shower available.
13. Area of rest such as easily accessible chair or sofa. If surgical site is a limb, availability of pillows to support and position extremity may be necessary.

C. Adaptive devices.

1. Dressing stick from occupational therapy department.
2. Sock aid.
3. Reacher.
4. Long-handled shoe horn.

D. Contact social services to arrange for devices needed postoperatively, as assessed preoperatively.

OUTPATIENT POSTOPERATIVE CARE

I. NURSING ACTIVITIES

A. Assist patient to a recliner or bed.
B. Assess operative site.
C. Take vital signs.
D. Offer pain medication.
E. Offer light diet (juice, tea, crackers).
F. Assist patient with ambulation.
G. Encourage patient to urinate.
H. Discontinue IV when tolerating oral fluids without difficulty and vital signs are stable.
I. Review written discharge instructions with patient and escort and give them a copy for home use.

II. DISCHARGE CRITERIA

A. Home readiness is the goal.
B. Ability to ambulate.
C. Minimal nausea, vomiting, and dizziness.
D. Tolerating liquids and snack.
E. Voiding without difficulty.
F. Pain is controlled on oral medication.
G. No IV sedation or analgesia within 1 hour prior to discharge.
H. Written discharge instructions and prescriptions given and understood.
I. Escort present.

III. HOSPITALIZATION

Patients may be hospitalized overnight due to uncontrolled pain, uncontrolled nausea and vomiting, inability to void, inability to ambulate, sleepiness, cardiac or respiratory complications, and an unavailable escort.

IV. DISCHARGE INSTRUCTIONS

A. Activity allowance.

1. Importance of rest emphasized.
2. Ambulation as determined by the surgeon.
3. No driving, operating machinery, or making important decisions for 24 hours.

B. Diet.

1. Resume preoperative diet as tolerated.
2. No alcoholic beverages for at least 24 hours.

C. Medications.

1. Analgesics as directed.

2. Anti-inflammatory medications as ordered by the physician with food.
3. Preoperative medications resumed. Consult medical provider as needed.
4. No aspirin unless otherwise directed by the surgeon.

D. Bathing restrictions.

1. General rule: do not get dressing wet.
2. Usually surgeon specified.

E. Wound care.

1. Ability to remove dressings and care for wound determined by the surgeon.
2. Instruct patient about neurovascular status checks, cast or device care, elevation of extremity, signs and symptoms of infection.

F. Complications/follow-up appointment with surgeon.

1. Call surgeon to report such complications as fever, difficulty voiding, persistent pain, nausea, vomiting, or headache, excessive bleeding.
2. Be sure to schedule follow-up appointment with surgeon within 2 weeks.
3. Expect a follow-up telephone call from the ambulatory surgery center. This call is to assess for any complications, reinforce discharge instructions, and evaluate care previously given by the center.

Bibliography

Aldrete, J.A., & Kroulik, D. (1970). A postanesthesia recovery score. *Anesthesia and Analgesia, 49*(6), 924-933.

Alexander, J.W., Fischer, J.E., Boyahian, M., et al. (1983). The influence of hair removal methods on wound infections. *Archives of Surgery, 118*(3), 347-352.

American Society of Anesthesiologists. (1999). *Practice guidelines for preoperative fasting and the use of pharmacologic agents to reduce the risk of pulmonary aspiration: Application to healthy patients undergoing elective procedures.* Illinois: Author.

American Society of Post Anesthesia Nurses. (1995). *Standards of perianesthesia nursing practice.* Thorofare, NJ: Author.

Association of Operating Room Nurses. (2000). *Standards of perioperative nursing practice. AORN standards and recommended practices for perioperative nursing.* Denver: Author.

Atkinson, L. (1996). *Berry & Kohn's operating room techniques* (8th ed.). St. Louis: Mosby.

Barash, P.G., Cullen, B.F., & Stoelting, R.K. (1993). *Handbook of clinical anesthesia* (2nd ed.). Philadelphia: Lippincott.

Berry, A.J., & Knos, G.B. (Eds.). (1995). *Anesthesiology.* Baltimore, MD: Willliams & Wilkins.

Burden, N. (Ed.). (1993). *Ambulatory surgical nursing.* Philadelphia: Saunders.

Cruse, P.J.E., & Foord, R. (1973). A five year prospective study of 23,649 surgical wounds. *Archives of Surgery, 107*, 206-210.

Defazio-Quinn, D.M. (Ed.). (1999). *Ambulatory surgical nursing core curriculum.* American Society of PeriAnesthesia Nurses.

Gregory, B. (1994). *Perioperative nursing series: Orthopaedic surgery.* St. Louis: Mosby.

Hoshowsky, V.M. (Ed.). (1995). *Orientation to the orthopaedic operating room.* Pitman, NJ: National Association of Orthopaedic Nurses.

Hoshowsky, V.M., & Reining, K.M. (1998). Perioperative considerations for the orthopaedic patient. In A.B. Maher, S.W. Salmond, & T.A. Pellino (Eds.). *Orthopaedic nursing* (2nd ed., pp. 261-295). Philadelphia: Saunders.

Hoshowsky, V.M., & Schramm, C.A. (1994). Intraoperative pressure sore prevention: An analysis of bedding materials. *Research in Nursing & Health, 17*, 333-339.

Litwack, K. (1995). *Post anesthesia care nursing* (2nd ed.). St. Louis: Mosby.

Litwack, K. (Ed.). (1999). *Core curriculum for perianesthesia* (4th ed.). Philadelphia: Saunders.

Longnecker, D.E., Tinker, J.H., & Morgan, E.G. (Eds.). (1998). *Principles and practice of anesthesiology* (2nd ed.). St. Louis: Mosby.

Mattocks-Whisman, F. (1996). Perioperative patient care. In S.W. Salmond, & N.E. Mooney, L.A. Verdisco (Eds.). *NAON: Core curriculum for orthopaedic nursing* (3rd ed.), (pp. 174-175). Philadelphia: W.B. Saunders Co.

Meeker, M., & Rothrock, J. (Eds.). (1999). *Alexander's care of the patient in surgery* (11th ed.). St. Louis: Mosby.

Miller, R.D. (Ed.). (2000). *Anesthesia* (5th ed., Vols. 1-2). Philadelphia: Churchill Livingstone.

National Association of Orthopaedic Nurses. (1992). *Guidelines for orthopaedic nursing.* Pitman, NJ: Author.

Phippen, M.L., & Wells, M.P. (Eds.). (2000). *Patient care during operative and invasive procedures.* Philadelphia: Saunders.

Roth, R.A. (Ed.). (1995). *Perioperative nursing core curriculum.* Philadelphia: Saunders.

Tetzlaff, J.E. (1995). *Clinical orthopedic anesthesia.* Boston: Butterworth-Heinenmann.

STUDY QUESTIONS

William Jones is a 20-year-old college football player scheduled to undergo a surgical arthroscopy of the right knee for a torn medial meniscus and anterior cruciate ligament reconstruction. (Questions 1-3)

1. During the preoperative interview, Mr. Jones appears tense and apprehensive about the surgery. Which of the following actions should the nurse take **first**?
   a. Teach Mr. Jones about the surgical procedure and postoperative recovery.
   b. Question Mr. Jones about his feelings regarding the surgery.
   c. Teach Mr. Jones about the preoperative activities and surgical procedure.
   d. Question Mr. Jones about his past medical history.

2. In the holding area, Mr. Jones tells the anesthesia provider that his father had a serious complication during surgery, but he doesn't know what it was. Which of the following complications is Mr. Jones most likely at risk for?
   a. Pseudocholinesterase deficiency.
   b. Aspiration
   c. Hypothermia.
   d. Malignant hyperthermia

3. Intraoperatively, Mr. Jones has a tourniquet applied to his operative extremity. Which of the following nursing actions would protect him from injury?
   a. Apply the tourniquet 2 inches above the knee.
   b. Apply the tourniquet high on the operative limb over foam padding.
   c. Apply the tourniquet high on the operative limb over cast padding.
   d. Apply the tourniquet 2 inches below the knee.

James Carson is a 70-year-old man who had a right total hip replacement 1 year ago. Today, he is scheduled to undergo a left total hip replacement under general anesthesia. (Questions 4-6)

4. Intraoperatively, Mr. Carson is placed in the lateral position. How should his nonoperative leg be positioned to prevent injury?
   a. Flexed at the hip and knee.
   b. Straight on top of pillows.
   c. Flexed at the knee only.
   d. Straight without pillows.

5. The circulating nurse is ready to apply the electrosurgical dispersive pad. Based on the surgical procedure and Mr. Carson's history, where should the dispersive pad not be placed?
   a. Left arm.
   b. Right arm.
   c. Right thigh.
   d. Back.

6. Postoperatively, Mr. Carson is taken to the PACU where the nurse notes that he is shivering. Mr. Carson's temperature is taken and is 93˚F. What should the nurse do next?
   a. Hang warm IV fluids.
   b. Apply a hot air warming blanket.
   c. Provide humidified oxygen.
   d. Monitor temperature every 30 minutes.

Sally Miller is a 45-year-old, 100 lb, female with an anteriorly herniated nucleus pulposus of L4-5. She is to undergo an anterior-posterior discectomy and fusion 1 month from now. Mrs. Miller has requested to donate her own blood prior to the procedure and to have her family donate blood as well. (Questions 7-9)

7. In regard to Mrs. Miller's autologous donation, which of the following rules apply?
   a. She is able to donate blood in amounts determined by body weight.
   b. She is unable to donate blood due to her low body weight.
   c. She may donate blood up to 48 hours prior to the procedure.
   d. She is unable to donate blood due to the type of surgical procedure.

8. Intraoperatively, Mrs. Miller's blood loss is 2 liters. Her blood is being collected via the cell saver for reinfusion at a later time. During the anterior portion of the procedure, the bowel is nicked. What infection control implication does this have for Mrs. Miller?
   a. Her wound is now a class 4.
   b. Her wound is now a class 1.
   c. Her wound is now a class 3.
   d. Her wound is now a class 2.

9. Mrs. Miller needs to receive blood. In what order should the blood be given?
   a. Cell saver, autologous, donor directed, bank.
   b. Autologous, donor directed, bank.
   c. Autologous, cell saver, donor directed, bank.
   d. Cell saver, donor directed, autologous.

10. To prevent peroneal nerve injury, where should padding be placed?
   a. Around the fibular head.
   b. Under the axilla.
   c. Around the lateral malleolus.
   d. Under the knees.

11. In the PACU, the nurse notes that a high-pitched crowing sound is coming from her patient. What is the probable reason for this noise?
   a. The patient is experiencing bronchospasm.
   b. The patient is experiencing aspiration.
   c. The patient is experiencing laryngospasm.
   d. The patient is experiencing obstruction.

12. In Phase 2 in the ambulatory surgery setting, patients are encouraged to?
   a. Sleep.
   b. Exercise.
   c. Defecate.
   d. Ambulate.

Chapter 6 Effects of Immobility

Marianne Genge Jagmin, PhD, RN, ONC

Contents

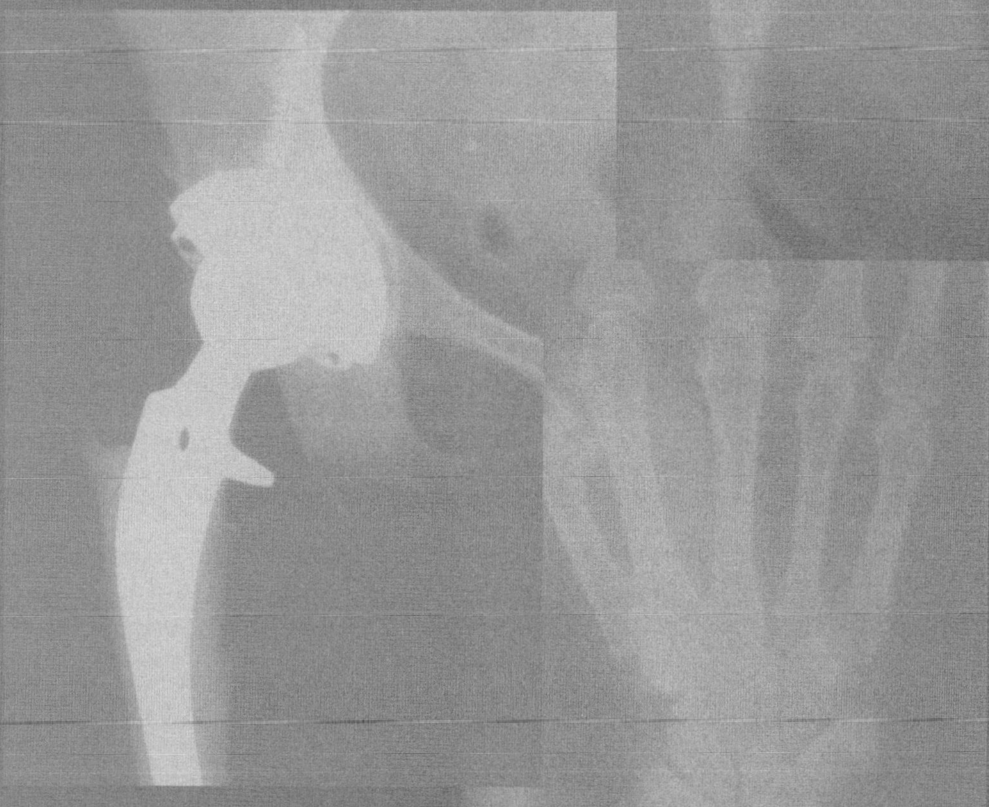

OBJECTIVES

At the completion of this chapter, the learner will be able to:

- Define immobility.
- Classify etiologies of immobility that orthopaedic patients might experience.
- Explain potential pathologic sequelae to immobility.
- Identify appropriate interventions for pathologic sequelae related to immobility.
- Develop nursing diagnoses related to pathologic sequelae of immobility.
- Identify appropriate nursing interventions for selected diagnoses for immobilized orthopaedic patients.
- Identify outcome criteria for immobilized patients.

KEY POINTS

- Immobility crosses all orthopaedic conditions, age groups, and health care settings.
- Care is directed toward identifying patients at risk and preventing the effects of immobility.
- Constant pressure of 70 mm Hg for longer than 2 hours leads to irreversible skin damage.
- Redness to a site for over 30 minutes after pressure has been removed indicates that a pressure area is developing and needs immediate treatment.
- Exercises may reduce some of the affects of deconditioning which occurs with bed rest.
- Decreased longitudinal stress on long bones of the upper and lower leg decreases bone density.
- Bone loss, which accompanies aging, is augmented by immobility and places the elderly patient at greater risk for stress fractures.

CHAPTER 6

EFFECTS OF IMMOBILITY

I. OVERVIEW

A. **Definition: immobility is defined as a state that either prevents or limits movement necessary to complete tasks within the environment. Immobility restriction may be generalized to the entire body or limited to an isolated area or areas. The extent and duration of immobilization together contribute to the degree that physiologic body systems are affected.**

B. **Etiology.**
   1. Environmental restriction: physical activity is limited due to external forces. Bodily movement is restricted due to either confinement to a specific area (bed rest) or application of restrictive devices (casts, traction, external devices).
   2. Physical or cognitive restriction: physical activity is limited due to internal forces. Movement is restricted by factors within the person (pain, impaired or lost motor function, critical illness, cognitive, social, or emotional instability).

C. **Pathophysiology.**
   1. Integumentary.
      a. Immobility fosters muscle disuse and decreased circulation to soft tissues.
      b. Prolonged pressure on a body area leads to disrupted nerve impulses and decreased circulation.
      c. Immobility and prolonged pressure on a body area may result in pressure ulcers.
         (1) Bony pressure points: occiput, spine of scapulae, spinous processes, lower sacrum, coccyx, ischial tuberosities, iliac crests, greater trochanter, patella, tibial tuberosity, fibular head, malleoli, heels, head of humerus, and elbows.
         (2) Tissues closest to bone are usually first to experience necrosis.
         (3) Prolonged pressures greater than normal, capillary pressures of 30 – 32 mm Hg arterial and 12 mm Hg venous, may lead to circulatory compromise and tissue necrosis.
         (4) Redness at a site for over 30 minutes, after pressure has been removed, indicates that a pressure area is developing.
         (5) Contributing factors.
            (a) Sensory and neurologic deficits.
            (b) Impaired blood circulation and edema.
               i. Interrupted vasomotor pathways related to shock, spinal shock, and flaccid paraplegia.
               ii. Peripheral arterial occlusion related to atherosclerosis and diabetes.
               iii. Venous engorgement related to edema; affects oxygenation and nutritional support of deprived tissues.
            (c) Low hemoglobin promotes tissue ischemia.
            (d) Nutritional status.
               i. Vitamins B and C are essential for tissue nutrition.
               ii. Circulation is affected by hypoalbuminemia, imbalance of nitrogen, sulfur, phosphorus, and calcium.
            (e) Infection and body temperature.
               i. Infection and fever increase metabolic rate and cellular metabolic deficiency.
               ii. Hypothermia in lower extremities may promote pressure ulcers in spinal cord injury patients.
               iii. Infected pressure ulcers can lead to systemic infections.
            (f) Moisture and/or body fluids trapped in linens predispose skin to maceration and breakdown.
            (g) Excretory waste and/or direct radiation can damage skin.
            (h) Shearing forces and friction can cause skin abrasion.
            (i) Sensitive areas at high risk for skin breakdown are scar tissue, skin grafts, areas of hematomas, and existing dermatologic problems (dermatitis psoriasis, seborrhea).
            (j) Common medications.
               i. Anticoagulants contribute to the hemorrhage of soft tissues and the hemmorrhage into soft tissue from other tissues.
               ii. Central nervous system depressants decrease movement during sleep.
               iii. Medications that may cause easy bruising and skin eruptions.
               iv. Diuretics can increase loss of fluid in cutaneous/subcutaneous tissues.
            (k) Age and trauma.
               i. Children exhibit the same problems as adults.
               ii. Skin loses elasticity as part of the aging process and results in the degeneration of elastic fibers as well as a reduced thickness and vascularity of dermis.

iii. Elderly and post-trauma patients present the highest risks for pressure ulcers.

2. Respiratory.
   a. Decreased metabolic processes due to immobility.
      (1) After 3 weeks of bed rest, the muscles work less efficiently and require about 26% less oxygen.
      (2) Cells that require less oxygen produce less carbon dioxide, causing respirations to become slower and more shallow in accordance with less demand for oxygen.
   b. Decreased respiratory movement.
      (1) Supine position causes the diaphragm to move cephalad, resulting in decreased thoracic size.
      (2) Quiet breathing while supine is due to abdominal muscle involvement rather than rib cage as when upright.
      (3) Decreased compliance of thoracic cage related to aging process.
      (4) Diminished strength in respiratory muscles with age possibly related to decrease in elastic recoil, increase in residual volume, and changes in skeletal muscle.
      (5) Counter-resistance of chair or bed against chest expansion.
      (6) Abdominal distention due to accumulation of feces, flatus, fluid.
      (7) Abdominal or chest binders, hip dressings, or casts.
      (8) Decreased muscle strength.
      (9) Narcotics, sedatives, or medications affecting the central nervous system can also affect rate and depth of respirations.
   c. Change in lung volumes.
      (1) Position change from upright to supine causes the lung to shift position 90 degrees.
      (2) All lung volume capacities, except tidal volume (TV), decrease with the largest change in the residual volume (RV).
      (3) Thoracic size decreases causing a decrease in functional residual capacity (FRC).
      (4) Closing volume (CV) (a volume at which the net forces of gravity, lung tissue elasticity, and properties of the airway are able to close small airways) may exceed FRC while the patient is recumbent and cause partial or complete closure of lung units involved in tidal breathing (atelectasis).
      (5) Total lung capacity is basically unchanged with advancing age.
      (6) Loss of elastic recoil of lung in the elderly causes CV to increase and thus increase the risk of atelectasis in the elderly.
   d. Decreased mobilization of secretions.
      (1) Decreased cleansing mechanism (coughing, changing of position and posture) fosters pooling of secretions.
      (2) Atelectasis interrupts mucociliary clearance of the airway resulting in pooling of secretions and increased bacterial growth distal to the obstruction.
      (3) Deep inspiration and rapid exhalation are required for coughing, but rapid exhalation is limited by abdominal musculature in the supine position.
      (4) Increased viscosity of secretions is due to dehydration from poor fluid intake and anticholinergic drugs.
      (5) Anesthetics, narcotics, and sedatives that decrease rate and depth of lung expansion and ventilation depress cough center and gag reflex.
      (6) Supine position permits gravity to pull mucus to dependent areas of the lung and interferes with efficiency of cilia, which sweep mucus from small bronchioles or trachea and larynx.
   e. Oxygen/carbon dioxide imbalance.
      (1) Increased carbon dioxide in blood is due to failure to expel it; tissue becomes hypoxic, as sufficient oxygen cannot be inspired.
      (2) Increased carbon dioxide concentration, initially, stimulates respirations via the respiratory centers in the pons and medulla, but this stimulus gradually weakens and carbon dioxide narcosis occurs.
      (3) Decreased oxygen concentration initially stimulates respirations via the aortic and carotid bodies, but this stimulus also becomes depressed.
      (4) Increased arterial and venous concentrations of carbon dioxide as carbonic acid ions create respiratory acidosis that can lead to respiratory or cardiac failure and death.
   f. Existing medical problems.
      (1) Children exhibit problems in respiratory system related to immobility similar to those in adults.
      (2) Age-related changes in lung tissue can be accelerated by frequent pulmonary infections, smoking, and exposure to environmental pollutants.

3. Cardiovascular.
   a. Orthostatic intolerance (postural hypotension).
      (1) Most common sign of cardiac deconditioning related to bed rest. Postural hypotension is a direct response to decreased blood volume (BV) and pooling of blood in lower extremities leading to a stroke volume (SV) insufficient to maintain cerebral perfusion.

(2) Horizontal position causes short-term increase in circulating BV.
(3) Circulating BV increase causes extracellular fluid to shift to the venous system, thus increasing venous volume.
(4) Increased venous volume increases blood pressure (BP), cardiac output (CO), SV, and heart rate (HR) and stimulates right arterial (RA) volume receptors, thus inhibiting antidiuretic (ADH) and aldosterone secretion resulting in diuresis of water and electrolytes.
(5) A compensatory decrease in plasma volume (PV) (8%-10% PV loss in first few days; 15%-20% PV loss over 2-4 weeks), HR, and BP also occur.
(6) During bed rest, a decrease in PV reduces cardiac filling, SV, and cardiac output.
(7) As a patient assumes an upright position, HR increases as a result of decreased SV and CO.
(8) An inadequate increase in sympathetic discharge fails to compensate for a greater postural reduction in SV.
(9) Maintaining an upright position may lead to syncope, tachycardia, nausea, and diaphoresis.
(10) Health status as well as other existing major trauma and/or disease processes contribute to how well a patient's cardiovascular system will tolerate major position changes.
(11) Elderly patients are more at risk for postural hypotension.
(12) Patients who take medications predisposing them to hypotension are also at a higher risk for postural hypotension.
(13) Patients with coronary artery disease (CAD) may experience angina when getting out of bed due to reduced diastolic filling, causing inadequate coronary blood supply.

b. Hemodynamic changes.
(1) Alteration in blood flow in supine position: 11% of total BV (about 500 cc) redistributes from lower extremities to central circulation due to change in vascular resistance and hydrostatic pressure changes.
(2) Blood redistributes primarily to lungs and increases pulmonary blood flow by 20%-30%.
(3) Less blood goes to the head and upper extremities.
(4) Increased central circulation leads to increased SV, which increases CO from a mean of 5-6 L/min standing to a mean of 7-8 L/min supine.
(5) Increased SV and CO lead to increased HR, peripheral vascular resistance (PVR), and a stable BP.
(6) Hemodynamic changes are maintained with prolonged bed rest, except the HR which increases by about 0.5 beats/minute/day.

d. Thrombophlebitis.
(1) Incidence increases with duration of bed rest.
(2) Bed rest results in compression of veins and thus venous stasis.
(3) Immobilization by cast or bed rest causes loss of normal muscle contractions.
(4) Decreased contractions of lower extremity muscles contribute to venous pooling.
(5) Venous pooling and dehydration, which often accompany immobility, cause blood to become more viscous and contribute to thrombus formation.
(6) Platelets tend to agglutinate after trauma.
(7) External pressure on veins restricts circulation and may also damage vein walls, thus placing patient at greater risk for the formation of a deep vein thrombus.

e. Valsalva maneuver.
(1) Valsalva maneuver is applied when patient uses upper extremities and trunk to move in bed.
(a) Thorax becomes fixed when breath is held.
(b) Breath is forced against closed glottis.
(c) Intrathoracic pressure rises and interferes with the entry of venous blood into the large veins.
(d) When breath is released, a surge of blood is delivered to the heart, causing tachycardia and changes in systolic blood pressure.
(e) Cardiac arrest may result if heart is not at an optimum level of function.
(2) Bedrest patients perform Valsalva 10-20 times per hour.
(3) People with a history of atherosclerotic cardiovascular disease on bed rest should be positioned with head of bed flat to reduce cardiovascular risks associated with Valsalva maneuver.

g. Exercise tolerance.
(1) A research study by Ferretti et al. (1998) found that after 42 days of bed rest, five male patients exhibited the following:
(a) Oxygen consumption and resting HR remained unchanged after bed rest.
(b) HR during exercise was higher after bed rest than before.
(c) SV was reduced both at rest and during exercise.
(d) CO was lower after bed rest both at rest and during exercise.
(e) Arterial oxygen concentration was lower after bed rest due to a reduction in hemoglobin.

(f) Oxygen delivery was lower after bed rest both at rest and during exercise.
(g) A down-regulation of the oxygen transport system follows bed rest.

(2) Cardiovascular changes previously mentioned induced by prolonged bed rest contribute to a decrease in maximal oxygen consumption (VO_2 max) and reserve capacity to do physical work.

(3) Exercise in an upright position or use of a sequential compression device that reduces venous pooling and simulates standing may prevent or reduce a decline in VO_2 max.

(4) Absence of orthostatic stress during bed rest is important for decrease in exercise tolerance.

(5) Immobility, or the total interruption of activity, is associated with reduced arterial distensibility. Daily activities are essential for maintaining arterial mechanical properties.

(6) The degree of deconditioning syndrome which can occur with bed rest can be manipulated by the duration and intensity of certain isotonic and isokinetic exercises.

4. Musculoskeletal.

a. Muscles generally experience disuse atrophy from decreased muscle load and activity. Skeletal muscle fiber size, diameter, and number of capillaries are all decreased.

(1) Muscle load and activity regulate the balance of protein synthesis and breakdown which maintain muscle mass and strength.

(2) Immobility decreases muscle load, activity, and protein synthesis and also increases protein breakdown, resulting in muscle disuse atrophy.

(3) Disuse atrophy.
(a) Muscle mass and strength loss as a result of inactivity.
(b) An adaptive mechanism in which cells survive in unfavorable conditions.

(4) Decreased muscle mass is related to lack of stress on muscle. Tension of one-third of the maximal capacity is required to maintain a muscle's mass.

(5) Immobilized muscle loses about 5% of its original strength per day and varies with degree of immobility.

(6) Muscle contraction 20%-30% of maximal strength is required to maintain muscle's strength.

(7) Muscle immobilized by a cast decreases linearly, with the greatest change in muscle occurring during week 1 of immobilization. The overall rate of muscle loss is determined by the number of contractions during time of immobilization.

(8) Immobilization for 1-2 months can cause a decrease of muscle size by one-half.

(9) Immobilization longer than 4 months can cause degeneration of nerve fibers to the degree that full recovery of muscle function is unlikely.

(10) Muscle immobilized in a shortened position exhibits specific changes.
(a) The muscle becomes contracted, fibrous tissue eventually replaces such muscle, and normal function is lost.
(b) The muscle experiences a decrease in weight exponentially from the 2nd to the 10th day.
(c) The muscle atrophies more quickly than muscles held stretched.

(11) Oxidative capacity of muscle mitochondria decreases, and muscles relax more in anaerobic pathways.

(12) Factors contributing to the degree of muscle atrophy include the following:
(a) Pre-immobilization muscle mass presents possible prognosis for post-immobilization state of muscle. Poor muscle mass will probably worsen and good muscle mass will recover better.
(b) Age and gender.
(c) Duration of immobilization.
(d) Length of stretch at which muscle was immobilized.
(e) Muscle fiber types and type of muscle.
(f) Fever and trauma cause increased metabolic needs which result in a rapid decline in muscle strength and endurance by accelerating protein catabolism.

b. Bones generally experience disuse osteoporosis with loss of bone matrix and minerals.

(1) Loss of bone matrix.
(a) Longitudinal stress on long bones of legs is decreased.
i. Osteoblasts form osseous matrix of bone and require stress of mobility and weight bearing for adequate functioning.
ii. Osteoclasts break down bone faster than osteoblasts can rebuild bone.
iii. Bone density is decreased.
iv. Complications: fractures, renal calculi, calcium depletion, and increased secretion of phosphorous and nitrogen.
v. 30% loss of bone must occur to be visualized on x-ray.
(b) Disuse osteoporosis is believed to be self-limited and balance between bone formation and resorption is

regained when bone mass has been reduced to a critical level.
(c) Contributing factors.
i. Poor pre-immobility degree of bone density.
ii. Cessation of menses.
iii. Pre-existing metabolic imbalances.
iv. Certain medications and medical conditions.
(d) Most visible in cancellous bone of metaphysis and epiphysis with first signs in epiphyseal and subchondral area.
(e) Common distal to fracture sites.
(f) Common in paralyzed people.
(g) Immobility fosters bones' sensitivity to parathyroid hormones.
(h) Bone formation is enhanced and within a short period, the situation is reversed during early immobilization.
(i) Contraction and relaxation of muscles promote blood flow into and out of bone like a pump.
(j) Muscle contraction produces electrical currents in bone. Bone end experiencing tension is compared to an anode; bone end being compressed is compared to a cathode.
(k) In children, bone becomes osteopenic (seen as "washed out" bone on x-ray) from disuse and lack of stress across the osseous tissue.
i. Process accelerated with neuromuscular diseases and osteogenesis imperfecta.
ii. Gradual return to activity important.
iii. May modify treatment to avoid the vicious cycle of increased fragility followed by recurrent immobilizing device.
(l) Bone loss that accompanies aging is augmented by immobility and places the elderly at a greater risk for stress fractures.
(m) Vicious cycle of increased fragility followed by recurrent fracture upon removal of immobilizing device may occur with elderly.
(2) Hypercalcemia.
(a) Hypercalcemia occurs when kidneys fail to excrete enough calcium.
(b) Immobility causes a negative calcium balance due to the mobilization of calcium from bone.
(c) Calcium loss probably due to lack of longitudinal pressure on weight-bearing bones rather than inactivity.
(d) Calcium loss averages about 200 mg/day while on bed rest.
(e) Calcium excretion is increased due to imbalance between osteoblastic and osteoclastic activity with osteoclasts breaking down bone faster than osteoblasts can build bone.
(f) Calcium excretion increases during first 4-7 weeks of bed rest, then plateaus or decreases, but stays higher than in ambulatory patients.
(g) Most frequently occurs in adolescent males who are physically active and in an active bone growth phase just prior to immobilization.
(h) Adults with Paget's disease and primary hyperthyroidism are at risk.
(i) Predisposing factor is rapid bone turnover prior to injury.
(j) Symptoms are headache, nausea, lethargy, weakness, emotional changes, and decreased glomerular filtration rate. Depression of neurons and smooth muscle, anorexia, nausea, vomiting which can lead to dehydration. With dehydration, kidneys cannot excrete enough calcium.
(k) 5 weeks after full activity, calcium levels return to normal.
(l) Crystalluria or ureteral stones seldom found.
(3) Elderly who have low bone mass prior to becoming immobile experience an increased risk of fractures due to bone calcium depletion. Even short-term immobility can be detrimental.

c. Joints generally experience alterations in synovial fluid with intra-articular degeneration, shortening of ligaments and tendons, and connective tissues changes resulting in some degree of joint contracture or decreased joint mobility.
(1) Altered flow of synovial fluid.
(a) Superficial layer of cartilage nourished by synovial fluid that clings to cartilage.
(b) Joint motion promotes an interchange of fluid between surface layers of articular cartilage and synovial fluid.
(c) Immobility prevents fluid diffusion into and out of cartilage in addition to compression and distention of cartilage.
(d) Cartilage extracellular fluid and thus nutrition stagnates and degenerative changes become permanent.
(2) Contracture of joint capsule and periarticular muscle.
(a) Joint capsule thickens and the synovia becomes hyperemic; fibrofatty proliferation of connective tissue in joint space.

(b) Inside the joint cavity connective tissue becomes abundant and causes adhesions limiting joint motion.
(c) Increased density of the connective tissue around the joint is due to failure to keep the latticework of tissue stretched open.
(d) Normal flexion and extension of muscle helps keep latticework open.
(e) Muscles bridging immobilized joint shorten.
(f) Problem is cyclic: with more contracture, there is more guarding of joint, less movement, and more contracture.
(g) A contracture occurs when there is lack of full passive range of motion of joint due to either joint, muscle, or soft tissue abnormality.

(3) Increased mobility or instability of a joint is related to lax ligaments.
(a) Laxity is caused by stretching of the muscle or decreased muscle tone.
(b) Joints are held in alignment by ligaments pulled tight via muscle tension.
(c) A joint not maintained in proper alignment may become unstable and painful.

(4) With age tissues become stiffer, thus decreasing joint mobility and increasing the risk of contracture in the elderly. Hips and knees are most prone to contractures.

5. Neurosensory.
a. Peripheral nerves do not degenerate with disuse but can be damaged by pressure or disruption of blood supply.
b. Improper positioning of casts or restraints can put undue pressure on nerves and blood vessels.
c. Frequent sites of nerve compression: peroneal nerve, radial nerve.

6. Metabolic.
a. Nitrogen balance.
(1) Decreased metabolic rate related to decreased energy requirements of cells and imbalances in metabolic processes.
(2) Negative nitrogen balance due to atrophy of muscle begins between the 6th and 10th day of immobilization.
(3) Anabolic processes decrease and catabolic processes increase with nitrogen excreted in urine.
(4) Loss of nitrogen exceeds nitrogen intake resulting in insufficient protein needed for muscle building and wound healing.
(5) Decreased nutritional intake, which often leads to decreased basal metabolic rate and a negative nitrogen balance associated with catabolism and a high calcium level.
(6) Persons in negative nitrogen balance may feel sluggish, anorexic, have a poor appetite for protein and become malnourished.

b. Thermoregulation.
(1) Temperature is elevated due to prevention of loss of body heat via conduction and radiation related to restrictive bed coverings.
(2) To lower body temperature, blood vessels dilate and the person perspires, contributing to loss of sodium, potassium, and chloride.

c. Endocrine.
(1) Supine position fosters production of adrenocortical hormones.
(2) Glucocorticoids affect fat, carbohydrate, and protein metabolism.
(3) Mineralocorticoids affect electrolyte balance (Na+, K+, Cl-).
(4) Activity of pancreas declines, as does patient's ability to tolerate sugar. Endogenous insulin loses its ability to lower serum glucose. These effects are often seen within 3 days.
(5) Usual diurnal pattern of metabolic processes is altered by persistent supine position.

7. Gastrointestinal.
a. Less energy is expended due to immobility.
b. Gastrointestinal functions of ingestion, digestion, and elimination are all affected; however, alterations in ingestion and elimination are most prominent.
c. Ingestion.
(1) Negative nitrogen balance occurs 6-10 days after immobilization from increased catabolic activity related to muscle atrophy.
(2) Prolonged negative nitrogen balance stimulates anorexia and decreased intake of nutrients.
(3) High-protein diet required.
(4) Need exists to meet basal metabolic requirements.
(5) Stress of immobility stimulates parasympathetic nerves. Dyspepsia, gastric stasis, distention, anorexia, diarrhea, or constipation may develop.

d. Elimination.
(1) Atrophy of primary muscles of defecation (abdominal, diaphragm, levator ani) contribute to difficulty with defecation associated with immobilized patients.
(2) Lack of exercise promotes general muscle weakness.
(3) Inactivity slows movement of feces into ascending colon and sigmoid.
(4) Suppression of defecation may lead to complete absence of defecation sensation and constipation may result.
(5) Position assumed during use of bedpan while recumbent is not conducive to defecation.
(6) Fecal impactions and fecalomas may develop after feces have been retained for

a long period. Symptom is passage of liquid stool around impaction.

(7) Cardiovascular accidents, hemorrhoids, ulcers, rectal prolapse, and heart block may occur as a person strains to have a stool.

(8) Mechanical bowel obstruction may be due to fecal impaction, accompanied by abdominal distention, dehydration, fluid and electrolyte imbalance, and dyspnea related to abdominal distention interfering with movement of diaphragm.

8. Urinary.
   a. Immobilization in the supine position is not conducive to optimal function of the urinary system.
   b. In the supine position, the hilus of the kidney is most superior and urine must be passed to the ureters against gravity.
   c. The renal pelvis may not empty completely when urine is being passed into the ureters because peristalsis may not be great enough to overcome gravity.
   d. Decreased muscle tone as a result of immobility may affect the tone of the primary muscle of micturition (detrusor), thus compromising the ability to empty the bladder
   e. Urinary stasis in the calyces may precipitate renal calculi or infection.
   f. Inability to relax perineal muscles and external sphincter in supine position prevents reflex action and contraction of detrusor muscle of bladder wall and micturition does not occur.
   g. Excessive stretch of bladder muscle may prevent sensation to void.
   h. With bladder distention, overflow may occur.
   i. Males with prostate hypertrophy may experience exacerbation of symptoms.
   j. Nephron function is not usually affected by immobility.
   k. During first few days of immobility urine output is increased due to increased kidney perfusion.
   l. Kidney excretes greater amounts of minerals and salts (sulfur, phosphorus, sodium, potassium, and calcium).
   m. Excretion of calcium is increased 2 days after immobility begins and reaches its maximum excretion in 5 days.
   n. Renal calculi due to immobility are composed primarily of calcium ("stones of recumbency").
   o. Factors contributing to stone formation are: urine stasis, alkalinity, increased phosphate concentration, and decreased urine volume.
   p. The paralyzed patient experiences a common triad of complications (hypercalciuria, renal stasis, and urinary tract infection) which lead to often large renal calculi.
9. Psychosocial/mental status.
   a. Effects of immobilization on children.
      (1) Forced inactivity in the form of immobility deprives a child of a means for dealing with stress.
      (2) Sensory deprivation in children leads to feelings of isolation, boredom, and being forgotten.
      (3) Behavioral changes are noted when a child experiences prolonged sensory deprivation: greater than normal anxiety, restlessness, difficulty problem solving, inability to concentrate, egocentrism, and sluggish intellectual and psychomotor functions.
      (4) Sensory and perceptual deprivation may lead to developmental delays.
      (5) Physical activity is an instrument for communication and a means of learning. Learning, motivation, drives, expectancies, and emotions all are affected by immobility.
      (6) Play is necessary for a child to cope better with hospitalization.
      (7) When children are able to see the reason for restraint (cast, IV), they are less likely to be resistant than when the reason is less obvious (bed rest in rheumatic fever).
   b. Effects of immobility on adults.
      (1) Immobility can lead to depression, noncompliance, and confusion.
      (2) Perceptual behaviors altered due to decreased interaction of the person with the environment.
      (3) Roles and activity are changed by immobility.
      (4) Interaction with the environment is essential for ego identity formation and this is limited by immobility.
      (5) Physical activity is an instrument for communication and a means of learning. Learning, motivation, drives, expectancies, and emotions all are affected by immobility.
   c. In the elderly, changes in affect, cognition, and perception can occur with bed rest. Affect changes include anxiety, fear, depression, and rapid mood swings. Perceptual distortions with bed rest range from daydreaming to hallucinations, difficulty concentrating, and loss of sense of time, somatic complaints, and noncompliant behavior.

II. ASSESSMENT (See therapeutic modalities and nursing interventions for systems assessment.)

III. COMMON THERAPEUTIC MODALITIES

A. Integumentary. Treatment guideline recommendations developed by the Agency for Health Care Policy and Research (AHCPR) address six areas: assessment; managing tissue loads; ulcer care; managing bacterial colonization and infection; operative repair; and education and quality improvement.

1. Assessment.

a. Basis for treatment. Includes location, stage, size of ulcer as well as presence of sinus tracts, undermining, tunneling, exudates, necrotic tissue, granulation tissue, and epithe-liazation.
b. Pressure ulcers are graded according to degree of severity or involvement.
    (1) Grade I: limited to epidermal and dermal layers.
    (2) Grade II: necrosis penetrates into subcutaneous layers.
    (3) Grade III: includes all subcutaneous layers to muscle and into muscle.
    (4) Grade IV: destruction of all soft tissue and penetration into bone.

2. Managing tissue loads: the goal is to have an environment conducive to soft tissue viability and healing of pressure ulcer.
    a. While in bed.
        (1) Patient should not be positioned on pressure ulcer or pressure points.
        (2) Head of bed should be low to prevent shear injury.
        (3) Pressure-reducing surfaces should be used to prevent further ulcers.
        (4) Static support surfaces should be used if patient can assume various positions and support is greater than 1 inch. Otherwise, use dynamic support.
        (5) Low air loss bed if Stage III or IV ulcers are on numerous sites.
    b. While in chair.
        (1) Reposition every 15 minutes.
        (2) If unable to change position frequently, should be on bed rest.
3. Ulcer care.
    a. Debridement.
        (1) Necrotic tissue debrided from the ulcer with attention to pain management.
        (2) Sharp debridement is most rapid.
        (3) Mechanical debridement includes:
            (a) Wet-to-dry dressings.
            (b) Hydrotherapy.
            (c) Wound irrigation.
            (d) Dextranomers (beads placed in ulcer bed to absorb bacteria, exudates, and other debris).
        (4) Enzymatic (when surgery is not feasible and there is no infection), i.e. collagenase.
        (5) Autolytic debridement used only in absence of infection. Synthetic dressing placed over ulcer and eschar self-digests via enzymes present in wound fluid.
        (6) No debridement of dry eschar free of edema, erythema, fluctuance, or drainage.
    b. Wound cleaning.
        (1) Initially and with every dressing change using a cleaning solution and minimal force.
        (2) Whirlpool used for pressure ulcers with much necrotic tissue and other tissue debris.
    c. Dressings
        (1) Ulcer bed should be kept moist but bordering skin should be kept dry.
        (2) Exudate should be controlled, preferably with colloid film dressings.
    d. Managing bacterial colonization and infection.
        (1) All stage II, III, and IV ulcers are infected.
        (2) Cultures should be obtained via needle aspiration.
        (3) Ulcer should be thoroughly cleansed.
        (4) Wound healing impaired if bacterial levels are greater than 10^5 organisms/gram of tissue or presence of osteomyelitis.
        (5) Measures to prevent cross contamination.
    e. Operative repair.
        (1) For stage III or IV ulcers.
        (2) Procedures include: direct closure, skin grafting, skin flaps, musculocutaneous flaps, free flaps.
        (3) Vigilant post-op care includes proper positioning and perfusion.
    f. Education and quality improvement.
        (1) Educational program for patient, family, and caregivers. Should include information regarding prevention to avert recurrence.
        (2) Program should be part of quality monitoring.

B. Respiratory.
1. Incentive spirometer.
2. Intermittent positive pressure breathing (IPPB).
3. In addition to turning, coughing, and deep breathing at least every hour.

C. Cardiovascular.
1. Monitor hemodynamic function.
2. Elastic support and/or sequential compression device applied to lower extremities.
3. Physical therapy for active and passive extremity exercise, unless contraindicated by other conditions.
4. Change of position (elevate head of bed, reverse Trendelenburg) to stimulate autonomic nervous system.
5. Fluid challenges.

D. Musculoskeletal.
1. Bone. Administration of anabolic steroids which have been shown to decrease urinary calculi formation by increasing the secretion of citric acid and decreasing the excretion of calcium.
2. Muscle. Physical therapy for muscle strengthening.
3. Joints. Physical therapy for joint range-of-motion (ROM). Splints/supports to maintain functional alignment.

E. Neurosensory.
1. Position patient for protection of desensitized areas.
2. Assess neurovascular status every 4 hours.
3. Re-orient patient as needed.

F. Metabolic.
1. Monitor vital signs.

2. Monitor serum electrolytes.
3. Diet to include high protein, high fluid.

G. Gastrointestinal.

1. Prophylactic high-fiber diet, increased fluid intake, and stool softener as needed if narcotics are also being administered.
2. Conservative treatment of bowel obstruction.
   a. Patient NPO.
   b. Intravenous fluids.
   c. Nasogastric suction.
   d. Enema.
   e. Rectal tube.
   f. X-rays to assess progress of decompression of distended colon.
3. Possible surgical intervention with bowel obstruction.

H. Urinary.

1. Cholinergic agent orally or subcutaneous injection if little or no urine output.
2. Renal calculi removal by surgical techniques if patient unable to pass stone.

I. Psychosocial/mental status.

1. Environmental stimuli.
2. Play therapy for children.
3. Appropriate referrals.
4. Provide socialization with peers, change environment when possible (take bed outside).
5. Allow for personalization of environment – pictures, own clothes, food from home, etc.

IV. NURSING DIAGNOSES, OUTCOMES, AND INTERVENTIONS

A. Integumentary.
Skin integrity, impaired (actual and potential).

1. Outcome: skin remains intact.
2. Interventions.
   a. Skin inspection should be performed minimally (once every shift) with specific attention to bony prominences. Findings should be documented.
   b. Turn and position often. Base frequency on patient's status/needs. Remind patient to do it him/herself if possible. Keep written record of times and position.
   c. Assess patient for pressure ulcer risk.
      (1) Standardized, well researched, risk assessment tool such as the Braden Scale should be used
      (2) As noted per the Braden Scale, the following subscales should be assessed for the patient's degree of risk:
         (a) Sensory perception.
         (b) Moisture.
         (c) Activity.
         (d) Mobility.
         (e) Nutrition.
         (f) Friction and shear.
   d. Use proper positioning: body weight evenly distributed, body alignment normal or neutral with as little stress as possible on body parts, and circulation not compromised by supportive devices (pillows, splints) or other equipment (casts, drains).
   e. Inspect skin over pressure points during each position change.
   f. Keep linens dry and wrinkle free.
   g. Practice regular toilet schedule individualized for patient to minimize incontinence.
   h. Use oscillating beds and alternating pressure mattresses.
   i. Avoid use of rubber rings and doughnuts. These compress larger areas around the pressure point and contribute to pressure ulcer growth.
   j. If a pressure ulcer should occur, react promptly.
      (1) Remove pressure.
      (2) Close portal of entry for infection.
      (3) Limit loss of serum proteins.
      (4) Provide high-protein diet to compensate for loss of protein.
      (5) Provide carbohydrates and fats in diet to maximize mobilization of proteins.
      (6) Consider debridement, wound cleansing, dressings, and infection control.
      (7) Frequent monitoring and assessment of treatment is essential.
      (8) Keep pressure off area.
   k. Key to management of skin integrity is prevention of complications.

B. Respiratory.
Breathing pattern, ineffective (actual and potential).
Airway clearance, ineffective (actual and potential).

1. Outcome: patient is afebrile without either respiratory congestion or distress.
2. Interventions.
   a. Auscultate lung fields at least every 8 hours.
   b. Use incentive spirometer at least 10 times every hour.
   c. Encourage turning and deep breathing every 2 hours.
   d. Turn patient per established schedule (q 2 hours) if condition permits.
   e. Encourage side-lying positions unless contraindicated.
   f. Encourage oral fluids. Avoid dehydration and use of anticholinergic drugs when possible.
   g. Assess for abdominal distention every 8 hours.
   h. Promote regular bowel/bladder practices per patient's usual schedule.
   i. Avoid over-sedation.

C. Cardiovascular.
Tissue perfusion, altered: cardiopulmonary.
Fluid volume excess.
Fluid volume deficit.

1. Outcomes:
   a. No evidence of venous thrombus formation or pulmonary embolus.
   b. Fluid balance maintained.
   c. Absence of acute orthostatic hypotension.
2. Interventions.

a. Assess vital signs every 8 hours.
b. Perform orthostatic blood pressure readings prior to ambulation as needed, every morning if possible.
c. Assess Homan's sign bilaterally every 8 hours.
d. Assess for thrombophlebitis every 8 hours.
e. Help patient practice active and passive range of motion exercises as well as isometric and isotonic exercises (ankle dorsi/plantar flexion; ankle rotation).
f. Promote self-care practices.
g. Apply elastic support hose and/or sequential compression devices to lower extremities.
h. Help patient change position frequently to alter intravascular pressure and stimulate neural reflexes of blood vessels and to help prevent hypotension.
i. Change patient's position from horizontal to nearly vertical by raising head of bed, reverse Trendelenburg, or by sitting patient in chair unless contraindicated.
j. Stress dynamic and static exercise while patient is immobilized to limit degree of deconditioning.
k. Teach patient to exhale rather than holding breath while moving in bed or defecating.
l. Avoid fatiguing patient.

D. Musculoskeletal.
Physical mobility, impaired.
Disuse syndrome, risk for.

1. Outcomes:
   a. No evidence of joint stiffness.
   b. No evidence of joint contracture.
   c. No evidence of joint laxity.
   d. Maintenance of muscle tone and/or strength.
   e. No evidence of fracture.
2. Interventions.
   a. Assess passive and active range-of-motion (PROM and AROM) every 8 hours.
   b. Assess ROM against resistance (muscle strength) in all joints every 8 hours.
   c. Mobilization of patient when feasible with weight bearing and activity.
   d. Exercise: isotonic (dynamic or isometric [static]) beyond muscle's ordinary level of activity to restore muscle bulk and strength.
   e. Use progressive resistive exercises.
   f. Use isometric exercises if joint inflamed.
   g. Teach importance of proper exercise.
   h. Maintain proper body alignment with special attention to joint support.
   i. Ambulate patient as often as possible.
   j. Change patient's position frequently, minimal every 2 hours.
   k. Encourage/assist with ROM.
   l. Place in whirlpool or warm bath during exercise.
   m. Encourage normal use of limb when possible.
   n. Use foot support to avoid footdrop.
   o. Support hand in position of function.
   p. Inspect muscles for impaired tone every 8 hours.
   q. Apply splints per order.
   r. Encourage significant others to participate in exercise plan.

E. Neurosensory.
Peripheral neurovascular dysfunction, risk for.

1. Outcome: peripheral neurovascular status intact.
2. Interventions.
   a. Position to promote neurosensory integrity.
   b. Avoid pressure in areas where nerves run superficially over bony prominences.
   c. Avoid pressure over brachial plexus.
   d. Maintain alignment of extremities that are paralyzed.
   e. Assess neurovascular status throughout body.

F. Metabolic.
Ineffective thermoregulation, potential.
Body temperature, altered: potential.
Fluid volume, deficient: actual/potential.

1. Outcomes:
   a. Maintains body temperature within normal limits.
   b. Maintains fluid and electrolyte balance.
2. Interventions.
   a. Monitor body temperature every 8 hours.
   b. Use lightweight bed clothing and bed cover to allow for loss of body heat by radiation.
   c. Maintain daily fluid and nutritional intake and output.
   d. Monitor serum electrolyte values.
   e. Maintain well-balanced diet with adequate intake. Consult dietician.

G. Gastrointestinal.
Nutrition, altered: less than body requirements.
Nutrition, altered: more than body requirements.
Constipation, clonic.

1. Outcomes:
   a. Absence of negative nitrogen balance and acute weight loss.
   b. No incidence of constipation or bowel obstruction.
2. Interventions.
   a. Promote high-carbohydrate, moderate-protein, well-balanced diet.
   b. Frequent small meals.
   c. Daily weights to assess weight loss/gain.
   d. Plan, with patient, a daily bowel program providing adequate time and privacy.
   e. Promote high-fiber diet.
   f. Encourage fluid intake. Minimum of 3L/day.
   g. Administer stool softeners and laxatives as needed.
   h. Assess bowel sounds every 8 hours.
   i. Check daily for abdominal distension.
   j. Assess digitally for fecal impaction as needed.

H. Urinary.
Urinary elimination, altered.

1. Outcomes:
   a. Balance between intake and output is maintained.
   b. Absence of renal calculi.
2. Interventions.

a. Monitor fluid intake and output daily.
b. Assess for bladder overflow.
 (1) Monitor frequency and amount of urination.
 (2) Assess for bladder distension.
 (3) Monitor for urine retention.
 (4) If unable to void, medication with cholinergic agent or catheterization may be necessary.
c. Encourage fluids.
 (1) Intake to 3L/day unless contraindicated.
 (2) Urine acidifying juices may be used to prevent calcium calculi; however efficacy is questioned.
d. Frequent turning and ambulation if possible.
e. Instruct patient on the cause of calculi formation.

I. Psychosocial/mental status.
Social interaction, impaired.
Diversional activity, deficient.

1. Outcomes:
 a. Maintains interaction with significant others and environment.
 b. Maintains orientation.
2. Interventions.
 a. Encourage visits by significant others.
 b. Mobilize patient as much as possible.
 c. Foster patient group activities.
 d. Provide positive reinforcement regarding progress in care, learning self-care procedures, etc.
 e. Provide glasses, hearing aids, etc.
 f. Keep clock and calendar in room.
 g. Re-orient patient as needed.
 h. Promote as normal a setting as possible (lights, activity).
 i. Involve patient in planning care.
 j. Encourage continued communication with family, work friends, etc.
 k. Problem solve with patient regarding coping mechanisms.
 l. Occupational therapy consult as needed.
 m. Play therapy for hospitalized children.
 n. Encourage crafts, reading, etc., according to patient's likes to provide diversion.

V. HOME CARE CONSIDERATIONS

A. Equipment considerations.

1. Special hospital beds might be considered to promote optimal positioning.
2. Assistive devices, such as slide boards, lifts, overbed trapezes, also should help foster patient safety.
3. Bedpan/commode should be available to promote proper (safe) elimination.

B. Caregiver considerations.

1. Primary caregiver needs to learn safe body mechanics when moving and/or positioning patients.
2. Home caregivers need to be aware of signs of complications related to immobility.
3. Caregivers should be aware of how to deal with complications related to immobility.
4. Caregivers should be aware of resources such as support groups, meal delivery services, and home health agencies.

C. Social supports: caregivers should be aware of support groups for families caring for ill relatives.

Bibliography

Agency for Health Care Policy and Research. (1992, May). *Pressure ulcers in adults: Prediction and prevention.* Clinical Practice Guideline. Quick Reference Guide for Clinicians No. 3. AHCPR Pub. No. 92-0047. Rockville, MD: Public Health Service, U.S. Department of Health and Human Services.

Agency for Health Care Policy and Research. (1994, December). *Pressure ulcer treatment.* Clinical Practice Guideline. Quick Reference Guide for Clinicians No. 15. AHCPR Pub. No. 95-0653. Rockville, MD: Public Health Service, U.S. Department of Health and Human Services.

Asher, R.A. (1947, October 14). The dangers of going to bed. *British Medical Journal, 967.*

Burke, M.M., & Laramie, J.A. (2000). *Primary care of the older adult: A multidisciplinary approach* (p. 292). St. Louis: Mosby.

Convertino, V.A. (1997). Caradiovascular consequences of bedrest effect on maximal oxygen uptake. *Medicine & Science in Sports and Exercise, 29*(2), 191-196.

Corcoran, P.J. (1991). Use it or lose – The hazards of bed rest and inactivity. *The Western Journal of Medicine, 154*(5), 536-538.

Faria, S.H. (1998). Assessment of immobility hazards. *Home Care Provider, 3*(4), 189-91.

Ferretti, G., Girardis, M., Moia, C., & Antonutto, G., (1998). Effects of prolonged bedrest on cardiovascular oxygen transport during submaximial exercise in humans. *European Journal of Applied Physiology & Occupational Physiology, 78*(5), 398– 402.

Freeland, A. (2000, June 5). *Pressure ulcers. The wound care information network* [Online]. Available: http://medicaledu.com/pres sure.htm

Giannattasio, C., Failla, M., Grappioto, A., Bigoni, M., Carugo, S., Denti, M., & Mancia, G. (1998). Effects of prolonged immobilization of the limb on radial artery mechanical properties. *Hypertension, 32*(3), 584-587.

Greenleaf, J.E. (1997). Intensive exercise training during bed rest attenuates deconditioning. *Medicine & Science in Sports and Exercise, 29*(2), 207-15.

Jagmin, M.G. (1998). In A.B. Maher, S.W. Salmond, & T.A. Pellino (Eds.), *Orthopaedic nursing* (2nd ed., pp. 92-114). Philadelphia: W.B. Saunders Company.

Krasnoff, J., & Painter, P. (1999). The physiological consequences of bed rest and inactivity. *Advances in Renal Replacement Therapy, 6*(2), 124-132.

Olson, E.V. (1967). The hazards of immobility. *American Journal of Nursing, 67*(4), 780-797.

Olson, E.V. (1990). The hazards of immobility. *American Journal of Nursing, 90*, 43-52.

Rubin, M. (1988). The physiology of bed rest. *American Journal of Nursing, 88*(1), 50-58.

Shoemaker, J.K., Hogeman, C.S., & Sinoway, L.I. (1999, October). Contributions of MSNA and stroke volume to orthostatic intolerance following bed rest. *American Journal of Physiology, 277*(4, Pt. 2), R1084-1090.

Wong, D.L. (1999). *The immobilized child.* In Whaley & Wong's Essentials of Pediatric Nursing (5th ed., pp. 1122-1126). St. Louis: Mosby.

STUDY QUESTIONS

Jennifer Smith, an 11-year-old gymnast, has spondylolisthesis and complains of increasing back pain and tight hamstring muscles. She was admitted for initial conservative treatment of bed rest 2 weeks prior to surgery. Following today's surgery, she is to spend 6 weeks in a back brace and on bed rest. (Questions 1-3)

1. Which of the following is most true about the impact of immobility on children in comparison to adults?
   a. Children are more prone to skin breakdown than adults.
   b. Immobility can lead to developmental delays in children.
   c. Adults are more prone to problems in the respiratory system related to immobility than children.
   d. In children, bones remain dense even though they experience disuse and lack of stress across the osseous tissue.

2. Children will be less likely to be resistant to immobilization when:
   a. Their parents are with them consistently.
   b. They are too sick to care.
   c. They are rewarded for being compliant.
   d. They are able to understand the reason for the restraint and/or immobility.

3. Which one of the following statements is most true about play and the immobilized child?
   a. Play often interferes with optimal healing.
   b. Play is beneficial to the immobilized child only when it is interactive.
   c. Play is needed for the child to better cope with hospitalization.
   d. Play is last on the list of priorities of nursing care of the immobilized child.

John Green, age 38, fell off a ladder while painting his house. He fractured his left femur and sprained his right wrist. The fracture was internally fixated and a long leg cast was applied. He will be sent home with crutches and his ambulatory status is non-weight-bearing for 6 weeks. (Questions 4-7)

4. Muscle immobilized by a cast:
   a. Decreases linearly in strength for the entire time it is immobilized.
   b. Decreases linearly in strength for 1 week, then after 1 week little strength is lost.
   c. Atrophies due to a decrease in muscle fiber size, length, and number.
   d. Atrophies due to a decrease in muscle activities and widens the muscle fibers.

5. Osteoblasts form the osseous matrix of bone and require:
   a. A diet high in calcium, ascorbic acid, and Vitamin D.
   b. Rest, immobilization, and a diet high in calcium and phosphorus.
   c. Stress of isometric contractions to multiply.
   d. Stress of mobility and weight bearing for adequate functioning.

6. While his leg is immobilized in the cast, Mr. Green's knee may experience:
   a. A degeneration of the joint capsule and patella.
   b. An altered flow of synovial fluid.
   c. Decreased laxity of the knee.
   d. Accumulation of calcium crystals in the joint space.

7. Mr. Green should be taught how to do neurovascular checks to his affected leg because:
   a. Peripheral nerves degenerate with disuse.
   b. Improper positioning of casts can put undue pressure on nerves and blood vessels.
   c. Immobility distorts peripheral sensory perception.
   d. The assessments will stimulate blood flow to the extremity.

Mrs. Brown, age 74, fell on a broken sidewalk and sustained a Smith fracture of the left wrist. She is status post-left mastectomy 10 years ago, pacemaker placement 1 year ago, and has mild Paget's disease. Her fracture was manually reduced in the emergency room and a short arm cast applied. She was instructed to wear a sling and not use the arm for 6 weeks. (Questions 8-10)

8. Mrs. Brown's fingers, hand, wrist, and lower arm may be weak following immobilization most likely because:
   a. Her diet was low in protein.
   b. Decreased muscle mass is related to too much stress on muscle.
   c. Immobilized muscle loses about 5% of its original strength per day and varies with degree of immobility.
   d. She did not follow the physician's orders.

9. Mrs. Brown may have to immobilize her wrist longer than 6 weeks because:
   a. She has osteoporotic bone like all elderly postmenopausal women.
   b. The normal treatment plan will need to be modified because of her Paget's disease.
   c. Treatment is modified to avoid the cycle of increased fragility and recurrent fracture after mobilization.
   d. The immobilization would augment calcium from the body and thus the onset of osteoporosis.

10. Mrs. Brown may develop contractures in her wrist, elbow, and shoulder, most likely because:
    a. Joint flexion/extension is needed to promote range of motion.
    b. Synovial fluid stagnates.
    c. Muscle fibers shorten.
    d. The ligaments become lax due to loss of muscle tone.

Ms. Green is 65 years old, 5 feet tall, and weighs 98 pounds. She sustained a pelvic fracture in a motor vehicle accident yesterday and is now post-surgery. She is placed on extended bed rest. She has a history of a kidney transplant, high blood pressure, cardiovascular disease, and is an insulin-dependent diabetic. (Questions 11-15)

11. Which of the following should the nurse be most concerned about in regard to renal calculi formation?
    a. Increased urine volume.
    b. Urine alkalinity.
    c. Decreased phosphate concentration.
    d. Sugar and protein in the urine.

12. How should Ms. Green be positioned to reduce cardiovascular risks associated with Valsalva's maneuver?
    a. Head of bed flat.
    b. Head of bed 45 degrees.
    c. Head of bed 90 degrees.
    d. The risks are just as great in any position.

13. In regard to fluid balance, one might observe which of the following in Ms. Green?
    a. Decreased urinary sodium excretion.
    b. Decrease in plasma volume about 300-500 cc.
    c. Net gain of body water.
    d. Excessive thirst and fluid intake.

14. While making her routine skin assessment of Ms. Green, the nurse notes a 2-inch in diameter reddened area on Ms. Green's sacrum as well as reddened areas on both of her heels. The nurse would document these areas as what type of pressure ulcer?
    a. Grade I.
    b. Grade II.
    c. Grade III.
    d. Grade IV.

15. The most important aspect of skin care and the key to the management of potential impaired skin integrity in the immobilized patient is to:
    a. Prevent complications in all patients regardless of age.
    b. Treat complications as soon as possible.
    c. Assess for risks of potential complications.
    d. Educate staff about the importance of frequent skin assessments.

Chapter 7 PAIN

Donna M. Barker, MS, RN, ONC
Karen A. Sikorski, MS, RN
Janet S. Tompkins, MS, Ed, MSN, ARNP-C
Phyllis Lisanti, PhD, RN

Contents

OBJECTIVES

At the completion of this chapter, the learner will be able to:

- Recognize the factors that influence pain behaviors and suffering.
- Identify common misconceptions of pain patterns, pain behaviors, and pain treatment of specific age groups addressed in chapter.
- Describe the assessment parameters for pain evaluation.
- Select appropriate analgesics, dosages, and routes for patients with pain across the lifespan, and with various types of pain.
- Compare nonpharmacologic interventions for acute, procedural, and chronic/cancer pain.

KEY POINTS

- The individual, as the expert in subjective phenomena, is to be believed regarding existence, severity, character, distribution, and exacerbating/relieving factors of pain.
- Consider pain the fifth vital sign for patient assessment and documentation.
- Physical, psychological, and pharmacologic methods of pain relief are effective, and a combined preemptive/preventive approach of these methods is the most effective.
- Most common continuing barriers in the management of pain are:
  - ♦ Failure to initially assess and reassess as appropriate
  - ♦ Failure to adequately treat pain
  - ♦ Lack of accountability for pain management
- Unrelieved pain continues to be prevalent for people with postoperative, cancer, and chronic pain.
  - ♦ > 50% of hospitalized patients have unrelieved pain due to under-medication.
  - ♦ 70%-90% of people with cancer (chronic malignant) pain report moderate to severe pain.
  - ♦ 25% of all cancer patients die in severe pain.

CHAPTER 7

PAIN

I. DEFINITIONS AND TYPES OF PAIN

A. Definitions.

1. Pain.
   a. The International Association for the Study of Pain (IASP) defines pain as "an unpleasant sensory and emotional experience associated with actual or potential tissue damage, or described in terms of such damage."
   b. According to M. McCaffery, the clinical definition of pain is "whatever the patient says it is, wherever he/she says it is, as severe as he/she says it is, lasting as long as he/she says it does."
   c. Opioid/opiate:
      (1) Natural or semi-synthetic medicines that relieve pain by binding to opioid receptors in the nervous system.
      (2) The word "opioid" is preferred due to negative connotations of the words "narcotic" or "drug."
   d. Addiction:
      (1) A psychological dependence on the use of substances or activities for their psychic effects, and is characterized by compulsive use.
      (2) Addiction should be considered if patients no longer have control over drug use, and continue to use drugs despite harm.
      (3) NOTE: People taking drugs for acute pain rarely become addicted. The percentage is < 1%.
   e. Pseudo-addiction:
      (1) Drug-seeking behavior that seems similar to addiction, but is really due to unrelieved pain.
      (2) The behavior stops once the pain is relieved, often through an increase in opioid dose.
      (3) Misunderstanding this phenomenon may lead the clinician to inappropriately stigmatize the patient with the label "addict."
      (4) In the setting of unrelieved pain, the request for increases in medication dose requires careful assessment, renewed efforts to manage pain, and avoidance of stigmatizing labels.
   f. Physical dependence:
      (1) The occurrence of withdrawal syndromes after opioid use is stopped, or quickly decreased without titration, or if an antagonist (naloxone) is administered.
      (2) It is not addiction.
      (3) Physical dependence is not a clinical problem:
         (a) If patients are warned to avoid abrupt discontinuation of the opioid.
         (b) A tapering-off regimen is used.
         (c) Opioid antagonist-drugs (including agonist-antagonist analgesics) are avoided.
   g. Tolerance.
      (1) Tolerance is needed for increased dosage of a drug to produce the same level of analgesia that previously existed.
      (2) Tolerance also occurs when a reduced effect is observed with a constant dose.
      (3) Analgesic tolerance is not always evident during opioid treatment, and is **not** addiction.
      (4) Often, tolerance is seen as "end of dose failure."
   h. Allodynia: pain due to a stimulus that does not normally provoke pain.
   i. Arthralgia: pain in a joint, usually due to arthritis or arthropathy.
   j. Balanced analgesia: multi-modal analgesia that combines a variety of approaches (regional techniques, opioids, and NSAIDs).
   k. Breakthrough pain:
      (1) Pain that increases above the pain that is controlled with continuous analgesia (incidental pain, spontaneous pain, and end-of-dose failure).
      (2) Requires "rescue dosing" with short-acting opioids.
   l. Hyperalgesia: increased response to a stimulus which is normally painful.
   m. Neuropathy:
      (1) Disturbance of function or pathologic changes in a nerve.
      (2) Characterized by numbness, tingling, "electric shock"-like pain.
      (3) Also described as jabbing, lancinating, or stabbing.
      (4) Can affect motor neurons, causing myelopathies.
   n. Preemptive analgesia:
      (1) Pain treatment before an anticipated onset of pain to prevent establishment of peripheral and central nervous system sensitization.
      (2) An example of preemptive analgesia is the use of epidural local anesthetic infusion prior to amputation of a limb in an attempt to prevent phantom limb pain.
   o. Complex Regional Pain Syndrome (CRPS):
      (1) Formerly known as Reflex Sympathetic Dystrophy (RSD).
      (2) Progressive and potentially severely disabling, often extremely painful condition affecting nerves, skin, muscles, blood vessels, and bones.

Table 7.1
Receptor Sites for Analgesia

Drug	Activity	Receptor Site
Morphine Methadone Codeine Fentanyl Meperidine Hydromorphone	Analgesia, respiratory depression, constipation, euphoria, tolerance	Mu Receptors
Butorphanol Buprenorphine Nalbuphine Pentazocine	Analgesia, sedation	Kappa Receptors
Butorphanol Pentazocine	Vasomotor stimulation, psychotomimetic effects	Sigma Receptors

p. Equianalgesia: the doses of different medications and routes needed to produce equal pain relief.
q. Potency: the intensity of the analgesic effect of a drug.

B. Types of pain.

1. Acute pain.
   a. Follows acute injury or disease.
   b. Evokes the stress response, and the classic physiological signs of stress may be present: diaphoresis, tachycardia, increased BP.
   c. Examples: fractured bone; postoperative pain.
   d. Expected to last < 6 months.
2. Chronic pain.
   a. Chronic malignant pain.
      (1) Pain associated with ongoing painful process.
      (2) Examples: cancer pain; rheumatoid arthritis.
   b. Chronic nonmalignant pain.
      (1) Pain in people whose tissue injury is nonprogressive or healed.
      (2) Examples: idiopathic low back pain; phantom limb pain; fibromyalgia.
   c. Chronic pain affects appetite, sleep, activities of daily living, relationships, concentration, depression, and can even cause suicidal ideation.
   d. Individuals with chronic pain can have acute and/or episodic pain in addition to the chronic process.
3. Somatic/nociceptive pain.
   a. Pain resulting from the ongoing activation of primary afferent neurons by various stimuli.
   b. Location of pain easily defined.
   c. Characteristics: sharp, stabbing.
4. Visceral pain.
   a. Occurs in tissues near center of the body.
   b. Location of pain vague.
   c. Characteristics: boring or dull.
5. Neuropathic.
   a. Arising from injured peripheral or central neural structures.
   b. Pain often follows peripheral distribution of nerve root.
   c. Characteristics: burning, numbness, tingling.
   d. Examples: radicular sciatic pain, phantom limb pain.

II. ANATOMY AND PHYSIOLOGY OF PAIN

A. Sources of pain in the musculoskeletal system.

1. In orthopaedics, pain is the most common symptom that motivates the patient to seek care.
2. The musculoskeletal system is made of diverse tissues: muscle, bone, tendon, ligament, articular cartilage, periosteum, and synovia. Of these, muscle, periosteum, ligament, and joint capsule respond to nociceptive impulses.
3. Periosteum is known to respond to both pressure and pain.
4. Bone pain can be induced by microfracture, repetitive motion/movement, and subsidence in arthritis, by periosteal elevation and distortion in infection or tumor, by vascular congestion and mechanical disruption.
5. Nociception refers to the stimulation of sensory nerve endings responding optimally to painful stimuli.
   a. Muscular nociception may be stimulated by chemoreceptors, such as metabolic byproducts of anaerobic activity, products of cell injury from trauma or ischemia, or chemical irritants, such as bradykinin or potassium.

b. Mechanoreceptors in muscle respond to stretch, pressure, or disruption.
c. Neuropeptides also sensitize muscle to pain.
6. Muscle pain may result from direct injury, which disrupts the tissue, or from indirect trauma, such as tears that occur as a result of athletic injuries (sprain or strain).
7. Inflammation and edema mediate pain responses.
8. Neural elements are subject to injury where they pass through the muscular compartments (as in compartment syndrome) and around bony prominences in the joints.

B. Pain perception requires afferent pain fibers of two types.

1. A delta.
   a. Largest in diameter.
   b. Most rapid conducting fiber.
   c. Myelinated.
   d. Sharp, stabbing, shooting pain.
2. C fiber.
   a. Smallest fiber.
   b. Slowest conducting fiber.
   c. Unmyelinated.
   d. Steady, slow, and constant pain.
3. Receptor sites are of three types (see Table 7.1).
   a. Mu receptors.
      (1) Mediate.
      (2) Supraspinal analgesia, respiratory depression, euphoria, physical dependence.
   b. Kappa receptors.
      (1) Mediate.
      (2) Spinal analgesia, no physical dependence, sedation.
   c. Sigma receptors.
      (1) Mediate.
      (2) Excitation, dysphoria, hallucinations.
4. Neurotransmitters: exert effects by interacting with receptors.
   a. Acetylcholine
   b. Norepinephrine
   c. Dopamine
   d. Serotonin
   e. Substance P.
   f. Enkaphalin (an endorphin thought to be a neurotransmitter).

C. Endorphins.

1. A group of endogenous polypeptides including the enkephalins, and alpha α, beta β, and gamma γ endorphins (beta being the most potent) which bind to opiate receptors.
2. They are secreted in response to fear, anxiety, and pain and raise the pain threshold, producing euphoria and sedation as well as analgesia.
   a. Like exogenous opiates, they are inhibited by naloxone and the body develops a tolerance to them, especially in response to uncontrolled stimuli.
   b. Thought to be part of the fight-or-flight stress response and are useful in promotion of analgesia and inhibition of pain-motivated behavior when the organism must defend itself.
   c. More effective for acute pain than chronic pain.

D. Autonomic nervous system (involuntary).

1. Controls activities of heart, viscera, glands, blood vessels, and smooth muscles.
2. Composed of sympathetic/parasympathetic systems.
3. Sympathetic and parasympathetic systems may act synergistically to innervate the same organ (eye, heart).
4. May act alone.
   a. Sympathetic: supplies uterus, kidneys, and arterioles.
   b. Parasympathetic: supplies glands of stomach, pancreas.

III. PHYSIOLOGIC EFFECTS ASSOCIATED WITH UNRELIEVED PAIN (See Table 7.2)

1. Negative physiologic and psychologic consequences.
2. Increase health care cost/lengthened hospital stays/increased use of health care.
3. Decreased patient satisfaction.
4. Increased complications (deep vein thrombosis [DVT] from decreased ability to ambulate due to pain).
5. Impact on quality of life.
6. Untreated acute pain sensitizes the nervous system leading to chronic pain.
7. Depressed immune response leading to delayed healing; cancer patients can experience more rapid growth of metastasis.
8. In fact, pain can KILL.
9. In the case of the elderly, consequences of unrelieved pain may lead to increased falls.

IV. EPIDEMIOLOGY OF PAIN

A. No other phenomenon is perhaps so universal, yet so personal, as pain. Cross-cultural studies have shown that there are both quantitative and qualitative differences between social and cultural groups, particularly in pain behaviors and reactions.

B. The following conclusions have been found in a review of multiple studies across the Anglo, Hispanic, and Asian populations:

1. Hispanic groups tend to be more emotional about pain than North American or English subjects.
2. Asians or Asian-Americans tend to be more stoic.
3. European Americans tend to have difficulty dealing with pain.
4. These responses may have either a negative and/or positive consequence in relation to pain.

C. A review of multiple cross-cultural studies of pain beliefs, perceptions, and responses among multiple cultural groups suggests the following:

1. The greatest cross-cultural variation is in the reactions and adaptations to pain, such as coping strategies.

Table 7.2
Harmful Effects of Unrelieved Pain

Domains Affected	Specific Responses to Pain
Endocrine	↑Adrenocorticotrophic hormone (ACTH), ↑cortisol, ↑antidiuretic hormone (ADH), ↑epinephrine, ↑norepinephrine, ↑growth hormone (GH), ↑catecholamines, ↑renin, ↑angiotensin II, ↑aldosterone, ↑glucagon, ↑interleukin-1; ↓insulin, ↓testosterone
Metabolic	Gluconeogenesis, hepatic glycogenolysis, hyperglycemia, glucose intolerance, insulin resistance, muscle protein catabolism, ↑lipolysis
Cardiovascular	↑heart rate, ↑cardiac output, ↑peripheral vascular resistance, ↑systemic vascular resistance, hypertension, ↑coronary vascular resistance, ↑myocardial oxygen consumption, hypercoagulation, deep vein thrombosis
Respiratory	↓flows and volumes, atelectasis, shunting, hypoxemia, ↓cough, sputum retention, infection
Genitourinary	↓urinary output, urinary retention, fluid overload, hypokalemia
Gastrointestinal	↓gastric and bowel motility
Musculoskeletal	Muscle spasm, impaired muscle function, fatigue, immobility
Cognitive	Reduction in cognitive function, mental confusion
Immune	Depression of immune response
Developmental	↑behavioral and physiologic responses to pain, altered temperaments, higher somatization, infant distress behavior; possible altered development of the pain system, vulnerability to stress disorders, addictive behavior, and anxiety states
Future pain	Debilitating chronic pain syndromes; postmastectomy pain, postthoracotomy pain, phantom pain, postherpetic neuralgia
Quality of life	Sleeplessness, anxiety, fear, hopelessness, ↓thoughts of suicide

May be duplicated for use in clinical practice. From McCaffery, M., & Pasero, C. (1999). *Pain: Clinical manual* (2nd ed., p. 24). St. Louis, MO: Mosby, Inc.

2. Incentives such as financial support tend to modify pain responses.
    a. These are more successful and less necessary if strong interpersonal support (from family and friends or from professionals) is available.
    b. This is especially true in regard to chronic pain with nonspecific causes.

V. ETHICAL PRINCIPLES OF PAIN MANAGEMENT

A. Autonomy.
1. The person's right to self-determination.
2. The nurse has the obligation to inform the patient of options and of the right to adequate pain control and the risks, benefits, and costs involved.

B. Beneficence.
1. The professional's responsibility to benefit the patient.
2. The safest and most reasonable way to relieve pain must be selected.
3. Unrelieved pain and high-tech life-support measures cause serious decrease in quality of life.
4. The movement toward physician-assisted suicide is largely due to inadequate relief of pain and suffering.

C. Non-malfeasance.
1. Nurse should avoid causing the patient harm and protect the patient from harm.
2. Adequate pain management has been shown to be the primary modality which relieves suffering in cancer and nonmalignant pain.

D. Veracity.
1. The use of a placebo for pain relief or to test for legitimacy of pain complaints abuses the relationship between the patient and caregiver and is indefensibly unethical.
2. Use of the placebo, even in cases of informed consent with research subjects, is coming under question.
3. It should be appreciated that all medications have a placebo effect as well as pharmacologic effect.

E. Justice: distribution of limited resources in a high-cost environment obligates the nurse to use the least costly method of relieving pain and to provide information regarding cost when discussing high-tech (PCA IV), costly modalities.

VI. PAIN MANAGEMENT

A. Goals of pain management.

1. Relieve pain, increase comfort.
2. Facilitate patient and family participation in recovery.
3. Increase function/ability to work or participate in activities of daily living.
4. Improve quality of life.
5. Promote a peaceful death.

B. Myths and barriers that hamper pain management (see Table 7.3).

1. Inadequate assessment or reassessment of pain.
2. Inadequate knowledge of pain management by both patients and health professionals.
3. Patient's reluctance to report pain due to fear of addiction.
4. Physician's reluctance to prescribe pain medication and nurse's reluctance to administer opioids.
5. Patient's fears of side effects.
6. Patient's and health professional's fear of addiction.
7. Lack of patient/health professional understanding that pain management is a right.
8. Institutional, procedural, and legal barriers.

C. Patients at risk for undermedication.

1. Females.
2. Children.
3. Elderly.
4. Minorities.
5. Cognitively impaired.
6. Chemically dependent.

D. Principles of pain management.

1. The person with the pain is the expert.
2. Perform a thorough pain assessment.
3. Believe the patient's report of pain.
4. Reassess after every change in dosage or drug and record the result.
5. Match the initial choice of drug to the intensity and type of pain.
6. Individualize the pain management plan to the patient.
7. Administer drugs orally whenever possible.
8. Use the simplest dosing schedule.
   a. Decrease number of pills.
   b. Increase patient compliance.
9. Avoid intramuscular (IM) administration because:
   a. IM injections hurt.
   b. IM drug absorption is not reliable.
10. Administer drugs around the clock (ATC) when pain is continuous (use patient-controlled analgesia [PCA] pumps when appropriate and available).
11. Give adequate doses; titrate to effect.
12. Give equianalgesic doses when changing from one medication to another, or from one route to another.
13. Increase opioid doses by percentages:
    a. Mild to moderate pain, 24%-50%.
    b. Moderate to severe pain, 50%-100%.
14. Make immediate release opioid available for break-through pain:
    a. 10%-20% of the 24-hour dose.
    b. Or, 1/4 to 1/3 of the 12-hour dose should be available every 1-2 hours.
15. Assess and plan for constipation for all patients receiving opioids.
16. NEVER use placebos to "test for pain."
17. Combine NSAIDs with opioids to decrease side effects and enhance opioids; the Agency for Healthcare Research and Quality (AHRQ) (formerly the Agency for Healthcare Policy and Research [AHCPR]) recommends combining NSAID and opioid for all postoperative pain unless contraindicated (see Tables 7.4 and 7.5).
18. Combine medications with non-drug interventions.
19. Combine analgesics for greater effect and fewer side effects than larger doses of a single medication. Examples:
    a. Acetaminophen + any other analgesic.
    b. Acetaminophen + any NSAID.
    c. Opioid + non-opioid (acetaminophen and/or NSAID) is recommended as a first choice for postoperative pain.
20. Recognize and treat side effects:
    a. Decrease opioid if possible.
    b. Try a different opioid.
    c. Use antiemetics.
    d. Note: respiratory depression is rare in people who have been receiving chronic opioid treatment.
21. AVOID meperidine: meperidine has a metabolite of nor-meperidine that lowers the seizure threshold.
22. When giving combination products, be aware of the ceiling dose of acetaminophen or NSAIDs.
23. Be aware of the development of physical dependence and prevent withdrawal.
24. Assume that surgery and other known-to-be-painful procedures will cause pain, and that pain has a negative impact on recovery.
25. COMMUNICATE the pain management plan to others; provide for continuity from one health care setting to another.

E. Management of pain in patients with addiction (see Table 7.6).

VII. ASSESSMENT

A. General concepts in assessing and managing patients in pain.

1. Pain is a subjective phenomenon with culturally-patterned, wide individual variations within the cultures. Assessment is necessary and valuable to:
   a. Help establish a diagnosis.
   b. Suggest intervention strategies.
   c. Follow progression or regression of a disease process.
   d. Promote communication between patient and health care provider.
   e. Assist in communication of a subjective experience into an objectively usable form.

Table 7.3
Pain Myths Across the Lifespan

Misconception	Fact	Special Considerations
Neonates-Preterm Infants 1. Nervous system is too immature to experience pain.	There is no evidence to confirm this and observation of neonates undergoing painful procedures or with known painful processes indicates this is not true.	Physiologic, paraverbal, and behavioral assessment is primary (e.g., Facial expressions and motor rigidity as well as crying).
2. Infants cannot safely be given centrally-acting analgesics.	Until about 1 month of age, clearance is delayed. Weight calibrated doses are necessary.	Frequent monitoring of vital signs. Use of neonatal pain scales.
Children 1. Children can tolerate more discomfort than adults.	Children under 4 years old have lower levels of endorphins. This suggests that the younger the child, the more pain is felt. Children may deny pain to avoid injections, be allowed privileges (playroom or going home), or to calm anxious parents.	Assessment as above plus: Preverbal child: 1. Use family's word for pain "ouchie" or "boo-boo." 2. Assessment tools useful (drawings of happy to screaming faces or cylinders "Empty to full with pain" as tools. Children can point to best descriptor of pain). 3. Observe changes in daily activity. Verbal Child: 1. Encourage verbalization by suggesting words to child. 2. Consult with parents about child's usual activity level.
2. Active children are not in pain.	Increased activity is frequently a sign of pain.	
Adolescents This age group cannot be trusted to report pain accurately.	May see medical or nursing personnel as authority figures and be reluctant to communicate for fear of being misunderstood. May need information about availability and appropriate use of pain management strategies.	This group can use standard pain assessment tools. Observe for inappropriate behavior (irritability/ withdrawal/ regression) and consult with parent about child's characteristic behavior as these may be signs of pain.
Adults 1. People often become addicted to narcotics while in the hospital.	Undertreatment of acute pain is a most common error. Tolerance and/or physical dependence may occur but can be managed by gradual withdrawal when painful process is alleviated. Addiction is a psychologic need for CNS active agents which predates an acute episode. Is not caused by analgesics.	"Clock-watching" is an indication of ineffective pain management.
2. Escalating doses will cause tolerance and eventual increase in side effects and can be dangerous.	Development of tolerance and side effects is widely individual. Respiratory depression is easily reversible with naloxone. Sedation may occur with elevation of dose but is usually transient, lasting a few days.	Monitor respiratory rate. Reaction to first doses of a narcotic is predictive of individual pattern of response.
3. Placebo responders do not have pain.	The fear of pain is a large component of the total pain experience. The patient's trust and confidence in the health care system and the individual health care provider is used inappropriately in placebo use.	The patient is to be believed.

Table 7.3 (continued)
Pain Myths Across the Lifespan

Misconception	Fact	Special Considerations
Elderly		
1. Older people must expect aches and pains.	Painful conditions are not part of the normal aging process and many common non-malignant processes are very painful but manageable. Use of trusted home remedies is often helpful.	The elderly are often reluctant to report because of cultural factors such as those encouraging stoicism or fear of rejection by youth-oriented society. Fear of drugs and addiction.
2. The elderly have less pain sensitivity.	This is not proven and this belief can increase anxiety and feelings of helplessness and loneliness in the elderly.	Change in activity patterns (giving up favorite activities, social occasions, etc.) are often most accurate indicators of pain in this group.
3. The elderly cannot tolerate centrally-acting medication.	Same principles apply through adulthood into very old age. Major difference: duration of analgesia (in the elderly, clearance may be delayed).	Dose must be titrated to effect. Start low and go slow. Usual starting dose 1/4 to 1/3 the usual starting dose.
4. Confusion postoperatively is due to the pain medication.	Confusion can be due to unrelieved pain.	Assume pain and trial pain relief measures.
5. Persons who can be distracted or can sleep do not have pain.	Distraction and sleep are coping mechanisms for some people.	Believe the patient's pain report and medicate around the clock.
6. Morphine is to be kept as a "last resort" – use should be avoided until later, and it has a toxic, lethal limited dosage.	Morphine can and SHOULD be used early in treatment. No dose ceiling for morphine exists.	Start low and go slow with the elderly. Titrate dose to effectively relieve pain with the least side effects.
7. It's best to wait as long as possible to get/take pain medication.	The longer the interval between doses, the more uncontrolled the pain.	Use around-the-clock dosages for best management. Use of long-acting opioids for chronic pain in the elderly most effective.

2. Factors affecting the degree of suffering.
   a. Cultural messages internalized by the patient are widely variable and influence pain behaviors.
   b. The health care provider's interpretation of pain.
      (1) Health care provider's socialization into the stoic mode regarding pain: the "silent sufferer."
      (2) Providers operate on principles of pain assessment.
         (a) Believing reports and other indicators of patients' pain.
         (b) An alternative is the belief that the provider knows when the patient has pain and needs medication.
      (3) Learned behavioral response to pain results from messages transmitted in the family milieu in which a child is socialized.
      (4) Self-awareness on the part of the caregiver of any personal biases regarding pain behaviors and the patient's orientation toward the experience of pain is essential to avoid stereotyping and misreading the patient's pain behaviors.
   c. Attributions of pain.
      (1) The process by which the patient consciously or unconsciously attributes the origin of pain to one of the following causes:
         (a) Benign (time-limited).
         (b) Malignant (life-threatening).
         (c) Disabling (lifestyle-threatening).
      (2) Example: patient misattributes acute back pain from a herniated nucleus pulposus to a tumor and presumes lifespan is now shortened.
      (3) Assess attributions and correct misinformation and/or encourage appropriate relief-seeking behavior.
         (a) Treat as a knowledge deficit.
         (b) Elicit the patient's underlying fears or suppositions.
   d. Meaning of pain.
      (1) The personalized interpretation of the

Table 7.4
Combining Analgesics

Acetaminophen + Any Other Analgesic = Acceptable Common Practice
Acetaminophen may be given along with any of the NSAIDs, opioids, or adjuvants.

Acetaminophen + NSAID = Acceptable, Common Practice
Acetaminophen may be given with any of the NSAIDs. Including acetaminophen usually adds analgesia without increasing side effects.

NSAID + NSAID = Not Recommended
This is not recommended. The additional pain relief is minimal and the risk of side effects is considerable.

Corticosteroid + NSAID = Caution
Prolonged administration of this combination increases the risk of side effects such as peptic ulcer.

Opioid + Nonopioid (Acetaminophen and/or NSAID) = Highly Recommended
Giving a nonopioid along with an opioid (either mu agonist or agonist-antagonist) is highly recommended. For all analgesic regimens, consider including a nonopioid, even if pain is severe enough to require an opioid. Many opioids given orally for mild to moderate pain, such as codeine and oxycodone, are compounded with a nonopioid, either aspirin or acetaminophen.

mu Agonist + Agonist-Antagonist = Rarely Appropriate
Very few situations exist when use of a mu agonist should be followed by an agonist-antagonist. This sequence may reverse analgesia of the mu agonist or precipitate withdrawal in a physically dependent patient. However, in an opioid-naive patient experiencing side effects such as itching or sedation from spinal opioids, nalbuphine is sometimes used to reverse these supraspinal side effects.

mu Agonist + mu Agonist = Usually Not Necessary
Few situations exist when more than one mu agonist should be administered to a patient. However, any or all of the mu agonists may be combined or given to the same patient. Side effects and analgesia simply will be additive.

Adjuvant + Opioid + Acetaminophen/NSAID = Often Appropriate for Chronic Pain, Sometimes Appropriate for Acute Pain
This combination may be very appropriate for a patient with chronic pain. (If the adjuvant analgesics provide a reasonably rapid onset of analgesia, this combination may be appropriate for acute pain.)

Adjuvant + Adjuvant = Sometimes Appropriate for Chronic Pain
An adjuvant from one group of drugs may be combined with an adjuvant from another group of drugs and is sometimes helpful in relieving chronic cancer pain or chronic noncancer pain. For example, there might be a patient who would benefit from a combination of all of the following: dexamethasone (Decadron®), a corticosteroid; dextroamphetamine (Dexedrine®), a psychostimulant, amitriptyline (Elavil®), a tricyclic antidepressant; and clonazepam (Klonopin®), an anticonvulsant.

May be duplicated for use in clinical practice. From McCaffery, M., & Pasero, C. (1999). *Pain: Clinical manual* (2nd ed., p. 116). St. Louis, MO: Mosby, Inc.

eventual consequences of pain.
(2) Example: to soldiers injured in battle, the injury may mean "a ticket home" and the pain may be almost a positive experience and possible subsequent disability relatively meaningless at the time of injury.

e. Diversional activities: distract patient from subjective discomfort.
f. Degree of stimulation of nociceptors.
   (1) Follows anatomic patterns.
   (2) There is not necessarily a direct relationship between nociception and suffering.
g. Psychologic state and traits.
h. Loss of work.
i. Physical disability.
j. Fear of death.
k. Financial concerns.
l. Social/familial functioning.

B. History.

1. The patient's reports or demonstrations of pain are the only essential criteria for the nursing diagnosis of pain.
2. Appropriate assessment strategies used correctly and consistently are necessary to assess varying characteristics of any pain.
   a. Intensity or severity of pain.
      (1) Numeric analog.
         (a) Patient is asked to score pain from 0-10, "0" means no pain and "10" means worst imaginable pain.
         (b) Individualized pain scales should be selected for patients in terms of age, cultural background, and medical condition.
         (c) Facilities should select a common pain scale (0-10 or 0-5) to use for the majority of patients so that pain and pain relief can be communicated to the health care team in a meaningful way.
      (2) Visual analog scale (VAS).
         (a) Patient is instructed to make an X on a horizontal or vertical (usually 10 cm long) line.
         (b) One end is identified as no pain and the opposite end as maximum imaginable pain.
      (3) Verbal analog: individual is asked to describe the pain by choosing from a list of verbal descriptors:
         (a) Simple: example is none, mild, moderate, severe.
         (b) Complex: example is McGill Pain Questionnaire and others where lists of descriptors are suggested for patients to select the most appropriate description of their experiences.
         (c) Verbal analogs presume a good grasp of the presenting language.
            i. Physical descriptors: aching, tingling, throbbing, burning, stab-

Table 7.5
Clinical Application of Balanced Analgesia

Definition of Balanced Analgesia
Balanced analgesia is a concept involving the continuous use of more than one method of controlling a patient's pain; continuous delivery of combined analgesic regimens. This may include more than one drug and more than one route of administration. Also referred to as multimodal (as opposed to unimodal) continuous analgesia. Usually refers to analgesia for acute pain, but the concept applies equally well to all other types of pain.

Clinical Examples of Balanced Analgesia
- Systemic NSAID = systemic opioid (ibuprofen PO + morphine PO)
- Systemic NSAID + epidural opioid and local anesthetic (ketorolac IV + fentanyl/bupivacaine epidurally)
- Local infiltration of anesthetic + systemic NSAID + systemic opioid (lidocaine infiltration of surgical site + ketorolac IV + IV PCA morphine)
- Regional block + systemic NSAID + epidural opioid and local anesthetic (epidural anesthetic during surgery; postoperatively epidural fentanyl/bupivacaine + ketorolac IV)

Examples of Improved Outcomes for the Patient with Acute Pain (Postoperative Pain or Trauma)
- Early ambulation
- Early enteral feeding
- Increased participation in recovery activities (coughing, physical therapy)
- Early discharge

May be duplicated for use in clinical practice. From McCaffery, M., & Pasero, C. (1999). *Pain: Clinical manual* (2nd ed., p. 120). St Louis, MO: Mosby, Inc.

bing, "electric shock."

ii. Affective descriptors: fearful, annoying, miserable, excruciating, cruel, etc.

(4) Children are presented with drawings of faces ranging from "happy face" to weeping face and asked to pick one that looks like they feel, or are shown pictures of a series of cylinders, or "glasses" empty to full with "pain" and asked to pick which one best shows their "glass of pain."

b. Location: "Where" it hurts on the visual analog "pain drawing?"

(1) Patient is presented with anterior and posterior views of silhouette drawings of the human figure. The silhouettes should be either androgynous or sex-appropriate for the patient.

(2) Patient is asked to mark on the drawing the location of the pain and sometimes the character of the pain. An example is one where a plus (+) sign shows aching and a negative (-) sign shows numbness/tingling.

(3) Patients usually relate well to this, finding it a satisfying way to communicate where it hurts, how it hurts, and (when combined with an intensity scale) how badly it hurts.

(4) Does not address the surface vs. deep aspect of pain locus, but this can be elicited by interview.

(5) Preverbal children can "point" to the pain on their own body or the drawing of the body.

c. Additional history data.

(1) Onset, duration of pain, and location of pain.

(2) Is pain intermittent or continuous?

(3) Pattern of exacerbations/remissions.

(4) Aggravating factors (position, fatigue, etc.).

(5) Alleviating factors: factors making the pain less intense, or better.

(6) Previous treatments and results.

(7) Functional capacity due to pain.

(a) The previous (pre-pain) level of functioning must be established.

(b) Lifestyle modifications necessary. The basic areas to be considered are:

i. Activities of daily living.

ii. Sexual functioning.

iii. Sleep.

iv. Work.

v. Leisure/sports.

vi. Interpersonal functioning.

vii. Appetite.

viii. Use of Brief Pain Inventory: asks patients to rate not only the pain and pain relief, but the impact of pain on their lives:

- Patients are asked to rate pain as worst, best, and average in last 24 hours.
- Interference with activity, mood, working ability, relations with other people, sleep, enjoyment of life are rated as well.

C. Physical examination.

1. Physical examination findings may be primary source in infants, developmentally delayed, demented, cognitively impaired, elderly, and chemically impaired individuals with a known or suspected painful process.
2. Findings on physical exam which are typically painful must be addressed, asked about.

a. Together with the patient:

(1) Select a pain assessment tool and teach the patient to use it.

(2) Note: patients may have more than one pain site and each should be evaluated and documented separately.

b. Assess pain with and without activity.

c. The least reliable parameters are physiologic vital sign changes. Though physiologic parameters of increased and decreased blood pressure may be indicative of acute pain close to onset, these

Table 7.6
Management of Pain in Patients with Active Addiction

General Guidelines That Apply to All Clinical Settings

1. If the patient acknowledges addiction or use of substances for nonmedical reasons, openly discuss this and encourage the patient to express any fears of how this may affect pain management and treatment by staff.
2. Accept and act on the patient's report of pain with appropriate assessment and treatment.
3. Aggressively manage pain: addiction treatment is not a priority when the patient has unrelieved pain.
4. Reassure the patient that staff is committed to providing aggressive and effective pain relief.
5. Develop with the patient a treatment plan for pain management. If feasible, provide the patient with a written copy.
6. Remind staff that (a) prescription of opioids to a known addict for the management of pain is not illegal, (b) persons with addictive disease may be relatively pain intolerant, and (c) that detoxification is an ineffective treatment for addictive disease.
7. Request consultation from an addiction specialist and a pain specialist so that both patient and staff know that support and guidance are available if needed.
8. Begin with nondrug or nonopioid analgesia. However, if pain relief is inadequate, add opioids. Begin with opioids when pain is moderate to severe.
9. If the patient is physically dependent on opioids, do not administer mixed opioid agonist/antagonists for analgesia (for example, nalbuphine) because withdrawal will be precipitated.
10. Assess patient's motivation for drug treatment; implement motivational interviewing strategies, and have treatment referral references on hand.

Inpatient Setting

1. Consider IV PCA as a method of administering opioid analgesics. PCA gives the patient more control and may reduce potentially confrontational interactions with staff. Monitor and adjust pump parameters because active addicts may require and safely receive larger doses than other patients.
2. For persons physically dependent on alcohol, sedative-hypnotics, or opioids, provide long-acting formulations of substitution medications to prevent emergence of withdrawal symptoms.
3. Monitor at least q4h for emergence of withdrawal symptoms from all drugs potentially abused by the patient, including alcohol, and treat aggressively and symptomatically.
4. When opioids are no longer needed for analgesia, taper them very slowly to minimize emergence of withdrawal symptoms; assess for presence of withdrawal symptoms at least q4h during analgesic taper; treat symptomatically.

Outpatient Setting

1. When opioid analgesics are required, select long-acting formulations such as transdermal fentanyl or controlled-release morphine. Less frequent dosing may increase the patient's adherence to the treatment plan. Also, drugs with a slow onset tend to have a low street value.
2. Administer analgesics ATC, giving the patient the specific times for taking medication, rather than saying "Three times a day."
3. Carefully document the treatment plan and provide the patient with a copy.
4. Provide the patient with whatever written information is available such as hours of operation, policies, methods of obtaining refills, and phone number(s), especially when the facility is not open.
5. At each visit, include the patient's analgesic use, pain severity and quality, level of function, and side effects. Record and discuss with the patient any behavior suggestive of inappropriate opioid use.

May be duplicated for use in clinical practice. From McCaffery, M., & Pasero, C. (1999). *Pain: Clinical manual* (2nd ed., p. 455). St. Louis, MO: Mosby, Inc

parameters must not be relied on for assessment.

d. All new pain must be evaluated, as it may be due to a complication (compartment syndrome or deep vein thrombosis).
e. Other areas of assessment include: are you experiencing any other symptoms (nausea, vomiting, diarrhea, constipation, itching, sleeplessness/confusion, urinary retention, or weakness)?
f. During all assessments, assess and document: (see Table 7.7).
   (1) Behavior changes.
   (2) Facial expressions.
   (3) Body language.
   (4) Other nonverbal cues.
g. All of the behaviors listed in Table 7.7 can be used to assess infants, the elderly, and cognitively-impaired patients.

3. Special population assessment.
   a. Elderly.
      (1) Establish a trusting, caring relationship that acknowledges suffering and demonstrates caring.
      (2) Content of assessing pain in the elderly is similar to that of younger individuals.
      (3) The amount of data collected must be adapted to meet the special needs of the elderly individual.
      (4) Strategies for pain assessment must be adapted for those with sensory, cognitive, or psychomotor deficits.
      (5) Behaviors indicative of pain in elderly (also those of preverbal children, Alzheimer's patients, withdrawn patients, and coma-

tose people) include:

(a) Facial expression.

(b) Motor activity or lack of; muscle rigidity/tension.

(c) Restlessness, guarding, etc.

(d) For suspected diagnoses, characteristic pains may be elicited. An example is straight leg raising test for lumbar radiculopathy.

(e) Vocalization (not necessarily verbal); may be crying out, moaning, etc.

(f) May use "proxy" pain ratings by family/familiar caregiver who knows the patient well and will interpret the behaviors, as they provide a caring relationship for the patient.

(6) Barriers to effective pain management in the elderly (see Table 7.8).

(7) Postoperative pain management in the elderly (see Table 7.9).

(8) Elderly patients need frequent assessment/reassessment of pain, and usually appreciate a scheduled approach to pain assessment and management.

b. Cognitively impaired patients.

(1) Self-report is still the most reliable indicator of pain; even patients with a substantial cognitive impairment may be able to use a pain rating scale.

(2) Repeat/reinforce use of a pain scale at least three times and allow patient enough time to respond.

c. Unconscious/comatose patients.

(1) DO NOT assume these patients are pain-free!

(2) If a reason exists to feel pain, a trial of analgesics can be diagnostic as well as therapeutic.

(3) If a patient who is unable to communicate needs a procedure known to be painful, treat the pain preemptively.

(4) Use of "proxy" pain ratings by family/friends who know the patient and his/her behavior well and can "interpret" behaviors and inform the staff.

Table 7.7
Behaviors Indicative of Pain

This list is a simple guide to behavioral assessment of pain in patients who are unable to provide a self-report of pain. It is not an exhaustive list.

Facial expressions: frown (wrinkled forehead), grimace, fearful, sad, muscle contraction around mouth and eyes.

Physical movements: restlessness, fidgeting, absence of movement, slow movements, cautious movements, guarding, rigidity, generalized tension (not relaxed), trying to get attention (beckoning someone).

Vocalization: groaning, moaning, crying, noisy breathing.

May be duplicated for use in clinical practice. From McCaffery, M., & Pasero, C. (1999). *Pain: Clinical manual* (2nd ed., (p. 95). St. Louis, MO: Mosby, Inc.

Table 7.8
Selected Barriers to Effective Pain Management in the Elderly

Barriers related to the elderly patient
- Fear of bothering, distracting, or angering caregivers.
- Belief that caregivers know pain is present and are doing all they can to relieve it.
- Hesitation to use unfamiliar equipment such as a patient-controlled analgesia pump.

Barriers related to the health care team
- Belief that elders cannot tolerate opioids.
- Persistent use of traditional as-needed IM injections.
- Belief that failure to express pain means absence of pain.
- Belief that pain perception decreases with age.

Barriers related to patient, family, and health care team
- Fear of addiction.
- Lack of understanding that pain management is a patient's right.
- Belief that pain is an inevitable consequence of aging, surgery, and hospitalization.
- Fear of side effects

Reprinted with permission: Ferrell & Ferrell. (1996). *Pain in the elderly* (p. 45). Seattle. WA: International Association for the Study of Pain.

VIII. NURSING DIAGNOSES, OUTCOMES, AND INTERVENTIONS

A. Coping, ineffective. Family coping, compromised.

1. Outcome.

a. Coping mechanisms are maintained.

b. Patient uses pain reduction strategies to decrease pain.

c. Patient will have the proper amount of exercise and rest.

2. Interventions.

a. Help patient recognize aggravating and alleviating factors.

b. Help patient and family determine if lifestyle modifications are necessary to control or relieve pain.

c. Teach patient physical, psychologic, and pharmacologic measures to control pain.

Table 7.9
Considerations in the Management of Postoperative Pain in the Elderly

• **Assume that surgery is painful and that pain will have a negative impact on recovery.** • **Use continuous multimodal, "balanced" analgesia.** ♦ Opioids with short half-life, but not meperidine. ♦ Acetaminophen and nonsteroidal anti-inflammatory drugs (NSAIDs) with short half-life. ♦ Local anesthetics (infiltrate wound, add to epidural opioid). • **Predict pain.** ♦ Consider preemptive analgesia. ♦ Use around-the-clock dosing, not as-needed (PRN). • **Use intravenous, intraspinal, or oral routes of administration, not intramuscular.** • **Use antiemetics (phenothiazines) only when indicated.** • **Supplement with nondrug methods.**

Reprinted with permission: Ferrell & Ferrell. (1996). *Pain in the elderly* (p. 47). Seattle, WA: International Association for the Study of Pain.

d. Emphasize communication among family members/supportive personnel as a coping strategy.
e. The use of alcohol and other self-medications (including over-the-counter pain medications) for pain control may be dangerous, especially when combined with prescription drugs. (See discussion of substance/chemical abuse presented earlier.)
f. Help the patient establish a balance between rest and activity as a strategy to minimize pain.
g. Allow patient as much control as possible and give choices in caregiving whenever possible.

B. Pain, chronic.
1. Outcomes.
   a. Patient decreased or relieved pain.
   b. Patient is able to identify factors that increase and decrease pain.
2. Interventions.
   a. Formation of a therapeutic partnership based on mutual trust is essential.
   b. Discuss appropriate pain strategies of pain management and provide information and advice.
   c. Help the patient choose among the alternative therapies and change these as pain needs change, and effectiveness is evaluated.
   d. Physical/nonpharmacologic.
      (1) Immobilization and support.
         (a) Support involved part.
         (b) Elevate injured part.
            i. Decreases vasocongestion/edema.
            ii. Prevents throbbing type pain, especially in extremities.
         (c) Immobilization of injured part: reduces pain by preventing further tissue damage.
      (2) Thermal interventions.
         (a) Cold application.
            i. Causes temporary slowing of neurotransmission.
            ii. Causes vasoconstriction and tends to inhibit swelling and inflammation.
            iii. In trauma, cold is used immediately to minimize swelling and acute pain.
            iv. Most effective when used for short periods (15-20 minutes) several times a day.
            v. Care must be taken to avoid thermal injuries.
         (b) Heat application.
            i. Causes temporary vasodilation, allowing increased blood flow to areas of vasoconstriction; facilitates removal of products of metabolism.
            ii. Comfort measure, as warmth is a reassuring quality.
            iii. Most effective when used for short periods (20-30 minutes).
            iv. Care must be taken to avoid thermal injuries.
         (c) Contraindications of the use of heat and cold applications.
            i. Patient history of orthostatic hypotension.
            ii. Over radiation therapy sites.
            iii. Allergy to cold (rare).
            iv. Patients with peripheral vascular disease.
            v. Decreased skin sensation in elderly.
      (3) Transcutaneous electrical nerve stimulation (TENS).
         (a) Device consisting of cutaneous stimulators connected to low voltage battery packs.
         (b) Useful in both acute and chronic pain.
         (c) Thought to work by competing with nociceptive impulses on the same conductive pathways.
      (4) Massage.
         (a) Comfort measure.
         (b) Hands-on technique which meets dependency/interactive needs.
         (c) Facilitates communication, relaxation, and stress reduction.
         (d) Relieves pain caused by muscle spasm if spastic muscle group is identified and skillfully massaged (except in areas where thrombus formation may be suspected.)
         (e) Contralateral massage: massage of opposite corresponding body part, especially effective with phantom limb pain.

(5) Assistive devices decrease stress on joints, decrease discomfort with ambulation.

e. Psychologic interventions.
  (1) Distraction.
    (a) Methods to divert attention from pain.
    (b) Examples of distraction are:
      i. Deep breathing during painful procedures.
      ii. Provision of television/radio/conversation/light reading/music.
      iii. Guided imagery.
  (2) Hypnosis (provided by a qualified health care provider).
    (a) Use in treatment of migraines, burns, terminal cancer, and severe pain or as appropriate for chronic orthopaedic conditions.
    (b) Self-hypnosis can be taught.
  (3) Therapeutic touch: transfer of energy from the person in the healing role to the person requesting/needing healing.
  (4) Relaxation techniques.
    (a) Especially helpful with anxiety/tension, which aggravates pain.
    (b) Breathing techniques combined with imagery is used.
    (c) Sleep does not necessarily mean the person is free of pain; rather it may be a mechanism for coping with pain.
    (d) Jaw relaxation.
      i. Let lower jaw drop down as if you were starting to yawn.
      ii. Rest your tongue in the bottom of your mouth.
      iii. Breathe slowly and evenly: inhale, exhale, rest.
    (e) Deep breathe/tense, exhale/relax, yawn for quick relaxation.
      i. Clench your fists and take a deep breath and hold it to the count of three.
      ii. Breathe out slowly and go limp.
      iii. Start to yawn.
  (5) Spiritual interventions.
    (a) Useful with patients who have a spiritual belief system.
    (b) Can provide a combination of distraction, relaxation, and quiet time.
  (6) Acupuncture (provided by a qualified health care provider).
    (a) Purpose of acupuncture is to restore equilibrium between yin and yang energy flows, to restore energy flow of the body to its proper rhythm.
    (b) May be used in conjunction with herbs, breathing, etc.
    (c) Western medical theory about acupuncture's effectiveness is that it stimulates endorphin production.
  (7) Imagery.
    (a) Cognitive strategy to alter the perception of pain.
    (b) Patient's focus may be on or away from the pain.
    (c) Biofeedback.
      i. Use of instrumentation to help patients monitor and increase their ability to influence psychophysiologic responses.
      ii. Used in combination with relaxation exercises for headache, low back pain, temporomandibular joint (TMJ) pain and other chronic pain syndromes.
      iii. Drawbacks: access to equipment and reimbursement issues.
  (8) Humor.
    (a) A method of pain management that was first proposed by Norman Cousins in 1976.
    (b) He reported anecdotally 2 hours free of pain after 10 minutes of laughter.
    (c) The use of laughter:
      i. Provides distraction.
      ii. Promotes communication with others and decreases loneliness (withdrawal from interaction is a common pain behavior).
      iii. Offers a method of coping with pain.
      iv Relaxes muscles, interrupting rigidity and spasm.
      v. Promotes endorphin production.
      vi. Stress relief.

IX. PRINCIPLES OF PHARMACOLOGIC MANAGEMENT

A. Individualize the regimen.

1. Consult World Health Organization (WHO) analgesic ladder for cancer/chronic pain relief.
2. Use pain scale to determine the step to begin.
   a. Step 1.
     (1) Addresses mild pain.
     (2) Nonopioid analgesic plus or minus an adjuvant analgesic (NSAID)
   b. Step 2.
     (1) Mild to moderate pain not relieved by a nonopioid.
     (2) Opioid for mild to moderate pain (Lortab®, Percocet®, Tylenol with Codeine No.3®, Vicodin®) plus or minus a nonopioid analgesic and/or adjuvant.
     (3) Note: if prescribing opioids, a stool softener/stimulator is needed to prevent constipation.

c. Step 3.
   (1) Moderate to severe pain.
   (2) Opioid for moderate to severe pain plus or minus a nonopioid, plus or minus an adjuvant.
   (3) Examples of opioids for moderate to severe pain: morphine, oxycodone, hydromorphone, fentanyl.
      (a) For chronic/cancer pain.
         i. Use of extended continuous/sustained release opioids is recommended, so that dosing intervals are more convenient.
         ii. When using extended/continuous/sustained opioids, teach patients not to chew, crush, or open the medication as this defeats the sustained release function.
         iii. Give these preparations at evenly spaced intervals (for example, every 12 hours).
      (b) Short half-life/("immediate release") opioids are used in combination with extended/continuous/sustained release opioids for breakthrough pain if/when needed, and should be ordered for "rescue dosing" whenever extended release opioids are used.
      (c) Recommended immediate release dosage in 10%-25% of the 24-hour sustained release dose, or 1/4 to 1/3 of the 12-hour dose.
      (d) Note: Use of > 2-4 doses of immediate release opioid in a 24-hour period indicates a need for reassessment of a potential increase in the 24-hour sustained release opioid dose.

3. Routes of administration.
   a. Oral route whenever possible.
      (1) Convenient.
      (2) Flexible.
      (3) Steady blood levels.
      (4) Can be patient-controlled analgesia by mouth.
   b. Intravenous (IV).
      (1) Quick onset of analgesia.
      (2) Candidates for IV route:
         (a) NPO patients.
         (b) Patients experiencing nausea/vomiting.
         (c) Patients who are unable to swallow.
         (d) Pre, intra, and postoperative patients.
         (e) Unconscious or cognitively-impaired patients.
      (3) Most frequent route used is patient controlled analgesia (PCA).
         (a) Bolus route.
         (b) Bolus and continuous infusion.
         (c) Continuous infusion.
   c. Subcutaneous.
      (1) Patient-controlled analgesia can be administered this way if no IV access.
      (2) Absorption is slower.
      (3) Dosage is the same as IV.
   d. Rectal.
      (1) Alternative route to oral used due to nausea/vomiting, inability to swallow, etc.
      (2) Dose varies, as does time for dose to be effective.
      (3) Sustained release products can be used rectally at approximately the same dosage as oral opioids.
      (4) Contraindicated in thrombocytopenic patients.
   e. Oral transmucosal.
      (1) Oral transmucosal fentanyl citrate (OTFC) used for conscious sedation, breakthrough pain. Use in the future possibly pre-procedural pain.
      (2) Preparation (Actiq®, looks like "candy" suckers) must be disposed of safely: watch opioid naive patients for oversedation.
   f. Buccal and sublingual:
      (1) Not often used.
      (2) Can be alternative route considerations.
   g. Transdermal.
      (1) Use in chronic pain:
         (a) Slow onset of action.
         (b) Takes 12-24 hours to provide adequate analgesia.
      (2) Difficult to titrate: use of immediate release opioid for breakthrough pain recommended.
      (3) Not for use in acute, or severe, increasing pain.
   h. Epidural.
      (1) Used for spine, thoracic, joint and major abdominal surgeries, for childbirth, and in children with cerebral palsy.
      (2) For acute pain, may be used as single or repetitive bolus, with or without continuous epidural by pump infusion, patient controlled analgesia (PCA).
      (3) For chronic pain, use of implanted infusion pumps, or external catheter and pump is becoming more frequent.
   i. Intramuscular (IM)
      (1) This route is to be AVOIDED.
      (2) Painful and can cause sterile abscesses of the muscle and soft tissue.
      (3) Can also cause damage to nerves if improperly administered.
      (4) Wide variation in dose absorption, thus ineffective in pain management either acute or chronic.
      (5) Most hospital patients have IV access.

4. Dosage.
   a. Titrate to effect to balance analgesia and side effects.
   b. Increase dose at onset/peak effectiveness of analgesic.

(1) Goal is to use the smallest dose that relieves the pain with the fewest side effects.
(2) Combination of opioids and NSAIDs most effective.

c. There is a ceiling on the analgesia provided by nonopioid and adjuvants. Tylenol® (acetaminophen) dosage limit is 4 grams (4,000 mg) in a 24-hour period.
d. There is *no* ceiling on the analgesia provided by mu-agonist opioids. Some cancer/chronic pain patients have had up to 40,000 IV units of morphine in 24 hours.

B. Optimize administration.

1. Stay ahead of the pain/pre-emptive analgesia.
2. Give analgesics *before* the last dose wears off.
3. ATC.
   a. ATC dosing is recommended for acute and chronic pain, such as postoperative pain.
   b. If pain is present > 12 hours per day, use ATC dosing.
   c. *Awaken patients at night* for their scheduled analgesic dose.
   d. Failure to awaken a patient for ATC dosing may cause an increase in pain as analgesic blood levels decrease.
4. PRN (*pro re nata*) equals "according to" or "as necessary."
5. PRN analgesics can be administered ATC if the patient is assessed to need analgesic intervention to control pain.
6. As pain decreases, assessment may indicate prn use.

C. Nurse's role.

1. Involve and teach patient and family about analgesic plan.
2. Titration of doses and dosage intervals.
3. Assessment and reassessment of pain level is essential.
4. Interdisciplinary pain management: clear communication between patient, nurse, physician, pharmacist, and family.
5. Assessment of the patient's pain with a standardized institution-wide pain tool. Use of pain logs and flow sheets.
6. Documentation in the patient record.
7. Assisting in establishing clinical guidelines for pain relief.
8. Persistence in attempting to achieve optimal pain management for all patients in pain/advocacy.
9. Provide for continuity of pain management.

D. Pharmacologic agents.

1. Peripheral-acting medicines: nonsteroidal anti-inflammatory drugs (NSAIDs) and Tylenol®, non-opioids.
   a. Anti-inflammatory, analgesic, and antipyretic in varying combinations.
   b. NSAIDs relieve pain by preventing production of prostaglandins. Prostaglandins are released from damaged cells and sensitize nociceptors to transmit pain impulses.
   c. Available as both over-the-counter and prescription preparations.
   d. Useful for pain in musculoskeletal system and postoperatively.
   e. Side effects include:
      (1) Physical effects.
         (a) Nausea.
         (b) Anorexia.
         (c) Gastritis.
         (d) GI bleeding.
         (e) Major GI bleeds are known to occur without any GI symptoms.
      (2) Can affect platelet aggregation: cause prolonged bleeding time and moderate elevation of partial prothromboplastin time (PTT).
      (3) Contraindicated for patients with chronic renal failure or aspirin allergy.
   f. Trial period of NSAIDs needed as individual patient response to NSAIDs varies (naproxen, piroxicam, indomethacin, ibuprofen).
   g. Cox-2 inhibitors.
      (1) Subset of NSAIDs and do not affect platelet aggregation.
      (2) Cox 2 specific drugs block the pain mediating prostaglandins at the Cox 2 receptor sites, but spare the Cox 1 inhibitors to release prostaglandin that protects the muscosal lining of the stomach.
      (3) Allergy to sulfa drugs prohibits some patients from use: example: Celebrex® (celecoxib).
      (4) Caution - watch brand names: Celebrex® sounds like Celexa® (citalopram), a psychiatric drug, and also like Cerebyx® (fosphentoin sodium), an anticonvulsant.
   h. Ketorolac (Toradol®).
      (1) Can be given orally, IV, or IM.
      (2) Used frequently as pre-emptive (pre-surgery) analgesia prior to orthopaedic procedures.
      (3) Not to be used > 5 days.
      (4) ATC dosage schedule most effective.
      (5) Use with opioid for best pain relief.
      (6) Dosing interval every 6 hours:
         (a) Maximum dose per day 40 mg orally and 120 mg IM/IV.
         (b) Usual IM/IV dose < 30 mg.
2. Central-acting mu-agonist opioid drugs. Block pain perception at the central nervous system level and block pain by bonding to receptor sites.
   a. Morphine sulfate is the "gold standard."
   b. Opioids used in moderate to severe pain of acute or chronic origin.
   c. Principle side effects:
      (1) Sedation.
      (2) Respiratory depression (rare with chronic use).
      (3) Pruritis.
      (4) Urinary retention.

Table 7.10
Naloxone Administration

1. Patients who require naloxone (Narcan®) usually meet all of the following criteria:
   - Unresponsive to physical stimulation
   - Shallow respirations or respiratory rate < 8 breaths/min.
   - Pinpoint pupils
2. Stop the administration of the opioid and any other sedative drugs. If given IV, maintain IV access.
3. Summon help. Ask a co-worker to prepare naloxone (see No. 4) and bring it to you. Remain with the patient and continue to attempt to arouse him/her.
4. Mix 0.4 mg (1 ampule) of naloxone and 10 ml of normal saline in a syringe for IV administration.
5. Administer the dilute naloxone solution IV very slowly (0.5 ml over 2 min) while you observe the patient's response (titrate to effect).
6. The patient should open his/her eyes and talk to you within 1-2 minutes. If not, continue IV naloxone at the same rate up to a total of 0.8 mg or 20 ml of dilute naloxone. If no response, begin looking for other causes of sedation and respiratory depression.
7. Discontinue the naloxone administration as soon as the patient is responsive to physical stimulation and able to take deep breaths when told to do so. Keep the syringe nearby. Another dose of naloxone may be needed as early as 30 minutes after the first dose because the duration of naloxone is shorter than the duration of most opioids.
8. Assign a staff member to monitor sedation and respiratory status and to remind the patient to deep breathe every 1-2 minutes until the patient becomes more alert.
9. Notify the primary physician and pain service. Document your actions.
10. Provide a nonopioid for pain relief.
11. Resume opioid administration at one-half the original dose when the patient is easily aroused and respiratory rate is > 9 breaths/min.

May be duplicated for use in clinical practice. From McCaffery, M., & Pasero, C. (1999). *Pain: Clinical manual* (2nd ed., p. 270). St. Louis, MO: Mosby, Inc.

NOTE: Table 7.10 provides the recommended titrate-to-effect procedure for administering naloxone (Narcan®) to reverse clinically significant respiratory depression. Giving too much naloxone or giving it too fast can precipitate severe pain, which is extremely difficult to control, and increase sympathetic activity leading to hypertension, tachycardia, ventricular dysrhythmias, pulmonary edema, and cardiac arrest. In physically dependent patients withdrawal syndrome can be precipitated; patients who have been receiving opioids for more than 1 week may be exquisitely sensitive to antagonists.

(5) Nausea and vomiting.
(6) Confusion/disorientation.
(7) Tolerance to opioid side effects develops before tolerance to opioids.

d. Examples of central-acting mu-agonist opioid drugs:
   (1) Pure mu-agonists: morphine sulfate, hydromorphone, meperidine, codeine.
   (2) Combination: opioid and NSAID: oxycodone, Vicodin® (hydrocodone bitartrate and acetominophen), Percodan® (oxycodone and aspirin), Percocet® (oxycodone and acetaminophen), and Darvocet-N 100® (propoxyphene napsylate and acetaminophen); synthetic: Ultram® (tramadol hydrochloride).
   (3) Exception:
      (a) There is no tolerance for constipation.
      (b) When administering opioids, it is good practice to also prescribe a stool softener/stimulant.

e. Meperidine has a dangerous metabolite, normeperidine, which accumulates in the body and causes side effects such as seizures, confusion, anxiety and hallucinations.
   (1) Darvocet-N100® (propoxyphene napsylate and acetaminophen) also has a metabolite that can cause similar symptoms.
   (2) Ultram® (tramadol hydrochloride) is not a pure mu-agonist, can cause severe nausea and vomiting, and needs slow titration.

f. As noted in the WHO analgesic ladder, combinations of peripherally-acting and centrally-acting analgesics and adjuvants may be used to manage pain.

g. Effects of opioids can be reversed with naloxone (Narcan®). Please refer to Table 7.10 for how to use Narcan®.

3. Antidepressants.
   a. Adjuvant analgesics used for chronic pain.
   b. Used to treat chronic pain because its use may delay in obtaining therapeutic serum levels.
   c. Have been shown to be effective in managing pain of arthritis, fibromyalgia, back pain, and neuropathic pain disorders.
   d. Antidepressant drugs are of two classes (tricyclic and "newer" antidepressants).
      (1) Tricyclic antidepressants
         (a) Tertiary amines examples are amitriptyline (Elavil®), clomipramine (Anafranil®), doxepin (Sinequon®), imipramine (Tofranil®).
         (b) Secondary amines examples: desipramine (Norpramin®) and nortriptyline (Pamelor®, Aventyl®).
      (2) Other antidepressants.
         (a) Effexor®, Desyerel®, Serzone®.
         (b) Selective serotonin reuptake inhibitors (SSRIs): Prozac®, Zoloft®, Paxil®.

(c) Tetracyclic: Ludiomil®.
(d) Aminoketone: Wellbutrin®.

4. Corticosteroids.
   a. Mechanism of action unknown and may decrease edema of damaged tissues to decrease pressure on pain nociceptors.
   b. Examples:
      (1) Prednisone.
      (2) Dexamethasone (Decadron®).
   c. Indications - used in:
      (1) Epidural injections.
      (2) Increased intracranial pressure.
      (3) Lymphedema.
      (4) Metastatic bone pain.
      (5) Neuropathic pain caused by infiltration or compression of peripheral nerves.
   d. Side effects:
      (1) Weight gain.
      (2) Increased blood pressure.
      (3) Osteoporosis.
      (4) Increased risk of infection.
      (5) Hyperglycemia.
      (6) Confusion.
      (7) Nausea and vomiting.
      (8) Abrupt cessation of steroid can increase pain severity.
5. $Alpha_2$: adrenergic agonists.
   a. Clonidine:
      (1) Used to treat:
         (a) Chronic headaches.
         (b) Reflex sympathetic dystrophy (RSD).
         (c) Chronic low back pain.
         (d) Neuropathic cancer pain.
         (e) Diabetic neuropathy.
         (f) Other neuropathic pain syndromes.
      (2) Side effects:
         (a) Sedation.
         (b) Decreased blood pressure.
      (3) Routes of usage:
         (a) Oral.
         (b) Transdermal.
         (c) Epidural.
   b. Anticonvulsant drugs:
      (1) Used for chronic lancinating (shooting) neuropathic pain.
      (2) Examples: Tegretol®, Neurontin®, Dilantin®, Klonopin®, Depakene®, and Baclofen®.
   c. Calcitonin:
      (1) Decreases bone pain, decreases rate of bone absorption/reabsorption (especially in osteoporosis).
      (2) Available in subcutaneous, IM, and nasal spray.
   d. Gallium nitrate:
      (1) An osteoclast inhibitor that may be used for malignant bone pain.
      (2) Further studies needed to prove effectiveness.
   e. Radiopharmaceuticals:
      (1) Used primarily for pain caused by metastatic bone disease.
      (2) Examples: phosphorus 32, strontium 89, samarium 153.
   f. Muscle relaxants:
      (1) Given by oral route.
      (2) Examples: Norflex®, Flexeril®, Robaxin®, Parafon Forte DSC®, and Soma Compound®.
   g. Benzodiazepenes:
      (1) Use for acute and chronic pain limited.
      (2) Used primarily for anxiety (short-term use) and conscious sedation.
   h. Topical analgesics:
      (1) Used in painful neuropathy syndromes (post-herpetic neuralgia), diabetic neuropathies) and osteoarthritis.
      (2) Examples: capsaicin (Zostrix®), EMLA® cream, lidocaine patches.
6. Muscle relaxants:
   a. Used in the treatment of musculoskeletal pain. (No evidence exists that skeletal muscle is actually "relaxed" in patients with muscle spasm or tension.)
   b. Best seen as alternatives to be used with opioid or nonopioid analgesics.
   c. Muscle relaxants are for acute short-term use only.
   d. Side effects:
      (1) Sedation, nausea, vomiting, dizziness, hallucinations, headache.
      (2) Safety tip: when helping patients to move or ambulate, use fall precautions.
   e. Examples are: Norflex® (orphenadrine), Flexeril® (cyclobenzaprine), Soma® (carisoprodol), Parafon Forte DSC® (chlorzoxazone), and Robaxin® (methocarbamol).
   f. Phenergan® (promethazine) and Vistaril® (hydroxyzine)
      (1) Often given erroneously in combination with opioid analgesics with the belief that they "potentiate" or make the opioid more effective, but there is no evidence to support this.
      (2) Studies show that promethazine actually increases pain sensitivity, and increases the amount of opioid needed to produce pain relief.
      (3) The doses of hydroxyzine needed to produce analgesia increase the risk of respiratory depression.
         (a) Hydroxyzine is not reversible by naloxone.
         (b) Hydroxyzine is also extremely irritating to tissue when injected, often producing a "burning" sensation.
7. Equianalgesic dosage (see Table 7.11).
   a. Use of conversion charts with equal analgesia dosage units for conversions from oral to IV, etc. Myth: IV route is more

Table 7.11
Equianalgesic Dose Chart

A Guide to Using Equianalgesic Dose Charts

- Equianalgesic means approximately the same pain relief.
- The equianalgesic chart is a guideline. Doses and intervals between doses are titrated according to individual's response.
- The equianalgesic chart is helpful when switching from one drug to another or switching from one route of administration to another.
- Dosages in this equianalgesic chart are not necessarily starting doses. They suggest a ratio for comparing the analgesia of one drug to another.
- The longer the patient has been receiving opioids, the more conservative the starting doses of a new opioid.

Opioid Mu Agonists	Parenteral (IM/SC/IV) (over 4 h)	Oral (PO) (over 4 h)	Onset (min)	Peak (min)	Duration (h)	Half-life (h)
Morphine	10 mg	30 mg	30-60 (PO) 30-60 (CR) 30-60 (R) 5-10 (IV) 10-20 (SC) 10-20 (IM)	60-90 (PO) 90-180 (CR) 60-90 (R) 15-30 (IV) 30-60 (SC) 30-60 (IM)	3-6 (PO) 8-12 (CR) 4-5 (R) 3-4 (IV) 3-4 (SC) 3-4 (IM)	24
Codeine	130 mg	200 mg NR	30-60 (PO) 10-20 (SC) 10-20 (IM)	60-90 (PO) UK (SC) 30-60 (IM)	3-4 (PO) 3-4 (SC) 3-4 (IM)	2-4
Fentanyl	100 g/h parenterally and transdermally 4 mg/h morphine parenterally; 1g/h transdermally morphine 2 mg/24 h orally	—	5 (OT) 1-5 (IV) 7-15 (IM) 12-16 h (TD)	15 (OT) 3-5 (IV) 10-20 (IM) 24 h (TD)	2-5 (OT) 0.5-4 (IV) 0.5-4 (IM) 48-72 (TD)	3-44 13-24 (TD)
Hydrocodone (as in Vicodin®, Lortab®)	—	30 mg NR	30-60 (PO)	60-90 (PO)	4-6 (PO)	4
Hydromorphone (Dilaudid®)	1.5 mg	7.5 mg	15-30 (PO) 15-30 (R) 5 (IV) 10-20 (SC) 10-20 (IM)	30-90 (PO) 30-90 (R) 10-20 (IV) 30-90 (SC) 30-90 (IM)	3-4 (PO) 3-4 (R) 3-4 (IV) 3-4 (SC) 3-4 (IM)	2-3
Levorphanol (Levo-Dromoran®)	2 mg	4 mg	30-60 (PO) 10 (IV) 10-20 (SC) 10-20 (IM)	60-90 (PO) 15-30 (IV) 60-90 (SC) 60-90 (IM)	4-6 (PO) 4-6 (IV) 4-6 (SC) 4-6 (IM)	12-15
Meperidine (Demerol®)	75 mg	300 mg NR	30-60 (PO) 5-10 (IV) 10-20 (SC) 10-20 (IM)	60-90 (PO) 10-15 (IV) 15-30 (SC) 15-30 (IM)	2-4 (PO) 2-4 (IV) 2-4 (SC) 2-4 (IM)	2-3
Methadone (Dolophine®)	10 mg	20 mg	30-60 (PO) UK (SL) 10 (IV) 10-20 (SC) 10-20 (IM)	60-120 (PO) 10 (SL) UK (IV) 60-120 (SC) 60-120 (IM)	4-8 (PO) UK (SL) 4-8 (IV) 4-8 (SC) 4-8 (IM)	12-190

Table 7.11 (continued)
Equianalgesic Dose Chart

Opioid Mu Agonists	Parenteral (IM/SC/IV) (over 4 h)	Oral (PO) (over 4 h)	Onset (min)	Peak (min)	Duration (h)	Half-life (h)
Oxycodone (as in Percocet®, Tylox®)	—	20 mg	30-60 (PO) 30-60 (CR)[9] 30-60 (R)	60-90 (PO) 90-180 (CR) 30-60 (R)	3-4 (PO) 8-12 (CR) 3-6 (R)	2-3 4.5 (CR)
Oxymorphone (Numorphan®)	1 mg	(10 mg R)	15-30 (R) 5-10 (IV) 10-20 (SC) 10-20 (IM)	120 (R) 15-30 (IV) UK (SC) 30-90 (IM)	3-6 (R) 3-4 (IV) 3-6 (SC) 3-6 (IM)	2-3
Propoxyphene (Darvon®)	—	—	30-60 (PO)	60-90 (PO)	4-6 (PO)	6-12
Agonist-antagonists Buprenorphine (Buprenex®)	0.4 mg	—	5 (SL) 5 (IV) 10-20 (IM)	30-60 (SL) 10-20 (IV) 30-60 (IM)	UK (SL) 3-4 (IV) 3-6 (IM)	2-3
Butorphanol (Stadol®)	2 mg	—	5-15 (NS) 5 (IV) 10-20 (IM)	60-90 (NS) 10-20 (IV) 30-60 (IM)	3-4 (NS) 3-4 (IV) 3-4 (IM)	3-4
Dezocine (Dalgan®)	10 mg	—	5 (IV) 10-20 (IM)	UK (IV) 30-60 (IM)	3-4 (IV) 3-4 (IM)	2-3
Nalbuphine (Nubain®)	10 mg	—	5 (IV) <15 (SC) < 15 (IM)	10-20 (IV) UK (SC) 30-60 (IM)	3-4 (IV) 3-4 (SC) 3-4 (IM)	5
Pentazocine (Talwin®)	60 mg	180 mg	15-30 (PO) 5 (IV) 15-20 (SC) 15-20 (IM)	60-180 (PO) 15 (IV) 60 (SC) 60 (IM)	3-4 (PO) 3-4 (IV) 3-4 (SC) 3-4 (IM)	2-3

May be duplicated for use in clinical practice. From McCaffery, M., & Pasero, C. (1999). *Pain: Clinical manual* (2nd ed., pp. 241-243). St. Louis, MO: Mosby, Inc

NOTE: Table 7.11 provides equianalgesic doses and pharmacokinetic information about selected opioid drugs.

Abbreviations:
ATC, around-the-clock; CR, oral controlled-release; h, hour; IM, intramuscular; IV, intravenous; g, microgram; mg, milligram; min, minute; NR, not recommended; NS, nasal spray; OT, oral transmucosal; PO, oral; R, rectal; SC, subcutaneous; SL, sublingual; TD, transdermal; UK, unknown.

potent than oral route – false.

b. Use of equianalgesic dosages increase the probability that dose route or drug changes will be accomplished without loss of pain control.

c. Equianalgesic dosing is:
   (1) Potency:
      (a) The intensity of the analgesic effect of the drug.
      (b) Example: morphine is more potent than meperidine as it takes only 10 mg of morphine to produce the same level of analgesia as meperidine 100 mg.
      (c) Because one drug is more potent than the other does not mean that it is more effective than the other.
      (d) All opioids (except codeine and propoxyphene) can attain the same level of effectiveness if given in the appropriate dose.
   (2) Equianalgesia: two doses are considered equianalgesic if they provide approximately the same amount of pain relief.

(3) When switching routes of drug delivery or changing to another opioid, consider the following questions:
(a) Is current medication the appropriate one?
(b) Is the current dose adequate?
(c) Is the current route appropriate?
(d) Is the current medication route appropriate?

X. ADMINISTRATION ROUTES

A. Oral route.

1. Scheduled ATC with rescue dose available for patients escalating or breakthrough pain.
   a. Provides consistent, serum steady state analgesia.
   b. Decreases anxiety and consequences of unrelieved pain.
   c. For acute/post-op/or chronic pain, use of long-acting opioid, with an immediate release (IR) opioid as a rescue dose.
2. PRN: least effective in acute pain situation when patient requests analgesia as pain is escalating; waits for dose to be administered, and then for analgesia to take effect.
3 Patient-controlled analgesia (PCA): patient self-administers oral opioid and maintains a record at the bedside.

B. Intramuscular.

C. Intravenous/subcutaneous PCA.

1. Effective for acute and chronic/cancer pain management when:
   a. Consistent serum analgesic concentration is needed.
   b. Parenteral route is necessary.
   c. Patient benefits by being in control.
2. Contraindications include:
   a. Sleep apnea.
   b. Cognitive inability to follow instructions to use PCA.
   c. Physical inability to access patient-administered dose device.
3. Advantages include:
   a. Ability to titrate to effect quickly.
   b. Maintain analgesic serum concentration especially with supplemental continuous infusion.
   c. Predictable absorption.
   d. Patient control.
4. Prescription includes:
   a. Medication and concentration.
      (1) Morphine sulfate.
      (2) Fentanyl.
      (3) Hydromorphone.
      (4) Meperidine (not recommended due to active metabolite nor-meperidine. Use > 48 hours not recommended).
   b. Loading dose(s) (boluses). If patient not comfortable, titrate increase to comfort.
   c. Mode: patient-administered (bolus) with or without continuous baseline infusion.
   d. Amount of patient-administered dose.
   e. Lockout interval (interval in which patient is unable to administer medication).
   f. Optional hourly or 4-hour cumulative dose limit.
5. Method.
   a. Selection.
      (1) Selecting a higher concentration (morphine 5 mg/ml rather than 1 mg/ml) decreases cost.
      (2) Uses nursing time more efficiently by decreasing the number of pump refills.
   b. Loading:
      (1) Doses must be adequate to achieve analgesia.
      (2) Doses given every 5 minutes are more effective than one large bolus dose.
   c. Addition of baseline infusion:
      (1) Promotes a steady-state during sleep and allows patient to achieve analgesia more quickly when awakened by pain.
      (2) Use of baseline/basal infusion requires more frequent assessment/reassessment for opioid-naive patients.
   d. Tolerance to opioids must be considered when determining analgesic dose.
      (1) Assess recent opioid history.
      (2) Question in pre-admitting or admitting data to help determine opioid dosage requirements.
   e. Patient must be assessed and reassessed:
      (1) Determine effective lockout interval for effective analgesia.
      (2) Use pharmacologic half-life of opioid used to determine lockout intervals.
   f. Hourly and 4-hour limits are encouraged as a safety feature.
      (1) Time limits may artificially limit the patient's ability to achieve or maintain analgesia when doses have been prescribed inadequately.
      (2) When limit is being reached consistently and analgesia is inadequate, consider increasing patient-administered dose and increasing or eliminating hourly or 4-hour limit.
   g Nurse/family controlled PCA administration: if patient is unable to administer PCA, dosages can be ordered ATC and administered by the RN or designated family member.
6. Patient education.
   a. Include family in patient teaching.
   b. Patient right to adequately relieve pain.
   c. Addiction rate is < 1% in patients using opioids for pain control.
   d. No one except the patient should press the button.
      (1) Nurse/family controlled PCA administration: if patient is unable to administer PCA.

(2) Dosages can be ordered ATC and administered by the RN or designated family member.

e. Assure that patient knows how PCA works, why it is effective, how to access doses, when to administer them, and side effects to report.

f. Teach patient to report any "new" or unrelieved pain.

g. Children who have attained the developmental level to operate the button and understand its use can use PCA.

h. Recommended patient assessment parameters for PCA include:

(1) Vital signs, especially respiratory rate.

(2) Use of a 0-10 pain scale.

(3) Use of a sedation scale.

(4) Frequent assessment/reassessment of pain level, and pain relief versus side effects.

(5) Refer to individual institution policy and procedure for assessment intervals.

i. Contraindications to PCA.

(1) Inability to press button or understand how PCA works.

(2) Unconscious, cognitively-impaired patients.

7. PCA safety issues.

a. Two RNs are required to set up and program the PCA pump and to check dosage and parameters.

b. These nurses need to be certified yearly to set up and program PCA pumps, and to set dosages and parameters.

c. Only the patient is to press the PCA button unless previous arrangements have been made. For example: the nurse or a responsible family member who has been taught about PCA may administer the doses.

D. Epidural analgesia.

1. Definition.

a. Administration of opioids and/or local anesthetic agents through an epidural catheter into the epidural space for acute/chronic/cancer pain when oral and parenteral routes are inappropriate or ineffective.

b. Analgesia is from the catheter insertion site down.

2. Contraindications include:

a. Coagulopathy.

b. Infection.

c. Immunosuppression.

d. Institutional restrictions.

e. Lack of patient/family willingness or resources to continue self-care at home when long-term analgesia is required by this route.

f. Difficult or contraindicated catheter placement.

3. Complications.

a. Epidural hematoma.

(1) Can occur following catheter insertion/removal.

(2) Require emergency decompression to prevent permanent deficits of paraplegia.

(3) Symptoms: increased unexplained constant back pain coupled with sensory and motor deficits.

b. Neurologic impairment:

(1) Occurs if catheter migrates to cerebrospinal fluid.

(2) NOT a common complication.

(3) Can result in hypotension, paraplegia, or respiratory depression.

c. Infection:

(1) Rare.

(2) Use strict aseptic technique during insertion and administration of medications.

d. Urinary retention:

(1) Monitor patient's ability to urinate.

(2) May need intermittent or Foley catheterization, or a decrease in local anesthetic concentration to lessen blockade of motor and sensory bladder nerves.

e. Nausea and vomiting: decreased concentration of opioid.

f. Hypotension/orthostatic hypotension:

(1) Result of sympathetic nerve blockade by epidural local anesthetics.

(2) If it occurs, bolus of 200-400 ml of crystalloid IV solution can be administered.

(3) Keep ephedrine, etc. available in the clinical area.

4. Advantages include:

a. Ability to titrate to effect quickly.

b. Long duration of opioid analgesia.

c. Selective effect of local anesthetic (LA).

d. Side-effect profile.

e. Minimal sedation.

f. Retention of cough reflex.

g. Earlier ambulation.

h. Decreased incidence DVT.

i. Increased gastrointestinal(GIT) motility.

5. Physician orders include:

a. Medication(s) and concentration(s).

(1) Opioids.

(a) Morphine sulfate.

(b) Fentanyl.

(c) Hydromorphone.

(d) Meperidine (see X. Administration Routes, C. Intravenius/subcutaneous PCA).

(e) Sufentanil.

(2) Local anesthetics.

(a) Lidocaine.

(b) Bupivicaine.

(c) Ropivicaine.

(c) Other: clonidine.

b. Continuous infusion rate of administration or intermittent administration dose and time interval.

c. Patient-administered dose and interval, if applicable.

d. Monitoring/assessment for opioids:

(1) Pain scale and patient rating.

(2) Sedation scale.
(3) Respiratory rate.
(4) Blood pressure.
(5) Motor and sensory function if local anesthetic used.
(6) See table for sample nursing guidelines for care of patient receiving epidural anesthesia.

e. Side-effect management.

6. Method.
a. The epidural catheter is inserted using aseptic technique percutaneously into the epidural space, covered with a transparent dressing and taped securely to the patient's back. (Correct catheter placement is determined by the anesthesia care provider.)
b. When preemptive analgesia is used, opioid is administered as surgery begins; the catheter also may be used to provide anesthesia during surgery.
c. The continuous infusion is typically initiated in the postanesthesia recovery unit (PACU).
d. Because the catheter is not sutured into place, frequent inspection of the dressing is necessary with assessment of the insertion site for redness, swelling, drainage, and tenderness.
e. For long-term analgesia:
(1) The epidural catheter can be permanently implanted with subcutaneous tunneling to the anterior lower abdomen for easy access.
(2) Use of a pain pump, or port with a refillable reservoir is the usual method of analgesia.
f. Tolerance to opioids must be considered when determining analgesic dose: the low dose of epidural opioid used to provide postoperative analgesia may not meet systemic requirements in the opioid-tolerant individual.

7. Safety issues for epidural analgesia.
a. Two nurses are required to program epidural pumps and to check dosage and parameters.
b. These nurses need to be certified yearly to set up and program epidural pumps and to set dosages and parameters.
c. Only one MD is to be responsible for all epidural orders on a patient, and standing orders need to be written per institution policy and procedure.
d. No other analgesics, hypnotics, or sedatives in addition to the epidural dosage are to be administered unless written by the MD responsible for the infusion.
e. Have an external pump dedicated to epidural infusion. If the pump is used for other infusions, it must be labeled clearly to avoid errors.

8. Patient education.
a. Include family in patient teaching.
b. Explain:
(1) How epidural analgesia works.
(2) Why it is effective.
(3) How to access doses (intermittent bolus administered by anesthesiologist, nurse, or patient-administered dose).
(4) What to expect when local anesthetic is used (numbness and weakness).
c. Teach patients to report side effects.
(1) Itching.
(2) Urinary retention.
(3) Nausea and vomiting.
(4) Constipation.
(5) Headache.
d. Teach patients to report ineffective analgesia or any "new" pain.

E. Regional analgesia.

1. Epidural steroid injection.
a. Usually used for pain treatment in patients with lower back and leg pain.
b. Method:
(1) Sterile preparation of the posterior lumbar site.
(2) Local anesthetic used to numb the site.
(3) Epidural needle then placed into the epidural space.
(4) A corticosteroid, or corticosteroid/local anesthetic solution is then injected.
c. Solution is used to bathe the spinal nerves and nerve roots to try and decrease swelling and inflammation.
d. Patient response may vary:
(1) Some may need as many as three injections in 2 week intervals.
(2) Some patients need only one injection for relief.
(3) For some patients, it doesn't work, and pain may increase.
(4) Only three injections per year is the usual "rule of thumb."
e. Nursing considerations: what to report.
(1) Diabetic patients' blood sugars may increase due to steroid use.
(2) Steroids can cross the placenta, so are contraindicated during pregnancy.
(3) Any changes in motor or sensory function post-injection.

2. Nerve blocks.
a. Local anesthetic solution is injected into a major nerve trunk. Produces both sensory and motor blockade.
b. Common types: brachial plexus: used for procedures involving the upper extremities.
c. Three approaches:
(1) Interscalene.
(a) Used for shoulder and arthroscopy procedures or chronic pain syndromes of upper extremities.
(b) Assess carefully for breath sounds post-procedure due to proximity of injection site to lungs.
(2) Supraclavicular.

(a) Used for chronic pain syndromes/procedures of lower arm contracture release or tendon repairs.
(b) Supraclavicular not often used due to increased potential for pneumothorax.
(3) Axillary.
(a) Same indications as supraclavicular.
(b) Less chance of pneumothorax.
(4) Femoral blockade – used for knee chronic pain/procedures of the knee.
(5) Ankle blockade.
d. Post-procedure assessment.
(1) Assess patient for:
(a) Return of neuromuscular function and sensation.
(b) Chronic pain.
(c) Amount of pain relief obtained.
(2) Hematoma formation at injection site. This is an emergency and needs immediate response.
(3) Possible allergic reactions/airway obstruction.
(4) Monitor vital signs and level of consciousness.
(5) Signs and symptoms of toxicity:
(a) First affect the CNS and then the cardiovascular system.
(b) Watch for drowsiness, restlessness, slurring of speech, muscular twitching, convulsions.
(c) Hypotension, bradycardia, heart block, and cardiac arrest can occur.
(6) Get oral analgesia on board BEFORE the block wears off.

3. Bier block – anesthesia commonly used for orthopaedic below the knee or elbow procedures.
a. Tourniquet applied to extremity being operated on at pressures > arterial flow.
b. Tourniquet time must be > 30-40 minutes to allow local anesthetic to be metabolized prior to being released into systemic circulation (toxic reactions can result); and no more than 90 minutes to prevent ischemic damage to the limb.
c. Assess for return of normal color, sensation, and capillary refill time.

F. Local anesthetic infusions.

1. Process.
a. Disposable spring-loaded 100 cc syringe filled with local anesthetic; can be a bulb syringe.
b. Set to infuse from 0.5 ml to 2 ml an hour into postoperative surgical site to assist in pain management.
2. Nursing considerations follow those of regional blocks.

G. Implantable long-term analgesia pumps.

1. Administration:
a. Implanted in subcutaneous pockets in the abdomen or side and provide continuous or intermittent infusion of preservative free opioid, opioid/local anesthetic.
b. Or adjuvant (clonidine) to provide a continuous and constant means of pain relief.
c. Patient will still require an immediate-release opioid/preparation for breakthrough pain to be prescribed.
2. Candidates include:
a. Chronic pain unsuccessfully treated with analgesic therapy.
b. Pain not appropriate for neurosurgical procedures.
c. Pain decreased midcervical dermatome.
d. Life expectancy greater than a few months.
3. Drawback.
a. Expensive for pump, drugs, and procedure.
b. Ability of patient and/or family to take on responsibility of care.
4. Safety.
a. Patient must notify Radiology prior to MRI that pump is in place.
b. Patient needs to know how to tell pump that needs to be refilled and how to troubleshoot problems.
c. Nursing role is to teach patient and family how to live with and manage pump. The nurse is a resource person.
d. Nurse must be certified to work with implanted pumps:
(1) Nurse most often refills reservoir.
(2) Nurse alters pump parameters with orders from prescribing physician
e. If patient expires, the pump alarm needs to be disabled.

XI. CONSCIOUS SEDATION

A. Purpose: provide safe and effective analgesia for patients during painful diagnostic/therapeutic procedures.

B. Definition: combinations of pharmacologic agents (Versed®, an amnesic drug given with morphine, an analgesic drug) given by one or more routes to minimally depress consciousness:

1. Provides satisfactory analgesia.
2. Allows the patient to maintain his/her airway.
3. Allows patient to respond to verbal commands and physical stimulation.

C. Goals.

1. Maintains consciousness.
2. Maintains own airway.
3. Can swallow and gag.
4. Responds to commands/stimulation.
5. Decrease anxiety and fear.
6. Pain relief acceptable.
7. Vital signs stable.
8. Patient cooperative through procedure.
9. Has amnesia through procedure.
10. Recovers safely

D. Medications.

1. Opioid analgesics.
a. Morphine sulfate.

b. Hydromorphone (Dilaudid®).
c. Fentanyl (Sublimaze®).
d. Meperidine (Demerol®).
2. Antianxiety/amnesic/muscle relaxants.
a. Versed® (midazolam).
b. Ativan® (lorazepam).
c. Valium® (diazepam).

E. Administration.

1. Continuously observe and document patient response blood pressure, respiratory rate, and O_2 saturation every 5 minutes.
2. Assess level of consciousness and mental status, skin color and condition, pain status every 5 minutes.
3. Maintain IV access
4. Observe institutional conscious sedation protocol.
5. 1:1 nurse/patient ratio for safety.

F. Post-procedure.

1. Continue to monitor vital signs, level of consciousness, pain level every 10-15 minutes for at least 1 hour after last drug given.
2. Inform MD if changes in vital signs or adverse responses.
3. Discharge criteria.
a. 1 hour has passed since last dose of sedative or analgesic.
b. Patient alert and oriented x3.
c. Vital signs stable.
d. O_2 saturation 95% or above.
e. Pain controlled.
f. Able to move/ambulate.
g. Responsible adult to drive patient home, and stay with patient for at least 2-3 hours, 24 hours if possible.
h. Review any/all discharge instructions per physician with the patient and family/caregiver.
i. Instructions for follow-up care and telephone contact numbers.
j. No major decision making for 24 hours.

XI. SPECIAL POPULATIONS

A. Individuals in special populations historically are undertreated for pain.

1. Cognitively-impaired patients.
2. Individuals with impaired communication (such as speak another language or deaf).
3. Conscious but unable to speak.
4. Individuals with a substance abuse history.
5. Previous long-term use of opioids.
6. Individuals at the extremes of the age distribution.

B. Pain in the elderly.

1. Review of the aging process:
a. Loss of weight.
b. Decrease total body water.
c. Decrease lean body mass.
d. Increase body fat.
e. Decrease small bowel surface area.
f. Decrease liver metabolism.
g. Memory and sensory impairment.
2. General medication use guidelines:
a. Make dosage adjustments.
b. When using opioids, "start low and go slow."
c. Titrate to effect.
(1) Start at 1/3 to 1/2 the usual adult dosage.
(2) Watch for polypharmacy, simplify drug regimen.
(3) Monitor for side effects.
3. Pain myths regarding the elderly (see Table 7.3).
a. Pain is a natural outcome of growing old: false. Pain is not an inevitable result of aging.
b. Pain perception decreases with age: false. There is no scientific basis for this.
c. If the elderly person doesn't report pain, they're not in pain: false. Patient could be feeling "don't want to bother/worry anyone."
d. Opioids are too "strong" to relieve pain in the elderly: false. Use a lower dose, start low, go slow, and titrate to effect.
e. Alzheimer's and cognitively-impaired elderly do not feel pain, and their reports are not to be believed: false. Assessment of these patients IS possible.
(1) Accept their report of pain, and treat it as you would a report from a non-cognitively impaired patient.
(2) Make at least three consistent attempts to use a pain scale.

C. Pain in children.

1. Insufficient treatment of pain in infants and children results from misconceptions and inadequate pain knowledge by medical staff.
2. Pain myths.
a. Infants are incapable of feeling pain: false. Data collected over the past 10-15 years support the fact that infants have the capacity for pain at birth.
b. Infants are not as sensitive to pain as children and adults: false (See above). Data support the fact that premature infants have an increased sensitivity to pain.
c. Infants are incapable of expressing their pain: false. Infants can verbalize their pain, and changes in facial expressions and behaviors are also indicators of pain.
d. Infants can't remember pain: false. Studies support evidence that past pain experiences influence present pain responses, thus emphasizing the need for good pain management throughout life.
e. Opioids and anesthetics can't be safely given to infants due to their inability to metabolize and eliminate drugs and their sensitivity to respiratory depression: false. If pharmacodynamics of analgesics are understood by the health professional and the infant is closely monitored in a setting where resuscitation is immediately available, analgesics can safely be administered for pain management of the infant.
3. Use of pediatric/neonatal pain scales which monitor behavior/facial expression.

D. Cognitively-impaired patients: unable to provide a self-report of pain.

1. Use behavioral assessment.
   a. Facial expressions:
      (1) Frown.
      (2) Sad expression.
      (3) Grimacing.
      (4) Fearful expression.
   b. Vocalizations:
      (1) Crying.
      (2) Moaning.
      (3) Groaning.
      (4) Noisy breathing.
      (5) Sighing.
   c. Physical movement:
      (1) Restless.
      (2) Confused.
      (3) Fidgeting.
      (4) Guarding of body parts.
      (5) Tension.
      (6) Rigid muscles.
      (7) Beckoning motions (trying to get attention).
2. Treat these patients comparatively as you would a non-cognitively impaired patient.

Bibliography

Agency for Health Care Policy and Research (AHCPR). (1992). *Acute pain management in infants, children, and adolescents: Operative and medical procedures.* AHCPR Publication No. 92-0020. Rockville, MD: U.S. Department of Health and Human Services.

Agency for Health Care Policy and Research (AHCPR). (1992). *Acute pain management operative or medical procedure and trauma.* AHCPR Publication No. 92-0032. Rockville, MD: U.S. Department of Health and Human Services.

Agency for Health Care Policy and Research (AHCPR). (1994). *Management of cancer pain.* AHCPR Publication No. 94-0592. Rockville, MD: U.S. Department of Health and Human Services.

American Academy of Pain Medicine and the American Pain Society. (1996). *Consensus statement: The use of opioids for the treatment of chronic pain.* Glenview, IL: American Academy of Pain Medicine and American Pain Society.

American Geriatrics Society. (1998). *Clinical practice guidelines: The management of chronic pain in older persons (pp. 635-651).* New York: The American Geriatrics Society.

American Pain Society (APS). (1999). *Principles of analgesic use in the treatment of acute and cancer pain (4th ed).* Glenview, IL: APS.

American Pain Society (APS). (1995). Quality improvement guidelines for the treatment of acute pain and cancer pain. *JAMA, 274*(23), 1874-1880.

American Society of Anesthesiologists Task Force on Pain Management, Chronic Pain Section (1997). Practice guidelines for chronic pain management. *Anesthesiology, 86*(4), 995-1004.

American Society of Pain Management Nurses (ASPMN). (1996). *ASPMN position statement: Use of placebos for pain management.* Pensacola, FL: ASPMN.

ASRA: Neuaxial anesthesia and anticoagulation consensus statements (2000). [On-line]. Available: www.asra.com/consensus/page5.shtml.

Auvil-Novak, S.E. (1999). The chronobiology, chronopharmacology, and chronotherapeutics of pain. *Annual Review of Nursing Research, 17,* 133-53.

Baltes-Messner, J., Van Den Largenberg, B., Koberstein, H., & Hollman, G. (1999). Pediatric sedation: The art and science. *Orthopaedic Nursing, 18*(5), 35-50.

Bieri, D., Reeve, R., Champion, G., et al. (1990). The faces pain scale for the self-assessment of the severity of pain experienced by children: Development and initial validation, and preliminary investigation for ratio scale properties. *Pain, 41,* 139-150. Amsterdam, The Netherlands: Elsevier Science NL.

Billig, T., & Weaver, K. (1997). Individualized doll therapy with children experiencing limb loss. *Orthopaedic Nursing, 15*(6), 50-55.

Borsook, D., LePel, A.A., & McPeek, B. (1996). *The Massachusetts General Hospital handbook of pain management.* Boston, MA: Little, Brown & Co.

Buck, M., & Paice, J.A. (1994). Pharmacologic management of acute pain in the orthopaedic patient. *Orthopaedic Nursing, 13*(4), 14-23.

Carey, S.J., Turpin, C., Smith, J., Whately, J., & Haddox, D. (1997). Improving pain management in an acute care setting. *Orthopaedic Nursing, 16*(4), 29-36.

Crutchfield, J., Zimmerman, L., Nieveen, J., Barnason, S., & Pozehl, B. (1996). Preoperative and post-operative pain in total knee replacement patients. *Orthopaedic Nursing, 15*(2), 65-72.

Cunningham, M.E. (1996). Becoming familiar with fibromyalgia. *Orthopaedic Nursing, 15*(2), 33-36.

Curtiss, C., & Schneider, J. (1999). How to improve outcomes in management of chronic pain: New directions for the use of opioids. *The Journal of Care Management,* 3-15.

Faries, J. (1998). Easing your patients' post-operative pain. *Nursing, 98,* 58-60.

Faucett, J. (1999). Chronic low back pain: Early interventions. *Annual Review of Nursing Research, 17,* 155-82.

Federation of State Medical Boards of the United States, Inc. (1998). *Model guidelines for the use of controlled substances for the treatment of pain (pp. 1-4).* Euless, TX: Federation of State Medical Boards of the United States.

B.R. Ferrel, & B.A. Ferrell. (1996). *Pain in the elderly.* Seattle: IASP Press.

Gianino, J.M., York, M.M., & Paice, J.A. (1996). *Intrathecal drug therapy for spasticity and pain.* New York: Springer.

Gordon, D.B., Dahl, J.L., & Stevenson, K.K. (1996). *Building an institutional commitment to pain management.* Madison: University of Wisconsin.

Gordon, D.B. (1998). Assessment and management of pain. In A.B. Maher, S.W. Salmond, & T.A. Pellino. *Orthopaedic nursing (2nd ed., pp.115-144).* Philadelphia: W.B. Saunders.

Halvorsen, P.B. (1999). Nonsteroidal anti-inflammatory drugs: Benefits, risks and Cox-2 selectivity. *Orthopaedic Nursing, 18*(6), 21-27.

Herr, K.A., Mobily, P.R., Kohout, F., & Wagennar, D. (1998). Evaluation of the faces pain scale for use with the elderly. *Clinical Journal of Pain, 14*(1), 29-38.

Johnson, J., Smith-Temple, J., & Carr, P. (1998). *Nurses guide to home health procedures.* Philadelphia: Lippincott.

Joint Commission on Accreditation for Health Care Organizations (JCAHO). (2000). *Standards for pain management.* Washington, DC: JCAHO.

Kester, K. (1997). Epidural pain management for the pediatric spinal fusion patient. *Orthopaedic Nursing, 16*(6), 55-62.

Kingery, W.S. (1997). A critical review of controlled clinical trials for peripheral neuropathic pain and complex regional pain syndromes. *Pain, 73*(2), 123-39.

Kost, M. (1998). *Manual of conscious sedation.* Philadelphia: W.B. Saunders Company.

Loeb, J.L. (1999). Pain management in long-term care. *American Journal of Nursing, 99*(2), 48-52.

Ludwig-Beymer, P. (1989). Transcultural aspects of pain. In J.S. Boyle & M.M. Andrews (Eds.), *Transcultural aspects of pain.* Glenview, IL: Little, Brown College Division, Scott Forsman & Co.

McCaffery, M., & Pasero, C. (1999). How can we improve the way we perform our pain assessments to meet the needs of patients from diverse cultures? *American Journal of Nursing, 99*(8), 18.

McCaffery, M., & Pasero, C. (1999). *Pain: Clinical manual, 2nd ed.* St. Louis, MO: Mosby, Inc.

McCaffery, M., & Vourakis, C. (1992). Assessment and relief of pain in chemically dependent patients. *Orthopaedic Nursing, 11*(2), 13-26.

Medical College of Wisconsin (1998). *Improving pain management in long-term care settings, palliative care program.* Milwaukee: Medical College of Wisconsin.

Miller, E.H., Belgrade, M.J., Cook, M., Bauman Portu, J., Shepherd, M., Sierzant, T., Sallman, P., & Fraki, S. (1999). Institution-wide pain management improvement through the use of evidence-based content, strategies, resources, and outcomes. *Quality Management in Health Care, 2,* 28-40.

Moore, R., & Brodsgaard, I. (1999). Cross-cultural investigations of pain. In I.K. Crombie, P.R. Croft, S.J. Linton, L. Resche, & M. Von Korff (Eds.), *Epidemiology of pain (pp. 53-79).* Seattle: International Association for the Study of Pain Press.

Neitzel, J.J., Miller, E.H., Shepherd, M.F., & Belgrade, M. (1999). Improving pain management after total joint replacement surgery. *Orthopaedic Nursing, 18*(4), 37-45.

Oerlemans, H.M., Oostendorp, R.A., de Boo, T., Perez, R.S., & Goris, R.J. (1999). Signs and symptoms in complex regional pain syndrom type I/reflex sympathetic dystrophy: Judgment of the physician versus objective measurement. *Clinical Journal of Pain, 15*(3), 224-32.

Paice, J.A. (1991). Unraveling the mystery of pain. *Oncology Nursing Forum, 18*(5), 843- 849.

Pascarelli, P. (1996). The role of the nursing during intravenous conscious sedation. *Orthopaedic Nursing, 15*(6), 23-25.

Pasero, C. (1999). *Self-directed learning program: Epidural analgesia for acute pain management.* Pensacola, FL: ASPMN.

Pasero, C., & McCafferey, M. (1996). In B.R. Ferrel & B.A. Ferrell, *Pain in the elderly.* Seattle: IASP Press.

Pasero, C., McCaffery, M., & Gordon, D.B. (1999). Build institutional commitment to improving pain management. *Nursing Management, 30*(1), 27-34.

Portenoy, R.K. (1996). Opioid therapy for chronic non-malignant pain: A review of the issues. *Journal of Pain and Symptom Management, 11,* 203-217.

Portenoy, R.K. (1997). *Pain in oncologic and AIDS patients.* Newtown, PA: Handbooks in Health Care.

Purdue Pharma, L.P. (1999). *Understanding key terms in pain management.* Norwalk, CT: L.P. Purdue Pharma.

Rapp, C.J., & Gordon, D.B. (2000). Understanding equianalgesic dosing. *Orthopaedic Nursing, 19*(3), 65-71.

Ronk, L.L. (1996). Spinal cord stimulation for chronic non-malignant pain. *Orthopaedic Nursing, 15*(5), 53-70.

Ruiz-Cavillo, E. (1993). Evaluation of the pain response by Mexican-American and Anglo-American women and their nurses. *Journal of Advanced Nursing, 18,* 451-459.

Ryder, E., & Sikorski, K. (1998). *Post-operative epidural analgesia with local anesthetics: A guide for nurses (pp. 1-20).* Westborough, MA: ASTRA USA, Inc.

Sanders, S.H., Brena, S.F., Spier, C.J., Beltrutti, D., McConnell, H., & Quintero, O. (1992). Chronic low back pain patients around the world: Cross-cultural similarities and differences. *Clinical Journal of Pain, 8*(4), 317-323.

Slowikowski, R.D., & Flaherty, S.A. (2000). Epidural analgesia for post-operative pain. *Orthopaedic Nursing, 19*(1), 23-32.

Snyder, M., & Chlan, L. (1999). Music therapy. *Annual Review of Nursing Research, 17,* 3-25.

Smith, S. (Ed.). (1999). *Orthopaedic nursing core competencies: Adult acute care.* Pitman, NJ: National Association of Orthopaedic Nurses.

Tompkins, J.S., Dunwoody, C.J., & Lisanti, P. (1996). Pain. In S.W. Salmond, N.E. Mooney, & L.A. Verdisco (Eds.) *NAON: Core curriculum for orthopaedic nursing (3rd ed., pp. 106-129).* Pitman, NJ: National Association of Orthopaedic Nurses.

Yetzer, E.A. (1996). Helping the patient through the experience of an amputation. *Orthopaedic Nursing, 15*(6), 45-49.

York, M., & Paice, J. (1998). Treatment of low back pain with instraspinal opioids delivered via implanted pumps. *Orthopaedic Nursing, 17*(3), 61-69.

Young, D. (1999). *Research-based protocol: Acute pain management.* Iowa City: University of Iowa.

Zang, S., & Bailey, N. (1997). *Home care manual making the transition.* Philadelphia: Lippincott.

STUDY QUESTIONS

Mrs. H., age 76, comes to the afternoon clinic with sudden onset of acute severe mid-thoracic spine pain which began the previous night while turning over in bed. The pain is exacerbated by any movement and even breathing. She has no history of back pain. The patient is 5 ft. 1/2 inches tall, weighs 89 pounds, is of small build, and is fair-skinned with positive family history of hip fracture (her older sister). She has never smoked but drinks wine with dinner. X-rays show T-6 compression fracture. She has tears in her eyes and has not eaten this morning though she took acetaminophen at the time of the pain onset. Mrs. H. states, "I know I'm being a baby about this. It's really not so bad." (Questions 1-4)

1. Which of the following should you consider when assessing Mrs. H's pain?
   a. Mrs. H. is elderly so she doesn't feel the pain as much as if she were younger.
   b. Mrs. H. needs to have an explanation of how crippling crush fractures can be.
   c. The acetaminophen is not effectively controlling the amount of pain.
   d. Mrs. H. is minimizing her pain and discomfort by being stoical.

2. Mrs. H.'s husband, who accompanies her, says, "You should have seen her last night! She screamed and cried and I thought she was dying. I wanted to call 911, but she wouldn't let me." From this comment, you could assume:
   a. She had been exaggerating to get her husband's attention and sympathy.
   b. Her husband is annoyed that they came to the clinic when she already feels better.
   c. Her endorphin response may be working but she is still in severe pain.
   d. Her husband should let her speak for herself because she is the one with pain.

3. At 2 weeks post-fracture, the home health nurse visits Mr. and Mrs. H. She finds their active teenage grandchildren visiting. Mrs. H. has given them lunch and gone for a walk with them. Mr. H. says she is always in too much pain to walk with him and "stays home watching soap operas on television all day." From this, the nurse can conclude:
   a. The sparkle is gone from their marriage and she is bored with him.
   b. Being with her grandchildren is the most important thing for Mrs. H.
   c. Mrs. H. is using the grandchildren as distraction for pain relief.
   d. Mrs. H. is less sensitive to pain because of her advanced age.

4. Mr. and Mrs. H. return to the clinic in 6 weeks as requested. She has been on one or two tablets of Tylenol with Codeine No.3® on a qid schedule with Elavil® 50 mg at h.s. (bedtime). She is feeling better and radiographs now show considerable healing. At this time you may anticipate:
   a. She can be changed to nonopioid medications in the daytime as tolerated.
   b. She will need inpatient detoxification from codeine.
   c. She should stop the medications now.
   d. She is addicted to the medications by now.

Mr. K. is a 45-year-old bricklayer who was injured on the job 1 year ago. He is receiving workers' compensation and, aside from health care matters (physician visits, physical therapy, etc.), he has been at home in his recliner because of severe leg and back pain from spinal stenosis and herniated nucleus pulposus. He has been taking 1-3 tablets of Percocet® every 4-5 hours. He also has been drinking a six-pack of beer and smoking 40 cigarettes per day, two lifelong habits. His wife has left him during the year because of his drinking and medication use, which have made him depressed and irritable. (Questions 5-8)

5. Mr. K.'s pain can be described as:
   a. Acute.
   b. Chronic nonmalignant.
   c. Chronic malignant.
   d. Holistic.

6. Mr. K. comes in for a laminectomy and fusion of the affected levels. For his postoperative medication, the most appropriate approach may be:
   a. Administer the same dose of Percocet® he has been taking at home.
   b. No opioids postoperatively since he is an active drug abuser.
   c. Percocet® , 2 tablets every 4 hours ATC and Toradol® 10 mg IM as needed.
   d. Percocet® , 2 tablets every 4 hour ATC and Toradol® 10 mg IM every 4 hours ATC.

7. The reason for the above plan is:
   a. The Percocet® has been effective and well tolerated.
   b. Giving Mr. K. more opioids will make it harder for him to detoxify from the drugs.
   c. If Mr. K. has the Percocet® , he shouldn't need much Toradol® .
   d. An addicted person needs a base level of the "substance" to be "normal" and a pain-relieving dose to cover the pain.

8. Mr. K. is discharged at 6 days postoperatively to a rehabilitation center as he lives alone without a reliable support system. In the rehabilitation center, efforts are begun to wean him off the opioids to Tylenol Extra Strength® ? This proves difficult to accomplish although he verbalizes wanting "to be clean" because his wife says she and their children will return. Mr. K.'s difficulties in weaning probably do not include:
   a. Lack of motivation.
   b. Continued postoperative pain.
   c. Physiological dependence.
   d. Psychological dependence.

Elizabeth T., age 6 years, had been injured and was brought to the emergency room by her family. She required open reduction and internal fixation of her right distal femur. (Questions 9-10)

9. In the post-anesthesia recovery room, Elizabeth screams loudly on transfer. From this, you can expect:
   a. She is in the post-anesthesia stage of excitement.
   b. She is looking for her mother.
   c. It is painful for her to be moved.
   d. She will have a problem getting along with the staff in pediatrics.

10. In the pediatric unit on her second postoperative day, Elizabeth enjoys the visit of a clown who dances and plays with the children. During the clown's visit Elizabeth laughs, sings, and eats ice cream. After the clown leaves, she cries and wants her mother to hold her. Your interpretation of this sequence of events is:
    a. She is spoiled and wants constant entertainment and attention.
    b. She is manipulating her mother to keep her from leaving.
    c. She is no longer distracted and is looking for relief from discomfort.
    d. The clown was too much stimulation for her.

Dr. R., a 35-year-old physician, is admitted for ORIF of a proximal wrist fracture. On admission to your post-anesthesia care unit for a 23-hour hospital stay, she has an epidural drip of hydromorphone with bolus doses programmed for breakthrough pain. (Questions 11-12)

11. What supplies would you keep at bedside?
    a. Extra hydromorphone for IM use.
    b. Naloxone.
    c. Neurologic evaluation instruments.
    d. Relaxation tapes.

12. Which of the following is **not** an advantage for using this type of analgesia for this patient?
    a. She will feel greater control of her pain management with the bolus doses.
    b. She will not be "clock-watching" if she knows she has breakthrough pain doses.
    c. There will not be wide variations in serum drug levels throughout the 23 hours.
    d. Hydromorphone has a metabolite which is known to cause excitement and dysphoria.

13. A method of cutaneous nerve stimulation that is an independent nursing action is:
    a. Acupuncture.
    b. Biofeedback.
    c. Pressure, rubbing, and massage.
    d. Application of counter-irritants.

14. Principal side effects of opioid/opiates do not include:
    a. Constipation.
    b. Sedation.
    c. Tolerance.
    d. Addiction.

15. Which of the following alternative therapies is theoretically based on the concept that it stimulates endorphin production?
    a. Imagery.
    b. Acupuncture.
    c. Distraction.
    d. Therapeutic touch/massage.

16. The "gold standard" drug for pain management is:
    a. Meperidine.
    b. Codeine.
    c. Morphine sulfate.
    d. Hydromorphone.

17. The preferred drug route for management of chronic pain is:
    a. IM.
    b. IV.
    c. Sub-q.
    d. PO.

18. The optimal route for analgesics is:
    a. Intravenous.
    b. Intramuscular.
    c. Oral.
    d. Transdermal.

19. Which of the following is **not** a barrier to effective pain management?
    a. Lack of health staff knowledge about pain.
    b. Reluctance of physicians to prescribe opioids.
    c. Fears of opioid addiction postoperatively.
    d. Patient's age and level of pain and discomfort.

Chapter 8 COMPLICATIONS

Nancy S. Morris, PhD, RN, CS

Contents

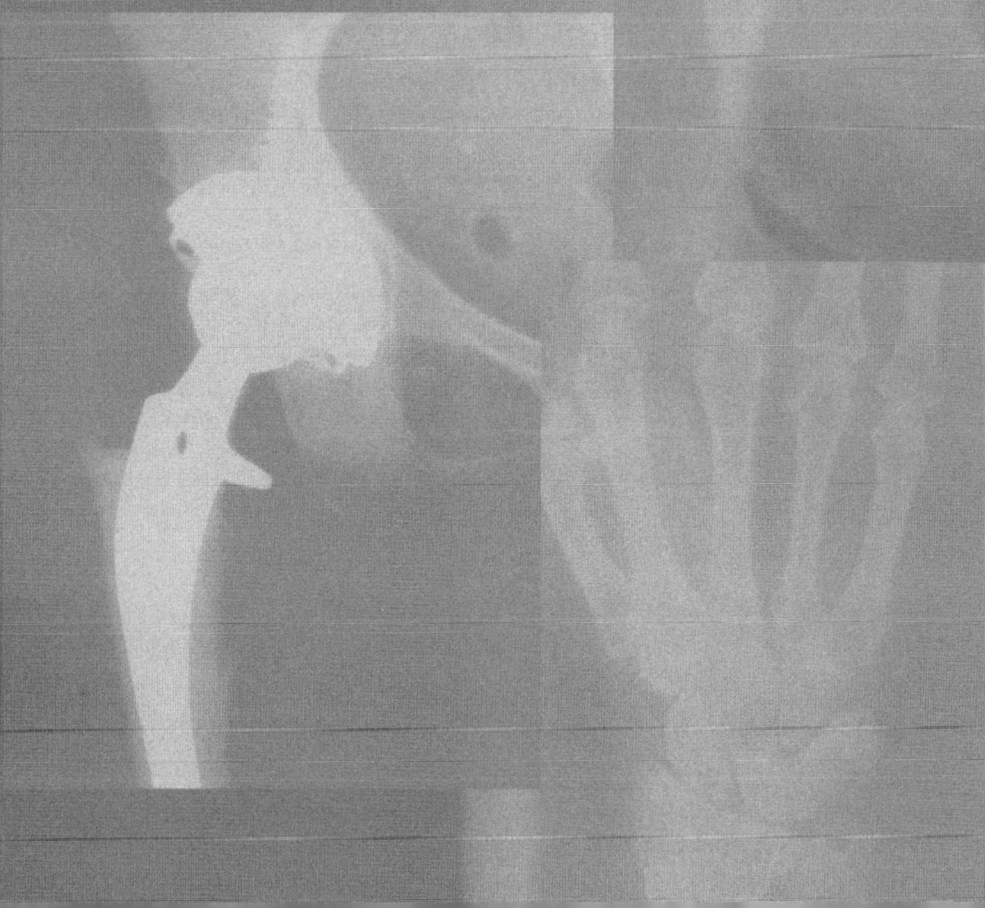

OBJECTIVES

At the completion of this chapter, the learner will be able to:

- Identify primary risk factors for complications associated with orthopaedic injuries and procedures.
- Discuss the key aspects of assessment for the following complications: acute confusion, impaired skin integrity, constipation, deep vein thrombosis, pulmonary embolism, compartment syndrome, fat embolism syndrome, hemorrhage, and nosocomial surgical site infection.
- Identify nursing interventions for the complications named above.
- Describe preventive measures to decrease the likelihood of the complications named above.
- Evaluate achievement of desired outcomes for the complications listed above.
- Initiate a discharge plan focusing on primary areas of concern for specific complications associated with orthopaedic conditions.

KEY POINTS

- Delineating risk factors and patient characteristics that may influence outcome achievement is a key component of providing high-quality nursing care.
- Confusion in a hospitalized adult creates concerns relating to the emotional status of the patient and family, safety, and dependence on others for self-care needs.
- Implementing a systematic approach to help patients establish and maintain normal bowel function after surgery with minimal dependence on medication is key.
- The immobility associated with many orthopaedic procedures place these patients at greater risk for pressure ulcer development.
- Preventive measures for venous thromboembolic conditions should begin preoperatively and be continued intraoperatively and postoperatively.
- An early clinical indicator of compartment syndrome is increasing pain unrelieved with appropriate analgesics and pain with passive stretching of the muscles in a given compartment.
- It is important to recognize symptoms early in preventing morbidity and mortality associated with fat embolism syndrome; therefore, awareness of risk factors and careful monitoring is essential.
- Ischemic tissue is infected easily and generally does not heal well, reinforcing the need for adequate local perfusion and oxygenation.

CHAPTER 8

COMPLICATIONS

GENERAL RISK FACTORS

I. INCREASED AGE
A. Risk begins to increase at 40 years of age.
B. Risk increases markedly after 60 years of age.

II. CO-MORBIDITY
A. Respiratory conditions.
B. Diabetes.
C. Immunosuppression.
D. Obesity.
E. Malnourishment.

III. DRUGS
A. Warfarin, corticosteroids, and NSAIDs may affect healing, bleeding, and coagulation.
B. Opioids may affect respiratory status and GI functioning.
C. Estrogen therapy and cigarette smoking increase risk of thromboembolism.

IV. ADDITIONAL RISK FACTORS
A. Mechanism of injury.
B. Open wounds.
C. Time between injury and stabilization of a fracture.
D. Postoperative mobility level.
E. Lack of social support.

ACUTE CONFUSION

I. OVERVIEW
A. Definition: an abrupt onset of a cluster of global, transient changes and disturbances in attention, cognition, psychomotor activity, level of consciousness, and/or sleep wake cycle.
B. Etiology.
1. Alterations in cerebral metabolism.
2. Impaired neurochemical transmission.

C. Risk factors.
1. Predisposing risk factors.
   a. Male gender.
   b. Age greater than 60 years.
   c. Prior cognitive dysfunction.
   d. Low functional status.
   e. High severity of illness/major organ failure.
   f. Anemia.
   g. Low serum albumin.
   h. Drug toxicity or drug-drug interaction.
   i. Drug or alcohol withdrawal.
   j. Infection.
2. Precipitating factors: physiologic.
   a. Low cardiac output.
   b. Low body temperature.
   c. High severity of illness.
   d. Acute metabolic imbalance.
   e. Fluid and electrolyte imbalance.
   f. Pain.
   g. Hypoxia.
   h. Infection.
   i. Overmedication.
   j. Malnutrition.
3. Precipitating factors: environmental.
   a. Sleep deprivation.
   b. Immobility.
   c. Sensory disturbance.
   d. Impaired communication.
   e. Social deprivation.

D. Pathophysiology.
1. Pathological mechanism involving lesions in cortical cholinergic systems and cerebral oxygen consumption probable.
2. Three areas of the brain most likely affected by acute confusion.
   a. Cortical and mid-brain structures responsible for thinking, perception, and memory.
   b. Reticular activating system responsible for attention and wakefulness.
   c. Autonomic system responsible for psychomotor and regulatory functions.

E. Incidence.
1. 20%-80% of hospitalized elderly; 20%-24% is the most frequently reported range.
2. 10%-50% among elderly postoperative patients.
3. Highest prevalence ranging between 24 and 72 hours after admission to a hospital.

F. Considerations across the lifespan.
1. Rare in children and young adults.
2. Most commonly seen with increased age.

G. Complications.
1. Longer length of hospitalization.
2. Increased mortality during and after hospitalization.
3. Discharge to a higher level of care.
4. Long-term care placement.
5. Increased risk for injury: falls.
6. Decreased functional status.

H. Prevention strategies.
1. Assess and meet personal hygiene needs.
2. Establish baseline mental status and reassess regularly.
3. Use prophylactic analgesics as indicated.
4. Assist with toileting as indicated.
5. Maintain an organized environment.
   a. Provide name tags for health care workers.
   b. Orient patient to room and unit.
   c. Place familiar items within patient's view
6. Provide meaningful sensory input.

a. Place clock and calendar within sight.
b. Ensure lighting is appropriate to time of day.
c. Encourage visits by family and friends.
7. Maximize independence.
a. Incorporate patient's usual routines into hospital day.
b. Encourage active participation of the patient.

II. ASSESSMENT

A. History.
1. Cognitive status – baseline and ongoing.
a. Mini-Mental State Examination.
b. Clinical Assessment of Confusion-A.
c. NEECHAM Confusion Scale.
2. Pain management.
3. Sleep disturbance.
4. Substance abuse.
5. Agitation, restlessness.

B. Physical examination.
1. Elevated temperature.
2. Low blood pressure.
3. Fingering, picking, or tremor (early cue).
4. Fluctuation in level of consciousness.
5. Poor skin turgor: dehydration.
6. Decreased urinary output: dehydration.

C. Diagnostic tests.
1. Complete blood count.
2. Serum albumin.
3. Metabolic profile.

III. COMMON THERAPEUTIC MODALITIES

A. Avoid drugs with anticholinergic effects.
B. Maintain hydration, perfusion, and oxygenation.
C. Ensure that nutritional requirements are being met.
D. Manage pain.
E. Correct metabolic imbalances.
F. Prescribe antipsychotic/sedative medications.

IV. NURSING DIAGNOSES, OUTCOMES, AND INTERVENTIONS

A. Thought processes, disturbed.
1. Outcomes.
a. Demonstrates intact cognitive ability.
b. Exhibits sound information processing.
c. Recalls immediate, recent, and remote information accurately.
d. Uses assistive and protective safety devices correctly.
2. Interventions.
a. Assess patient's behavior at least daily.
b. Re-orient patients in a consistent manner.
c. Minimize disruption to the usual diurnal biologic rhythms.
d. Provide companionship.
e. Provide calendars, clocks, and newspapers.
f. Ensure easy access to glasses, hearing aids, and other functional devices.
g. Administer antipsychotic/sedative medications as indicated.

B. Sleep pattern, disturbed.
1. Outcomes.
a. Achieves usual sleep routine.
b. Feels rested upon awakening.
2. Interventions.
a. Implement measures to relieve pain.
b. Provide as much exercise as allowed.
c. Reduce anxiety through patient education.
d. Orient to hospital environment.
e. Reduce corridor noises and noise from roommate.
f. Administer antipyschotic/sedative medications as indicated.

C. Injury, risk for.
1. Outcomes.
a. Environmental risk factors are monitored.
b. Personal behavioral risk factors are monitored.
c. Patient does not sustain an injury.
2. Interventions.
a. Maintain the safety of the environment.
(1) Assess client hourly.
(2) Orient patient to physical arrangement of room.
(3) Place client in room close to nurse's station.
(4) Leave door to client room open at all times.
(5) Provide adequate lighting for increased visibility.
(6) Place patient's articles within easy reach.
(7) Maintain bed in low position.
(8) Consider use of non-restraint device such as bed alarm system.
(9) Use half or three-quarter side rails on beds when indicated.
(10) Avoid unnecessary rearrangement of physical environment.
(11) Ensure equipment is maintained appropriately (locks on wheels of bed and wheelchairs).
(12) Evaluate the need and institution policy on use/nonuse of restraints.
b. Fall prevention.
(1) Assist unsteady individual with ambulation.
(2) Provide assistive devices (walking belt, walker) to steady gait.
(3) Assist with toileting at frequent, scheduled intervals.
(4) Use alarm systems (ankle/wrist bracelets, bed/wheelchair alarms) as appropriate.
(5) Select rooms with open doorways and proximity to nurses to allow for frequent observation.
(6) Collaborate with other health care team members to minimize side effects of mediacations that contribute to:
(a) Orthostatic hypotension.
(b) Unsteady gait.
(c) Sedation.
(7) Respond promptly to call bells, requests from patients.
(8) Examine the need for the least restrictive safety restraint.

V. HOME CARE CONSIDERATIONS

Acute confusion should be resolved before discharge from hospital.

PRESSURE ULCER

I. OVERVIEW

A. Definition: any lesion caused by unrelieved pressure that results in damage of underlying tissue.

1. Stage I: nonblanchable erythema of intact skin.
2. Stage II: partial thickness skin loss involving epidermis and/or dermis.
3. Stage III: full thickness skin loss involving damage or necrosis of subcutaneous tissue that may extend down to, but not through, underlying fascia.
4. Stage IV: full thickness skin loss with extensive destruction, tissue necrosis, or damage to muscle, bone, or supporting structures.

B. Etiology.

1. Reduced tissue oxygenation due to sustained pressure.
2. Reduced tissue oxygenation due to disruption of the microvasculature by shearing forces.

C. Risk factors.

1. Impaired mobility/prolonged immobility.
2. Increased age.
3. Moisture/incontinence.
4. Depression.
5. Dehydration.
6. Nutritionally compromised (malnutrition and obesity).
7. Altered tissue perfusion.
8. Hypotension.
9. Edema.
10. Altered level of consciousness.
11. Altered sensory perception.
12. Medications (adrenocortical steroids, sedatives, analgesics, hypotensive drugs, antineoplastic drugs).
13. Length of surgical procedure (2.5 hours or more).
14. Pathologic conditions (neurologic deficits, diabetes).

D. Pathophysiology.

1. Mean skin capillary pressure in healthy people is 25 mm Hg.
2. Severe or prolonged circulatory interference (external compression with pressures > 30 mm Hg) will occlude blood vessels leading to anoxia and cell death in surrounding tissues.
3. Reduced tissue oxygenation due to sustained pressure and disruption of the microvasculature by shearing forces is main determinant of pressure ulcer formation.

E. Incidence.

1. Incidence in the acute care setting ranges from 2.7%-29.5%.
2. Incidence increases to 12%-66% for surgical patients.
3. Orthopaedic patients at higher risk due to imposed mobility restrictions.

F. Considerations across the lifespan.

1. Can affect individuals across the lifespan.
2. Increased age is an independent risk factor.

G. Complications.

1. Osteomyelitis.
2. Septicemia.
3. Significant tissue necrosis requiring surgical intervention.
4. Development of scar tissue.
5. Need for amputation.
6. Body image disturbance.
7. Increased length of stay.
8. Potential for amputation.

H. Prevention strategies. Identify at-risk individuals.

1. Assess skin daily.
2. Assess nutritional status.
3. Maintain and improve tissue tolerance to pressure to prevent injury.
   a. Keep skin clean with mild cleansing agent.
   b. Moisturize dry skin gently.
   c. Avoid massage over bony prominences.
   d. Protect intact skin with moisture barrier ointment or skin protective barrier wipe/spray.
   e. Correct fluid and nutritional deficiencies and supplement dietary intake as appropriate.
4. Protect against adverse effects of external mechanical forces (pressure, friction, and shear).
   a. Use proper positioning, transferring, and turning techniques.
   b. Apply lubricants, protective films, protective dressings, and protective padding.
   c. Consider smooth mattress cover (nylon) to prevent friction.
   d. Reposition immobilized patient at least every 2 hours.
   e. Position shifts in chair every 15 minutes.
   f. Use positioning devices as indicated.
   g. Use draw sheet/lifting devices to help reposition patient.
   h. Limit the amount of time the head of the bed is elevated above 30 degrees to minimize friction/shearing.
   i. Elevate knees slightly to prevent sliding in bed.
   j. Use pressure reduction or pressure relief support surfaces on bed and chair (mattress overlays, low air loss beds, air fluidized beds).
   k. Increase mobility.

II. ASSESSMENT

A. History.

1. Adequacy of nutrition/dietary intake.
2. Independence with mobility.
3. Control of elimination.
4. Intactness of sensations.

B. Physical examination.

1. Conduct risk assessment daily (Braden Scale, Norton Pressure Ulcer Prediction score).
2. Evaluate skin turgor, color, integrity – especially over bony prominences.
3. Monitor capillary refill regularly.
4. Conduct nutritional assessment, pre-albumin, and albumin level.

5. Evaluate sensation.
6. Determine mobility level.
7. Assess blood pressure.

C. Diagnostic tests.

1. Serum pre-albumin and albumin.
2. Complete blood count.
3. Serum glucose as indicated.

III. COMMON THERAPEUTIC MODALITIES

A. Maintain oxygenation.

B. Prevent/treat fever.

C. Avoid hypotension.

D. Choose dressing appropriate to wound type.

E. Debride (mechanical, chemical, autolytic, use of sharps) necrotic tissue.

F. Use normal saline with wet-to-dry dressing changes.

G. Maintain serum glucose levels between 80 and 125mg/dl.

IV. NURSING DIAGNOSES, OUTCOMES, AND INTERVENTIONS

A. Skin integrity, impaired (Stage I or II pressure ulcer).

1. Outcomes.
   a. Adequate nutritional intake.
   b. Intact peripheral tissue perfusion.
   c. Epithelialization of wound.
   d. Maintenance of skin integrity.
   e. Risk control strategies in place.
2. Interventions.
   a. Correct fluid and nutritional deficiencies.
   b. Turn/reposition the immobilized patient at least every 2 hours.
   c. Facilitate small shifts of body weight.
   d. Use appropriate devices to keep heels and bony prominences off the bed.
   e. Use pressure reduction or pressure relief support surfaces on bed and chair (mattress overlays, low air loss beds, air fluidized beds) as appropriate.
   f. Use draw sheet/lifting devices to help reposition patient.
   g. Select a topical treatment/appropriate dressing that maintains a moist wound healing environment.
   h. Monitor for signs and symptoms of infection.
   i. Initiate consultation services of a enterostomal therapy nurse as needed.

B. Tissue integrity, impaired (Stage III or IV pressure ulcer).

1. Outcomes.
   a. Adequate nutritional intake.
   b. Intact peripheral tissue perfusion.
   c. Epithelialization of wound.
   d. Maintenance of skin integrity.
   e. Risk control strategies implemented.
2. Interventions.
   a. Correct fluid and nutritional deficiencies.
      (1) Adequate protein important for wound healing and immune system functioning.
      (2) Vitamins A, C, and E, and the minerals zinc and iron important for wound healing and to decrease risk of infection.
   b. Turn/reposition the immobilized patient at least every 2 hours.
   c. Facilitate small shifts of body weight.
   d. Use appropriate devices to keep heels and bony prominences off the bed.
   e. Use pressure reduction or pressure relief support surfaces on bed and chair (mattress overlays, low air loss beds, air fluidized beds), as appropriate.
   f. Use draw sheet/lifting devices to help reposition patient.
   g. Select a topical treatment/appropriate dressing that maintains a moist wound healing environment.
   h. Monitor for signs and symptoms of wound infection.
   i. Initiate consultation services of an enterostomal therapy nurse as needed.

C. Infection, risk for.

1. Outcomes.
   a. Remain free from signs and symptoms of infection.
   b. Patient/caregiver able to describe signs and symptoms of infection.
   c. Risk control strategies in place.
   d. Adequate nutritional intake.
   e. Epithelialization of wound without infection.
2. Interventions.
   a. Ensure diet adequate in protein, zinc, iron, and vitamins A, C, and E.
   b. Adhere to universal precautions.
   c. Monitor CBC, serum protein, serum albumin, culture results as appropriate.
   d. Ensure appropriate wound care technique.
   e. Teach patient/caregiver wound care.
   f. Teach patient/caregiver signs and symptoms of infection.

V. HOME CARE CONSIDERATIONS

A. Teach patient/caregiver to prevent undue pressure.

B. Teach patient/caregiver signs of skin breakdown.

C. Emphasize value of handwashing.

D. Teach patient/caregiver wound care.

E. Ensure appropriate disposal of used dressing materials.

F. Teach patient/caregiver signs and symptoms of infection.

CONSTIPATION

I. OVERVIEW

A. Definition: a state in which an individual's pattern of elimination is characterized by hard, dry stool which results from a delay in passage of food residue.

B. Etiology.

1. Inability to perceive gastrocoloic reflex.
2. Loss of rectal tone and sensitivity.

3. Delay in passage of food residue.

C. Risk factors.

1. Immobility.
2. Deficiency of dietary fiber.
3. Dehydration.
4. Side effects of medications.
5. Altered dietary intake.
6. Fecal impaction.
7. Stress.
8. Ignoring of the gastrocolic reflex.
9. Change in environment and routine.

D. Pathophysiology.

1. Reflex contraction of the rectum and relaxation of the anal sphincter is normally initiated when feces enter the rectum.
2. Defecation triggered by brainstem from input from pelvic organs and cortex.
   a. Visceral efferent nerves cause colonic propulsion and internal anal sphincter relaxation.
   b. Somatic efferent nerves inhibit contraction of the striated muscle of the pelvic floor.
3. Consistently ignoring gastrocolic reflex may lead to adaptive change in rectal tone and sensitivity.
   a. Decrease in rectal sensation and an increase in rectal capacity allows a large amount of stool to collect in rectum, leading to fecal impaction.
   b. Patient unable to defecate because he/she cannot detect presence of feces in rectum until mass becomes too large to expel.
4. Immobility decreases colonic activity and may lead to atrophy of the primary muscles of defecation.

E. Incidence.

1. Difficult to ascertain due to different definitions of constipation.
2. Inconsistent self-report of constipation.

F. Considerations across the lifespan.

1. Common dysfunction among:
   a. All age groups.
   b. Both sexes.
   c. All educational and socioeconomic levels.
2. Highest occurrence is among individuals 65 years or older.

G. Complications.

1. Abdominal discomfort, nausea, vomiting.
2. Hemorrhoids.
3. Impaction.
4. Intestinal obstruction.
5. Headache.
6. Decreased appetite.

H. Prevention strategies.

1. Promote adequate fluid intake/prevent dehydration.
2. Encourage high-fiber diet.
3. Avoid constipating medications.
4. Use stool softeners in high-risk patients (post-surgery and immobilized).
5. Promote environmental support (easy access to toilet, privacy).
6. Encourage passive and active exercise.
7. Simulate home routine.

II. ASSESSMENT

A. History.

1. Decreased defecation frequency.
2. Passage of hard, dry stool.
3. Straining at stool.
4. Painful defecation.
5. Rectal pressure.
6. Impaired appetite.
7. Headache.
8. Abdominal pain.
9. Decreased fluid intake.
10. Diet low in fiber/roughage.
11. Use of medications with constipation as side effect.

B. Physical examination.

1. Hard, dry stool.
2. Abdominal tenderness.
3. Abdominal gaseous or fluid distention.
4. Palpable mass in lower abdomen.
5. Hypoactive or hyperactive bowel sounds.
6. Fecal impaction palpated on digital rectal exam.

C. Diagnostic tests.

1. Flat plate abdominal x-ray in select circumstances.
2. Further diagnostic studies usually limited to chronic constipation.

III. COMMON THERAPEUTIC MODALITIES

A. Laxative agent for short-term use.

1. Bulk-forming agents.
2. Stimulant irritant cathartics.
3. Saline cathartics.
4. Lubricants.
5. Stool softener.

B. Enemas for acute constipation and fecal impaction.

C. Suppositories to empty lower bowel.

D. Adequate fluid intake.

E. High-fiber diet.

IV. NURSING DIAGNOSES, OUTCOMES, AND INTERVENTIONS

A. Constipation.

1. Outcomes.
   a. Regular bowel elimination.
   b. Mobility level sufficient for toileting.
2. Interventions.
   a. Evaluate bowel function daily.
   b. Encourage patients to follow the same defecation routine they have at home.
   c. Provide privacy and promote use of toilet/commode.
   d. Offer warm fluids to initiate gastrocolic reflex.
   e. Encourage physical activity and mobility as appropriate.
   f. Encourage dietary selections of foods high in fiber with goal of 25 g/day for adults.
   g. Encourage adequate fluid intake (48-64 ounces/day).

V. HOME CARE CONSIDERATIONS

A. Resume regular bowel routine.

B. Minimize use of medications that have constipation as a side effect.

C. Change in fluid and fiber intake as appropriate.

D. Consider stool softeners especially if using narcotic analgesics.

HEMORRHAGE

I. OVERVIEW

A. Definition: the abnormal and excessive loss of blood related to internal or external bleeding.

B. Etiology.

1. Interruption to the blood vessel integrity.
2. Shift in balance of clotting mechanisms.

C. Risk factors.

1. Patient-related.
   a. Coagulation disorder.
   b. Low preoperative platelet count.
   c. Excessive anticoagulation.
   d. Tumor growth impinging blood vessels.
   e. Hepatic disease.
   f. Medication use (anti-inflammatory and anticoagulants).
   g. Infection.
   h. Gastrointestinal ulcers.
2. Injury-related.
   a. Fractured bone interrupting the blood vessel integrity.
   b. Foreign body interrupting the blood vessel integrity.
   c. Significant soft tissue damage.
3. Procedure-related.
   a. Anatomic aspects of selected surgical procedures.
   b. Technical aspects of selected surgical procedures.

D. Pathophysiology.

1. Abnormalities of the blood vessel walls.
   a. Intrinsic factor related to inborn abnormality.
   b. Extrinsic factors related to nature of injury or result of treatment modality.
2. Abnormal clotting mechanisms.
   a. Intrinsic factor related to inborn abnormality.
   b. Extrinsic factors related to nature of injury or result of treatment modality.

E. Incidence.

1. Higher incidence in:
   a. Revision arthroplasty.
   b. Multi-level anterior/posterior spine procedures.
   c. Multi-trauma.
2. Higher incidence in patient with identified risk factors.
3. Lower incidence of blood loss with uncemented hip/knee prostheses.

F. Considerations across the lifespan.

1. Occurs across the lifespan.
2. Undiagnosed coagulation disorders more a concern among children.

G. Complications.

1. Shock.
2. Edema of subcutaneous tissue and visceral organs consequence of high-volume crystalloid therapy.
3. Disseminated intravascular coagulation (DIC).
4. Death.

H. Prevention strategies.

1. Preoperative period.
   a. Evaluate laboratory tests (Hgb, Hct, PT, APTT, platelet count).
   b. Reverse anticoagulated patients preoperatively (vitamin K).
   c. Discontinue patient use of aspirin, NSAIDs, vitamin E, and warfarin before surgery if possible.
   d. Recombinant human erythropoietin may be given to allow autologous blood donation in patients with anemia.
   e. Use of pneumatic antishock garments if multitrauma patient.
   f. Autologus blood donation for elective surgery.
2. Intra-operative period.
   a. Use hypotensive anesthesia keeping blood pressure 20 mm Hg below average preoperative blood pressure to minimize blood loss during surgery.
   b. Monitor laboratory tests (Hgb, Hct, PT, APTT, INR, platelet count, fibrinogen assay, arterial blood gases) as indicated.
   c. Use fibrin tissue adhesive in total knee arthroplasty.
   d. Initiate cell savage systems.
   e. Pneumatic antishock garments as appropriate.
   f. Use of electrocautery, tourniquets, and direct pressure.
   g. Hypothermia.
3. Postoperative period.
   a. Monitor laboratory tests (Hgb, Hct, PT, APTT, INR, platelet count, fibrinogen assay, arterial blood gases) as indicated.
   b. Use and monitor cell savage systems.
   c. Continue with vitamin K, if appropriate.

II. ASSESSMENT

A. History.

1. Nature and extent of injury/health problem.
2. Verbalization of actual blood loss.
3. Anxiety.
4. Dizziness.
5. Weakness.
6. History of coagulation disorder.
7. History of other pathologic-related conditions.

B. Physical examination.

1. Pallor.
2. Cool, moist skin.
3. Tachycardia, possibly irregular pulse.
4. Decreased blood pressure with a narrowed pulse pressure.
5. Rapid and shallow breathing.
6. Decreased urine output.
7. Abnormal drainage from drains or wounds.
8. Frank bleeding from wound or surgical incision.

9. Restlessness.

C. Diagnostic tests.

1. Complete blood count.
2. Coagulation studies.
3. Check urine for blood – if source of bleeding not known.
4. Check stool for blood – if source of bleeding not known.

III. COMMON THERAPEUTIC MODALITIES

A. Restore and maintain adequate blood volume.

1. Blood transfusion (homologous or autologous blood).
   a. Plasma-poor red cells (RC) to correct oxygen carrying capacity.
   b. Fresh frozen plasma (FFP) to treat associated hypofibrinogenemia.
   c. Packed red blood cells (PRBC), platelets, and whole blood (WB) may be used.
   d. Autologus blood.
      (1) Preopoerative: pre-donated autologous deposits.
      (2) Intraopoerative: salvage by cell saver.
      (3) Postoperative: salvage by autotransfusion system.
      (4) See Chapter 5, Perioperative Patient Care.
2. Intravenous fluids.
   a. Crystalloids (lactated Ringer's solution or normal saline). Cumulative volume of crystalloids is usually 4-5 times greater than the actual blood loss.
   b. Colloids (albumin, hydroxyethyl starches, dextran, and gelatin preparations).

B. Maintain sufficient oxygen carrying capacity.

C. Secure hemostasis.

1. Direct pressure if source of bleeding easily noted.
2. Elevate bleeding extremity above heart level.
3. Resuturing or surgical intervention.
4. Vitamin K or clotting factor replacement.
5. Arteriography and instillation of autologuous or synthetic clotting material when surgical intervention contraindicated (closed pelvic fracture).

D. Intraoperative and postoperative blood salvage.

E. Replace lost iron reserves: iron supplementation.

IV. NURSING DIAGNOSES, OUTCOMES, AND INTERVENTIONS

A. Anxiety.

1. Outcome: effective use of coping strategies to manage anxiety.
2. Interventions.
   a. Provide factual information regarding condition and treatment.
   b. Encourage verbalization of feelings, perceptions, and fears.
   c. Be physically available to the patient.
   d. Touch patient to express concern, support, as appropriate.
   e. Use a calm, reassuring approach.
   f. Stay with the patient to promote safety and reduce fear.

B. Peripheral neurovascular dysfunction, risk for.

1. Outcomes.
   a. Peripheral tissue perfusion will be maintained.
   b. Vital signs are stable.
   c. Fluid balance is restored.
2. Interventions.
   a. Monitor neurovascular status at least every 2 hours.
   b. Monitor and replace fluid volume as indicated.
   c. Monitor hemoglobin and hematocrit.
   d. Monitor vital signs.

C. Fluid volume, deficient.
Fluid volume, excess.

1. Outcomes.
   a. Fluid balance is maintained.
   b. Peripheral pulses are palpable.
   c. Hematocrit is within normal limits.
   d. Blood pressure is within expected range.
2. Interventions.
   a. Monitor vital signs:
      (1) Pulse (slow or bounding/dysrhythmic).
      (2) Respirations (any signs of tachypnea, labored/shallow breathing, rales/rhonchi).
      (3) Blood pressure (low or elevated).
   b. Monitor hematocrit, electrolytes, blood urea nitrogen (BUN), creatinine.
   c. Administer fluid replacement as indicated.
   d. Administer blood products as appropriate.
   e. Monitor urinary output:
      (1) Maintain accurate intake and output.
      (2) Note amount of each voiding (very large or minimal amount).
      (3) Note color of urine (very dark or very light).
      (4) Check specific gravity (increased or decreased).
   f. Monitor skin:
      (1) Turgor (decreased).
      (2) Color (pale or flushed).
      (3) Moisture (dry or diaphoretic).
      (4) Eyeballs (sunken).
      (5) Fontanelles of infants (depressed).
      (6) Tongue (furrowed/dry).
      (7) Mucosa (lips, gums: dry).
   g. Note if neck veins collapsed/distended when patient is lying flat.

D. Tissue perfusion, ineffective: peripheral.

1. Outcomes.
   a. Circulation to extremities is maintained.
   b. Peripheral pulses are palpable.
   c. Vital signs are stable.
   d. Fluid balance is maintained.
2. Interventions.
   a. Monitor peripheral circulation (pulses, edema, capillary refill, color, temperature of extremity).
   b. Consider supplemental oxygenation.
   c. Monitor fluid status.
   d. Administer fluid replacement as indicated.
   e. Administer blood products as appropriate.

V. HOME CARE CONSIDERATIONS

A. Formulate a plan for post discharge follow-up.

B. Continue iron supplementation as appropriate.

C. Coordinate referrals relevant to care as appropriate.

PULMONARY EMBOLISM (PE)

I. OVERVIEW

A. **Definition: a pulmonary embolus (PE) is a clot or other hemostatic plug that has dislodged from its primary site and traveled via venous circulation to the right heart. Once there, it then enters the pulmonary circulation causing a partial or complete obstruction of one or both branches of the pulmonary artery or its subdivisions.**

B. **Etiology.**
   1. Local venous trauma.
   2. Migration of a venous thrombus.

C. **Risk factors.**
   1. Patient related.
      a. Age: risk increases after age 40; even greater risk after age 60.
      b. Previous thromboembolism.
      c. Physical/pathological conditions.
         (1) Congestive heart failure.
         (2) Cardiomyopathy and pericarditis.
         (3) Stroke.
         (4) Venous insufficiency.
         (5) Obesitiy.
         (6) Varicose veins.
         (7) Anasarca.
         (8) Polycythemia rubra vera.
         (9) Nephrotic syndrome.
         (10) Inflammatory bowel disease.
      d. Hypercoagulability.
         (1) Pregnancy.
         (2) Estrogen therapy.
         (3) Malignancy.
         (4) Use of oral contraceptive.
         (5) Sickle cell disease.
         (6) Dehydration.
      e. Deficiencies in clotting cascade (antithrombin III, protein C, protein S, fibrinogen, factor V Leiden, or plasminogen).
      f. Lupus anticoagulant.
   2. Procedure related.
      a. Venous stasis.
         (1) Immobilization.
         (2) Surgery > 30 minutes.
         (3) Obstruction or compression of the iliac or femoral veins.
      b. Postoperative infection.
      c. Vascular injury.
         (1) Surgery:
            (a) Orthopaedic (pelvic, hip, spine, or lower extremity).
            (b) Large abdominal or pelvic tumors.
            (c) Gynecologic surgery.
         (2) Re-operation.
         (3) Trauma.
         (4) IV therapy.
         (5) IV drug abuse.
      d. General restoration.

D. **Pathophysiology.**
   1. Venous thrombus either undergoes lysis, becomes organized, or becomes dislodged and carried in the circulation as an embolus.
   2. When a significant portion of the pulmonary arterial bed is obstructed, blood flow distal to the embolus is either partially or totally occluded.
   3. A ventilation/perfusion mismatch occurs increasing physiologic dead-space ventilation and resulting in unoxygenated blood.
   4. Atelectasis occurs due to loss of surfactant contributing to hypoxemia.
   5. The increased pulmonary vascular resistance caused by the PE leads to pulmonary hypertension and increased right ventricular workload.
   6. All of these events lead to hypoxia and the clinical manifestation of PE.

E. **Incidence.**
   1. Estimated 600,000 yearly.
   2. Accounts for approximately 5% of sudden deaths in the hospital setting.
   3. Usually occurs within 48-72 hours of injury or surgery.
   4. PE may not be preceded by a symptomatic DVT.
   5. Actual incidence difficult to ascertain as many PE are undiagnosed. A high index of suspicion is required to achieve an accurate diagnosis.
   6. Commonly taught triad of symptoms characteristic of PE (dyspnea, pleuritic chest pain, and hemoptysis) appears in combination in approximately 28% of patients.

F. **Considerations across the lifespan.**
   1. PE uncommon in children.
   2. Children may present with minimal objective findings on preliminary testing supporting the value of risk factor assessment and high index of suspicion in select cases.
   3. Warfarin contraindicated during pregnancy.

G. **Complications.**
   1. Pulmonary infarction.
   2. Atelectasis.
   3. Right ventricular failure.
   4. Death.

H. **Prevention strategies.**
   1. Identify patient at risk.
   2. Administer pharmacologic interventions.
      a. Prophylactic anticoagulation for high-risk patients.
         (1) Aspirin.
         (2) Unfractionated or low molecular weight heparin.
         (3) Warfarin.
      b. Additional prophylactic approaches for high-risk patients.
         (1) Danaparoid.
         (2) Dermatan sulfate.
         (3) Dextran.
         (4) Hirudin and analogues.
         (5) Thrombin inhibitors.
         (6) Antiplatelet substances.
   3. Encourage nonpharmacologic interventions.

a. External pneumatic compression devices.
b. Graduated compression stockings.
c. Foot impulse pump.
d. Early ambulation.
e. Frequent plantar flexion and dorsiflexion of the foot, ankle, and toes.
f. Deep breathing exercises to help the large veins empty by increasing negative pressure in the thorax.

4. Surgical interventions.
   a. Prophylactic inferior vena cava filter in select high-risk patients.
   b. Epidural/spinal anesthesia instead of general anesthesia when feasible.
   c. Non-cemented prostheses when possible.
5. Keep the patient well hydrated.

II. ASSESSMENT

A. History.

1. Nonspecific symptoms.
2. Pleuritic chest pain.
3. Sudden onset shortness of breath.
4. Anxious/apprehensive.
5. Sense of impending doom.

B. Physical examination.

1. Neurologic.
   a. Apprehensive.
   b. Restlessness.
   c. Confusion.
   d. Anxiety.
2. Respiratory.
   a. Dyspnea.
   b. Cough.
   c. Hemoptysis.
   d. Abnormal respiratory rate/pattern.
   e. Decreased breath sounds.
   f. Abnormal breath sounds (crackles, wheezes).
   g. Hypoxia.
3. Cardiac.
   a. Tachycardia.
   b. Palpitations.
   c. Split S2.
   d. Abnormal blood pressure (hypotension).
   e. Syncope.
4. Vascular.
   a. Distended neck veins.
   b. Positive hepatojugular reflex.
5. Integumentary.
   a. Cool or warm skin temperature.
   b. Diaphoresis.
   c. Pallor, cyanosis, sluggish capillary refill.
   d. Fever.

C. Diagnostic tests.

1. Arterial blood gases: early respiratory alkalosis and later respiratory acidosis.
2. Chest x-ray: useful to rule out other causes of symptoms and to compare with ventilation-perfusion (V/Q) scan.
3. Electrocardiogram: inverted t-wave segments indicate hypoxemia.
4. V/Q scan: highly sensitive in ruling out a PE.
5. Pulmonary angiography: sensitivity of 98% and specificity of 96%.
6. D-Dimer assays: nonspecific but negative predictive value of 91.4%.
7. Spiral CT scans: equal sensitivity/specificity as compared to pulmonary angiography for third-order vessels.

III. COMMON THERAPEUTIC MODALITIES

A. Oxygen therapy acutely: mechanical ventilatory assistance may be indicated.

B. Anticoagulation: heparin therapy initially and then transition to warfarin 48-72 hours before discontinuing heparin.

C. Thrombolytic therapy to lyse clots (urokinase, streptokinase, recombinant human tissue-type plasmin). Contraindicated if recent surgery.

D. Emergency surgical embolectomy if evidence of hemodynamic and/or respiratory instability.

IV. NURSING DIAGNOSES, OUTCOMES, AND INTERVENTIONS

A. Gas exchange, impaired.

1. Outcomes.
   a. Adequate gas exchange with no respiratory compromise.
   b. Peripheral tissue perfusion maintained.
   c. Pulmonary tissue perfusion maintained.
2. Interventions.
   a. Airway management.
      (1) Position patient to maximize ventilation potential.
      (2) Encourage slow, deep breathing; turning; and coughing.
      (3) Assist with incentive spirometry as appropriate.
   b. Cough enhancement.
      (1) Encourage patient to take a deep breath, hold it for 2 seconds, and cough two or three times in succession.
      (2) Instruct patient to inhale deeply, bend forward slightly, and perform three or four huffs.
      (3) Instruct patient to follow coughing with several maximal inhalation breaths.
   c. Oxygen therapy.
   d. Respiratory monitoring.
   e. Vital sign monitoring.

B. Knowledge, deficient.

1. Outcomes.
   a. Knowledgeable about purposes of treatment modalities.
   b. Understands follow-up care regarding anticoagulation.
2. Interventions.
   a. Discuss activity level and any restrictions.
   b. Explain treatment modalities.

C. Anxiety.

1. Outcomes: effective coping strategies to manage anxiety.
2. Interventions.
   a. Provide factual information regarding condition and treatment.

b. Encourage verbalization of feelings, perceptions, and fears.
c. Be physically available to the patient.
d. Touch patient to express concern and support, as appropriate.
e. Use a calm, reassuring approach.
f. Stay with the patient to promote safety and reduce fear.
g. Assist patient with relaxation exercises.

D. Tissue perfusion, ineffective: cardiopulmonary.

1. Outcomes.
   a. Adequate gas exchange with no respiratory compromise.
   b. Peripheral tissue perfusion maintained.
   c. Pulmonary tissue perfusion maintained.
   d. Vital signs not compromised.
   e. Arterial blood gases within normal range.
2. Interventions.
   a. Administer oxygen therapy.
   b. Monitor respirations.
   c. Monitor vital signs.
   d. Encourage good ventilation (use of incentive spirometry, cough and deep breath every 2 hours).
   e. Administer anticoagulants as appropriate (heparin initially followed with warfarin 48-72 hours before discontinuing heparin).
   f. Monitor laboratory values (PTT, INR, blood gases, hemoglobin).
   g. Provide for adequate hydration.

E. Role performance, ineffective.

1. Outcomes.
   a. Physical needs provided for by caregiver as necessary.
   b. Mutual recognition and acceptance of temporary support.
2. Interventions.
   a. Caregiver support.
   b. Mutual goal setting.
   c. Coping enhancement.

V. HOME CARE CONSIDERATIONS

A. Ensure knowledge of anticoagulation therapy.

1. Purpose and duration of anticoagulation for 3-6 months.
2. Need for and frequency of monitoring INR levels.
3. Potential drug-food interactions with foods high in vitamin K including:
   a. Mayonnaise.
   b. Broccoli/brussels sprouts/cabbage.
   c. Collard greens/endive/kale/lettuce.
   d. Green scallion.
   e. Parsley/spinach/turnip greens/watercress.
4. Potential drug-drug interactions most commonly seen with:
   a. Adrenergic stimulants/antidepressants/psychostimulants.
   b. Analgesics/anesthetics/narcotics, NSAIDs/hypnotics/salicylates.
   c. Antiarrhythmics, antibiotics, anticonvulsants.
   d. Antimalarial agents/antineoplastics/thyroid drugs/oral diabetes agents.
   e. Beta-adrenergic blockers/diuretics/MAO inhibitors.
   f. Hepatotoxic drugs/hypolipidemics/uricosuric agents.
   g. Steroids/vitamins/alcohol.
5. Risk of bleeding and strategies to reduce risk.
   a. Take warfarin at the same time each day.
   b. Keep eating habits and activities similar every day.
   c. Have INR measured as recommended.
   d. Notify health care provider of any change in medications, including use of over-the-counter medications.
   e. Notify health care provider of any illnesses, bleeding in urine or stool, or cuts that don't stop bleeding easily.
   f. Consider wearing a Medical Alert bracelet.
6. May need protamine sulfate or vitamin K as an antidote.

B. Ensure understanding of necessary follow-up.

1. Need for regular monitoring of INR.
2. Importance of informing all health care providers that patient is taking an anticoagulant.
3. Formulate a plan for post-discharge follow-up.

FAT EMBOLISM SYNDROME (FES)

I. OVERVIEW

A. Definition: fat embolism syndrome is the presence of fat globules in the pulmonary circulation system. The globules were most likely released into the system from bone marrow and tissue and then became entrapped in the circulation system of the lung capillaries causing a blockage of blood circulation. There may also be occlusions of small vessels that supply the brain, kidneys, and other organs.

B. Etiology.

1. Manipulation in the medullary canal during stabilization of a fracture or during endoprosthetic surgery leads to an increase of the intramedullary pressure.
2. High intramedullary pressure, especially in long bones, is the main causative factor for fatty marrow release into the circulation.
3. Multi-fractures and crush injuries, especially those caused by high-energy forces.

C. Risk factors.

1. Fracture of a long bone (femur, tibia, ribs, fibula, or pelvis).
2. Intramedullary reamed and unreamed nailing after femoral fracture or metastases.
3. Total joint replacements of the hip or knee with high-volume prostheses or bilateral procedures.
4. Multiple trauma.
5. Hypovolemic shock following traumatic injury.
6. Sepsis.
7. Disseminated intravascular coagulation (DIC).
8. Reduced cardiopulmonary physiologic reserve.
9. Pathologic fractures.
10. Patent foramen ovale.

11. Delayed open reduction internal fixation.
12. Shock.

D. Pathophysiology.

1. Mechanical theory.
   a. Fat embolized by direct entry of fat into the blood stream.
      (1) Fracture of bone disrupts the intramedullary compartment releasing fat cells to venous circulation.
      (2) Injured adipose tissue release fat cells to venous circulation.
   b. Cerebral signs and petechiae caused from obstruction of capillaries in the brain and skin.
   c. Hypoxia and progressive respiratory distress caused by obstruction of vessels in the lungs.
2. Biochemical theory.
   a. Increase in circulating fatty acids.
      (1) Agglutination of endogenous or exogenous plasma fat leads to an increase in fatty acids.
      (2) Lysis of triglycerides may occur at the time of injury mobilizing free fatty acids.
      (3) Release of catecholamines after major injuries may increase the amount of circulating free fatty acids.
      (4) Interaction of C-reactive protein with triglycerides may lead to increased formation of fat globules.
   b. Fatty acids cause endothelial damage and are directly toxic to pneumocytes.
3. Effects of bone marrow/fat on the lung (target organ of the FES).
   a. Acute mechanical obstruction of pulmonary arteries can cause right heart failure.
   b. An inflammatory cascade of mediator-related local effects of released bone marrow leads to endothelium damage of the pulmonary vessels.
      (1) Causes interstitial pulmonary edema.
      (2) Leads to adult respiratory distress syndrome (ARDS).
   c. Free fatty acids increase capillary permeability and contribute to pulmonary edema.
   d. Free fatty acids inactivate lung surfactant causing patchy alveolar collapse leading to decreased oxygen diffusion from alveoli to lung capillaries.
   e. Hypoxia and paradoxical emboli through an open foramen ovale or pulmonary shunts causes cerebral decompensastion.

E. Incidence.

1. Higher incidence with fractures of a long bone (femur, tibia, ribs, fibula, and pelvis).
2. Higher incidence with more than one bone fracture.
3. Higher incidence with hip and knee joint replacements, especially bilateral procedures.
4. FES has an occurrence rate of:
   a. 2% occurrence after femoral fractures.
   b. 0.5%-3.5% after single long-bone fractures.
   c. 0.1% after hip and knee replacements.
   d. Up to 10% in joint replacement after femoral neck fractures.
   e. 5%-10% after multiple fractures.
   d. Up to 90% in multiple trauma patients.
5. FES may occur within hours of injury:
   a. Typically the signs and symptoms of FES do not appear until at least 6-12 hours after time of injury.
   b. Primary symptoms (overt form) occur within 24-72 hours of injury.
   c. Subclinical form appears 72 hours after injury.
   d. A fulminate form occurs within hours after injury and may quickly progress rapidly to death.

F. Considerations across the lifespan.

1. Uncommon in children.
2. Most common in young males due to susceptibility to trauma.

G. Complications.

1. Hypoxemia.
2. Respiratory distress syndrome (ARDS).
3. Disseminated intravascular coagulation.
4. Congestive heart failure.
5. Coma.
6. Prolonged hospitalization.
7. Death.

H. Prevention strategies.

1. Prevent excessive movement of long-bone fractures with early splinting and immobilization.
2. Hydrate to avoid hypovolemia and prevent circulatory instability.
3. Drain fracture hematoma early.
4. Corticosteroid use is controversial.
5. Minimize delay to surgical fixation of fractures (best if done within 24-48 hours).
6. Surgical considerations.
   a. Careful intramedullary lavage before placement of prosthesis to decrease debris available for embolization.
   b. Use of osteotomes or high-speed burr drills produce a lower embolic load than ultrasonic tools.
   c. Venting of the femoral canal to decompress the medullary canal before pressurization.
   d. Use of bone-vacuum cementing technique with total hip arthroplasty.
   e. Use of pneumatic tourniquet during elective surgeries.
   f. Intermittent blood gas analyses during regional anesthesia.
   g. Continuous capnometry during general anesthesia.

II. ASSESSMENT

A. History.

1. Clinical presentation varies widely from subtle symptoms to profound respiratory failure.
2. Time of injury.
3. Extent of injury.
4. Pleuritic chest pain
5. Palpitations.

6. Symptoms associated with hypoxia.
   a. Apprehension.
   b. Restlessness.
   c. Mental status changes.
   d. Agitation
   e. Anxiety

B. Physical examination.

1. Integumentary.
   a. Petechiae of the skin and mucosa (conjunctivae, axillae, anterior side of chest and neck, around the navel and in the mouth) present in 50%-60% of patients.
   b. Fever.
   c. Jaundice.
2. Cardiac system: tachycardia.
3. Respiratory system.
   a. Increasing respiratory distress, use of accessory muscles.
   b. Dyspnea.
   c. Tachypnea.
   d. Rales and rhonchi.
4. Neurologic system.
   a. Restlessness.
   b. Apprehension.
   c. Agitation.
   d. Irritability.
   e. Confusion.
   f. Somnolence.
   g. Lethargy.
   h. Loss of consciousness.
5. Genitourinary system.
   a. Oliguria.
   b. Proteinuria.
   c. Hematuria.

C. Diagnostic tests.

1. Characteristic serum laboratory results consistent with FES.
   a. Hematocrit/hemoglobin decreased suddenly with onset of symptoms.
   b. Platelets decreased.
   c. Calcium decreased.
   d. Serum lipase increased initially.
   e. Free fatty acids increased.
   f. Cortisol increased.
   g. Glucagon increased.
   h. Catecholamines increased.
   i. Erythrocyte sedimentation rate increased.
   j. Prolonged thrombin and prothrombin time.
   k. Blood gas analysis: PaO_2 may drop to less than 60 mm Hg, PaC O_2 may rise > 55 mg Hg as a result of respiratory acidosis (pH < 7.3).
2. Chest x-ray shows a diffuse snowstorm pattern.
3. Electrocardiogram with nonspecific changes.
4. MRI-T2-weighted imaging sensitive for cerebral fat embolism.

III. COMMON THERAPEUTIC MODALITIES

A. Primarily supportive interventions.

1. Initiate oxygen therapy; intubation and ventilatory support as indicated.
2. Provide fluid volume replacement.
3. Ensure appropriate airway management.
4. Steroid use is controversial but may be helpful in overt and subclinical forms of FES.

B. Intensive care unit monitoring.

IV. NURSING DIAGNOSES, OUTCOMES, AND INTERVENTIONS

A. Gas exchange, impaired.

1. Outcomes.
   a. Adequate gas exchange with no respiratory compromise.
   b. Peripheral tissue perfusion maintained.
   c. Pulmonary tissue perfusion maintained.
2. Interventions.
   a. Airway management:
      (1) Position patient to maximize ventilation potential.
      (2) Encourage slow, deep breathing; turning; and coughing.
      (3) Assist with incentive spirometry as appropriate.
   b. Administer oxygen therapy.
   c. Monitor respiratory patterns.
   d. Monitor vital signs.
   e. Elevate head of bed.
   f. Monitor hemaglobin/hematocrit results.
   g. Administer blood transfusions as needed.

B. Breathing pattern, ineffective.

1. Outcomes.
   a. Adequate movement of air into and out of the lungs.
   b. Stable vital signs.
   c. Use of effective coping strategies to manage anxiety.
   d. Effective respiratory efforts without respiratory compromise.
2. Interventions.
   a. Airway management.
      (1) Position patient to maximize ventilation potential.
      (2) Encourage slow, deep breathing; turning; and coughing.
      (3) Assist with incentive spirometry as appropriate.
   b. Reduce anxiety.
   c. Provide mechanical ventilation.
   d. Administer oxygen therapy.
   e. Monitor respiratory patterns.
   f. Monitor vital signs.
   g. Position to maximize ventilatory efforts.

C. Tissue perfusion, ineffective: cardiopulmonary.

1. Outcomes.
   a. Adequate gas exchange with no respiratory compromise.
   b. Peripheral tissue perfusion maintained.
   c. Pulmonary tissue perfusion maintained.
   d. Vital signs not compromised.
   e. Arterial blood gases within normal range.
2. Interventions.

a. Administer oxygen therapy.
b. Monitor respiratory patterns.
c. Monitor vital signs.
d. Encourage good ventilation (use of incentive spirometry, cough and deep breathe every 2 hours).
e. Administer anticoagulants as appropriate (heparin initially followed with warfarin 48-72 hours before discontinuing heparin).
f. Monitor laboratory values (PTT, INR, blood gases, hemoglobin).
g. Provide for adequate hydration.

D. Role performance, ineffective.

1. Outcomes.
   a. Physical needs provided for by caregiver as necessary.
   b. Mutual recognition and acceptance of temporary support.
2. Interventions.
   a. Caregiver support.
   b. Mutual goal setting.
   c. Coping enhancement.

E. Anxiety.

1. Outcomes: use of effective coping strategies to manage anxiety.
2. Interventions.
   a. Provide factual information regarding condition and treatment.
   b. Encourage verbalization of feelings, perceptions, and fears.
   c. Be physically available to the patient.
   d. Touch patient to express concern, support, as appropriate.
   e. Use a calm, reassuring approach.
   f. Stay with the patient to promote safety and reduce fear.

V. HOME CARE CONSIDERATIONS

A. Formulate a plan for post discharge follow-up.

B. Coordinate referrals relevant to care as appropriate.

DEEP VEIN THROMBOSIS (DVT)

I. OVERVIEW

A. Definition: Deep vein thrombosis (DVT) is the occurrence of a clot in a deep vein in the lower extremity.

1. A thrombus is the formation of a fibrin clot within a blood vessel, typically the deep veins of the lower extremity.
2. Phlebitis is the inflammation of a vein.
3. Thrombophlebitis describes a condition in which there is both a clot and inflammation.

B. Etiology.

1. Stasis of venous flow.
2. Injury to the endothelial.
3. Hypercoagulability of the blood.

C. Risk factors.

1. Age: risk increases after age 40; even greater risk after age 60.
2. General anesthesia.
3. Postoperative infection.
4. Vascular wall injury.
   a. Surgery (especially of pelvis, hip, or lower extremity).
   b. Re-operation.
   c. Trauma.
   d. Previous thromboembolism.
   e. IV therapy.
   f. IV drug abuse.
   g. Smoking.
5. Venous stasis.
   a. Immobilization.
   b. Surgery > 30 minutes.
   c. Obstruction or compression of the iliac or femoral veins.
      (1) Large abdominal or pelvic tumors.
      (2) Obesity.
      (3) Pregnancy.
   d. Congestive heart failure.
   e. Shock.
   f. Varicose veins.
   g. Stroke.
   h. Cardiomyopathy.
   i. Pericarditis.
   j. Anasarca.
6. Hypercoagulability.
   a. Pregnancy.
   b. Estrogen therapy.
   c. Malignancy.
   d. Sickle cell disease.
   e. Dehydration.
   f. Polycythemia rubra vera.
   g. Deficiencies in clotting cascade (antithrombin III, protein C, protein S, fibrinogen, factor V Leiden, or plasminogen).
   h. Lupus anticoagulant.
   i. Nephrotic syndrome.
   j. Inflammatory bowel disease.

D. Pathophysiology.

1. Endothelial injury, a hypercoagulable state, and venostasis upset the normal balance between blood-clotting activators and inhibitors.
2. Circulating coagulation proteins generate thrombin, which helps convert fibrinogen to fibrin.
3. Fibrin forms a mesh-like substance that traps plasma, platelets, and other blood cells to form a fibrin nidus.
4. As the nidus grows, it develops into a thrombus.
5. Clinical symptoms appear when thrombus is large enough to impede blood flow in one of the large vessels.

E. Incidence.

1. Most common sites are anterior and posterior tibial vein, the peroneal veins, the popliteal vein, the saphenous vein, and the femoral vein.
2. Can also occur in the upper extremity but this is less common.
3. 45%-70% incidence after hip and knee surgery.
   a. Increases with bilateral surgeries.

b. Decreases when epidural anesthesia used with arthroplasty as compared with general anesthesia.
c. Lower incidence with non-cemented prosthesis.
4. Multiple trauma patients.
5. Acute paraplegics are at risk and unable to feel the sensory symptoms.

F. Considerations across the lifespan.
1. DVT uncommon in children.
2. Increased risk of DVT during pregnancy (warfarin therapy is contraindicated)

G. Complications.
1. Pulmonary embolism.
2. Postphlebitic syndrome.
3. Heparin-induced thrombocytopenia.

H. Prevention strategies.
1. Identify patient at risk.
2. Pharmacologic interventions.
   a. Prophylactic anticoagulation for high-risk patients.
      (1) Aspirin.
      (2) Unfractionated or low molecular weight heparin.
      (3) Warfarin.
   b. Additional prophylactic approaches for high-risk patients.
      (1) Danaparoid.
      (2) Dermatan sulfate.
      (3) Dextran.
      (4) Hirudin and analogues.
      (5) Thrombin inhibitors.
      (6) Antiplatelet substances.
3. Nonpharmacologic interventions.
   a. External pneumatic compression devices.
   b. Graduated compression stockings.
   c. Foot impulse pump.
   d. Early ambulation.
   e. Frequent plantar flexion and dorsiflexion of the foot, ankle, and toes.
   f. Deep breathing exercises to help the large veins empty by increasing negative pressure in the thorax.
4. Surgical interventions.
   a. Prophylactic inferior vena cava filter in select high-risk patients.
   b. Epidural/spinal anesthesia instead of general anesthesia when feasible.
   c. Non-cemented prostheses when possible.

II. ASSESSMENT

A. History.
1. Determine history of recent surgical procedure.
2. Identify any risk factors specified in the preceeding DVT section I., C.
3. Assess pain for pattern consistent with DVT.
   a. Aching, mild, or severe pain.
   b. Constant, not intermittent in nature.
   c. Movement and/or weight bearing aggravates pain.
4. Inquire about unilateral swelling of extremity.

B. Physical examination.
1. Increased warmth of extremity.
2. Unilateral swelling of extremity.
3. Erythema of extremity.
4. Tenderness to palpation.
5. Palpable, tender venous cord in popliteal fossa suggestive of popliteal DVT.
6. Positive Homan's sign – not specific or sensitive to DVT and present in < 1/3 of symptomatic patients.

C. Diagnostic tests.
1. Contrast venography.
2. Doppler ultrasonagraphy with compression.
3. MRI.
4. Radionuclide venography.
5. Scintigraphic scanning.
6. Radionuclide scintigraphy.
7. Venous pressure measurements.

III. COMMON THERAPEUTIC MODALITIES

A. Full dose anticoagulation with unfractionated heparin or low molecular weight heparin followed with warfarin.

B. Goal of international normalized ratio (INR) of 2.0-3.0.

C. Analgesics for pain management.

IV. NURSING DIAGNOSES, OUTCOMES, AND INTERVENTIONS

A. Pain, acute.
1. Outcomes.
   a. Reports pain level satisfactory.
   b. Uses analgesics appropriately.
   c. Engages in nonpharmacologic techniques.
2. Interventions.
   a. Assess pain level.
   b. Initiate pharmacologic measures to relieve pain (avoid aspirin and NSAIDs).
   c. Initiate nonpharmacologic measures to relieve pain.
      (1) Elevate extremity.
      (2) Apply moist heat.
      (3) Use distraction techniques.

B. Knowledge, deficient.
1. Outcomes.
   a. Knowledgeable about risk factors and preventive measures.
   b. Knowledgeable about prescribed activity and anticoagulation medications.
   c. Understands follow-up care regarding anticoagulation.
2. Interventions.
   a. Teach about risk factors and preventive measures.
   b. Discuss activity level and any restrictions.
   c. Explain prevention and treatment modalities:
      (1) Pneumatic compression devices.
      (2) Graduated compression stockings.
      (3) Foot impulse pump.
      (4) Range-of-motion exercises.
      (5) Anticoagulation medications.

C. Tissue perfusion, ineffective: peripheral.
1. Outcomes.
   a. Resolution of swelling.

b. Distal peripheral pulses strong and symmetrical.
c. Successful pain management.
2. Interventions.
a. Monitor peripheral circulation (pulses, edema, capillary refill, color, temperature of extremity).
b. Assess pain level.
c. Initiate pain relieving measures.
d. Administer anticoagulant therapy as appropriate (heparin initially followed with warfarin within 48-72 hours before stopping heparin).
e. Monitor laboratory values (PTT, INR, CBC, platelets) as appropriate.
f. Elevate involved extremity to decrease swelling.

V. HOME CARE CONSIDERATIONS

A. Ensure knowledge of anticoagulation therapy.
1. Purpose and duration of anticoagulation for 3-6 months.
2. Need for and frequency of monitoring INR levels.
3. Potential drug-food interactions with foods high in vitamin K including:
a. Mayonnaise.
b. Broccoli/brussels sprouts/cabbage.
c. Collard greens/endive/kale/lettuce.
d. Green scallion.
e. Parsley/spinach/turnip greens/watercress.
4. Potential drug-drug interactions most commonly seen with:
a. Adrenergic stimulants/antidepressants/psychostimulants.
b. Analgesics/anesthetics/narcotics, NSAIDs/hypnotics/salicylates.
c. Antiarrhythmics, antibiotics, anticonvulsants.
d. Antimalarial agents/antineoplastics/thyroid drugs/oral diabetes agents.
e. Beta-adrenergic blockers/diuretics/MAO inhibitors.
f. Hepatotoxic drugs/hypolipidemics/uricosuric agents.
g. Steroids/vitamins/alcohol.
5. Risk of bleeding and strategies to reduce risk.
a. Take warfarin at the same time each day.
b. Keep eating habits and activities similar every day.
c. Have INR measured as recommended.
d. Notify health care provider of any change in medications, including use of over-the-counter medications.
e. Notify health care provider of any illnesses, bleeding in urine or stool, or cuts that don't stop bleeding easily.
f. Consider wearing a Medical Alert bracelet.
6. May need protamine sulfate or vitamin K as an antidote.

B. Ensure understanding of necessary follow-up.
1. Need for regular monitoring of INR.
2. Importance of informing all health care providers that patient is taking an anticoagulant.
3. Formulate a plan for post-discharge follow-up.

COMPARTMENT SYNDROME

I. OVERVIEW

A. Definition: a condition in which increased progressive pressure within a confined space (muscle compartment) compromises the circulation and the function of tissues within that space.

B. Types.
1. Acute compartment syndrome.
a. Medical emergency, as can be limb threatening.
b. Generally occurs following trauma.
2. Chronic (exertional) compartment syndrome.
a. Overuse injury primarily of the lower extremity.
b. Induced by exertion and relieved by rest.
3. Crush syndrome.
a. Systemic manifestation of prolonged muscle compression and compartment syndrome.
b. Aggressive treatment necessary to prevent prolonged multiorgan failure and death.

C. Etiology.
1. Decreased compartment volume (size).
a. Closure of fascial defects.
b. Application of excessive traction to fractured extremities.
2. Increased compartment content.
a. Bleeding of a vascular injury due to a fracture or a coagulation defect.
b. Increased capillary permeability due to postischemic swelling, trauma, intense use of muscles, burns, intra-arterial drug injection, snakebite.
c. Increased capillary pressure due to intense use of muscles, venous obstruction, edema.
d. Diminished serum osmolarity.
e. Other causes: infiltrated infusion, pressure transfusion, leaky dialysis cannula, muscle hypertrophy, popliteal cyst.
3. Externally applied pressure.
a. Tight cast, dressing, brace, air splint, or antishock trousers.
b. Lying on limb.
c. Trapped under heavy object with prolonged pressure.

D. Risk factors.
1. External compression forces exert pressure and decrease the size of a specific anatomic compartment.
a. Tight cast, dressing, brace, air splint, air trousers.
b. Prolonged compression to an extremity.
c. Traction.
2. Internal compression force from increased content within a confined compartment can raise the internal pressures.
a. Bleeding.
b. Edema.
3. Additional contributing factors.
a. Acute trauma.
b. Fracture.

c. Infection.
d. Tibial nailing.
e. Insensate extremity.
f. Significant venous obstruction.
g. Significant infiltration of an IV site.
h. Frostbite.
i. Venomous bites.

4. Specific for chronic (exertional) compartment syndrome.
   a. Intensive exercise.
   b. Prolonged weight-bearing physical activity.

E. Pathophysiology.

1. Compartments are enveloped by tough inelastic facial tissue.
   a. Swelling of muscle increases pressure and reduces capillary blood perfusion.
   b. Failure of microcirculation occurs when local blood flow is unable to meet the metabolic demands of the tissue leading to tissue hypoxia and cell death.
2. Ischemia-edema cycle.
   a. Tissue swelling leads to compression of vessels and nerves.
   b. Significant swelling causes muscle ischemia.
   c. Ischemic muscles release histamine leading to capillary dilation and increased capillary permeability.
   d. Capillary dilation and increased capillary permeability lead to increased edema and further decrease in perfusion and oxygenation of vital tissues.
   e. Increased lactic acid production causes more anaerobic metabolism and increased blood flow.
   f. Increased blood flow raises the tissue pressure, leading to a cycle of increasing compartmental pressure.
3. The tissue pressure level at which perfusion is sufficiently impaired as to threaten cell viability varies according to the age and circulatory status of the patient.
4. Muscle damage is irreversible after 4-8 hours of ischemia and nerve damage is irreversible after 8 hours of ischemia if the pressure is not relieved.

F. Incidence.

1. Acute compartment syndrome.
   a. Incidence most prevalent within first week after injury.
   b. Compartments most commonly affected (see Table 8.1).
      (1) Leg (anterior, lateral, superficial posterior, and deep posterior).
      (2) Forearm (superficial flexor, deep flexor, and extensor).
      (3) Upper arm (deltoid and biceps).
   c. Hand (interosseous), buttock (gluteal), thigh (quadriceps), and abdomen are affected less frequently.
2. Chronic (exertional) compartment syndrome.
   a. Often occurs bilaterally.
   b. Equal incidence in males and females.
   c. Anterior compartment affected most frequently.
3. Crush syndrome.
   a. Incidence related to extent of injury.
   b. Reported more commonly in major disasters.

G. Considerations across the lifespan.

1. Cell viability in children is compromised at a lower compartmental pressure than in adults, so intervention becomes mandatory when the compartmental pressure has risen to within 30 mm Hg of the mean arterial pressure.
2. Diagnosis of increased compartmental pressure in a child is clinically demanding as it requires patient cooperation, which may be lacking in the scared, irritable, or preverbal child.
3. The agitated child with increasing analgesia requirements requires a thorough evaluation to rule out compartment syndrome.
4. Standard double-ported 18G needle used for invasive monitoring is too large for use in children; consider single-ported needles.
5. Acute applies to all age groups, similar incidence in adults and children.
6. Chronic generally found in young, active individuals.

H. Complications.

1. Volkmann's contracture, a rapidly developing flexion deformity of the wrist and fingers, with loss of power, resulting from fixed contracture of the flexor muscles of the forearm.
2. Objective sensory and motor deficit.
3. Infection.
4. Rhabdomylolysis.
5. Myonephropathic syndrome.
6. Amputation.
7. Limb deformity/contracture.
8. Acute renal failure.
9. Contractures.

I. Prevention strategies.

1. Acute compartment syndrome.
   a. Avoid excessive external pressure to area of concern.
   b. Monitor for early symptoms of a tight cast, splint, dressing.
      (1) Increased pain.
      (2) Increased swelling.
      (3) Numbness.
      (4) Paresthesia.
   c. Provide adequate hydration to maintain mean arterial blood pressure.
   d. Measure intracompartmental pressure when initial signs or symptoms of compartment syndrome are recognized.
2. Chronic (exertional) compartment syndrome.
   a. Avoid aggravating activities.
   b. Cross-training with low-impact activities.

II. ASSESSMENT

A. History.

1. Acute: progressive pain out of proportion to what is anticipated.

a. First and most important symptoms are subjective.
b. Pain assessment:
(1) Primary symptom is increasing pain out of proportion to the injury.
(2) Pain unrelieved by appropriate narcotics.
(3) Pain is described as deep, throbbing, persistent, and usually localized to the area of the compartment. Sometimes pain is experienced as diffuse pain.
(4) Immobilization is unsuccessful in relieving the pain which correlates with increasing compartment pressure.
c. Sensory assessment:
(1) Numbness and tingling, specifically associated with nerve in an affected compartment, may indicate onset of decreased tissue perfusion.
(2) May experience paresthesia like "pins and needles," "feeling of being asleep."
d. Onset of symptoms.
(1) Precipitating factors: nature and extent of injury.
(2) Aggravating factors: cast, traction, splint, positioning, swelling.
(3) Relieving factors: analgesics, position change, cast splitting, loosening bandage/splint.

2. Chronic: bilateral pain is present in 90% of patients.
a. Discomfort described as aching, tightness, or squeezing in the affected limb.
b. Relationship of symptoms to activity. Time period following cessation of exercise in which symptoms disappear.
c. Previous injuries or immobilization.

3. Crush syndrome.
a. Cause and duration of limb compression.
b. Position of extremity during crush.
c. Pain may be described as deep, unremitting, and poorly localized.

B. Physical examination.

1. Acute (see Table 8.1).
a. Inspection.
(1) Increased tenseness of skin swelling and increasing erythema are an early sign of increasing pressure within compartment.
(2) Tenseness of skin and pallor are a later sign of increased compartment pressures.
b. Pain assessment: pain with passive stretching of muscles in a given compartment is an early clinical indicator of ischemia.
c. Neurovascular assessment.
(1) Sensory exam: decreased sensation, tingling, paresthesia all indicative of decreased perfusion.
(2) Motor exam: a decrease in and loss of motor strength and motion is a late sign of ischemia.
(3) Vascular examination.
(a) Pallor, cool temperature, and slow capillary refill are early signs of decreased tissue perfusion.
(b) Absence of pulse is a very late sign of decreased tissue perfusion.
d. Palpable tightness of the compartment.

2. Chronic.
a. Inspection and palpation:
(1) No generalized swelling.
(2) Muscle hernia (soft tissue mass more pronounced with active dorsiflexion of the foot).
b. Vascular examination usually normal.
c. Isolated muscle weakness dependent on compartment involved.
d. Numbness and paresthesias rare.

3. Crush syndrome.
a. Inspection and palpation: tense, swollen extremity may be present.
(1) Swelling may be absent in the presence of dehydration and peripheral vasoconstriction from shock.
(2) Cool, clammy skin with hypovolemia.
(3) Accompanying skin changes: erythema, bullae, vesicles.
b. Alteration in urinary output.

C. Diagnostic tests.

1. Laboratory tests.
a. Serum: elevated CPK, LDH, and SGOT all indicative of muscle damage.
b. Urine: myoglobin in urine indicative of muscle damage.

2. Measurement of intracompartmental pressures with pressure monitor.
a. Normal compartment pressure between 0-8 mm Hg.
b. Differential pressure (difference between diastolic BP and compartment pressure) of 30 mm Hg is necessary to perfuse the compartment.
c. Compartment pressures of 30-45 mm Hg are high enough to cause tissue necrosis if the diastolic blood pressure is not high enough to perfuse the compartment.

3. Measurement methods.
a. Injection technique: measures the amount of pressure via a pressure transducer, which requires an injection of a small amount of fluid into the compartmental tissue through a needle. A steady state reading is not achieved.
b. Wick method: strands of wettable material extending into the compartment tissue from a fluid-filled catheter connected to a pressure transducer measure tissue pressure.
c. Continuous infusion technique: utilizes a needle inserted into compartment tissue while a slow continuous infusion of nonheparinized saline is maintained. Pressure within needle is monitored with a standard blood pressure transducer.

4. Acute.

Table 8.1
Assessment of Neurovascular Integrity of the Major Compartments of the Upper and Lower Extremities

Compartment	Muscles	Nerve	Assess Tender-ness	Assess Sensation	Assess Motion	Assess for Pain with Passive Stretch
Upper Extremity						
Superficial Flexor	Pronator teres, flexor carpi radialis, palmaris longus, flexor carpi ulnaris, flexor digitorum superficialis	Median	Volar Forearm	Tip of index finger	Oppose thumb and little finger	Extend the thumb
Deep Flexor	Flexor digitorum profundus, flexor pollicis longus, pronator quadratus	Ulnar	Volar Forearm	Tip of little finger	Abduct all fingers	Adduct the fingers
Extensor	Extensor carpi radialis longus and brevis, extensor carpi ulnaris, extensor digitorum, extensor indicis, extensor digiti minimi, abductor pollicus longus, extensor pollicis longus and brevis, supinator	Radial	Dorsal Forearm	Web space between thumb and index finger	Extend wrist and with hyper-extension of thumb and wrist, hyperextend the four fingers at the MCP joints	Flex the thumb and fingers
Lower Extremity						
Anterior	Tibialis anterior, extensor hallucis longus, extensor digitorum longus, peroneus tertius	Deep peroneal	Anterior aspect lower leg	Web space between great toe and second toe	Dorsiflex foot and extend toes	Plantar flex the foot and flex toes
Lateral	Peroneus longus, peroneus brevis	Super-ficial peroneal	Lateral aspect lower leg	Dorsum of foot	Evert the foot	Invert the foot
Superficial Posterior	Gastrocnemius, soleus, plantaris	Sural and tibial	Between tibia and Achilles tendon	Lateral aspect fifth toe	Plantar flex foot and invert foot	Dorsiflex and evert the foot
Deep Posterior	Popliteus, flexor hallucis longus, flexor digitorum longus, tibialis posterior	Tibial	Between tibia and Achilles tendon	Medial and lateral surfaces of the soles of the foot	Plantar flex foot, flex toes, and invert foot	Dorsiflex foot, extend toes, and evert foot

a. Continuous monitoring used in comatose, unresponsive, or uncooperative patients.
b. In alert patients, one-time pressure monitoring and ongoing evaluation of signs and symptoms may be used.

5. Chronic:
   a. Diagnosis confirmed by identifying a positive clinical pattern of muscle compartment pain with exercise and measurement of compartment pressures.
   b. Compartment pressures chronically elevated with resting pressure of 15-30 mm Hg and postexercise pressures above 30 mm Hg.
   c. Magnetic resonance imaging (MRI) may be ordered to assess muscle density changes.
   d. 99T cm-methoxyisobustyl isonitrile (99Tcm-MIBI) scintiraphy.
   e. Thallium stress testing.
6. Crush syndrome:
   a. CT scan.
   b. MRI.
   c. Muscle biopsy.
   d. Compartment pressure monitoring.
   e. Serum lab studies (9CPK, LDH, SGOT, electrolytes).
   f. Urine for myoglobin.

III. COMMON THERAPEUTIC MODALITIES

A. Acute compartment syndrome

1. Relieve sources of pressure: bivalve cast, remove splint, remove or loosen constrictive bandage, release or decrease traction.
2. Elevate extremity at heart level: elevation above the heart reduces the arterio-venous pressure gradient and may further compromise local blood flow.
3. Provide adequate hydration to maintain mean arterial blood pressure.
4. Monitor compartment pressures (continuous or intermittent).
5. Provide supplemental oxygen to ensure optimal saturation.
6. Monitor serum levels of CPK, LDH, and SGOT and urine values of myoglobin.
7. Decompress compartment surgically via fasciotomy if compartment pressures remain elevated and ischemia is a threat.
   a. Tourniquet is not used during decompression procedure.
   b. Envelopes are opened along the length of the muscle compartment.
   c. After decompression, the skin is left open to prevent "rebound" compartment syndrome.
   d. Passive range of motion is done daily on the affected joint per physician order.
   e. In 3-5 days, the wound is examined surgically and necrotic tissue is debrided, or the edges are gradually approximated with surgical tape over 1-2 weeks.
   f Skin graft may be needed to achieve closure.
8. Amputation may be necessary if severe neuromuscular damage occurs.

B. Chronic compartment syndrome.

1. Conservative management.
   a. Orthotics for sports shoes.
   b. Reduce/eliminate aggravating activity.
   c. Nonsteroidal anti-inflammatory drugs.
   d. Referral to physical therapy.
2. Surgical compartment decompression.
   a. Fasciotomy.
   b. Fasciectomy.

C. Crush syndrome.

1. Interventions as noted for acute compartment syndrome as appropriate.
2. Supportive care for rhabdomyloysis, renal failure, and coagulopathies.

IV. NURSING DIAGNOSES, OUTCOMES, AND INTERVENTIONS

A. Peripheral neurovascular dysfunction, risk for.

1. Outcomes.
   a. Peripheral tissue perfusion will be maintained.
   b. Arterial blood pressure will be at least 30 mm Hg higher than compartment pressure.
2. Interventions.
   a. Monitor neurovascular status at least every 2 hours.
   b. Maintain elevation of extremity at heart level (elevation reduces the arterio-venous pressure gradient).
   c. Assess for inadequate pain management.
   d. Monitor and encourage hydration.
   e. Monitor compartment pressures (continuous or intermittent) if high risk.
   f. Communicate and collaborate with physician in a timely manner if signs and symptoms of compartment syndrome appear.

B. Pain, acute.

1. Outcomes.
   a. Reports pain level satisfactory.
   b. Uses analgesics appropriately.
   c. Engages in nonpharmacologic pain management techniques.
2. Interventions.
   a. Administer analgesics.
   b. Assess for constrictive cast, dressing, or splint and relieve pressure if excessive.
   c. Initiate nonpharmacologic pain management techniques as appropriate.
   d. Control environmental factors that may influence the patient's response to discomfort.
   e. Elevate extremity to heart level.
   f. Educate patient about medications and treatments.

C. Infection, risk for.

1. Outcome: patient will remain free of infections
2. Interventions.
   a. Use sterile techniques in caring for wound: wet to dry dressings.
   b. Assess quality of decompression wound as needed. (Skin closure usually occurs 3-6 days after surgical decompression.)
   c. Administer prophylactic antibiotics per orders.

d. Assess for signs of infection (elevated temperature).
e. Obtain blood and wound cultures if infection is suspected.
f. Continue assessment for signs and symptoms of increased compartment pressure.
g. Avoid constrictive postoperative dressing.

V. HOME CARE CONSIDERATIONS

A. Considerations if patient had a fasciotomy.
1. Teach patient/caregiver wound care.
2. Teach patient/caregiver signs and symptoms of infection.

B. Ensure accommodation in the home if patient has activity restrictions.

C. Formulate a plan for post-discharge follow-up.

DELAYED UNION/NONUNION

I. OVERVIEW

A. Definition.
1. Delayed union is a continuation of or increase in bone pain and tenderness beyond a reasonable healing period. Healing of the fractures is slowed but not completely stopped.
2. Nonunion occurs when fracture healing has not taken place 4-6 months after the fracture occurs and spontaneous healing is unlikely.

B. Etiology.
1. Distraction of fracture fragments associated with delayed union.
2. Infection.
3. Insufficient blood supply to fracture site.
4. Uncontrolled repetitive stress on the fracture site.

C. Incidence.
1. Varies by fracture location.
2. Varies by fracture type.
3. Varies by initial treatment modality.

II. ASSESSMENT

A. History.
1. Type of fracture/location/soft tissue interposition.
2. Initial type of immobilization.
3. Adherence to initial restrictions/weight-bearing limitations.
4. Smoking history and use of NSAIDs, steroids, or calcium channel blockers (associated with slower healing).
5. Pain assessment.

B. Physical examination.
1. Tenderness with palpation.
2. Motion at the fracture site.

C. Diagnostic tests.
1. Serial x-rays.
2. CT scan.

III. COMMON THERAPEUTIC MODALITIES

A. Bone grafting.
1. Allografts or autografts.
2. Cortical or cancellous.

B. Internal fixation.

C. External fixation.

D. Electrical bone stimulation.
1. Direct, invasive.
   a. Requires surgical placement of cathode, anode, and generator.
   b. Fracure immobilized with cast, brace, or external fixation.
   c. No active participation of patient required.
   d. Contraindicated with osteomyelitis.
2. Indirect, noninvasive.
   a. Treatment coil or transducer applied to cast or skin over fracture site and connected to portable battery pack.
   b. Requires active patient participation.
   c. Treatment time ranges from 2-10 hours per day for 3-6 months.
   d. Contraindicated with certain types of demand pacemakers.

E. Pulsed, low-intensity ultrasound.

IV. NURSING DIAGNOSES, OUTCOMES, AND INTERVENTIONS

A. Physical mobility, impaired.
1. Outcomes.
   a. Safe ambulation with assistive device as necessary.
   b. Pain free joint motion.
2. Interventions.
   a. Teaching: use of assistive device (crutches, cane, walker, etc.).
   b. Teaching: prescribed exercises.
   c. Teaching: prescribed activity level/weight bearing status.
   c Pain management

B. Knowledge, deficient.
1. Outcomes.
   a. Knowledge about purpose and use of electrical bone stimulation.
   b. Complies with recommended use of electrical bone stimulation and activity/mobility restrictions.
2. Interventions.
   a. Teaching: purpose and use of electrical bone stimulation.
      (1) Understanding relationship of immobilization, weight-bearing, and stimulator use.
      (2) Changing electrodes.
      (3) Attaching battery packs.
      (4) Attaching power source.
      (5) Problem solving equipment issues.
   b. Mutual goal setting.
      (1) Develop a regimen to maximize success with use of bone stimulator, activity restrictions, and use of immobilization device.
      (2) Encourage verbalization of feelings, perceptions, and fears.

V. HOME CARE CONSIDERATIONS

A. Use of electrical bone stimulation associated with monthly follow-up visits to monitor incision, generator, output, records of time used, and assessement of immobilzation and progress with bone healing.

B. **Invasive direct-current stimulation requires outpatient procedure for removal of generator and cathode lead once union achieved or power source exhausted (8 months).**

C. **Determine availability of home support for lengthy healing and recuperation period.**

NOSOCOMIAL SURGICAL SITE INFECTIONS (SSI)

I. OVERVIEW

A. **Definition: superficial incision, deep incision, or organ/space surgical site infections that occur within 30 days after operative procedure (within 1 year if an implant is in place).**

B. **Etiology.**
  1. Break in integrity of skin.
  2. Bacterial contamination.

C. **Risk factors.**
  1. Intrinsic factors.
    a. Patient characteristics.
      (1) Young (< 1 year) or advanced age.
      (2) Nosocomial infection other than SSI (urinary tract infection, pneumonia).
      (3) Substance abuse including tobacco.
      (4) Obesity.
      (5) Malnutrition.
      (6) Diabetes.
      (7) Rheumatoid arthritis.
      (6) Hypovolemia.
      (7) Chronic steroid use.
      (8) NSAID use.
      (9) Chemotherapy recipient.
      (10) Latent infection.
      (11) Low socioeconomic status.
      (12) Prolonged inactivity.
    b. Injury characteristics.
      (1) Extent of tissue trauma.
      (2) Presence of foreign material.
      (3) Wound classification.
  2. Extrinsic factors.
    a. Preoperative factors.
      (1) Preoperative stay over 4 days.
      (2) Preoperative shave > 1 day prior to surgery.
      (3) Inadequate immobilization of a fractured bone.
    b. Intraoperative factors.
      (1) Positive intraoperative wound culture.
      (2) Perioperative antibiotics.
      (3) Use of drains and packings.
      (4) Primary versus secondary closure.
      (5) Duration of surgery.
      (6) Surgeon expertise.
      (7) Use of drapes.
      (8) Glove punctures.
      (9) Irrigation.
    c. Postoperative factors.
      (1) Cold ambient temperature.
      (2) Insufficient fluid replacement.
      (3) Hypertension.
      (4) Inadequate analgesia.
      (5) Compromised blood perfusion.
      (6) Low oxygenation.
      (7) Inadequate aseptic technique.

D. **Pathophysiology.**
  1. Microcirculation damage from surgical incision or traumatic injury.
    a. Increased demand for oxygen due to hemostasis and inflammation.
    b. Platelets aggregate and release chemoattractants and growth factors.
    c. Subsequent coagulation occludes vessels and prevents exsanguination but also widens the area of impaired circulation.
    d. Microcirculation further stressed with bradykinin, complement, and release of histamine by mast cells.
    e. Epithelial cells move and replicate in response to growth factors and oxygen tension.
    f. Epithelization occurs most rapidly in hydrated, well-oxygenated tissues.
  2. Peripheral vasoconstriction, which results from central sympathetic control of subcutaneous vascular tone, is an important impediment to maintaining oxygen supply in wounds.
  3. Exogenous infection possible following contamination during the postoperative period.

E. **Incidence.**
  1. Mean SSI rate for orthopaedic procedures is 2.3%.
  2. Rate of infection after total hip arthroplasty is approximately 1% over the lifetime of the prosthesis.
  3. Rate of infection after arthroscopy ranges from 0%-3%.

F. **Considerations across the lifespan.**
  1. Affects all ages.
  2. Risk factors noted above increase risk.

G. **Complications.**
  1. Osteomyelitis.
  2. Septicemia.
  3. Re-operation for debridement.
  4. Increased length of stay.
  5. Death.

H. **Prevention strategies.**
  1. Adherence to universal precautions and aseptic techniques in all clinical settings.
  2. Preoperative strategies.
    a. Optimize cardiopulmonary function.
    b. Control hypertension.
    c. Prevent sympathetically induced peripheral vasoconstriction (maintain blood volume, control pain, alleviate anxiety, keep patient warm).
    d. Replenish nutritional deficits.
    e. Minimize unnecessary movement of fractured bones.
    f. Improve or maintain blood sugar control.
  3. Intraoperative strategies.
    a. Give antimicrobial prophylaxis.
      (1) Single dose of appropriate antibiotic 30 minutes before skin incision.
      (2) Additional antibiotic doses if surgery is longer than 3 hours, major blood loss

occurs, or an antimicrobial with a short half-life is used.
  b. Adhere to strict aseptic technique.
  c. Handle soft tissues gently.
  d. Debride devitalized bone and soft tissues.
  e. Ensure stable fixation of fractures.
  f. Keep patient warm to avoid vasoconstriction.
  g. Elevate PaO_2.
  h. Close wound without excessive tension.
  i. Ensure quality operating room ventilation system.
4. Postoperative strategies.
  a. Provide adequate analgesia.
  b. Keep patient warm to avoid vasoconstriction.
  c. Maintain hydration.
  d. Control blood pressure and serum glucose levels.
  e. Assess and provide for nutritional needs.
  f. Adhere to aseptic technique with dressing changes.
  g. Wash hands thoroughly.
  h. Give microbial therapy as indicated.

II. ASSESSMENT

A. History.
1. Increased pain.
2. Increased warmth over wound/incision.
3. Verbalization of odor from wound/incision.
4. Fever/chills.
5. Intrinsic risk factors.

B. Physical examination.
1. Erythema around incision/wound.
2. Edema around incision/wound.
3. Increased temperature around incision/wound.
4. Purulent exudate from incision/wound.
5. Elevated body temperature.
6. Poor wound healing.
7. Notable malodor from incision/wound.

C. Diagnostic tests.
1. Complete blood count (WBC increased with infection).
2. Erythrocyte sedimentation rate elevated with infection.
3. C-reactive protein elevated with infection.
4. Wound culture.
5. Hemoglobin

III. COMMON THERAPEUTIC MODALITIES

A. Local wound care.

B. Systemic/oral antibiotics.
1. Consider results of microbiologic culture.
2. Distinguish between surface colonization and invasive infection.

C. Monitor and ensure adequate perfusion and oxygenation.

D. Provide for optimal nutritional intake.
1. High protein and sufficient calories to prevent a catabolic-induced decline in lean muscle mass, which can further impair wound healing.
2. Vitamins A, C, and E, and the minerals zinc and iron are important for wound healing and to decrease risk of infection.

IV. NURSING DIAGNOSES, OUTCOMES, AND INTERVENTIONS

A. Infection, risk for.
1. Outcomes.
  a. Resolution of infection.
  b. Knowledge of treatment for diagnosed infection.
  c. Knowledge of signs and symptoms of infection to monitor for recurrence.
  d. Ability to describe activities to increase resistance to infection.
2. Interventions.
  a. Ensure appropriate wound care technique.
  b. Administer antibiotic therapy, as appropriate.
  c. Promote appropriate nutritional intake.
    (1) Adequate protein important for wound healing and immune system functioning.
    (2) Vitamins A, C, and E, and the minerals zinc and iron are important for wound healing and to decrease risk of infection.
  d. Adhere to universal precautions.
  e. Teach patient/caregiver about medications and wound care.
  f. Teach patient/caregiver signs and symptoms of infection.

B. Pain, acute.
1. Outcomes.
  a. Reports pain level satisfactory.
  b. Uses analgesics appropriately.
  c. Engages in nonpharmacologic techniques.
2. Interventions.
  a. Assess pain level.
  b. Initiate pharmacologic measures to relieve pain.
  c. Initiate nonpharmacologic pain management techniques.
  d. Control environmental factors that may influence the patient's response to discomfort.

C. Nutrition, imbalanced: less than body requirements.
1. Outcomes.
  a. Patient will maintain body weight.
  b. Patient will consume adequate nutrition required to combat infection.
2. Interventions.
  a. Maintain a well-balanced diet.
  b. Increase intake of vitamin C and protein required for healing.
  c. Maintain adequate fluid and fiber in the diet.
  d. Obtain foods based on patient's choice.

V. HOME CARE CONSIDERATIONS

A. Teach the patient/caregiver how to care for the wound.

B. Teach patients the signs and symptoms of infection and how to take his/her temperature.

C. Emphasize the value of handwashing.

D. Ensure appropriate disposal of used dressing materials.

E. Develop strategies with patient/caregiver to enhance compliance with prescribed medication regimen.

F. Formulate a plan for post-discharge follow-up that includes appointments and appropriate times to

notify physician.

G. **Coordinate referrals relevant to wound care as appropriate.**

H. **Instruct on diet appropriate for the healing process.**

Bibliography

Anderson, F.A., & Wheeler, H.B. (1995). Venous thromboembolism. *Clinics in Chest Medicine, 16,* 235-251.

Andrychuk, M.A. (1998). Pressure ulcers: Causes, risk factors, assessment, and intervention. *Orthopaedic Nursing, 17*(4), 65-81.

Baba, R., & Razak, M. (1998). Contributing factors in non-union of the humeral shaft fracture and the results of treatments. *Medical Journal of Malaysia, 53SA*: 42-51.

Bergstrom, N., Braden, B., Kemp, M., Champagne, M., & Ruby, E. (1998). Predicting pressure ulcer risk: A multisite study of the predictive validity of the Braden Scale. *Nursing Research, 47*, 261-269.

Blackman, P. G. (2000). A review of chronic exertional compartment syndrome in the lower leg. *Medicine & Science in Sports & Exercise, 32-3S,* 4-10.

Bulger, E.M., Smith, D.G., Maier, R.V., & Jurkovich, G.J. (1997). Fat embolism syndrome, a 10-year review. *Archives of Surgery, 132,* 435-439.

Csokasy, J. (1999). Assessment of acute confusion: Use of the NEECHAM Confusion Scale. *Applied Nursing Reserch, 12*, 51-55.

Dalen, J.E., & Hirsh, J. (1995). Prevention of venous thromboembolism. *Chest, 108*(Suppl.), 312S-334S.

DeBaun, B.J. (1998). Prevention of infection in the orthopedic surgery patient. *Nursing Clinics of North America, 33*, 671-684.

DeBoer, A.S., Mintjes-de Groot, A.J., Severijnen, A.J., van den Berg, J.M., & van Pelt, W. (1999). Risk assessment for surgical-site infections in orthopedic patients. *Infection Control & Hospital Epidemiology, 20*(6), 402-407.

Edwards, P.D., Miles, K.A., Owens, S.J., Kemp, P.M., & Jenner, J. R. (1999). A new non-invasive test for the detection of compartment syndromes. *Nuclear Medicine Communications, 20*, 215-218.

Eftychiou, V. (1996). Clinical diagnosis and management of the patient with deep venous thromboembolism and acute pulmonary embolism. *Nurse Practitioner: American Journal of Primary Health Care, 21*(3), 50, 52, 58.

Folstein, M.F., Folstein, S.E., & McHugh, P.R. (1975). Mini-mental state: A practical guide for grading the cognitive state of patients for clinicians. *Journal of Psychiatric Research, 12*, 189-198.

Giannoudis, P.V., MacDonald, D.A., Matthews, S.J., Smith, R.M., Furlong, A.J., & De Boer, P. (2000). Nonunion of the femoral diaphysis. The influence of reaming and non-steroidal anti-inflammatory drugs. *Journal of Bone & Joint Surgery, 82B*, 655-658

Hager, C.A., & Brncick, N. (1998). Fat embolism syndrome: A complication of orthopaedic trauma. *Orthopaedic Nursing, 17*(2), 41-46, 58.

Heine, T.A., Halambeck, B.L., & Mark, J.B. (1998). Fatal pulmonary fat embolism in the early postoperative period. *Anesthesiology, 89*(6), 1589-1591.

Hiippala, S. (1998). Replacement of massive blood loss. *Vox Sanguinis, 74*(Suppl. 2), 399-407.

Hofmann, S., Huemer, G., & Salzer, M. (1998). Pathophysiology and management of the fat embolism syndrome. *Anaesthesia, 52*(Suppl. 2), 35-37.

Horan, R.C., Gaynes, R.P., Martone, W.J., Jarvis, W.R., & Emori, T.G. (1992). CDC definitions of nosocomial surgical site infections, 1992: A modification of CDC definitions of surgical wound infections. *Infection Control and Hospital Epidemiology, 13*, 606-608.

Jagmin, M.G. (1998). Postoperative mental status in elderly hip surgery patient. *Orthopaedic Nursing, 17*(6), 32-42.

Johnson, M., & Mass, M. (1997) (Eds.). *Nursing outcomes classification* (NOC). Boston: Mosby.

Levy, O., Martinowitz, U., Oran, A., Tauber, C., & Horoszowski, H. (1999). The use of fibrin tissue adhesive to reduce blood loss and the need for blood transfusion after total knee arthroplasty. *The Journal of Bone and Joint Surgery, 81A*(11), 1580-1588.

Kosiak, M. (1959). Etiology and pathology of ischemic ulcers. *Archives of Physical Medicine and Rehabilitation, 40*, 62-68.

Kracun, M.D., & Wooten, C.L. (1998). Crush injuries: a case of entrapment. *Critical Care Nursing Quarterly, 21*(2), 81-86.

Maklebust, J. (1999). Interrupting the pressure ulcer cycle. *Nursing Clinics of North America, 34*, 861-671.

Mars, M., & Hadley, G. P. (1998). Raised compartmental pressure in children: A basis for management. *Injury, 29*(3), 183-185.

Mayr, E., Frankel, V., & Ruter, A. (2000). Ultrasound--an alternative healing method for nonunions? *Archives of Orthopaedic & Trauma Surgery, 120,* 1-8.

McCloskey, J.C., & Bulechek, G. M. (Eds.). (2000). *Nursing interventions classification* (NIC) (3rd edition). Boston: Mosby.

Morris, N.S. (1999). Complications associated with orthopaedic surgery. In National Association of Orthopaedic Nurses (Ed.), *An introduction to orthopaedic nursing* (2nd ed.). Pitman, NJ: National Association of Orthopaedic Nurses.

North American Nursing Diagnosis Association. (2001). *Nursing diagnoses: Definitions and classification*. Philadelphia: North American Nursing Diagnosis Association.

Neelon, V., Champagne, M., Carlson, J., & Funk, S. (1996). The NEECHAM confusion scale: Construction, validation, and clinical testing. *Nursing Research, 45*, 324-330.

Panel for the Prediction and Prevention of Pressure Ulcers in Adults. (1992, May). *Pressure ulcers in adults: Prediction and prevention.* Clinical Practice Guideline, Number 3. AHCPR Publication No. 92-0047. Rockville, MD: Agency for Health Care Policy and Research, Public Health Service, U.S. Department of Health and Human Services.

Pellino, T.A., Polacek, L.A., Preston, M.A.S., Bell, N.L., & Evans, R.L. (1998). Complications of orthopaedic disorders and orthopaedic surgery. In A.B. Maher, S.W. Salmond, & T. A. Pellino (Eds.), *Orthopaedic nursing* (2nd ed., pp. 212-260). Philadelphia: Saunders.

Pitto, R.P., Koessler, M., & Kuehle, J.W. (1999). Comparison of fixation of the femoral component without cement and fixation with use of a bone-vacuum cementing technique for the prevention of fat embolism during total hip arthroplasty. *Journal of Bone and Joint Surgery, 81A*, 831-843.

Read, N.W., Celik, A.F., & Katsinelos, P. (1995). Constipation and incontinence in the elderly. *Journal of Clinical Gastroenterology, 20,* 61-70.

Ross, D.G. (1996). Chronic compartment syndrome. *Orthopaedic Nursing, 15*(3), 23-27.

Ryaby, J.T. (1998). Clinical effects of electromagnetic and electric fields on fracture healing. *Clinical Orthopaedics & Related Research. 355S*, 205-215.

Schultz, A., Bien, M., Dumond, K., Brown, K., & Myers, A. (1999). Etiology and incidence of pressure ulcers in surgical patients. *AORN Journal, 70*, 434, 437-440.

Swain, R., & Ross, D. (1999). Lower extremity compartment syndrome. When to suspect acute or chronic pressure buildup. *Postgraduate Medicine, 105*(3), 159-162, 165, 168.

Tapson, V.G., & Witty, L.A.(1995). Massive pulmonary embolism, diagnostic, and therapeutic strategies. *Clinics in Chest Medicine, 16*, 329-340.

ten Duis, H.J. (1997). Review: The fat embolism syndrome. *Injury, 28*, 77-85.

Vermeersch, P. (1997). Validation of the structure for the "Clinical assessment of confusion-A." *Nursing Research, 46*(4), 208-212.

Vickery, G. (1997). Basics of constipation. *Gastroenterology Nursing, 20*(4), 125-128

Von Schroeder, H.P. & Botte, M.J. (1998). Crush syndrome of the upper extremity. *Hand Clinics, 14,* 451-456.

STUDY QUESTIONS

1. On the third postoperative day, post-total knee replacement, the nurse notices that 64-year-old Mr. Albert has eaten very little of his lunch. He complains of a headache, a stomach ache, and even though he is passing flatus, he feels bloated. Although he ate breakfast, he has no appetite now. Based on this limited information, which of the following complications is the most likely?
   a. Paralytic ileus.
   b. Bowel obstruction.
   c. Constipation.
   d. Depression.

Mary Brown, a 55-year-old female who has diabetes and arthritis was involved in a car accident and sustained an acetabular and a pelvic fracture which required a 3-hour surgical procedure to repair. You note from her medical records she takes insulin once a day for her diabetes, ASA® 10 grain twice a day and PRN for her arthritis pain, Premarin® 0.625 mg once a day, and has a family history of heart condition. (Questions 2-3)

2. In the immediate postoperative period, which of the following postoperative complications is Mary most likely to develop?
   a. Thrombophlebitis.
   b. Fat embolism.
   c. Hemorrhage.
   d. Compartment syndrome.

3. As you continue to care for Mrs. Brown, you must be alert that she is at high risk to develop which of the following complications?
   a. Pulmonary embolism.
   b. Delayed union.
   c. Decubitus ulcers.
   d. Deep vein thrombosis.

Bob Suppa, a 42-year-old-male, is day 1 post-rodding of his fractured femur. He is apprehensive, restless, and complaining of chest pain and difficulty catching his breath. He is tachypenic (28), tachycardic (120), and is becoming confused. (Questions 4-6)

4. Bob's restlessness and impending confusion is likely due to:
   a. Pain.
   b. Hypoxia.
   c. Tachycardia.
   d. Cardiac failure

5. Which of the following would not be appropriate as an immediate diagnostic test?
   a. Blood gases.
   b. Lung scan.
   c. PT/PTT.
   d. Enzyme studies.

6. Bob's symptoms are most consistent with:
   a. Deep vein thrombosis.
   b. Hemorrhage.
   c. Fat embolism.
   d. Mild heart attack.

Dorothy is a 40-year-old obese female who is 5 days post-operative following right total hip arthroplasty. She has been very difficult to ambulate and frequently refuses physical therapy. Today upon awakening, she began to complain of increased swelling in her operative leg and tightness of the skin. She has been treated with Percocet®, Coumadin®, and Keflex® over the past 24 hours. Valium® was added on the third postoperative day when it was discovered that she had thrombophlebitis. (Questions 7-9)

7. What factor is not a risk factor for thrombophlebitis development?
   a. Her weight.
   b. Her lack of ambulation.
   c. Her surgery.
   d. Her drinking.

8. The most common assessment finding in a patient with a deep vein thrombosis is:
   a. Fever of undetermined origin.
   b. Homans sign.
   c. Throbbing trunk pain.
   d. Sudden swelling in one extremity

9. What nursing intervention is not appropriate for a patient with a confirmed diagnosis of deep vein thrombosis?
   a. Sequential compression device.
   b. Anticoagulant therapy.
   c. Elevation of extremities.
   d. Application of warm moist heat.

Max is a 35-year-old businessman who was found unconscious in his apartment with a tourniquet around his upper arm and drug paraphernalia scattered around him. The tourniquet was tightly applied. His fingers were dusky, but blanched when touched. He was admitted to the intensive care unit for drug overdose, but upon awakening began to complain bitterly of pain in his right forearm, the same arm where the tourniquet was found. You suspect compartment syndrome. He has had no changes in his laboratory findings – CBC, electrolytes, and urinalysis are all normal. (Questions 10-12)

10. Which of the following questions would be the most important to ask those who have been caring for him to confirm your suspicion of compartment syndrome?
    a. "Has the patient complained of numbness?"
    b. "Has a venogram been ordered and performed?"
    c. "If you move his fingers, does he express pain?"
    d. "How brisk is his nail bed blanch?"

11. A compartment monitor is applied. A compartment monitor is used to measure:
    a. Vascular pressure.
    b. Tissue pressure.
    c. Fluid pressure.
    d. Motor neuron activity.

12. The diagnosis of compartment syndrome is confirmed. The nursing management includes:
    a. Monitoring the compartment pressure.
    b. Checking neurovascular signs every shift.
    c. Elevating extremity above heart level.
    d. Applying a pressure dressing to the affected extremity.

Martha, a 36-year-old teacher sustained a tibial fracture 9 months ago when she fell off her bicycle. She was treated by closed reduction and casting. Although she has followed all instructions regarding living with a cast and caring for a cast, her x-rays still show insufficient callus to remove the cast. Her physician has diagnosed the problem as being a delayed union and applied a electric bone stimulation (EBS) device. (Questions 13-14)

13. What factor is most likely to cause delayed bone union following a fracture?
    a. Inadequate intake of calcium.
    b. A cast that is too tight.
    c. Not enough weight-bearing activities.
    d. Insufficient blood supply to the fracture site.

14. What is the most important nursing care you can provide for Martha?
    a. Checking for alterations in circulation, sensation, and motion in the leg.
    b. Monitoring the number of hours the EBS is on and hours the EBS is off.
    c. Assessing the amount of pain she is having during the "on" time.
    d. Teaching Martha and her family about the use and purpose of the EBS.

Chapter 9 INFECTIONS

Karen E. Zorn, BSN, RN, ONC

Contents

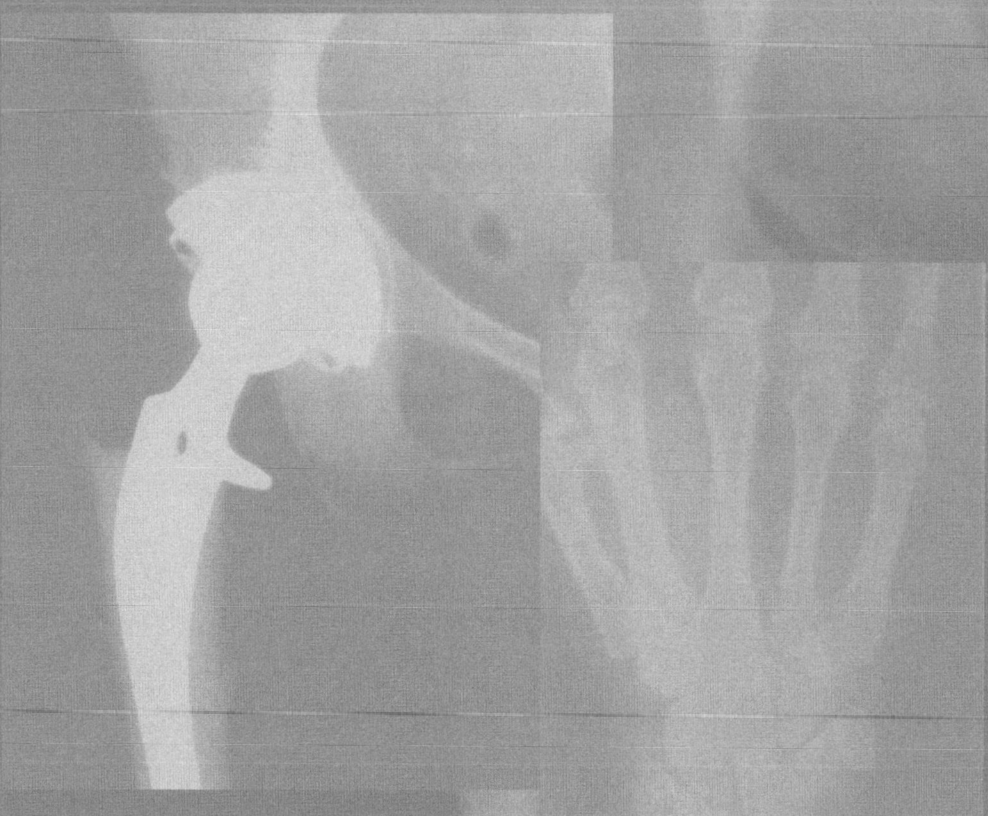

OBJECTIVES

At the completion of this chapter, the learner will be able to:

- Identify the infectious disease processes most common in orthopaedic practice.
- Identify microorganisms commonly responsible for orthopaedic infections.
- Identify host characteristics and procedures that place the patient at risk for developing infection.
- Identify common diagnostic and therapeutic modalities used to treat infections in orthopaedic patients.

KEY POINTS

- Adherence to and compliance with antibiotic treatment regimens are extremely important.
- Handwashing and aseptic technique help to diminish the risk of infection.
- Assessment for infection should be included in all phases of care. Signs and symptoms of infection require prompt evaluation.
- With state-of-the-art techniques most orthopaedic infections can be treated effectively and salvage function.

CHAPTER 9

INFECTIONS

OSTEOMYELITIS

I. OVERVIEW

A. Definition.

1. Osteomyelitis is a disease in which there is infection of the bone or surrounding tissues.
2. The infection may involve the periosteum, the cortex, the medullary canal, or all layers of the bone.
3. The infection may be acute or chronic.
   a. Acute osteomyelitis refers to cases presenting for initial therapy in which signs and symptoms have been present for a short duration and there is an absence of bony destruction.
      (1) Symptoms are generally more prominent than those of chronic osteomyelitis.
      (2) Most often hematogenous in origin but can occur secondary to a contiguous focus of infection.
   b. Chronic osteomyelitis refers to those cases in which symptoms have been present for longer than 3 months or in which initial therapeutic regimens have failed.
      (1) Infection usually occurs from exogenous injury.
      (2) Systemic symptoms are generally mild and periodic in nature secondary to the low-grade infection and the attempt by the body to wall off the infection.
      (3) Chronic osteomyelitis is generally classified by the Cierny/Mader classification system which specifies the stages of the infection based on the anatomic site combined with physiologic status.
         (a) Classification system: anatomic site.
            i. Stage I: superficial.
            ii. Stage II: medullary.
            iii. Stage III: localized.
            vi. Stage IV: diffuse.
         (b) Classification system: physiologic class.
            i. A-Host: normal systemic defenses, metabolic capabilities, and vascularity.
            ii. B-Host: local, systemic, or combined wound healing deficiencies.
            iii. C-Host: minimal disability present, anticipated high morbidity or poor prognosis for cure.

B. Etiology.

1. Acute osteomyelitis.
   a. Generally secondary to transient bacteremia which may be in conjunction with minor trauma, but the source of the bacteremia is frequently not known.
   b. Generally occurs from a hematogenous or endogenous spread through the vascular system into the bone or synovial tissue.
   c. Immune compromise secondary to diabetes, renal failure, sickle cell, alcoholism or IV drug abuse is usually present in adults who develop acute osteomyelitis.
   d. Over the age of 5, the most common bacteria isolated is *Staphylococcus aureus* followed by *Staphylococcus epidermidis*.
   e. Under the age of 3, *Haemophilus influenza* is the most common pathogen.
2. Chronic osteomyelitis.
   a. Generally secondary to an exogenous source such as trauma or surgical manipulation of the bone, but can be secondary to bacteremia.
   b. Can be caused by any microorganism, most common bacteria isolated are *Staphylococcus aureus*, followed by *Staphylococcus epidermidis*, and Pseudomonas; less common infecting organisms are fungi, viruses, and mycobacterium.
   c. Usually confined to the site of trauma.

B. Pathophysiology.

1. Acute osteomyelitis.
   a. Initiated by the spread of microorganisms through the vascular system into the medullary cavity.
   b. In children:
      (1) The infection generally occurs in the metaphyseal region close to the epiphysis.
      (2) Anatomy in these areas have small-end arterial loops which turn acutely to meet large veins. The arterial loops are responsible for sluggishness and turbulence in the blood vessels, which can allow bacteria to precipitate.
   c. The metaphyseal vessels contain minimal macrophages to control bacteria.
   d. Once the infection is present, cellulitis of the marrow develops.
      (1) As the infection advances, breakdown of the bacteria and white cells results in increasing exudates in the marrow causing increasing pressure within the medullary canal.
      (2) As the pressure increases there is compromise of the vasculature of the medullary canal, resulting in further necrosis.
      (3) Eventually the infection can pass through the cortex into the subperiosteal region due to the osteoclastic activity produced by the inflammation.
      (4) By lifting the periosteum the blood supply to the underlying cortex is disrupted, resulting in further necrosis and cortical de-vascularization.

(5) Once cortical devascularization is present, the infection usually becomes chronic.

e. Mild trauma is associated with approximately one-third of cases.

f. In infancy and adulthood the metaphyseal vessels cross the epiphysis allowing the bacteria to cross to subchondral bone, resulting in a greater incidence of septic joints and in childhood disruption of the growth plate.

g. Periosteal elevation and resultant cortical devascularization is unusual in adults: although the periosteum is thinner it is more firmly attached to the cortex.

2. Chronic osteomyelitis.
   a. Most commonly initiated by bacterial contamination from trauma or during surgical manipulation.
   b. During the initial trauma, bacteria is directly inoculated into the local wound.
      (1) The initial trauma causes devascularized and necrotic bone, periosteum, or soft tissue, allowing the bacteria to multiply without alerting the host.
      (2) The initial trauma may mask the early signs allowing the infection to continue to progress.
   c. Once the infection is recognized, the body attempts to eradicate it by walling the necrotic area off from the live bone with granulation tissue creating what is called a "sequestrum."
      (1) As the host defense progresses, the granulation tissue initially formed around the infected area changes to an avascular fibrous membrane further isolating the infection.
      (2) Reactive bone then forms around the infection and necrotic tissue, creating an involucrum in a further attempt to protect the host.
   d. The isolation of the bacteria by these mechanisms protects the body from systemic infection but prevents the host defenses and antibiotics from effectively combating the bacteria.
   e. The bacteria continue to produce toxins causing breakdown of the surrounding soft tissue and bone.
   f. Only on rare occasions does the infection spread outside the initial area of trauma.

C. Incidence.

1. Acute osteomyelitis.
   a. 1:5,000 incidence in children under 13.
   b. Two times more frequent in boys probably secondary to active play and resultant minor trauma.
   c. 40% of cases occur in children younger than 20 years old, 35% in adults over 50 years old.
   d. Can involve any bone but usually involves the long bones in children. Femur and tibia account for approximately 50% of childhood cases.
   e. In adults most common in the spine, pelvis and small bones.
   f. Present in multiple sites 10%-15% of the time.
2. Chronic osteomyelitis.
   a. Approximately 1%-3% of hospital admissions are for osteomyelitis.
   b. Incidence after orthopaedic surgery is 0.5%-1.8%.
   c. Most common following open fracture with direct contamination of the wound.
   d. Can occur in any bone. Most common in the long bones especially the tibia, which is the most common site of open fracture.

D. Considerations across the lifespan.

1. If growth plates involved, may develop progressive limb-length discrepancies and deformities.
2. Recurrences are possible even years after initial treatment.

E. Complications.

1. Loss of function of the joints above or below the infection secondary to pain or immobility.
2. Leg-length discrepancies or deformities.
3. Renal insufficiency or hearing loss secondary to nephrotoxic or ototoxic antibiotics.

II. ASSESSMENT

A. History.

1. Presenting symptoms.
   a. Acute osteomyelitis.
      (1) Dependant on age.
      (2) Infants may have minimal symptoms secondary to a poor inflammatory response by the immature immune system. The presenting symptoms in infants may range from irritability when the affected limb is touched to pseudoparalysis or signs of sepsis.
      (3) Young children usually present with localized pain or refusal to use the affected limb. As the infection progresses signs of inflammation are present. Effusions in adjacent joints can occur.
      (4) Older children and adolescents usually present with significant localized pain and tenderness. Fever and chills may occur.
      (5) Adults may present with symptoms ranging from vague pain to severe pain with obvious signs of sepsis.
   b. Chronic osteomyelitis.
      (1) Systemic symptoms are generally mild.
      (2) Characterized by remissions and exacerbations.
      (3) May range from localized mild pain at the infection site to severe pain in the entire extremity.
      (4) Soft tissue abscesses and draining sinuses may occur.
      (5) If draining sinuses are present purulent drainage with surrounding erythema can occur, large wounds may extend down to expose necrotic bone and hardware.
      (6) Once the sinus develops and drains it may resolve until pressure again builds up.
2. Medical history.

a. Acute osteomyelitis.
   (1) May include recent history of systemic bacterial or viral infection.
   (2) Recent history of mild trauma (bruising).
   (3) Puncture wounds.
   (4) Adults may have history of immune compromise secondary to diabetes, renal failure, drug abuse, vascular insufficiency, poor nutrition or tobacco use.
b. Chronic osteomyelitis.
   (1) Trauma or surgical manipulation of the extremity.
   (2) Previous history of acute osteomyelitis treated or not.
   (3) Continuous or intermittent symptoms.
   (4) May have history of immune compromise.

B. Physical examination.

1. Findings as variable as the presenting symptoms.
2. Fever common in acute osteomyelitis, uncommon in chronic osteomyelitis.

C. Diagnostic tests.

1. Acute osteomyelitis.
   a. Routine x-rays generally show no changes in the early phase, it takes 10-14 days after the start of infection for x-rays to detect bone lysis. Used to rule out other causes.
   b. Sedimentation rate: generally elevated.
   c. CBC: leukocytosis.
   d. Blood cultures: positive 50%-60% of the time.
   e. Bone scan: usually positive in the area of infection.
   f. Aspiration or bone biopsy for culture of the affected area.
2. Chronic osteomyelitis.
   a. Routine x-rays: bone and soft tissue changes.
   b. Sedimentation rate: mildly to severely elevated.
   c. CBC: generally minimal, if any elevation in WBC, may show anemia of chronic disease.
   d. C-reactive protein: will be elevated and return to normal after treatment faster than the sedimentation rate.
   e. Blood cultures: negative.
   f. CT scans: delineate changes in the bone, can identify sequestrums and involucrum.
   g. MRI: useful to delineate the marrow and soft tissue changes.
   h. Cultures of any drainage or sinus.

III. COMMON THERAPEUTIC MODALITIES

A. Acute osteomyelitis.

1. Antibiotics once appropriate cultures have been obtained.
   a. Antibiotics may start out as broad spectrum but should be tailored to the specific organism once sensitivities are obtained.
   b. Generally 4-6 weeks of parenteral antibiotics based on the response monitored by physical signs and laboratory tests.
2. Surgical drainage of soft tissue and bone abscesses may be necessary.
3. Hyperbaric oxygen therapy: may be used as an adjunctive therapy in patients with immune compromise.

B. Chronic osteomyelitis.

1. Surgical disease: will not resolve with antibiotics alone.
   a. The principles of osteomyelitis surgery are to remove all nonviable material from the wound, including hardware and dead bone, to stabilize the bone if necessary, and to obliterate the dead space.
   b. If necessary the soft tissue envelope is restored with myoplasties or free tissue transfers.
2. Antibiotic beads:
   a. Beads, either made of bone cement or biodegradable may be used at the site, to provide a local depot of antibiotics and antibiotic levels not achievable systemically.
   b. Beads should be in a sealed wound to avoid contamination and possible superinfection.
3. Antibiotics based on culture sensitivities.
   a. Duration is debatable but should be based on the anatomic type and host classification. B-Hosts or compromised individuals will need a longer antibiotic course.
   b. Monitoring of antibiotic blood levels is important to assure adequate levels and reduce toxicity.
4. Once the infection has resolved reconstruction can proceed.
5. Hyperbaric oxygen therapy may be used as an adjunctive therapy in those who are immune compromised, either systemically or locally at the site.
6. Referral to specialty center if unable to resolve.

IV. NURSING DIAGNOSES, OUTCOMES, AND INTERVENTIONS (See Table 9.1)

V. PRACTICE SETTING CONSIDERATIONS

A. Hospital.

1. Teach appropriate use of mobility aids prior to discharge.
2. Teach importance of taking antibiotics as prescribed and for the entire course as ordered.
3. Instruct in proper wound, dressing, and pin care as needed.

B. Office.

1. Promote appropriate physical therapy.
2. Reinforce instructions for care given in hospital.
3. Referral to specialty center if unable to resolve.

C. Home care.

1. Reinforce activity instructions.
2. Reinforce wound dressing and pin care to patient and family.
3. Instruct patient and family in importance of clean technique and handwashing to reduce spread of infection.
4. Make sure patient and family understand that the infection is not contagious.

Table 9.1
Nursing Diagnoses, Outcomes, and Interventions for Patients with Infections

Nursing Diagnoses	Outcomes	Interventions
A. Pain	• Determines a comfort/function goal. • Describes how unrelieved pain will be managed. • Reports that pain management regimen relieves pain.	• Ask patients to describe past experiences with pain and the effectiveness of measures used to control it. • Describe adverse effects of unrelieved pain. • Determine current medication use. • Discuss patients' fears of under-treated pain, overdose, or addiction.
B. Fear	• Verbalizes known fears. • States accurate information about the situation. • Demonstrates coping behaviors to reduce fear.	• Assess source of fear. • Discuss fears with patients and help to distinguish between real and imagined threats to their well-being. • Provide accurate information. • Explain all procedures to patients in ways they understand.
C. Physical mobility, impaired	• Demonstrates use of adaptive equipment to assist with mobility. • Meets defined goals of mobility.	• Observe for cause of mobility impairment. • Monitor ability to tolerate mobility. • Consult with physical therapy to improve mobility.
D. Role performance, altered	• States personal strengths. • Acknowledges problems contributing to inability to carry out normal role. • Accepts physical limitations regarding role and considers ways to accomplish those goals within the limitations. • Identifies realistic perception of role.	• Allow patient to express feelings about role change. • Reinforce strengths and effective coping skills. • Identify ways to compensate for physical disabilities.
E. Skin integrity, impaired	• Retains or regains integrity of skin. • Describes measures to prevent injury to the skin. • Demonstrates measures to heal skin and prevent re-injury.	• Assess site of skin impairment and determine etiology. • Monitor patients' skin care practices. • Assess mobility-related risk factors. • Assess patients' nutritional status and refer as needed.
F. Infection, risk for	• States symptoms of infection of which to be aware. • Demonstrates appropriate hygienic measures such as handwashing to prevent spread of infection. • Demonstrates appropriate care of infection-prone site.	• Observe and report signs of infection. • Encourage proper diet, fluid intake, and rest to bolster immune system. • Use proper handwashing techniques. • Follow standard precautions for dealing with bodily fluids. • Provide appropriate site care for all indwelling lines.

SEPTIC ARTHRITIS

I. OVERVIEW

A. Definition: invasion of the synovium and joint space by microorganisms, leading to an inflammatory response.

B. Etiology.

1. Hematogenous spread to the joint is most common and usually affects people with underlying medical or surgical illnesses.
2. Can be spread by direct inoculation from puncture wounds from either trauma or surgical intervention.
3. Extension into the joint from a contiguous site of infection, such as in childhood acute osteomyelitis, can also lead to septic arthritis.
4. Any microorganism can cause the sepsis.
   a. In the immune-compromised patient bacteria that is usually not pathogenic frequently causes the infection.
   b. *Staphylococcus aureus* is the most common organism isolated.
   c. Streptococcus is also common.
   d. *Haemophilus influenza* is the most common organism in young children.
   e. *Neissreia gonorrhoeae* is most common in sexually active young adults.

C. Pathophysiology.

1. The microorganisms arrive in the joint through hematogenous, contiguous, or direct extension routes.
2. Once the microorganism is present it causes intense local reaction, including hyperemia, vascular congestion, and synovial proliferation.
3. As the infection progresses destruction of the cartilage occurs due to inhibition of the chondrocytes, pressure necrosis, and the release of proteolytic enzymes from the breakdown of the bacteria.
4. As the synovium proliferates it also causes enzymatic digestion of the articular cartilage.

D. Incidence.

1. In infancy and early childhood:
   a. Septic arthritis occurs twice as common as does osteomyelitis.
   b. Incidence is highest in the first 2 years of life.
2. Any joint may be affected:
   a. Hip and knee are most commonly affected in childhood.
   b. The knee is the most commonly affected joint in adults.
3. Only one joint is usually involved.
4. Polyarticular involvement occurs about 9% of the time: and is usually in elderly patients or those treated for rheumatoid arthritis with steroids.
5. Gonococcal infection generally occurs in young, healthy, sexually active adults.

E. Considerations across the lifespan.

1. May develop arthritis or bony ankylosis secondary to loss of cartilage.
2. Children may develop limb-length deformities or discrepancies.
3. Patients with septic arthritis of the hip may develop later avascular necrosis of the femoral head.

F. Complications.

1. Destruction of articular cartilage.
2. Progression to chronic infection.
3. Loss of joint function.

II. ASSESSMENT

A. History.

1. Presenting symptoms.
   a. Pain, often exaggerated with motion.
   b. Swelling, erythema, and heat of the involved joint; in early stages these symptoms may be minimal.
   c. Systemic symptoms such as fever, chills, and malaise may accompany the joint pain.
2. Medical history.
   a. Childhood: recent infection at another site including upper respiratory infection, impetigo, otitis media, or recent history of trauma to the involved joint.
   b. Adult: family or patient history of rheumatoid arthritis, recent history of uninvolved joint sepsis, recent history of acute illness including gonorrhea, hepatitis, or rubella.

B. Physical examination.

1. Lower extremity involvement: antalgic gait or inability to walk.
2. Upper extremity: guarding of the affected extremity.
3. Synovial effusion and varying degrees of erythema depending on the duration of infection prior to exam.
4. Tenderness and increased warmth of the joint.
5. Limitation of both active and passive motion.

C. Diagnostic tests.

1. X-rays: joint effusion and soft tissue swelling, later synovial thickening.
2. Synovial fluid aspiration: shows elevated leukocytes with 90% or more polymorphonuclear neutrophils (PMNs).
3. Cultures of the joint fluid: if caused by organisms other than gonococcus are usually positive.
4. Sedimentation rate and C-reactive protein: elevated.

III. COMMON THERAPEUTIC MODALITIES

A. Antibiotic therapy based on the culture results, start empirically prior to culture results if suspicion is high.

B. Drainage of the purulence either by aspiration, arthroscopic, or open surgical drainage.

C. Rest and immobilization of the affected extremity until the acute symptoms resolve.

D. Rehabilitation of the joint once the acute symptoms resolve, continuous passive motion (CPM) machine may be useful.

IV. NURSING DIAGNOSES, OUTCOMES, AND INTERVENTIONS (See Table 9.1)

V. PRACTICE SETTING CONSIDERATIONS (See Osteomyelitis: Practice Setting)

PROSTHETIC JOINT INFECTION

I. OVERVIEW

A. Definition: infection surrounding a prosthetic replacement.

1. Stage I: early postoperative infection (< 4 weeks postoperative).
2. Stage II: acute hematogenous infection (< 4 weeks duration).
3. Stage III: late chronic infection (> 4 weeks duration).

B. Etiology.

1. Direct inoculation of bacteria into the wound either:
   a. During the surgical procedure.
   b. From sepsis contiguous to the prosthesis.
   c. Contamination from infected postoperative hematoma.
   d. Delayed wound healing.
   e. Suture abscesses prior to sealing of the deep layers of the closure.
2. Hematogenous spread from transient bacteremia.
   a. Bacteremia may occur from obvious sources of infection such as pneumonia, urinary tract infections (UTIs), dental caries, gum disease, dermatitis.
   b. Transient bacteremia may occur during invasive procedures such as colonoscopy, urinary catheterization, and dental cleaning.
3. Common organisms isolated are *Staphylococcus aureus*, *Staphylococcus epidermis*, Streptococcus, Pseudomonas, and *Escherichia coli*.
4. Compromising factors.
   a. Prior surgery at the site, soft tissue loss, vascular insufficiency to the extremity, prior radiation to the wound area, fistula formation, or active infection present longer than 3-4 months.
   b. Compromise secondary to malnutrition, cardiac or pulmonary insufficiency, renal failure, diabetes, immune compromise, systemic inflammatory disease, alcoholism, smoking, or chronic indwelling catheters.

D. Pathophysiology.

1. Microorganisms introduced into the viable tissue create local edema, necrosis, and inflammation reducing local circulation.
2. Bacterial toxins accumulate and increase the local acidity. As the acidity increases the phagocytes die releasing enzymes and creating further tissue destruction.
3. Foreign bodies such as prosthetic devices and methylmethacrylate (bone cement) allow small inoculum of bacteria to flourish out of the reach of the normal defenses of the body.
4. In the presence of foreign bodies certain bacteria, such as Staphylococcus and Pseudomonas produce glycocalyx, or biofilm, a fibrous material that further protects the organism from the host defenses.

D. Incidence.

1. 1%-3% of all prosthetic joints develop sepsis.
2. Use of perioperative prophylactic antibiotics, clean air systems in the operating room (OR), and body exhaust suits help reduce the infection rate.

E. Considerations across the lifespan.

1. Each prosthetic revision increases the chance of subsequent sepsis and generally increases bone loss.
2. Compromising factors increase with age.

F. Complications.

1. Loss of joint or joint function.
2. Chronic osteomyelitis.
3. Renal compromise or hearing loss secondary to antibiotics.

II. ASSESSMENT

A. History.

1. Presenting symptoms: pain with or without other signs of infection.
2. Medical history.
   a. Previous sepsis.
   b. Night sweats.
   c. Postoperative wound drainage.
   d. Recent invasive procedures.
   e. Draining sinuses.
   f. Immune compromise.

B. Physical examination.

1. Depends on the virulence of the organism and host factors.
2. Pain in the region of the prosthesis, particularly with compression.
3. Decreased range of motion.
4. Erythema, edema, and/or increased warmth locally.
5. Wound drainage.

C. Diagnostic tests.

1. Arthrocentesis:
   a. Fluid is aspirated prior to the initiation of antibiotic therapy.
   b. Fluid is sent for culture and cell count.
   c. Fluid is positive in 60%-70% of infected joints.
2. Surgical biopsy for definitive diagnosis.
3. Sedimentation rate and C-reactive protein: elevated.
4. X-rays: show loosening or cyst formation.
5. Bone scan: can rule out infection if negative.
6. Gallium scan: increased uptake in mechanical loosening or infection.

III. COMMON THERAPEUTIC MODALITIES

A. Acute infections.

1. Diagnosed and treated within 72 hours can sometimes salvage the joint with appropriate antibiotics, arthrotomy, or arthroscopy with copious irrigation.
2. Exchange of the polyethylene components at the time of the irrigation can also increase the chances for resolution.

B. Chronic infections.

1. Can be managed by surgical removal of the prosthesis and the surrounding necrotic and nonviable tissue including the cement and devitalized bone.
2. Prosthesis can then be replanted in a one stage or delayed two-stage procedure.

C. Type and duration of antibiotics determined by the infecting agent and the host status.

D. Success rates depend on the virulence of the bacteria and the experience and surgical skill of the surgeon.

IV. NURSING DIAGNOSES, OUTCOMES, AND INTERVENTIONS (See Table 9.1)

V. PRACTICE SETTING CONSIDERATIONS

A. See Osteomyelitis: practice setting considerations.
B. Referral to specialty center if unable to resolve.

BONE AND JOINT TUBERCULOSIS (TB)

I. OVERVIEW

A. Definition.
1. An infectious disease from hematogenous spread of *Mycobacterium tuberculosis* causing destruction of the bones and joints.
2. An extrapulmonary form of TB occurring following lymphohematogenous spread from a primary lung lesion.
3. Musculoskeletal TB is not communicable to others.

B. Etiology.
1. *Mycobacterium tuberculosis* is transmitted through the airborne route.
2. Infection develops in the lungs.
3. The mycobacterium spreads hematogenously through the bloodstream to the bones or synovial lining of joints.

C. Pathophysiology.
1. Onset is usually insidious with a long history of mild or moderate joint or bone pain.
2. Only 50% of patients with bone or joint TB have active pulmonary TB.
3. Mycobacterium causes:
   a. An inflammatory reaction, followed by the formation of granulation tissue.
   b. The organism does not produce enzymes to destroy the cartilage but rather the granulation tissue eventually erodes the cartilage and the bone.
4. In advanced disease, abscesses may form around the joint eventually draining through the skin and producing secondary bacterial contamination.
5. In spinal TB:
   a. The disc space quickly narrows, followed by destruction of the vertebral bodies.
   b. The anterior body generally collapses producing gibbus type deformities and with multiple vertebra involvement significant kyphosis.

D. Incidence.
1. Cases of TB have increased in the United States secondary to the increase in acquired immune deficiency (AIDS). As the rate of TB increases so will the rate of skeletal TB.
2. TB of the spine (Pott's disease) is most common.
   a. Lower thoracic and upper lumbar lesions are more common in adults.
   b. Upper thoracic is more common in children.
3. Hip, knee, ankle, sacroiliac joint, shoulder, and wrist are in that order the most commonly affected joints.
4. Monoarticular in 80%-90% of cases.
5. Of those patients with pulmonary TB only approximately 1% will develop skeletal TB.
6. TB is more common in those of Asian or African descent.

E. Considerations across the lifespan.
1. Risk of developing TB and subsequent skeletal TB are increased with:
   a. Extremes of age (very old and very young).
   b. Immunosuppression.
   c. Malnutrition.
2. Infants and children are at increased risk for developing skeletal TB due to vascularity of bone.
3. Spinal and bone deformities can occur following skeletal TB in children and adults.

F. Complications.
1. Loss of joint function.
2. Fractures secondary to osteoporosis.
3. Bone and joint deformities.
4. Chronic pain and possible paralysis from untreated spinal TB.

II. ASSESSMENT

A. History.
1. Presenting symptoms.
   a. Mild to moderate joint or bone pain.
   b. Joint effusions.
   c. Systemic symptoms, such as night sweats or weight loss.
   d. Spinal deformity.
2. Medical history.
   a. History of pulmonary TB or household exposure.
   b. Night sweats.
   c. Weight loss.
   d. Immune compromise.
   e. Joint effusions.

B. Physical examination.
1. Synovial thickening.
2. Possible joint effusion.
3. Mildly increased warmth.
4. Severe muscle atrophy surrounding the joint.
5. Limitation of motion – especially in later infection.
6. Alterations in posture, gibbus deformities or kyphosis of the spine.

C. Diagnostic tests.
1. X-rays.
   a. Severe osteoporosis of the surrounding bone, even early in the infection.
   b. Soft tissue swelling but preservation of the cartilage until late disease.
2. Tuberculin skin test: usually positive, unless immune compromised.
3. Arthrocentesis: 20,000-100,000 WBC with 50%-60% polys.
4. Sedimentation rate: elevated.
5. CBC: WBC normal or slightly elevated.
6. Culture of synovial fluid: usually positive for *Mycobacterium tuberculosis* but may take 6-8 weeks for results.

7. Biopsy for definitive diagnosis: positive for caseating granuloma.

III. COMMON THERAPEUTIC MODALITIES

A. Antibiotic therapy using a multi-drug regimen for TB.

1. The earlier the diagnosis is made and treatment initiated the better the outcome.
2. Multiple drug regimens are used because the tubercle bacilli tend to mutate to drug-resistant forms if not initially killed.
3. The same drugs used to treat pulmonary TB are effective for bone and joint TB.
   a. INH and rifampin are generally given in combination with either ethambutol or streptomycin for a period of 6-24 months.
   b. Isoniazid (INH), rifampin, and streptomycin are bactericidal for actively dividing extracellular TB.
   c. INH and rifampin are bactericidal for TB in the closed caseous membranes.
   d. Pyrazinamide, rifampin, and INH are bacteriocidal for TB in the macrophages.
   e. Because of the slow-growing nature of the TB and its ability to mutate, treatment is a combination of drugs that is effective against TB in all phases of its lifespan.
   f. Compliance with a full course of treatment is necessary to gain cure, to prevent the emergence of drug resistance, and to stop the transmission of disease.

B. Surgical intervention may be used to establish diagnosis, drain abscesses, or to stabilize joints.

1. With spinal TB if spontaneous fusion does not occur surgical fusion may be necessary.
2. Synovectomy is sometimes done to remove a large nidus of infection.

IV. NURSING DIAGNOSES, OUTCOMES, AND INTERVENTIONS (See Table 9.1)

V. PRACTICE SETTING CONSIDERATIONS

A. Cases of TB must be reported in accordance with state public health law.

B. Drug resistance is almost always secondary to inadequate drug therapy.

C. Patients must be monitored for toxic side effects of medications.

SKIN AND SOFT TISSUE INFECTIONS

I. OVERVIEW

A. Definition.

1. Impetigo: superficial infection of the skin characterized by pustules.
2. Folliculitis:
   a. Minor infection of the hair follicle.
   b. Can progress to inflammatory nodules called furuncles.
3. Cellulitis: inflammation of the skin and subcutaneous tissue.
4. Pyomyositis: acute bacterial infection of skeletal muscle.
5. Clostidial myonecrosis (gas gangrene): acute infection of the soft tissue and muscle quickly causing muscle necrosis.
6. Necrotizing fascitis:
   a. Acute infection of the fascia and surrounding muscle.
   b. Can quickly become life threatening.

B. Etiology.

1. Staphylococcus and streptococcus are the most common bacteria in skin and soft tissue infections, but a multitude of organisms can be responsible.
2. Impetigo.
   a. Generally caused by streptococcal organisms.
   b. May develop at site of previous abrasions or insect bites.
3. Folliculitis.
   a. Caused by normal skin flora bacteria, such as staphylococcus.
   b. Usually occurs in areas of friction and sweat gland activity.
4. Cellulitis:
   a. Frequently caused by streptococcus organisms but may be caused by multiple organisms.
   b. Usually occurs in areas of venous stasis or areas where lymphatic drainage is blocked.
   c. Erysipelas.
      (1) A type of cellulitis that frequently occurs at the site of free tissue transfers, especially in the leg.
      (2) It is due to the lack of lymphatic drainage in the flap and thus inability to clear transient streptococcus organisms.
5. Pyomyositis.
   a. Generally caused by *Staphylococcus aureus* (95%).
   b. Usually occurs after deep nonpenetrating trauma to the involved muscle.
6. Clostridial myositis.
   a. Caused by gas-forming anaerobic bacteria, usually *Clostridium perfringens*.
   b. Gram stain will show gram positive rods.
   c. Other organisms can produce myonecrosis but they generally do not advance as rapidly or produce the toxins.
   d. Frequently occurs secondary to puncture wounds.
7. Necrotizing fascitis:
   a. Generally caused by streptococcus but can be caused by other organisms.
   b. Infection usually develops at the site of a minor trauma and then quickly spreads to the surrounding fascia producing putrification of the fascia.

C. Pathophysiology.

1. Skin lesions such as minor abrasions, burns, IV sites, and decubitis ulcers may become secondarily infected.

2. Infections can be mild or life threatening depending on:
   a. Virulence of the organisms.
   b. Portal of entry.
   c. Health status of the host.

D. Incidence.

1. Rates of skin and soft tissue infections in the general population range from 1.1%-6%.
2. Infections range from very mild requiring little if any treatment to those with life-threatening consequences.

II. ASSESSMENT

A. History.

1. Poor nutrition.
2. Breaks in skin integrity.
3. Recent trauma, including surgery, to the involved area.

B. Physical examination.

1. Common findings:.pain, erythema, edema, fluctuance, or drainage.
2. In cellulitis and infections of the muscle and fascia, fever, chills, and general malaise may also be present.
3. Localized muscle pain may progress quickly to swelling and induration.
4. In gas gangrene, the bacteria produce toxins that necrotize the muscle and release gas, producing the classic symptoms of:
   a. Swelling with purple or bronze discoloration.
   b. Bullae.
   c. Watery discharge.
   d. In later stage crepitation, due to the gas within the tissues.
5. In deep muscle infections and necrotizing fascitis:
   a. Appearance of the skin may not indicate the true extent of the infection.
   b. Patients can quickly become toxic.
   c. Pain is usually severe.

C. Diagnostic tests.

1. Culture of drainage if present.
2. Aspiration for culture of deep abscesses.
3. MRI: to visualize the extent of muscle and fascia involvement.
4. CBC: WBC will be elevated, significantly with myonecrosis.

III. COMMON THERAPEUTIC MODALITIES

A. Local or oral antibiotics for mild infections.

B. Systemic antibiotics started, empirically based on the organisms that commonly cause the diagnosis, and then adjusted to the specific organism once culture and sensitivities are available.

C. Serial surgical debridements to remove all nonviable tissue followed by gradual closure once no further necrosis is present.

D. Fasciotomy as necessary to reduce compartment pressures caused by deep abscesses within the muscle.

E. Hyperbaric oxygen therapy to inhibit the toxins and to maintain viable tissue.

F. General supportive care including mechanical ventilation as needed.

G. Nutritional support by parenteral means if necessary.

IV. NURSING DIAGNOSES, OUTCOMES, AND INTERVENTIONS (See Table 9.1)

V. PRACTICE SETTING CONSIDERATIONS

A. Hospital.

1. Instruct in proper wound care and dressing changes.
2. Instruct in importance of regaining or maintaining adequate nutritional intake.

B. Office.

1. Reinforce instructions for care given in hospital.
2. Promote appropriate mobility.

C. Home.

1. Reinforce proper wound care.
2. Reinforce importance of maintaining proper nutrition.
3. Instruct patient and family on importance of compliance with antibiotic regimen.
4. Advise patient and family to assess skin regularly and report any signs of onset of infection.

NOSOCOMIAL INFECTIONS

I. OVERVIEW

A. Definition.

1. Nosocomial infections are infections acquired within a hospital or health care institution.
2. Common sites of nosocomial infection are:
   a. Urinary tract.
   b. Surgical wounds
   c. Lower respiratory tract.
   d. Bloodstream
3. Majority of the infections become clinically apparent while the patient is still hospitalized.

B. Etiology.

1. Endogenous sources: patient's own bacterial flora.
2. Exogenous sources:
   a. Health care workers.
   b. Contaminated equipment.
   c. Other patients.
3. *Escherichia coli*, gram-negative rods, and Group D *Enterococci* are most common in urinary tract infections.
4. *Pseudomonas aeruginosa* and *Staphylococcus aureus* most common in hospital-acquired pneumonia.
5. Staphylococcal organisms and gram-negative bacteria responsible for most nosocomial bacteremias and septic phlebitis.
6. An increasing number of nosocomial bacteria are becoming resistant to conventional antibiotics secondary to the overuse and misuse of antibiotics.
   a. *Methicillin-resistant Stapylococcus aureus* (MRSA).
   b. *Methicillin-resistant Staphylococcus epidermidis* (MRSE).
   c. *Vancomycin resistant Enterococci* (VRE).

C. Pathophysiology.

1. Urinary tract infections (UTI) are:
   a. Most common nosocomial infection.
   b. Bacterial infections develop in 2%-4% of the cases.
   c. Risk factors for UTI increase with:
      (1) Catheterizations.
      (2) Length of time the catheter is in place.
      (3) Being female.
      (4) Loss of a closed system.
2. Surgical wound infections may be superficial or deep.
   a. Risk factors include:
      (1) Length of preoperative hospitalization.
      (2) Surgical time.
      (3) Operating room traffic.
      (4) Nutritional status.
      (5) Inappropriate antibiotic prophylaxis.
   b. Routes of bacterial entry can be direct contamination or hematogenous spread.
3. Lower respiratory tract infections are associated with significant morbidity and mortality.
   a. Risk factors:
      (1) Include age > 70 years.
      (2) Chronic lung disease.
      (3) Mechanical ventilation.
      (4) Immunosuppression.
      (5) Surgery.
      (6) Fall and winter seasons.
   b. Routes of bacterial entry can be by:
      (1) Aspiration of gastric contents.
      (2) Inhalation of contaminated solutions in nebulizers.
      (3) Direct introduction of pathogens by suction catheters and endotracheal tubes.
4. Bacteremia is commonly associated with central and peripheral venous catheters.
   a. Risk factors include:
      (1) Type and location of venous catheter.
      (2) Length of time catheter is in place.
      (3) Immunosuppression.
   b. Routes of entry can be intraluminal by contaminated solutions and extraluminal by bacteria that colonize the catheter entry site.
5. Antibiotic-resistant bacteria are associated with:
   a. Longer or more frequent hospitalizations.
   b. Prolonged illness.
   c. Immunosuppression
   d. Use of more toxic antibiotics.
   e. Risk factors include:
      (1) Prior antibiotic therapy.
      (2) Intensive Care Unit (ICU) stay.
      (3) Presence of invasive devices such as IVs, catheters, and endotracheal tubes.

D. Incidence.

1. Approximately 5% of all hospital admissions will develop nosocomial infections.
2. Increasing number of nosocomial infections are caused by antibiotic-resistant bacteria.

II. ASSESSMENT

A. History: presenting symptoms, dependant on site of infection.

B. Medical history.

1. History of recent hospitalization or surgical intervention.
2. History of indwelling catheters, IVs, or endotracheal tubes.

C. Physical examination: findings indicative of the presenting infection.

D Diagnostic tests.

1. Cultures: usually positive, may be antibiotic-resistant bacteria.
2. Sedimentation rate and C-reactive protein: elevated.
3. X-rays useful to diagnose pneumonia.

III. COMMON THERAPEUTIC MODALITIES

A. Appropriate antibiotic therapy based on culture sensitivities.

B. Symptomatic treatment.

C. Prevention of further spread by appropriate isolation.

D. Surveillance for nosocomial infections to identify unusual occurrence or a rise in the incidence of infection.

IV. NURSING DIAGNOSES, OUTCOMES, AND INTERVENTIONS (See Table 9.1)

V. PRACTICE SETTING CONSIDERATIONS

A. Hospital.

1. Maintain appropriate isolation.
2. Instruct family in isolation techniques to prevent further spread.

B. Home care considerations.

1. Instruct family in importance of handwashing and aseptic technique.
2. Reinforce importance of completing antibiotic therapy.
3. Instruct family and patient in signs and symptoms of infection and to report those symptoms immediately.

Bibliography

Cannale, S.J., & Bently, J.H. (1995). *Operative pediatric orthopaedics* (2nd ed.). New York: Mosby-Year Book, Inc.

Cierny, G., Levin, L.S., & Perry, C.R. (1999). *Musculoskeletal sepsis: acute wound management.* Instructional Course Lectures Handout. Rosemont, IL: American Academy of Orthopaedic Surgeons.

Cierny, G., & Zorn, K.E. (1996). Arthrodesis of the tibiotalar joint for sepsis. *Foot and Ankle Clinics, 1*(1), 177-197.

Everts, C.M. (1990). *Surgery of the musculoskeletal system.* New York, NY: Churchill Livingston Inc.

Foglar, C., & Lindsey, R.W. (1998). C-reactive protein in orthopaedics. *Orthopaedics, 21*(6), 687-692.

Gaine, W.J., Ramamohan, N.A., Hussein, N.A., Hullin, M.G., & McGreath, S.W. (2000). Wound infection in hip and knee arthroplasty. *The Journal of Bone and Joint Surgery, 82*(4), 56-565.

Glover, T.L. (2000). How drug-resistant microorganisms affect nursing. *Orthopaedic Nursing, 19*(2), 19-27.

Jaurequi, L.E. (1995). *Diagnosis and management of bone infections.* New York, NY: Marcel Dekker, Inc.

Ladwig, A. (1999). *Nursing diagnosis handbook.* Saint Louis, MO: Mosby, Inc.
Maher, A.B., Salmond, S.W., & Pellino, T. (Eds.). (1994). *Orthopaedic nursing.* Philadelphia: Saunders.
McLaren, A.C., & Spooner, C.E. (1996). Salvage of infected total knee components. *Clinical Orthopaedics and Related Research, 331*,146-150.
McPherson, E.J. Tontz, W., Pataskis, M., Woodsome, C., Holton, P., Norris, L., & Shurfelt, C. (1999, March). Outcome of infected total knee utilizing a staging system for prosthetic joint infection. *The American Journal of Orthopaedics*, 161-165.
Patzakis, M.J. (1994). Symposium: Current concepts in the management of osteomyelitis. *Contemporary Orthopaedics, 28*(2), 157-185.
Saadeh, C. (1998). The erythrocyte sedimentation rate: Old and new clinical applications. *Southern Medical Journal, 91*(3), 220-225.
Walenkamp, G.H. (1997). Chronic osteomyelitis. *Acta Orthopaedics Scandinavia, 68*(5), 497-506.

STUDY QUESTIONS

Four-year-old Tommy presented to the emergency room with a 2-week duration of abnormal posture and tenderness to his back. On exam, his back muscles were rigid. An MRI revealed marked kyphosis of the spine due to destruction of vertebrae. He was diagnosed with Pott's disease based on clinical findings and a positive PPD skin test (> 10 mm). (Questions 1-4)

1. It has been determined that tuberculosis is limited to Tommy's spinal vertebrae. Children are believed to be at increased risk of developing skeletal tuberculosis because they:
   a. Are more likely to be calcium deficient.
   b. Have increased vascularity of bones due to growth.
   c. Are generally more active and more predisposed to open fractures.
   d. Are exposed to children from a variety of backgrounds at school.

2. The most significant intervention to prevent tuberculosis in children is to:
   a. Have them wear a mask in public.
   b. Do annual PPD skin testing.
   c. Test children with tuberculosis contact.
   d. Get children vaccinated with BCG.

3. All of the following are true regarding Tommy's treatment plan **except:**
   a. Prescribe the standard antituberculosis drugs in dosage and duration of time.
   b. His mother may stop giving him his medications when his symptoms subside.
   c. Medications may be altered during the course of treatment based on sensitivity results.
   d. Baseline hepatic function should be established.

4. In educating the family prior to Tommy's discharge home, it is **most** important to stress:
   a. The need for annual chest x-ray on all household contacts.
   b. That Tommy comply with the full course of antituberculosis treatment.
   c. The importance of good nutrition and exercise for Tommy.
   d. The need to stop medication when his symptoms stop but only if he develops stomach irritation.

Sara, a 70-year-old woman, presents with right hip joint pain, decreased range of motion of the hip, and fever of 1-week duration. One year ago she had a right total hip replacement. (Questions 5-6)

5. The treatment plan for Sara includes removal of prosthesis, debridement of devitalized tissue, administration of parenteral antibiotics, and delaying reimplantation. Which of the following interventions would not be an appropriate option for Sara?
   a. Placement of antibiotic impregnated beads at the time of debridement.
   b. Use of antibiotic impregnated cement at time of reimplantation surgery.
   c. Use of skeletal traction to preserve joint space and leg length.
   d. Hip immobilization in a spica cast and continuing with parenteral antibiotics.

6. Infections of total joint prosthesis may occur following:
   a. Hematogenous spread of the pathogen from another foci.
   b. Contamination at the time of surgery.
   c. Direct inoculation of the joint space.

Dennis Reardon, age 21, sustained injuries in a motorcycle accident requiring surgery and an open reduction of a right femur fracture. He received prophylactic antibiotics at the time of surgery. Ten days after surgery he developed a fever of 103°; he had chills, and edema and erythema at the operative site. The site was also producing serosanguineous drainage. (Questions 7-9)

7. The most common organism involved in osteomyelitis is:
   a. *Staphylococcus aureus.*
   b. *β-hemolytic streptococci.*
   c. Clostridium.
   d. Enterobacter.

8. Antibiotic treatment is recommended for:
   a. 1 week.
   b. 2 weeks.
   c. 4-6 weeks.
   d. 6 months.

9. Prolonged IV antibiotic therapy would put Dennis at increased risk for:
   a. Chronic osteomyelitis.
   b. Colonization with antibiotic-resistant bacteria.
   c. Nosocomial infection of the circulatory system.
   d. Secondary infection of the operative site.

Mary, age 40, presented to her physician with a painful left knee. She had surgery to this knee 5 years ago due to trauma but has been symptom-free until recently. On exam, the knee is swollen, warm, and painful. Joint fluid was obtained which was cloudy, 70,000 wbc/cc with predominance of polys (> 80%). (Questions 10-13)

10. The organism most commonly isolated causing septic arthritis in adults > 30 years old is:
    a. *Staphylococcus aureus.*
    b. *Escherichia coli.*
    c. Candida.
    d. *Hemophilus influenzae.*

11. Risk factor(s) for the development of septic arthritis in Mary's case was:
    a. Her gender and the length of time since the trauma.
    b. Prior surgery to knee.
    c. Aspiration of joint fluid.
    d. Age and trauma.

12. The most common organism causing septic arthritis in people < 30 years is:
    a. *Neisseria gonorrhoea.*
    b. *C trachomatis.*
    c. *Pseudomonas aeryginosa.*
    d. *Escherichia coli.*

13. You would instruct Mary to:
    a. Stop antibiotics and call her physician if there is no improvement or if symptoms worsen.
    b. Stop antibiotic therapy 1 day after all symptoms have resolved.
    c. Complete the fully prescribed antibiotic course without any interruption.
    d. Stop antibiotics after 5 days of therapy if there are signs of improvement.

Cory, a 27-year-old man, suffered a compound fracture to the left forearm after falling from the roof to the ground while making repairs to his home. After treatment, he did well and was discharged home. Two weeks later, he presented in the emergency room with complaints of acute pain over the fracture site. His wife reported confusion and a change in mental status. Physical assessment revealed T 100 F, BF 132, RR 22. The fingers of the left hand were cold and edematous. The cast was removed. The wound had a foul odor and was edematous. Tissue palpitation was crepitant with a crunchy, "bubbly" sensation. (Questions 14-15)

14. What is the most likely cause of these symptoms?
    a. "Cast syndrome."
    b. Volkmann's ischemia contracture.
    c. *Clostridium perfringens* gas gangrene.
    d. Nerve damage.

15. Management of this condition would include
    a. Vigorous cardiovascular stability action.
    b. Surgical exploration and antibiotic therapy.
    c. Antibiotics and obtaining blood and wound cultures.
    d. Amputation and blood thinning medications.

Chapter 10 Therapeutic Modalities

Cathleen E. Kunkler, BSN, RN, CNA, ONC

Contents

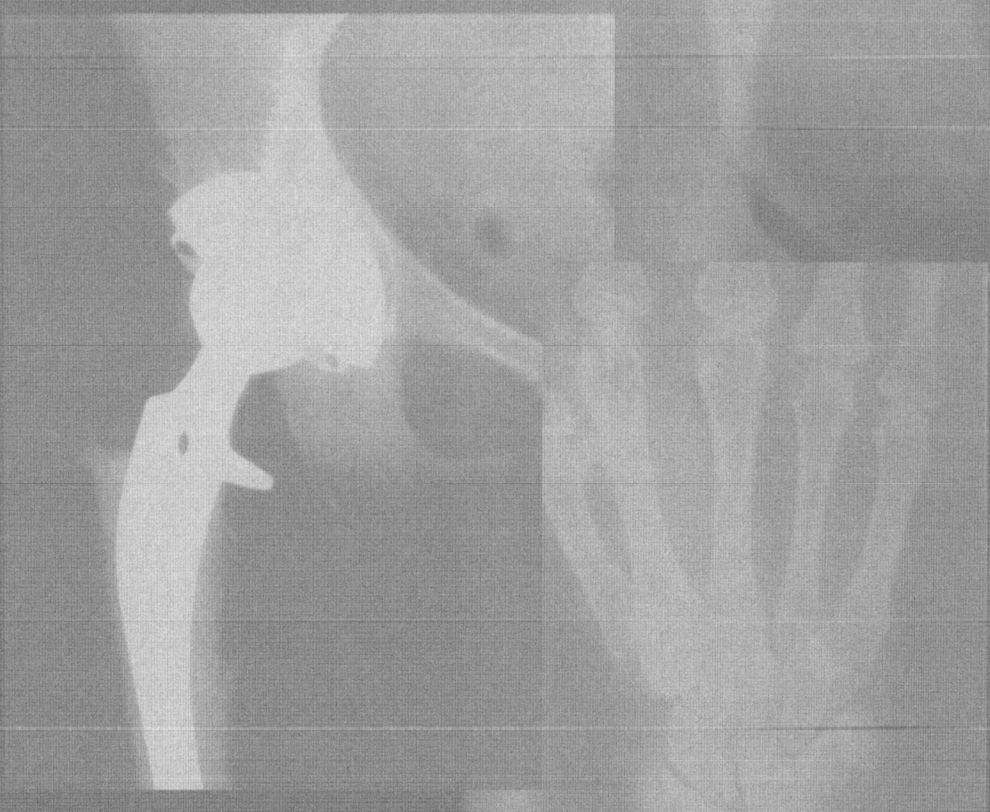

OBJECTIVES

At the completion of this chapter, the learner will be able to:

- Describe the purpose and indications for use of the treatment modality.
- Describe the mechanism of action and principles of use of the treatment modality.

KEY POINTS

- Elevation of extremity to decrease edema:
    - ♦ Hand higher than elbow
    - ♦ Elbow higher than shoulder
    - ♦ Ankle higher than knee
    - ♦ Knee higher than hip
- Pin tract care/external fixator care for neurovascular changes.
- Avoid pressure over bony prominences.
- Document appropriate use of treatment modalities.
- The procedure for doing stairs: Going upstairs using crutches, lead with the unaffected leg and follow with the crutches and affected foot moving together. Coming downstairs, the crutches and affected leg lead and then unaffected. Remember, "up with the good, down with the bad."
- There are no "one size fits all" ambulatory devices; fit devices to the individual.
- Assess patients for difficulty in adhering to bracing.

CHAPTER 10

THERAPEUTIC MODALITIES

CASTS

I. OVERVIEW

A. **Definition: a cast is a temporary circumferential immobilization device.**

B. **Functions.**
   1. Immobilization.
   2. Prevents or corrects deformities.
   3. Maintains, supports, and protects realigned bone.
   4. Promotes healing and early weight bearing.

C. **Casting materials.**
   1. Natural.
      a. Plaster of Paris.
         (1) Powdered calcium sulfate crystals incorporated into a bandage (roll of tape).
         (2) Use is diminishing.
   2. Synthetic materials.
      a. Polyester/cotton knit.
      b. Thermoplastic: open weave polyester polymer fabric tape.
      c. Fiberglass:
         (1) Knitted fiberglass tape permeated with a water-activated polyurethane resin.
         (2) Most commonly used.
      d. Fiberglass-free, latex-free polymer.
         (1) Polyester substrate with extensible yarns incorporated into tape.
         (2) Use with known or suspected latex allergy or with allergy prone individuals.
   3. Hybrid: combination of plaster of Paris beneath layers of fiberglass.
   4. Additional supplies.
      a. Gloves.
      b. Stockinette and webril or cast padding.
      c. Liner such as Gore-Tex® barrier for moisture absorption.
      d. Blunt-end bandage scissors.
      e. Cast saw.
      f. Duckbill cast bender.
      g. Cast spreader.
      h. Cast shoe/walking heels.

D. **Types of casts.**
   1. Upper extremity.
      a. Short arm.
      b. Long arm.
      c. Hanging long arm.
      d. Long arm cylinder.
      e. Thumb spica.
   2. Lower extremity.
      a. Short leg.
      b. Long leg.
      c. Leg cylinder.
      d. Short and long abduction boots.
      e. Abduction cast (Petri/A-frame).
      f. Total contact cast.
         (1) Well-molded, minimally padded cast that has contact with entire plantar aspect of foot/toes and lower extremity.
         (2) Post amputation to shrink and mold residual limb.
   3. Body casts.
      a. Spinal body vest with or without straps.
      b. Risser and Pantaloon Risser.
      c. Minerva jacket.
      d. Airplane or shoulder spica.
      e. Turnbuckle.
      f. Unilateral, one-and-a-half, and bilateral hip.
      g. English walking.

E. **Advantages of casts for immobilization.**
   1. Relative ease of application.
   2. Requires minimal care.
   3. Protects the tissue.
   4. May not require hospitalization.
   5. Patient can generally be active and mobile.
   6. New materials quick setting and lightweight.

F. **Considerations across the lifespan.**
   1. Fractures in children usually require a shorter period of immobilization.
   2. Pediatric patients have poor pain acknowledgment that may mask potential complications.
   3. Pediatric patients require more astute assessment of cast loosening and neurovascular changes due to changes in edema.
   4. The frail skin of the elderly requires extra padding, especially over bony prominences.

G. **Complications.**
   1. Neurovascular compromise.
   2. Incorrect fracture alignment.
   3. Skin breakdown from pressure.
   4. Compartment syndrome.
   5. Cast syndrome/superior mesenteric artery syndrome (SMAS).
      a. Occurs only with body spica casts.
      b. Compression of duodenum anteriorly and aorta and vertebral column posteriorly in superior mesenteric artery causes decrease in blood supply to bowel, which results in hemorrhage and necrosis of GI tract.
      c. Risk/contributing factors.
         (1) Body cast or hip spica cast: avoid lumbar lordosis during cast application.
         (2) Extensive supine positioning/recumbency.
         (3) Hyperextension of lumbar spine.
         (4) Spinal instrumentation and distraction.
      d. Sign and symptoms.
         (1) Vague abdominal pain, pressure, and distention.

(2) Nausea and projectile vomiting.
(3) Bowel obstruction.
(4) May occur days or weeks after cast application due to weight loss of retroperitoneal fat after immobilization.

e. Treatment of SMAS.
(1) Bivalve, window, or remove cast.
(2) Decompress stomach with NG tube and continuous or intermittent suction as needed.
(3) NPO and intravenous hydration.
(4) Change position from supine to prone if possible.
(5) Surgery to release ligament of Treitz.
(6) If untreated can be fatal.

II. ASSESSMENT

A. History: focuses on previous acute injury; or chronic, developmental, or congenital condition that required casting. Also includes any other treatments by casting.

1. Assess the effects of casting on patient's lifestyle.
   a. Hand dominance.
   b. Home situation.
   c. Previous ambulatory status.
2. Support systems.

B. Physical examination.

1. Complete physical examination with special emphasis on the extremity or area of the body requiring immobilization by casting.
2. Compare affected extremity with unaffected extremity when possible.
3. Compare each assessment with previous assessments.
4. Pre-casting.
   a. Determine general peripheral vascular status.
   b. Assess neurovascular status for:
      (1) Color.
      (2) Temperature.
      (3) Capillary filling.
      (4) Pulses.
      (5) Any sensory disturbances:
         (a) Burning.
         (b) Decreased sensation.
         (c) Numbness.
      (d) Paresthesia.
      (6) Motion.
      (7) Pain.
      (8) Edema.
   c. Assess skin integrity, including:
      (1) Scars.
      (2) Open lacerations.
      (3) Pressure ulcers.
      (4) Bruises.
      (5) Varicosities.
      (6) Open wounds.
      (7) Peripheral vascular disease.
      (8) Atrophy.
      (9) Rashes.
      (10) Poor hygiene.
   d. Alignment of the affected body part.
   e. Abdominal and urologic characteristics of area to be covered by cast, including:
      (1) Bowel sounds.
      (2) Abdominal or bladder distention.
      (3) Softness upon palpation.
      (4) History of nausea and vomiting.
      (5) Elimination patterns.
   f. Respiratory characteristics of area to be covered by cast, including:
      (1) Respiratory rate.
      (2) Quality of breath sounds.
   g. Muscle strength and reflexes.
   h. Jewelry removal.
   i. Nail polish removal.
5. Post-casting.
   a. Determine peripheral vascular status.
   b. Assess neurovascular status above and below cast.
   c. Note the shape and size of cast to determine if cast becomes deformed or broken before dry.
   d. Assess skin integrity around edges of cast.
   e. Check position of the casted body part.
   f. Check for drainage on cast.
   g. Note any odor from cast.
   h. Determine patient's comfort in cast.
   i. Assess patient's response to presence of cast.

III. COMMON THERAPEUTIC MODALITIES

A. Pre-casting.

1. Determine type of cast to be used.
2. Use premedication as necessary.
   a. Muscle relaxants.
   b. NSAIDs.
   c. Analgesics.

B. Cast application.

1. General anesthesia may be indicated in some cases.
   a. Positioning, stability.
   b. Uncooperative patient.
      (1) Age.
      (2) Spasticity.
      (3) Fear.
      (4) Discomfort.
2. General principles.
   a. Protect skin/bony prominences under cast.
      (1) Stockinette.
      (2) Webril
      (3) Padding.
   b. Select appropriate casting material; proper water temperature for preparation of casting material.
   c. Proper alignment of joints in position of function.
   d. Provide abdominal opening (window), if patient is in body cast.

C. Post-casting.

1. Analgesics/NSAIDs.
2. Activity orders: isometrics of quad sets and gluteal sets 10 times each and every hour.
3. Amount of elevation: "Hands above the heart and toes above the nose."

a. Hand higher than elbow.
b. Elbow higher than shoulder.
c. Foot higher than knee.
d. Knee higher than hip.

4. Ice, rest, compression, elevation as above.
5. Univalve/bivalve/remove cast (with signs of neurovascular compromise, compartment syndrome).
6. Notify physician.

D. Sling usage with upper extremity casts.

1. Place in sling until edema or tenderness subside.
2. Support weight of casted hand and wrist in slightly flexed position to prevent shoulder muscle strain.
3. A sling greatly reduces neck fatigue and elbow and wrist pressure.
4. Commercially made slings are available or slings can be cut from canvas.
5. Basic design is to give comfort and support by spreading weight of upper extremity evenly across neck and shoulders, but should not obstruct access to check neurovascular status.
6. With canvas, make a triangular sling, pin at both sides of back of neck (rather than knotted over cervical spine) to prevent pressure.
7. Remove sling to rest extremity and to wash sling, if necessary.

E. Change cast indications.

1. Inspect incision.
2. Looseness due to reduced edema, slides off extremity.
3. Increased complaints of pain, tightness, or looseness.
4. Excessive wetness; excessive trauma to cast.
5. Foreign object placed in cast.
6. Poor original application.

F. Cast removal.

1. Support joints above and below injury when removing cast.
2. Caution patient about:
   a. Cast saw noise.
   b. Saw cuts by vibrations.
   b. Cast dust inhalation.
   c. Ear and eye protection.
3. Continue to provide support to joints above and below affected joint.
4. Wash skin gently with mild soap and water, don't try to remove all of the dead skin.
5. Lubricate skin with protective emollient, lotion, cream, or ointment.

IV. NURSING DIAGNOSES, OUTCOMES, AND INTERVENTIONS

A. See Table 10.1.

B. Injury, potential.
Skin integrity, impaired.

1. Outcomes.
   a. No evidence of skin irritation.
   b. A clean dry cast is maintained with no loss of integrity.
   c. Neurovascular integrity maintained.
   d. No evidence of refracture or dislocation/subluxation.
2. Interventions.

a. Prevent/monitor skin and cast complications.
(1) Pre-casting.
(a) Examine skin before cast application for:
i. Bruises.
ii. Rashes.
iii. Varicosities.
iv. Peripheral vascular problems.
v. Poor turgor.
vi. Atrophy.
vii. Open wounds.
viii. Lacerations.
(b) Notify physician of abnormalities.
(c) Record on patient's chart.
(d) Assess tetanus status and need for prophylaxis.
(e) Prior to cast application:
i. Cleanse part or parts of body to be casted.
ii. Cut stockinette to extend several inches beyond cast to allow for finishing the edges (petal).
iii. Pad well over bony prominences.
(2) Casting.
(a) Reduction of fracture site performed by physician, nurse practitioner, or physician assistant.
(b) Cover skin surfaces with padding and/or stockinette.
(c) Apply dampened plaster rolls/synthetic cast tapes smoothly and evenly.
(d) Overlap each turn of plaster roll by approximately one-half its width so that no two turns directly overlap, which could cause undue pressure in that area.
(e) Cover joint areas while in moderate or full flexion by using partially overlapping figure 8 turns.
(f) Incorporate longitudinal strips of wet plaster if additional strength is needed for support around joints.
(g) If cast will not need trimming, petal edges while casting by turning down the ends of the stockinette over the plaster, then covering the turned-down edges with plaster/synthetic casting material to hold the stockinette in place and create a smooth edge against skin.
(h) Application with cast tape similar to plaster. Cast tape adheres to previous turn and is stable in approximately 15 minutes.
(3) Post-casting.
(a) Elevate extremity to heart level.
(b) Trim edges of cast to prevent roughness; tape rough edges if needed.
(c) Petal edges with transpore tape or moleskin if stockinette edge is not used. (Always petal edges of spica cast around perineal opening to prevent soiling.)

Table 10.1
Common Nursing Diagnoses, Outcomes, and Interventions

Diagnoses	Outcomes	Interventions
A. Physical mobility, impaired	• Performs ROM exercises, passive and active, and muscle-setting exercises. Ambulates with an assistive device if required for weight-bearing restrictions.	• Assessment. 1. Assess the amount of movement or limitations imposed by the injury, therapeutic modality. 2. Assess the ROM of unaffected muscles. 3. Assess ambulatory status with or without assistive devices. • Promote muscle strength and joint function. 1. Teach patient purposes and regimens for ROM exercises and muscle-setting exercises to unaffected tissues. - Quadriceps, triceps, biceps, and gluteus setting exercises. 2. Physical, occupational, and massage therapies. • Assist in positioning/movement. 1. Turn patient to relieve pressure on tissues and increase perfusion. 2. Initially assist with transfer and ambulation to assess abilities, balance, gait, strength, coordination. • Promote safety within parameters of decreased mobility. 1. Side rails up to avoid loss of balance or falls. 2. Alert patient to safety hazards in home, work, or school. • Promote healthy nutritional intake including protein and calcium to promote healing.
B. Skin integrity, impaired	• Skin remains intact. No odors or excess drainage from skin surfaces, pin sites. Adequate perfusion.	• Assessment. 1. Assess all skin surfaces surrounding the therapeutic modality and bony prominences for evidence of integrity or pressure areas. 2. Assess for evidence of circulatory compromise: whiteness, bluish discoloration, excessive redness. 3. Assess therapeutic modality for rough edges, tightness, excessive itching. d. Assess for odors or drainage. • Maintain skin integrity. 1. Gently apply lotion and massage around bony prominences, but not directly over reddened areas.

Common Nursing Diagnoses, Outcomes, and Interventions

Diagnoses	Outcomes	Interventions
B. Skin integrity, impaired (continued)	• Skin remains intact. No odors or excess drainage from skin surfaces, pin sites. Adequate perfusion. (continued)	2. Reposition patient every 2 hours and PRN. 3. Keep bed linens clean, dry, and wrinkle-free. 4. Do not use powder or talc as it tends to collect moisture and irritate the skin. 5. Check peripheral pulses under elastic bandages: if unable to palpate, loosen bandages. 6. Check skin under elastic bandages for areas of breakdown, blistering, or redness. 7. Perform pin site care per protocol. 8. Evaluate alignment and fit of therapeutic modality. a. Note swelling, edema which may compromise neurovascular functioning. b. For circular fixators, check the opposite extremity for lacerations or skin breakdown. 9. See Chapter 6, Effects of Immobility.
C. Peripheral neurovascular dysfunction, risk for	• Neurovascular status is maintained. Capillary refill is 1-3 seconds. Peripheral pulses present and strong. Color is pink or normal as compared to unaffected extremity.	• Perform neurovascular assessment bilaterally. 1. Color. 2. Temperature of tissues. 3. Edema. 4. Pain. 5. Capillary refill. 6. Motor function. 7. Sensory function. 8. Peripheral pulses (if non-palpable, use Doppler). • Maintain alignment and integrity of immobilized extremity. 1. Position and elevate extremity ("Hands above the heart and toes above the nose") as tolerated. a. Assess for compartment syndrome. (1) Pain out of proportion to the injury. (2) Pain on passive muscle stretch. (3) Pallor of extremity. (4) Paresthesia, numbness. (5) Pulselessness.

Table 10.1 (continued)
Common Nursing Diagnoses, Outcomes, and Interventions

Diagnoses	Outcomes	Interventions
C. Peripheral neurovascular dysfunction, risk for (continued)	• Neurovascular status is maintained. Capillary refill is 1-3 seconds. Peripheral pulses present and strong. Color is pink or normal as compared to unaffected extremity. (continued)	b. Evaluate readiness of emergency equipment such as cast cutter, cast spreader. (1) Evaluate setup and function of therapeutic modality. (2) Ice bags to injured tissues to reduce edema. (3) Heat after 48-72 hours. (Avoid with bruises, crushing injuries, and fractures because of increased bleeding tendencies). (4) For child in traction, draw line on sheet and tell him/her not to slip below.
D. Pain, acute	• Pain is diminished or relieved by pain management protocol.	• Pain assessment 1. Intensity. 2. Location. 3. Type. 4. Timing. 5. Aggravating or alleviating factors. 6. Disabilities from pain. 7. Patient's understanding and meaning given to pain. 8. Presence of muscle spasms. 9. Pre-verbal child's facial expressions. • Physical measures to control pain. 1. Reposition patient to relieve pressure. (Note change in severity and pattern of pain with repositioning.) 2. Turn patient if permitted to relieve soreness, spasms, and pain. 3. Have patient use trapeze to shift self to more comfortable position and to relieve pressure on posterior tissues. 4. Massage and lubricate sore muscles. • Psychologic/cognitive measures to control pain; distraction techniques. 1. Explain the reasons for muscle spasms and pain that may be present. 2. Relaxation/distraction techniques. 3. Diversional activities and recreation.

Table 10.1 (continued)
Common Nursing Diagnoses, Outcomes, and Interventions

Diagnoses	Outcomes	Interventions
D. Pain, acute (continued)	• Pain is diminished or relieved by pain management protocol. (continued)	• Pharmacologic measures to control pain. 1. Narcotic analgesics may be required in the post-fracture state. 2. Aspirin/NSAIDs to decrease inflammation. 3. Muscle relaxants.
E. Self-care, deficient 1. Bathing/hygiene 2. Dressing/grooming 3. Eating 4. Toileting	• Regain independence in self-care as permitted by therapeutic modality.	• Assessment of ability to perform self-care activities and availability of persons to assist with individual's self-care. • Explain the modifications or limitations imposed by the cast, traction, fixator, brace, orthoses.
F. Diversional activity deficit; social interaction, impaired	• Participate in activities using muscles and joints as able. Interact appropriately with visitors and others.	• Assessment of: 1. Activity likes and dislikes. 2. Muscle strength and weaknesses for particular games or activities. 3. Physical abilities or limitations. 4. Concerns about moving while using therapeutic modality. • Assist patient to engage in active diversional activities that use unaffected muscles and joints. 1. Avoid passive activities that lessen muscle use and lessen muscle strength. 2. Encourage patient to work with hobbies, personal interests. 3. Encourage visits from family and friends or with other patients to lessen feelings of isolation, loneliness, or confinement. 4. Observe for age-appropriate behaviors and possible regression. 5. Observe for disuse syndrome.
G. Self-concept, disturbed; hopelessness; body image, disturbed; sleep pattern, disturbed	• Regain a positive outlook, body concept. • Effectively deal with feelings of hopelessness and lack of control/power. • Establish acceptable sleep pattern.	• Assess for: 1. Reaction to illness. 2. Reaction to therapeutic modality. 3. Reaction to activity restrictions. 4. Reaction to changes in body image. 5. Ability to get sufficient rest and sleep to participate and cooperate in treatment plan.

Table 10.1 (continued)
Common Nursing Diagnoses, Outcomes, and Interventions

Diagnoses	Outcomes	Interventions
G. Self-concept, disturbed; hopelessness; body image, disturbed; sleep pattern, disturbed (continued)	• Regain a positive outlook, body concept. Effectively deal with feelings of hopelessness and lack of control/power. Establish acceptable sleep pattern. (continued)	• Listen to the patient's expression of concerns and feelings. 1. Encourage verbalization of feelings. 2. Psychosocial evaluation. 3. Determine effective coping mechanisms used in past difficult situations. • Positively reinforce movement toward wellness, gains in functional capacity. 1. Stress the positives, not what is absent or cannot be done. 2. Teach self-care techniques to increase independence, self-confidence and patient control over illness/injury.
H. Injury, risk for	• Free from complications of immobility. • No injury sustained from actual therapeutic modality.	• Check mechanics of cast, traction (ropes, pulleys, weights, etc.), fixators, brace, orthoses. 1. Maintain proper alignment. 2. Reposition PRN. 3. See Chapter 6, Effects of Immobility.

(d) Cleanse residue from cast materials off patient's skin after application is complete.
(e) Instruct patient not to place foreign objects beneath cast.
(f) Note amount of bleeding on cast (circling may or may not be considered helpful due to porosity of cast materials), and apply ice bags to lessen bleeding.
(g) Observe for respiratory or cardiac distress in patients with a cast jacket.
i. Have cast cutter available and be aware of quickest method to remove cast jacket to initiate cardiopulmonary resuscitation (CPR).
ii. Have wrench taped to jacket.

b. Maintain cast integrity.
(1) Plaster casts.
(a) Leave cast uncovered and open to air to dry.
(b) Place cast on firm, smooth surface with pillow (without rubber or plastic) under joints to prevent flattening of plaster or entrapment of heat.
(c) Reposition patient, alternating from supine, prone, and lateral side to side when possible every 2-4 hours to promote drying. (Avoid putting any pressure on toes.)
(d) Drying period of large plaster casts may be 48-72 hours depending on humidity and temperature.
(e) Drying may be aided by use of fans.
(f) Explain warmth felt by patient as plaster sets and dries.
(g) Support and move cast with palms of hands instead of fingers to prevent indentations in plaster.
(h) Turn patient, supporting major joints. Do not use abductor bars to turn patient in a spica cast.
(i) Weight bearing, if ordered, is not recommenced until the cast is completely dry.
(j) When turning, inspect the cast for cracks, softening, or excessive flaking. (Report these areas to physician and document in the patient's record.)
(k) Do neurovascular assessment of extremities, based on institutional policy (such as every 15 minutes X-2 hours, every 30 minutes X-2 hours, every 2 hours X-4 hours, every 4

hours X-8 hours, and then every 8 hours, if N/V signs remain normal).

(l) Keep cast dry.
  i. Cover with a plastic bag securely closed at the top when showering or bathing.
  ii. Avoid rain or other sources of moisture.

(m) Cleanse soiled plaster with a mild powdered cleanser and a slightly dampened cloth and pat dry completely, only when necessary.

(2) Synthetic casts.
  (a) Dry completely by blotting cast with towels and using hand blower on cool or warm setting to thoroughly dry cast and lining to prevent skin maceration/burns and alterations in cast integrity. (Warmth will be felt by patient due to chemical reaction from synthetic cast curing.)
  (b) May weight bear in 30 minutes per order.
  (c) Surface of cast is rough, so caution needs to be taken to protect opposite limb and furniture from scratches.
  (d) May be immersed in water depending on casting material and physician's permission.
  (e) Flush out well with clear fresh water after bathing or swimming to remove mild soaps or chlorine residue.

c. Monitor/prevent ongoing complications.
  (1) Inspect the skin around the edges of cast for redness or skin irritation.
    (a) Monitor areas over bony prominences for pressure or burning sensation.
    (b) Skin may be massaged and cooled with alcohol.
  (2) Assess cast for:
    (a) Any smell or drainage that may indicate a pressure sore or wound infection beneath the cast.
    (b) Feel cast for abnormally warm areas.
  (3) Perform neurovascular checks to ascertain local effects of cast on tissues.
    (a) Capillary refill.
    (b) Color of skin.
    (c) Temperature of skin.
    (d) Presence and amount of edema.
    (e) Comfort/sensations of casted area.
    (f) Mobility of tissues contiguous to the encasted tissues.
    (g) Pain.
    (h) Changes in function experienced.

C. Cast syndrome, potential (for patient with body spica cast).

1. Outcome: patient exhibits no signs or symptoms of fluid volume deficit/cast syndrome.
2. Interventions: prevent fluid loss from cast syndrome for patients in body spicas.
   a. Be sure abdominal window is adequate.
   b. Observe patient for prolonged nausea and projectile vomiting; record and report to the physician.
   c. Auscultate bowel sounds, palpate abdomen, assess abdominal distention and rebound tenderness.
   d. Monitor electrolytes and abdominal diagnostic tests.
   e. Keep patient NPO if nausea and vomiting occur.
   f. Monitor and record any N/G tube drainage.
   g. Monitor and record intravenous fluid replacement therapy.
   h. Reposition patient. If patient is able to tolerate prone position, this may provide some relief from pressure.
   i. Cast removal may be considered by the physician if condition does not improve.
   j. Surgical intervention may be considered by the physician if condition continues.
   k. After nausea and vomiting subside and bowel sounds are present, gradually increase diet.

D. Ineffective breathing pattern, potential.

1. Outcomes.
   a. Normal breath sounds in all quadrants.
   b. Performs deep breathing and coughing exercises.
2. Interventions.
   a. Assess respiratory function in patients with a body or spica cast and in immobilized patients.
   b. Teach and encourage deep breathing and coughing exercises.
   c. Help patient change position every 2 hours and PRN to increase perfusion.

E. Injury, potential (refracture/dislocation/subluxation following cast removal).

1. Outcomes.
   a. Patient complies with activity restrictions.
   b. No evidence of refracture/dislocation/subluxation.
2. Interventions.
   a. Explain to patient that muscles and joints in cast will be weak and sore and that use and movements should be initiated moderately with rest periods.
   b. May use analgesic/NSAIDs for soreness, pain, or inflammation.
   c. Explain to patient that it takes twice as long to regain full function as the limb was in the cast.
   d. Elevate affected extremity frequently after cast removal to prevent edema.
   e. Discuss activity restrictions, exercises for muscle strengthening, and methods to avoid refracture and dislocation after cast removal.

V. HOME CARE CONSIDERATIONS

A. Provide patient/family teaching.

1. Give patient information and instruction related to signs and symptoms of complications to watch for

(severe pain, burning, numbness, tingling, skin discoloration, swelling, paralysis, foul odor, warm spots, elevated temperature, soft areas and cracks, pallor, and coolness of fingers and toes).
2. Instruct patient to keep extremity elevated when possible.
3. Instruct patient in skin care.
4. Instruct patient in care of cast to maintain integrity.
5. Instruct patient to notify physician of any abnormalities.
6. Explain atrophy that may occur with casting and the need to continue exercises, both active and passive, as permitted by physician.
7. Instruct in activity level and use of ambulatory devices, if indicated.
8. Instruct in comfort measures.
9. Instruct patient/family in proper application and elevation of an extremity in a sling.

B. Discuss sexual activities and positions, if needed.

C. Observe the patient's mobility.
1. Ambulation.
2. Stair climbing.
3. Transfers.

D. Decrease anxiety related to cast removal.
1. Explain use of cast saw; potential small cuts and/or heat burns.
2. Inform patient that skin beneath cast may be scaly and tender. Advise on use of lotions, creams, or ointments.
3. Instruct on activity level in immediate removal period.

TRACTION

I. OVERVIEW

A. Definition: the application of a pulling force to an injured or diseased part of the body or an extremity while a countertraction pulls in the opposite direction.

B. Purposes.
1. Reduce fractures and/or subluxations/dislocations and maintain alignment.
2. Decrease muscle spasm associated with low-back pain or cervical whiplash and relieve pain.
3. Correct, lessen, or prevent deformities/contractures.
4. Promote rest of a diseased or injured part; provide immobilization to prevent soft tissue damage.
5. Promote active and passive exercise.
6. Expand a joint space during arthroscopic procedure or prior to joint reconstruction.

C. Mechanisms.
1. Static: promotes immobilization (continuous).
2. Dynamic: promotes movement (intermittent).
3. Running traction: exerts a pull in one plane (straight).
4. Balanced suspension: allows patient movement without change in the pull of traction.

D. Basic principles of maintaining effective traction.
1. Provide countertraction (using part of the patient's body, bed positioning, or pull of weights in opposite direction).
2. Prevent friction by NOT:
   a. Tucking in top linens.
   b. Allowing foot-plate to rest against the bed.
   c. Allowing shearing of elbows or heels against linen.
3. Other ways to prevent friction are:
   a. Avoiding clamps, hooks, etc. resting against the bed frame.
   b. Making sure weights move freely through pulleys:
      (1) Clear footboard.
      (2) Suspend weights off floor.
   c. Traction knots are not near the pulleys or at the patient attachment point.
4. Maintain line of pull established by physician (usually neutral unless otherwise specified).
5. Maintain continuous or intermittent traction as required by physician's order and type of traction.
6. Safely transfer with halo traction due to altered field of vision.

E. Classifications.
1. Skin.
   a. Attaches to skin and soft tissue, providing a light pull.
   b. May be removed and reapplied intermittently as per physician orders.
   c. 5-8 pounds of weight (1-5 pounds for children) maximum for arms and legs to prevent occlusion of small blood vessels.
   d. Weight is applied with skin adherent strips, cervical head halters, ace wraps, or commercial encircling devices (foam splints, traction boots, pelvic belts).
   e. If weight is distributed over larger areas (pelvic), more weight can be used.
   f. Weight is distributed evenly over largest possible body surface to prevent uneven pull and skin breakdown.
   g. Maintained for relatively short periods.
   h. Used for:
      (1) Stabilization of fractured bones prior to repair with surgery or skeletal traction.
      (2) Relief of muscle spasms.
      (3) Immobilization of joints/bones with inflammatory conditions to relieve pain.
      (4) Prevention of flexion contractures.
2. Skeletal.
   a. Attaches directly to bone and provides a strong, steady, continuous pull.
   b. Pin insertion sites:
      (1) Distal femur.
      (2) Proximal tibia.
      (3) Proximal ulna.
   c. Weight is applied with:
      (1) Steinmann's pins or Kirschner wires to extremities.
      (2) Halo or tongs to the head.
   d. A range of 15-40 pounds of weight is commonly used depending on:
      (1) Injury/pathology.

(2) Body size.
(3) Degree of muscle spasm.

e. Traction should not be removed without physician's order.
f. Skeletal traction is frequently used in conjunction with balanced weighted suspension.

3. Manual.
   a. Applied with hands.
   b. Steady pull maintained.
   c. Used during:
      (1) An emergency.
      (2) Casting.
      (3) Fracture reduction.
      (4) Halo application.

F. Considerations across the lifespan.

1. Type of traction used may depend on patient's age. (Bryant's traction only used on children younger than 3 who weigh less than 35 pounds).
2. Teaching should be appropriate for patient's developmental level (use of play therapy for children).
3. Emphasis on independence/control in age groups for whom these issues are crucial (adolescents).
4. Increased risk of complications (especially complications related to immobility and acute or temporary confusion) in elderly population.
5. Developmental delays if prolonged therapy.

G. Complications.

1. Neurovascular compromise.
   a. Muscle or nerve weakness, numbness or tingling.
   b. Temporary increase in pain, muscle spasms, numbness, tingling, loss of sensation.
2. Inadequate fracture alignment.
   a. Post-treatment arthritis if muscles and joints malaligned in full extension with skin traction.
   b. Thrombosis or pulmonary emboli.
   c. Fat emboli syndrome.
   d. Skin integrity impairment.
      (1) Skin traction.
         (a) Skin breakdown over bony prominences.
         (b) Loss of skin attachment (epidermis from subcutaneous tissue).
      (2) Skeletal traction.
         (a) Pin tract infection.
         (b) Development of pressure ulcers (sacrum, coccyx, heels, trochanters, spine, scapulae, elbows, ears).

II. ASSESSMENT

A. History: focuses on previous acute injury; or chronic, developmental, or congenital condition that required traction. Also includes previous history of treatment with traction.

B. Physical examination.

1. Complete physical examination with special emphasis on extremity or area of body requiring treatment with traction.
2. Compare affected extremity with unaffected extremity when possible.
3. Compare each assessment with previous assessments and compare side to side.
   a. General peripheral vascular status.
   b. Assess neurovascular status for:
      (1) Color.
      (2) Temperature.
      (3) Capillary filling.
      (4) Pulses.
      (5) Sensation.
      (6) Motion.
      (7) Pain.
      (8) Edema.
   c. Assess skin integrity, including:
      (1) Scars.
      (2) Open laceration.
      (3) Pressure ulcers.
      (4) Bruises.
      (5) Rashes.
      (6) Other skin disorders.
      (7) Poor hygiene.
      (8) Any history of diabetes or vascular disease.
   d. Alignment of affected part of body.
   e. Abdominal and urologic characteristics, if patient is immobile, including:
      (1) Bowel sounds.
      (2) History of nausea and vomiting.
      (3) Abdominal or bladder distention.
      (4) Elimination patterns.
      (5) Softness upon palpation.
6. Respiratory characteristics of patient if immobile, including:
      (1) Breath sounds.
      (2) Respiratory rate and quality.

C. Diagnostic tests.

1. X-rays to establish injury or condition.
2. X-rays after traction applied to establish realignment of bone and progression of healing.

III. COMMON THERAPEUTIC MODALITIES

A. Pre-medicate as necessary prior to traction application.

B. Apply traction.

1. Skin traction, in many cases, is applied by nurse or technician.
2. General anesthesia may be used in some cases.

C. Post-traction application. Orders as specified for:

1. Amount of traction weight.
2. Activity and exercise.
3. Pin care.
4. Ice application.
5. Positioning.
6. Analgesics/NSAIDs.

IV. NURSING DIAGNOSES, OUTCOMES, AND INTERVENTIONS

A. See Table 10.1.

B. Physical integrity, impaired.

1. Outcomes.
   a. Mechanisms of traction maintained.

b. Countertraction maintained by keeping patient pulled up in bed.
c. Patient maintains desired position and alignment to promote healing.
d. No evidence of skin breakdown or neurovascular impairment.

2. Interventions.
   a. Maintain mechanics of traction.
      (1) Inspect traction apparatus each shift and PRN.
      (2) Tighten all bolts on frame and on parts of equipment.
         (a) IV-type basic frame.
         (b) "Four poster" Balkan frame.
         (c) Three-bar frame.
      (3) Secure all slipknots with tape.
      (4) Observe for frayed ropes.
      (5) Confirm amount of weight.
      (6) Check that ropes run freely through pulleys and are not restricted by bed linens. (Use only new traction cord.)
      (7) Keep weights hanging freely. Do not remove or lift weights when moving patient. Weights should never hang over patient.
   b. Provide nursing care for patient with adherent skin traction.
      (1) Apply commercial skin traction tapes or strips of moleskin or adhesive lengthwise to either side of affected extremity.
         (a) Be sure tapes extend far enough beyond extremity.
         (b) Do not go beyond tibial tubercle to prevent pressure on peroneal nerve.
      (2) Wrap extremity with Ace© bandage using a spiral or figure-8 configuration. Should cover longest surface possible for even distribution of pull.
      (3) Be sure spreader bars are wide enough to prevent pressure on bony prominences and neurovascular compromise.
      (4) Inspect traction for sliding and wrinkles and palpate over taped area each shift. Document any tenderness or skin breakdown.
      (5) Reapply skin traction if it becomes nonfunctional.
      (6) Remove skin traction for skin care as permitted by physician.
      (7) Inspect, massage, and lubricate skin with gel or ointment, especially around edges of traction.
         (a) Powder, lotion, and creams are not recommended.
         (b) Note any redness, skin irritation, burning sensation, drainage, or foul odor.
      (8) Reposition patient as permitted by traction and physician's orders.
      (9) See Table 10.2 for nursing considerations for specific types of traction.
   c. Provide nursing care for patients with skeletal traction.
      (1) Provide pin site care per protocol.
      (2) Weights should not be lifted or removed; can cause severe muscle contraction with displacement of the fracture fragments.
      (3) Neurovascular checks.
      (4) Observe for edema.
      (5) Teach patient to perform range of motion (ROM) and muscle strengthening exercises.
         (a) Isotonic and isometric exercises to reduce complications.
         (b) Encourage use of trapeze to reposition self in bed.
      (6) Prevent foot drop:
         (a) Keep forefoot and ankle in neutral position with or without the aid of a splint.
         (b) Do not gatch knees of bed.
      (7) Psychological issue of immobility, dependence, body image, and reduced self-esteem.
      (8) See Table 10.2 for nursing considerations for specific types of traction.
   d. Prevent the hazards of immobility relative to the respiratory, gastrointestinal, integumentary, and vascular systems.
   e. Maintain desired position and alignment to promote healing.
      (1) Be aware of proper positioning and alignment for specific types of traction.
      (2) Use appropriate restraints for uncooperative patients.
      (3) Reevaluate patient's position to note continued alignment, increase or decrease in symptoms of soreness, pain, muscle spasms.

V. HOME CARE CONSIDERATIONS

A. Coordinate with hospital and community resources for transport from hospital to home; set up traction in home.

B. Factors that promote successful home traction therapy.

1. Patient/family/caregiver competence, physical and psychosocial ability.
2. 24-hour commitment of caregivers.
3. Patient commitment to home traction therapy and compliance.
4. Available support network.
5. Availability of home care services; staff's comfort with traction.
6. Physical layout of home, able to accommodate bed with traction set up.
7. Patient/family receptiveness to education and performance of special duties.

C. Teach patient and/or responsible family member.

1. Setup of traction apparatus.
2. Application/removal of traction.
3. Signs and symptoms of complications:
   a. Neurovascular compromise.
   b. Skin breakdown.
   c. Bowel and bladder alterations.
   d. Respiratory compromise.

Table 10.2
Nursing Considerations According to Type of Traction

Type of Traction	Indications	Nursing Considerations
1. Halo • Skeletal	• Cervical and high thoracic fractures, subluxations, dislocations, fusions, scoliosis, maintain stability during surgery	a. Provide continuous pull. If pin loosening or penetration occur, apply manual traction and support sides of head with sandbags or apply Philadelphia collar. Notify physician immediately. b. Incorporate signs and symptoms of cranial nerve impairment with neurovascular assessments. c. Observe for eye movements, pupillary changes, blurred vision, photosensitivity, difficulty with swallowing, speech, or tongue control. d. Administer pin care every shift. e. Log roll. f. Muscle setting exercises and active range of motion in appropriate joints. g. Provide distraction or social/ recreational activities. h. Provide emotional support.
2. Cervical head halter • Skin	• Severe sprains, strains, torticollis, mild cervical trauma	a. Observe for pain and pressure in the ears, temporomandibular joint (TMJ), chin, and occiput. b. Add a soft, thin, foam pad beneath chin. c. Perform baseline cranial nerve assessment and document baseline findings. d. Men should be clean shaven when possible. e. May be set up so head is kept in a straight position or so that head of bed can be elevated depending on the patient's condition. As long as the patient's spinal column remains in correct alignment, patient is able to change position, with assistance. f. Use of small cervical pillow determined by the patient's condition. g. Elevate HOB 20-30 degrees for correct alignment. h. Traction removed for meals if permitted by physician. i. Intermittent cervical skin traction is sometimes used, physician orders.
3. Side arm traction/90-90 upper extremity traction • Skin or skeletal	• Supracondylar fractures of the elbow, humerus, and shoulder	a. Do not change position in bed (back lying position) or position of the head of bed. b. Tilt patient toward affected extremity. c. Maintain 90-90 traction with shoulder and forearm flexed or shoulder abducted and elbow flexed. d. Countertraction can be applied by placing shock blocks under the traction side of the bed.

Table 10.2 (continued)
Nursing Considerations According to Type of Traction

Type of Traction	Indications	Nursing Considerations
3. Side arm traction/90-90 upper extremity traction • Skin or skeletal (continued)	• Supracondylar fractures of the elbow, humerus, and shoulder (continued)	e. Observe for radial, ulnar, and median nerve pressure, numbness and tingling of one or more fingers; decreased ability to oppose thumb and fingers (signs of Volkmann's ischemic contracture). f. Patient can use his/her feet to lift buttock for bedpan, skin care, and changing the bed. g. Back and skin care for the upper portion of the body is accomplished by pressing down on the mattress. h. 2-3 weeks callus formation may be sufficient to allow for spica cast application. i. Provide emotional support and teaching about the traction and future care management. j. Provide social and recreational activities.
4. Dunlop traction • Skin or skeletal	• Supracondylar fractures of the elbow • Humerus	a. See side arm traction. b. Used with children. c. Check for Volkmann's ischemic contracture.
5. Pelvic sling • Skin	• Pelvic fractures	a. Sling compresses sides of pelvis. b. Provide good perineal and lower back care. c. Check for foot drop, voiding difficulties, perineal irritations, skin breakdown, correct size, fit, and application of sling. d. Maintain sling beneath lower back with cheek of buttocks elevated 1-2 inches from the bed. e. Clarify orders for lifting and turning.
6. Pelvic traction • Skin	• Muscle spasms associated with low back pain, ruptured disc	a. Apply the pelvic belt across the patient's lower abdomen, making sure it is on the pelvis and that it does not go above the iliac crest or umbilicus, and directly on the patient's skin, when possible. b. Make sure of the correct size. c. Amount of weight varies from 15-40 pounds, depending on patient's size and amount of muscle spasms. d. Assure there is even/straight pull along thighs/knees to the spreader bar or weight attachment. e. William position (supine with 15-20 degrees elevation of the knees and 30-45 degree elevation of the head) preferred. If necessary bed flat when side lying. f. Observe skin for irritation, heat and redness and massage iliac crests. g. Instruct patient to ask for assistance to remove weights and belt, if allowed bathroom privileges.

Table 10.2 (continued)
Nursing Considerations According to Type of Traction

Type of Traction	Indications	Nursing Considerations
7. Bryant traction • Skin	• Developmental dysplasia of the hip (DDH) • Femur fracture in child younger than 2-3 years of age, weighing less than 30-35 pounds	a. Make sure patient's buttocks just clear the mattress, with hips flexed 90 degrees and knees extended. b. Assure that spreader bar keeps pressure from being applied to malleoli. c. Be sure traction is taken down daily (every shift and PRN) to provide skin care of both extremities. d. Child may be positioned either parallel or perpendicular to head and foot of bed. If positioned perpendicular, then caregiver may bring child out of bed to hold in arms and feed. e. Toddlers may need to be restrained to prevent "flipover." f. Family may be taught to provide care for home Bryant traction, a 2-4 week period with 2-4 pounds of weight, followed by hip spica cast if necessary.
8. Buck extension • Skin	• Fractures of the hip for short term, hip contractures, muscle spasms from surgery (hip/knee) or arthritic conditions of hip/knee	a. Keep patient's heels off the bed. Use pillow and/or heel protectors. b. Avoid pressure on the dorsum of the foot and over the head of the fibula or malleolus. c. Assess for peroneal nerve palsy. d. 5-7 pounds weight effective. e. Countertraction may be applied by elevating the foot of bed to prevent sliding down and shearing or by slightly elevating knee gatch. f. The leg in traction should be on the mattress *without* a pillow under the leg. g. Place rolled towel or padded sand bag along the external surface of knee to prevent external rotation of affected leg. h. If on an unrepaired fracture, do not release the traction. i. Teach patients to use trapeze and unaffected foot/leg to lift themselves in assisting with bed pan use, skin care, and linen changes. j. In most instances, head of bed may be elevated for meals, but not for continuous positioning.
9. Russell traction • Skin	• Fractured hip • Short-term use fractured femur not amenable to internal fixation • Fracture tibia/fibula	a. Modification of Buck with the addition of a sling under the femur, not affected knee, to provide more comfort and less rotation. b. Hips and knees slightly flexed 30 degrees or less and immobilized.

Table 10.2 (continued)
Nursing Considerations According to Type of Traction

Type of Traction	Indications	Nursing Considerations
9. Russell traction • Skin (continued)	• Fractured hip • Short-term use fractured femur not amenable to internal fixation • Fracture tibia/fibula (continued)	c. Make sure the sling is smooth and doesn't apply pressure in the popliteal space or the head of the fibula. Due to arrangement of the pulleys, the pull of the traction is double the amount of weight applied. d. The arrangement of the ropes, pulleys, and knee sling distributes the pull more effectively throughout the entire limb, therefore less injurious to skin. e. Back-lying position.
10. Adjunct to traction: balanced suspension with Thomas splint and Pearson attachment	• Device that supports the extremity and overcomes the force of gravity. • Use: used with skin or skeletal traction for femur or tibial fractures not amenable to internal fixation, for acetabular fractures, for maintaining joint space following removal of a prosthesis, and for hip/knee contractures. Can be used alone for exercise, to maintain elevation, to support dependent part, and/or to maintain correct alignment.	a. Pad ischial ring; check increased pressure in groin and knee areas. b. Neurovascular assessment. c. Position the extremity in sling to keep pressure off the heel and Achilles tendon to not carry weight of lower extremity. d. Pearson attachment parallels knee. e. Prevent foot drop; use footboards. f. If bed in semi-Fowler's, lay flat at least 20 minutes every shift to prevent hip flexion contracture. g. Assure no external rotation of extremity to prevent peroneal nerve palsy. h. Perform quadriceps muscle setting exercises and heel cord exercises 10 times per hour while awake and PRN.

e. Cardiac compromise.
f. Infection.
g. Whom to contact.

4. Neurovascular checks.
5. Adult positioning and activity limitations.
6. Pediatric positioning in bed, high chair, infant seat, lap, and playpen (dependent on traction apparatus).
7. Modifications in/assistance with activities of daily living (ADL).
8. Skin care.
9. Pin care.
10. Pain management.

D. Referral for periodic visits from public health nurse, PT/OT as appropriate.

E. Discuss need for diversionary activities.

EXTERNAL FIXATORS

I. OVERVIEW

A. Definition: external fixation is a versatile method of immobilization that employs percutaneous transfixing pins/wires in bone attached to a rigid external frame. Allows a wide range of anatomic correction, both congenital and acquired.

B. Types: external fixators are classified according to the design of the principle components, and there are six basic types of frame configurations.

1. Unilateral frame: fixation on one side of limb
2. Bilateral: rigid bar on both sides of limb connected to full pins that transfix the bone, or 1/2 pins.
3. Quadrilateral: four bars, two on each side of limb connected to pins that transfix the bone.
4. Semicircular: bars that incompletely encircle limb.
5. Triangular: pins are placed on two or more planes.
6. Circular: modular 1/2 rings assembled to circle limb transfixed by small wires.

C. Basic elements: external fixators vary in appearances but have similar purposes.

1. Anchor frames in main bony fragments (pins/wires).
2. Provide longitudinal support (rods).
3. Connect pins/wires to supporting frames.

D. Factors that affect selection of external fixation.

1. Age.
2. Affected bone/limb.
3. Existence of multitrauma.
4. Severity of local soft tissue injury.
5. Complexity of congenital or acquired deformity/defect.
6. Personal preference and clinical experience of surgeon.
7. Patient's ability for self care.

E. Indications.

1. Simple fracture fixation (open and closed).
2. Complex fracture fixation with extensive soft tissue injury.
3. Correction of bony or soft tissue defects/deformities; ligamentotaxis (comminuted epiphyseal fracture).
4. Pseudoarthroses (false joint) of long bone (congenital and acquired) develops at site of former fracture.
5. Nonunion.
6. Malunion.
7. Limb length discrepancies.
8. Stabilization of joint arthrodesis (ankylosis) or fixation of a joint.
9. Circumstances in which urgent transport is needed and/or facilities for internal fixation are not available.

F. Contraindications.

1. Patients in whom cooperation or mental competence is lacking.
2. Fracture will heal with more conservative treatment.
3. Fracture is best treated with internal fixation.
4. Diabetes, steroids due to increased potential for pin tract infection.

G. Advantages of external fixation.

1. Skeletal stability proximal to or a distance from site of injury.
2. Rigid fixation with compression to ensure primary bone healing.
3. Free access to injured site for primary and secondary procedures; facilitate vascular and soft tissue reconstruction.
4. Great versatility in treating a wide variety of bone and soft tissue lesions, access open wounds, reduce sepsis.
5. Ability to stabilize injuries extending across two or more adjacent limb segments, reduce blood loss with pelvic fixation.
6. Adjustability of alignment, length, and mechanical properties.
7. Ability to use simultaneously and/or sequentially with internal fixation and other methods of skeletal stabilization.
8. Minimal interference with adjacent joints.
9. Potential early mobilization of limb and patient from non/partial to full weight bearing.
10. Maintains bone and muscle bulk.
11. Facilitates nursing care.
12. Patient-centered device, patient comfort.
13. Immediate fracture fixation.
14. Reduced complications associated with immobilization.
15. Less scarring than with internal fixation.

H. Complications: complications associated with external fixators can be classified as:

1. Clinical.
   a. Improper insertion of pin/wires causing damage to joint space or iatrogenic treatment/diagnostic neurovascular injuries.
   b. Compartment syndrome; less incidence than with open reduction internal fixation (ORIF).
   c. Joint stiffness or contractures.
   d. Pin-tract infections.
   e. Obstruction of injury access by fixator frame.
   f. Improper use of lengthening.
      (1) Too fast – early union/nonunion
      (2) Too slow – early consolidation/union.
   g. Delayed healing (nonunion/malunion).
   h. Loss of alignment or correction.
   i. Epiphyseal plate disturbance where new bone forms along the plate.
2. Mechanical.
   a. Component failure from misuse.
   b. Inadequate mechanical frame properties.
   c. Malfunction or breakage of components.
3. Multifactorial.
   a. Mismatch of clinical needs and frame selection.
   b. Pin problems (drainage, loosening, infection).
   c. Delayed or inhibited bone consolidation or regeneration.
   d. Unrealistic expectations.
   e. Lack of experience.
   f. Lack of long-term treatment planning.

II. ASSESSMENT

A. History.

1. Description of an acute injury, chronic, developmental, or congenital condition requiring external fixation.
2. Assess effects of external fixation on patient's lifestyle.
3. Normal level of function, weight-bearing status, ROM.
4. Ability to use supportive devices and adapt to limits of external fixator.
5. Means of transportation.
6. Pain history and means used to control or cope.
7. Previous infections.
8. Neurovascular status.
9. Medical/surgical history (endocrine/metabolic) concerning present conditions under treatment.

B. Physical examination.

1. Focus is on affected extremity for:
   a. Pain.
   b. Pallor.
   c. Paresthesia.
   d. Paralysis.
   e. Pulse.
   f. Presenting condition.
   g. Leg-length discrepancy.
2. Appearance and placement of pin/wires.
3. Stability of patient upon admission.
4. Bed position and alignment of affected limb.

C. Diagnostic tests.
1. Radiographs.
2. CT scan.
3. Neurovascular studies.
4. Physical/occupational therapy evaluation.

III. THERAPEUTIC MODALITY CONSIDERATIONS

A. Evaluate for type of external fixation/determine immediate and long-term treatment plans.
B. Apply external fixator.
C. Distraction optimal rate is 1-1½ mm/day divided into four equal doses in children. Adult distraction rate is ¾ mm day in three divided doses.
D. Level of activity and its progression with short- and long-term goals.
E. Physical therapy and occupational therapy needs.
F. Care of the device, with dressing changes, ROM, pin/wire care instructions for immediate and home care.
G. Pain management.
H. Discharge planning and follow-up care.

IV. NURSING DIAGNOSES, OUTCOMES AND INTERVENTIONS

A. See Table 10.1.
B. Injury, potential.
Physical mobility, impaired.
1. Outcomes.
   a. Patient adjusts to altered gait patterns/weight-bearing status.
   b. Evaluates self for safety relative to self-injury from dizziness, disturbed balance, and vertigo which could result in a fall.
2. Interventions.
   a. Teach patient safety maneuvers to balance self with frame and assistive device to prevent falls.
   b. Teach safe use of assistive devices.
   c. PT/OT referral.

C. Impaired skin integrity, potential.
1. Outcomes.
   a. No evidence of pin necrosis or infection.
   b. Minimal serous drainage from pin sites.
2. Interventions.
   a. Observe for early signs and symptoms of pin tract infection:
      (1) Discharge.
      (2) Warmth.
      (3) Redness.
      (4) Note any odor.
      (5) Color.
      (6) Serous drainage in small amount is normal until "tenting" occurs:
         (a) Skin forms a tent-like attachment.
         (b) Seals around the pin/wire insertion site sealing wound.
   b. Perform pin care noting any pin-skin motion or tension on pins/wires, loosening of pins.
      (1) Solution of half-strength peroxide with normal saline.
      (2) Solution determine by institutional policies.
   c. Note any redness, swelling about pins/wires, tightness of skin around pins; warmth of extremity.
   d. Perform wound care as directed under sterile conditions.
   e. Culture for suspected pin tract infection for appropriate antibiotic regimen.
   f. Monitor skin tears as external fixator is adjusted to correct a deformity/defect or limb lengthening. Wires/pins must pull through soft tissue to correct problem; these usually heal quickly as pin/wire motion is at slow rate and rhythm.
   g. Check integrity of fixator; a loose frame can cause friction and pin-skin motion, causing pain, infection, and inability to do physiotherapy.
   h. Mark external fixator with nail polish, tape, or some other means to indicate where daily/weekly adjustment of frame is necessary to achieve goals. (Not needed if it has a clicking mechanism.)
   i. Teach patient and significant other to perform frame integrity check, pin/wire care, and/or wound care.

V. HOME CARE CONSIDERATIONS

A. Patient and family teaching to include:
1. Pin site care.
   a. Solution of half-strength peroxide with normal saline, followed by rinse with distilled or nursery water.
   b. Use cotton tip applicator only once. New applicator for each pin.
   c. Proceed from skin out and remove "tenting" crusting.
2. After 1-2 weeks, shower daily with antibacterial, non-emollient soap.
3. Signs and symptoms to report to physician.
   a. Loosening/movement of pins.
   b. Increase in drainage from pin site.
   c. Redness, soreness, pain, itching, compromised neurovascular status.
   d. Fever.
   e. Change in neurovascular status.
4. Reinforce information regarding purpose of fixator and treatment goals.
   a. Elevate leg to heart level.
   b. Frequent stretch breaks to prevent joint stiffness.
5. Frame integrity check.
6. Distraction or compression technique when indicated; active and passive ROM.

B. Discuss sexual functions/needs in light of immobility and placement of external fixator.
C. Discuss appropriate adaptive clothing/devices.
1. Velcro, snaps, ties, non-skid socks, shoes.
2. Tub mat and shower chair.
3. Wheelchair or wagon for children.

D. Smoking causes vasoconstriction and may interfere with healing.
E. School or work adaptations for prolonged absence.

CONTINUOUS PASSIVE MOTION (CPM) MACHINE

I. OVERVIEW

A. Definition: a technique for applying continuous range of motion to a joint using a stationary electronically controlled machine.

B. Indications.

1. Passive motion has been shown to stimulate healing of articular cartilage.
2. CPM has been shown to reduce the development of adhesions during healing.
3. Used in a variety of situations involving healing of articular cartilage in joints.
    a. After total joint arthroplasty, synovectomy, open meniscectomy, incision and drainage of septic joint, arthrotomy, capsulotomy, joint debridment.
    b. Tibial plateau fractures.
    c. Supracondylar fractures.
    d. ORIF intraarticular fractures.
    e. Patellectomy, synovectomy for rheumatoid arthritis, knee manipulation.
    f. Joint contractures (in hemophiliacs), adhesive capsulitis, ligamentous repair, restricted motion secondary to adhesions.
    g. Finger flexor tendon repair.

C. Complications.

1. Since this technique is most effective when it is continuous (6-22 hours daily).
    a. Patient is only allowed out of machine for limited periods.
    b. Patient is at risk for problems related to immobility and bed rest.
2. Increased bleeding at surgical site.

D. Advantages.

1. Reduces disuse atrophy.
2. Provides early mobilization to enhance healing and tissue remodeling.
3. Reduces capsular contracture, maintains articular cartilage.
4. Reduces joint effusions and associated pain, and joint hemiarthrosis.
5. Reduce total knee arthroplasty (TKA) postoperative hospitalization, amount of time required to attain ROM goals, incidence of postoperative knee manipulation.

II. ASSESSMENT

A. History.

1. Emphasis on description of acute injury, chronic, developmental, or congenital.
2. Previous history of treatment with CPM.
3. Assess hand dominance if upper extremity involved.

B. Physical examination: emphasis on extremity to be treated with CPM and on body systems most affected by immobility.

1. Neurovascular status of involved extremity.
2. Skin integrity of involved extremity.
3. Condition of involved joint, including:
    a. Color.
    b. Swelling.
    c. Tenderness.
    d. Condition of surgical incision, if present.
4. General peripheral vascular status.
5. General skin integrity.
6. Elimination, nutritional, and sleep patterns,.
7. Respiratory characteristics including respiratory rate and quality of breath sounds.

III. COMMON THERAPEUTIC MODALITIES

A. Degrees of flexion and extension to be used.

B. Schedule for being in and out of CPM machine.

C. Document time patient spends in machine.

D. Proper positioning of the extremity so that the joint is over the area of flexion and extension of CPM.

IV. NURSING DIAGNOSES, OUTCOMES, AND INTERVENTIONS

A. See Table 10.1.

B. Powerlessness.

1. Outcomes: patient participates in self-care and decision making regarding regimen.
2. Nursing interventions.
    a. Organize environment to facilitate patient's independence while in CPM machine.
    b. Allow patient as much control as possible over time out of CPM machine.
    c. Provide information to alleviate anxiety related to purpose and understanding of CPM machine.
        (1) Run machine through one complete cycle before leaving patient alone. Answer patient's questions about the machine.
        (2) Demonstrate technique or immediate discontinuance of CPM for emergent situations (sharp, sudden acute pain).

V. HOME CARE CONSIDERATIONS. Teach patient and/or family.

A. Correct application and use of CPM machine.

B. Signs and symptoms of complications.
1. New or increased joint swelling, increased redness, tenderness or itching.
2. Unusual pain or fever.

BRACES/ORTHOTICS/ORTHOSES

I. OVERVIEW

A. Definition: external appliance that applies forces to or removes forces from the body in a controlled manner to enhance function and mobility, control of motion, and provide pressure relief.

B. Indications.

1. Maintain or correct position.
2. Improve function, facilitate mobility.
3. Correct and prevent anatomic deformities.
4. Aid in control of involuntary muscle movement; prevent increased muscle imbalance and provide support.

5. Maintain surgical correction; protect during postoperative healing process.
6. Facilitate normal movement patterns; assist muscle in re-education.
7. Transfer strength from one joint to another.
8. Reduce axial load, friction, and shear.
9. Relief of pain by limiting motion or weight bearing.
10. Immobilize and protect weak, painful, or healing musculoskeletal segments.

C. Bracing/splinting:

1. Bracing and/or splinting is an individualized treatment modality.
2. Patient's brace/splint may be designed by orthotist or occupational therapist.
3. A variety of braces, immobilizers, and splints are commercially available.

D. Major types.

1. Orthoses.
   a. AFO (ankle foot orthosis): short leg brace.
      (1) Prevent equinus deformity with peroneal palsy or mechanical weakness.
      (2) Accommodate foot deformities, relieve pressure, enhance comfort though custom shoes, shoe modifications, inserts, orthotics.
   b. KAFO (knee ankle foot orthosis): long leg brace used to stabilize the hip, knee, or ankle joints.
   c. HKAFO (hip knee ankle foot orthosis): long leg brace with pelvic band used to stabilize the pelvic and lower extremity joints
   d. CTLSO (cervical thoracic lumbar sacral orthosis): Milwaukee brace.
   e. TLSO (thoracic lumbar sacral orthosis): Boston brace.
   f. Scottish rite brace (Lovell): hip abduction orthosis.
   g. Knee immobilizer, de-rotation or hinged orthosis used to support cruciate or collateral ligament injuries.
   h. Ilfeld splint: hip abduction orthosis used to control selected hip motions to prevent recurrent dislocations.
   i. A-frame orthosis: hip abduction orthosis.
   j. Pavlik harness: newborn to 3 months.
2. Splints.
   a. Static:
      (1) Resting pan.
      (2) Cock-up.
      (3) Thumb spica.
         (a) No moving parts; hold movable part in functional position.
         (b) Immobilize for pain management.
   b. Dynamic:
      (1) Tenodesis.
      (2) Outrigger.
      (3) Hinged elbow
         (a) Static base plus one or more moving parts; provides desired mobility to joints.
         (b) Enhance upper extremity function.

E. Considerations across the lifespan.

1. Assess routinely for fit during rapid growth periods.
2. Assess routinely for condition of brace/splint during active stages of childhood/adolescence.
3. Monitor compliance closely during adolescent period due to self-concept concerns (compliance with schedule of wear and activity limitations).
4. Begin a child with 1-2 hours of brace wear and gradually progress to 2-4 hour intervals.
5. Wear clean, wrinkle-free, white sock, t-shirt or other liner beneath brace; avoid powders and lotions, toughen sensitive skin areas with alcohol.
6. Monitor skin integrity and neurovascular assessment carefully in geriatric patients.
7. Changes may be required with growth or following reconstructive surgery.
8. Changes may be required as one muscle regains strength (AFO – cut back to orthotic).

F. Complications.

1. Prolonged immobility in brace/splint may cause decreased ROM or contractures.
2. Skin breakdown, pressure ulcers.
3. Neurovascular compromise.
4. Calluses, pressure sores, verruca.
5. Inappropriately applied brace/splint may worsen deformity.

II. ASSESSMENT

A. History: focuses on previous acute injury; or chronic, developmental, or congenital condition that required bracing or splinting. Also includes prior experiences with braces or splints.

1. Prior compliance with brace or splint.
2. Knowledge of reasons for bracing, care of, application of, schedule of wear.
3. Age/developmental considerations: regarding compliance, potential for brace wear or damage, potential for skin breakdown.

B. Physical examination: complete musculoskeletal and neurological examination with focus on:

1. Neurovascular status.
2. Skin integrity.
3. Mental/emotional status.
4. Nutritional status.
5. Elimination status.
6. Brace fit.

III. COMMON THERAPEUTIC MODALITIES

A. Determine type of brace to be used: physician in conjunction with occupational or physical therapist and orthotist.

B. Determine amount of activity.

C. Determine desired position and amount and type of movement permitted.

IV. NURSING DIAGNOSES, OUTCOMES, AND INTERVENTIONS

A. See Table 10.1.

B. Skin integrity, impaired.

1. Outcome: patient's skin remains in good condition.
2. Interventions: teach patient and/or significant others:
   a. Correct application of brace/splint; positioning, ties and straps flat, no contact with skin.
   b. Care of brace (cleaning, oiling, drying).
   c. Assessment of skin integrity.
   d. Reporting of rubbing or pressure from brace.
   e. Pressure areas.
   f. Special attention should be given to insensate extremities.
   g. Contact person if brace/splint breaks or becomes unuseable.

C. Noncompliance, potential for.

1. Outcomes.
   a. Verbalizes prescribed schedule of wear and allowed activities.
   b. Verbalizes understanding of purpose of bracing/splinting, follow-up care.
   c. Verbalizes understanding of potential problem areas and appropriate management of problems.
2. Nursing interventions. Teach patient/significant other:
   a. Rationale behind bracing/splinting.
   b. Prescribed schedule of wear.
   c. Activities permitted while in brace.
   d. Brace fit, brace condition.
   e. Function, mobility in brace/splint.
   f. Position in brace/splint.

V. HOME CARE CONSIDERATIONS (Identify barriers to adherence with bracing.)

AMBULATING DEVICES AND TECHNIQUES

I. OVERVIEW

A. Indications.

1. Assistive devices and techniques for using them are selected on basis of factors:
   a. Patient's overall strength.
   b. Ability to use specific muscle and joints.
   c. Amount of weight bearing allowed.
2. People with conditions affecting the hips, pelvis, or lower extremities.

B. Weight-bearing status.

1. Non-weight bearing (NWB): no weight borne by affected extremity.
2. Touch-down weight bearing (TDWB): foot (toe touch) makes contact with floor but no weight is supported.
3. Partial weight bearing (PWB): 25-50% of patient's weight borne on affected extremity.
4. Weight-bearing as tolerated (WBAT): amount of weight borne dictated by patient's pain and tolerance.
5. Full weight bearing (FWB): no limitations, full weight borne by affected extremity.

C. Crutches.

1. Types.
   a. Axillary crutches:
      (1) Most commonly used.
      (2) Adjustable wooden or metal.
      (3) Has the patient's weight borne on the hands and wrists.
      (4) Usable for all five crutch walking gaits
   b. Forearm crutches with a platform:
      (1) No axillary bar, but it does have a platform for the forearm with a strap to keep the forearm in place and a handgrip for the hands.
      (2) Elbows are kept at a constant 90-degree angle while using the crutches
      (3) Permits weight bearing to be distributed over the forearm rather than on the wrist and hands.
      (4) Individuals may need assistance in attaching the arm straps.
      (5) Usually a 2-point or 4-point gait is used.
   c. Forearm Loftstrand (also sometimes called Canadian) crutches.
      (1) No axillary bars, but they do have cuffs/bands that fit around forearms, allowing the person to release the handgrips without dropping the crutches.
      (2) Cuffs should fit comfortably around the forearms below the elbows.
      (3) Permit weight bearing on the wrists and hands.
      (4) Provide less stability but are less cumbersome and easier to use than axillary crutches, especially on stairs without a railing.
      (5) Usually a 2-point or 4-point gait is used
2. Measurement for crutches.
   a. One method is to determine the patient's height and subtract 40 cm (16 inches).
   b. If the patient has to be measured in bed:
      (1) Have patient lying supine and bed flat.
      (2) Measure from the anterior fold of the axilla to the sole of the foot.
      (3) Then add 5 cm (2 inches).
   c. If the patient is able to sit without back support:
      (1) Patient sits up and abducts both arms straight out from the body.
      (2) Then have the patient flex one arm at the elbow.
      (3) Measure across the patient's back from the fingertip on the one hand to the elbow on the other.
      (4) The back is not to be bowed or flexed.
      (5) Can also be used with patient standing.
   d. If the patient can stand: measure 3.75 to 5 cm ($1\frac{1}{2}$ to 2 inches) below the axillary fold to a point on the floor 10 cm (4 inches) in front of the patient and 15 cm (6 inches) laterally from the small toes.

e. The handgrips should be adjusted to allow the elbows to be at 30 degrees of flexion when the patient is standing.

3. Gaits.
   a. 4-point gait:
      (1) Supported/partial weight bearing is permitted on both legs.
      (2) Safest gait and gives maximal balance because there are always three points of contact with the floor.
      (3) It is a slow gait because it requires constant shifting of weight.
      (4) Crutches and feet move in alternately sequence.
         (a) Right crutch (most right handed people start with the right).
         (b) Left foot.
         (c) Left crutch.
         (d) Right foot.
         (e) Continue to repeat the sequence.
   b. 2-point gait:
      (1) Partial bilateral weight bearing is permitted on both legs.
      (2) Faster than the 4-point gait because there are only two points of contact with the floor at one time.
      (3) Crutch and foot move together in the sequence.
         (a) Right leg and left crutch move forward simultaneously.
         (b) Then left leg and right crutch move forward simultaneously.
         (c) Continue to repeat the sequence.
   c. 3-point gait:
      (1) No weight bearing to partial weight bearing on affected leg.
      (2) Fast gait that requires the most strength and balance.
      (3) Patient must be able to support their entire body weight on their arms.
      (4) Crutch and foot sequencing.
         (a) The weakest foot (no weight bearing or toe touch weight bearing) and both crutches move forward simultaneously.
         (b) The stronger leg then moves forward, while the person's body weight is supported on the crutches (affected leg may be used for balance if partial weight bearing is allowed).
         (c) Continue to repeat the sequence.
   d. Swing-to and swing-through gaits:
      (1) Usually used when both of the patient's lower extremities are weak or paralyzed.
      (2) Patient may or may not be wearing long leg braces.
      (3) Swing-to gait is used by patients who not only have weakened leg muscles but also have poor abdominal and back muscles, which make it more difficult to regain and maintain balance once they have moved forward.
      (4) Swing-through gait is used by patients who are better able to stabilize themselves.
      (5) Sequencing of the gaits.
         (a) Starting point with feet together and crutches at sides.
         (b) Both crutches move forward at the same time
         (c) Patient lifts the body by transferring the weight to the crutches.
         (d) Swing-to gait: swings the body weight up to the crutches.
         (e) Swing-through gait: swings the body weight through and past the crutches.
         (f) Both gaits: straighten and stabilize the body before once more moving the crutches forward.
   e. Alternate 4-point sweep-through gait: for patients with concurrent visual and neuromuscular disability provides exploration of upcoming terrain by crutches before they are placed in traditional reciprocal position.
      (1) Both crutches just lateral to the foot, advance left crutch obliquely to the right just above the ground and place in front of right foot.
      (2) Sweep left crutch horizontally along ground from right to left until located in front of left foot.
      (3) Advance right foot until opposite left crutch.
      (4) Advance right crutch obliquely to the right just above the ground and place in front of left foot.
      (5) Sweep right crutch horizontally along ground from right to left until located in front of left foot.
      (6) Advance left foot until opposite right crutch.

4. Procedure for going up and down stairs using crutches:
   a. Going up stairs:
      (1) Walk forward to about a half-step width away from the stairs.
      (2) Place weight on the hands and lift the stronger or unaffected leg up to the next step. (Arms need to be strong enough to support the patient's body weight during the move.)
      (3) Once the foot is safely on the next step, the affected or weaker leg and crutches are advanced.
      (4) Continue the sequence.
      (5) If there is a handrail, the patient places both crutches in one hand, grasps the handrail, and then follows the same sequence.
   b. Going down stairs:
      (1) Walks to the forward edge of the top step.
      (2) Advances the crutches and the weaker or affected leg to the next lower step by tilt-

ing the pelvis and bending the unaffected leg at the knee and hip.
(3) Once the crutches are safely placed on the lower step, the stronger or unaffected leg is advanced.
(4) If there is a handrail, both crutches are held in one hand and the rail with the other while going through the above procedure.
c. Two memory devices to help the patient remember the sequence:
(1) Strong leg goes up first and comes down last.
(2) Up with the good and down with the bad.

D. Walker.

1. Provides more support and stability than crutches.
a. Facilitates partial weight bearing or full non-weight bearing.
b. Enhance stability with poor balance.
c. Reduce risk for falls.
d. Decreased cardiopulmonary function.
2. Patient should lift the walker, set it ahead, and step up to it.
a. Neither walker nor feet should slide.
b. Use supportive footwear and footwear with good soles.
3. In pediatrics, a reverse walker is sometimes used for patients with cerebral palsy to encourage standing up straight.
4. Types of walkers.
a. Stationary walker:
(1) Has four legs with rubber tips and no movable parts.
(2) 4-point, 2-point, 3-point, and swing-to gaits can be used.
b. Folding walker:
(1) Has the same basic design as the standard walker except that it is hinged.
(2) Allows the sides to fold when not in use.
(3) Sides to swing out and lock into place when opened.
(4) 4-point, 2-point, 3-point, and swing-to gaits can be used.
c. Gliding walker:
(1) Has metal plates on the tips instead of rubber and can be pushed or slid.
(2) Commonly used by the elderly.
(3) 4-point, 2-point, and 3-point gaits can be used.
d. Wheeled or rolling walker:
(1) Has wheels on the front legs that lock when pressure is applied.
(2) Commonly used by the more frail elderly.
(3) 4-point, 2-point and 3-point gaits can be used.
e. Reciprocal walker:
(1) Has a hinge mechanism that allows one side to be advanced ahead of the other.
(2) Believed to be more stable than a stationary walker.
(3) Commonly used by the elderly.
(4) 4-point and 2-point gaits can be used.
f. Hemiwalker:
(1) A modification designed for someone who has the use of only one arm.
(2) Handgrip is placed in the center front of the walker.
(3) Allows for maneuvering the walker with one hand, using a step gait.

E. Cane.

1. Canes are used to:
a. Provide support.
b. Aid in greater balance.
c. Relieve pressure on weight-bearing joints.
2. Least stable of the assistive devices for ambulation.
3. A cane is used on side opposite affected leg (or on the good side) and helps support body weight as affected/weaker leg is moved forward.
4. Two canes may be used like crutches when both lower extremities are weakened.
5. Types of canes:
a. Standard cane:
(1) Has a small base of support.
(2) Comes with C-curve or T-top.
b. Quad/tripod canes: provides a wide base of support through the number of legs projecting from the base of the cane.
c. Walkane:
(1) Provides greater stability than a quad cane and looks like a cross between a cane and a walker.
(2) Lighter and smaller than a walker.
(3) More versatile than a hemiwalker.
(4) More stable than a cane.
(5) The base is too large to be used on stairs.
6. Correct fit:
a. Patient's elbow must be flexed to a 25-30 degree angle.
b. Handle should approximate greater trochanter for correct alignment.
c. If patient has the cane, measure distance from wrist crease to the floor.
d. Keep rubber tips in good condition to prevent slippage.

F. Transfer techniques: focus is to frame potential benefits within a goal-directed approach to mobility rather than focus on the transfer technique itself.

1. Independent:
a. Requires no assist.
b. Transfer and ambulation performance is safe.
2. Standby assist of one:
a. Requires only verbal cuing or direct visual observation.
b. Clinician ready to assist if need arises.
3. Contact guard of one:
a. Patient has poor balance and judgement.
b. Clinician places hand on patient and provides support if needed.
4. Physical assist:

a. Patient may require minimal to maximal physical assistance of one or more clinicians.
b. Support devices (such as transfer belts) or mechanical devices may be used.

5. Total assist:
   a. Complete assistance of two or more clinicians.
   b. Mechanical devices (electric or hydraulic lifts) required to complete transfers.

G. Considerations across the lifespan.

1. Age may affect choice of assistive device (older adults may not have sufficient upper body strength and balance to use crutches).
2. Safety considerations may vary with age of patient (school-age children and adolescents may tend to "overdo" or avoid using assistive devices; elderly patients may have visual impairments that make them unable to see potential hazards).
3. Social stigma of aging; elderly may tend not to use as is a sign of declining health. The perception of temporary versus permanent affects compliance of use. Women tend to use before men.
4. Nurse's approach as a "tool for living" can facilitate compliance.
5. Elderly may cover need to use mobility aid/device and withdraw from society. Physician "order" may facilitate compliance.
6. Walker more likely used before cane as walker is used after hip fracture or total joint arthroplasty (TJA) and is associated with healing process, not old age and frailty.

II. ASSESSMENT

A. History: focuses on acute injury; or chronic, developmental, or congenital condition requiring ambulatory devices.

1. Assess effects of use of ambulatory devices on patient's lifestyle and environment.
2. Determine prior ambulatory status.

B. Physical examination: major emphasis is placed on assessment of musculoskeletal and neurologic systems.

1. Overall physical strength.
2. Pain, stiffness, motion of joints, especially knees, elbows, wrists, hands and fingers.
3. Strength of quadriceps, triceps.
4. Stability, balance.

III. COMMON THERAPEUTIC MODALITIES

A. Determine amount of weight bearing permitted.

B. Evaluate type of aid and make appropriate adjustments.

IV. NURSING DIAGNOSES, OUTCOMES, AND INTERVENTIONS

A. See Table 10.1.

B. Injury, potential for.

1. Outcomes.
   a. Assistive devices are of correct height/length.
   b. Patient demonstrates appropriate/safe gait using assistive devices.
   c. Home environment is free of safety hazards.
2. Interventions.
   a. Measure assistive devices/patient for correct fit.
      (1) Crutches.
         (a) While patient is lying down (wearing shoes to be used for ambulation), the crutch should reach from anterior fold of axilla diagonally out to a distance 6 inches from heel.
         (b) Another method of fitting crutches is to measure distance from anterior fold of axilla to heel plus 2 inches.
         (c) Handgrips should be positioned so that elbows are flexed 15-30 degrees. When patient is using crutches, tops should be 1 to $1\frac{1}{2}$ inches below the axilla (two fingers can be inserted between crutch and axilla).
         (d) Improper fit may result in crutch palsy or back strain.
      (2) Walker: should be high enough so patient does not have to bend over or lean forward to use it.
      (3) Cane: patient's elbow should be flexed 24-30 degrees when holding the cane.
   b. Teach patient/family:
      (1) When using crutches, bear weight on hands NOT through axilla.
      (2) Proper use of assistive devices.
      (3) Gait recommended with assistive device.
      (4) Use on stairs.
   c. Environmental safety precautions taken.
      (1) Clear environment.
      (2) Provide rubber tips for assistive devices. Replace rubber tips at first sign of wear.
      (3) Make sure patient has a sturdy, secure pair of shoes for ambulation.
      (4) Have patient dangle legs sitting on edge of bed prior to getting up.
      (5) Scatter rugs removed.
      (6) Sit in chairs with armrests. To facilitate easier access may use wooden blocks to increase height of low-position chairs.
         (a) Feel chair at back of legs, grip handpieces of both crutches with one hand on the unaffected side.
         (b) Using other hand on chair armrest, lower self into chair.
         (c) To get up, slide forward to chair edge and place both crutches on unaffected (stronger) side.
         (d) Lean forward and push off using hand on affected (weaker) side.

V. HOME CARE CONSIDERATIONS

A. Help patient assess home environment.

B. Assist in planning modifications to make home environment safe.

C. Remove furniture or cords that might cause tripping, remove scatter rugs, make sure floors are dry.

WHEELCHAIRS

I. OVERVIEW

A. Definition: a chair mounted on wheels especially for the use of physically challenged persons.

B. Indications.

1. Lack of stamina to walk distances.
2. Aid to promote independence and enhance mobility of individual with musculoskeletal injury or progressive disease process.
3. Inability to weight bear during injury-healing process.

C. Wheelchair use.

1. Based on physical and emotional preference and/or needs.
2. Useful adjunct in the recovery process to allow increased psychosocial participation of the individual.
3. Allows the individual to expend his/her energy to optimally perform activities of daily living, while still affording an ability to lead an active life.

D. Types.

1. Styles.
   a. Manual.
      (1) Standard weight.
      (2) Lightweight and ultra lightweight.
      (3) Sport and recreational.
      (4) Heavy duty for patients over 250 pounds.
      (5) Tilt multi-positioning.
      (6) Pediatric.
   b. Power: motorized/battery operated.
   c. Geriatric chair.
2. Materials.
   a. Canvas.
   b. Wooden.
   c. Metal.
3. Features.
   a. Armrests: stationary or removable.
   b. Leg rests: removable, adjustable (swings out and elevates).
   c. Collapsibility, rigid versus folding, for ease of transport.
   d. Attached swing away tables on gerichairs.
   e. Reclining positions on many models.
   f. Safety locks to prevent motion during transfers.

E. Considerations across the lifespan.

1. Assess for routine maintenance needs to ensure safety of use.
2. Ensure safety of use through proper instruction to patient and caregivers
3. Use chair appropriate to age of patient.
   a. Pediatric patient requires a small wheelchair.
   b. Elderly patient may require a geriatric wheelchair.
4. For adolescent or young adult emphasize the importance of not "popping wheelies."

F. Complications.

1. Thrombosis related to decreased mobility.
2. Skin breakdown, pressure ulcers.
3. Injury related to improper use.

II. ASSESSMENT

A. History.

1. Mobility requirements of patient: work or school attendance that may be easier when combining use of an assistive device and a wheelchair.
2. Overall strength of patient.
3. Socialization needs of patient.
4. Assess psychological impact that wheelchair use may have on patient. (Elderly may view negatively whereas younger patient may look upon wheelchair as being "really neat" and special for short-time use.)

B. Physical examination.

1. Ability for patient to sit erect.
2. Able to physically wheel chair or use motorized chair without assistance.
3. Caregiver support to push wheelchair and maintain safety.

III. COMMON THERAPEUTIC MODALITIES

A. Determine appropriateness and length of time for wheelchair use.

B. Investigate rental versus purchase options.

IV. NURSING DIAGNOSES, OUTCOMES, AND INTERVENTIONS

A. Injury, potential for.

1. Outcomes.
   a. Proper use and safety precautions.
   b. Uses correct transfer techniques to/from chair.
2. Interventions.
   a. Wheelchairs are of correct size for patient.
      (1) Fit patient to correct chair.
         (a) Pediatric.
         (b) Adult: standard, wide, geriatric.
      (2) Teach patient/family proper use of wheelchair and safety precautions:
   b. Patient demonstrates safe transfer technique to/from chair.
      (1) Place wheelchair parallel to bed/chair and lock.
      (2) Use a transfer belt to ensure additional safety, if patient cannot weight bear.
      (3) Patient should be wearing slippers or non-skid footwear.
      (4) Assist to standing position, pivot, and then sit in wheelchair.
      (5) For patient with a cast, one person can hold casted leg while a second individual helps patient with stand pivot transfer.
   c. A hoyer lift can also be used to place patient in wheelchair.
   d. Patients unable to weight bear, a wheelchair with removable arms placed parallel to the bed and a sliding transfer board help get them out of bed (OOB).
   e. Always remember to lock the wheels and to support the patient's lower extremities.
   f. Environment is free of safety hazards.

V. HOME CARE CONSIDERATIONS

A. Provide patient/family teaching.

B. Observe transfer technique for demonstration of safety understanding.

C. Facilitate acquisition of wheelchair from a loan closet, rental medical supply company, or direct purchase.

D. Ascertain if caregiver transportation can accommodate the space required of a wheelchair, and if they can physically lift to place in vehicle.

E. Home environmental check for:

1. Smooth flooring, preferably with nonresilient hard finish.
2. Large doorways.
3. Low countertops.
4. Adequate lighting.
5. May require home renovations, if use is for extended period.
6. External ramp access may be required.

Bibliography

Addamo, S., & Clough, J. (1998). Modalities for mobilization. In A. Maher, S. Salmond, & T. Pellino (Eds.), *Orthopaedic nursing 2nd edition* (pp. 323-350). Philadelphia: WB Saunders Company.

Adkins, L. (1997). Cast changes: Synthetic versus plaster. *Pediatric Nursing, 23*(4), 422-427.

Aminzadeh, F., & Edwards, N. (1998). Exploring senior's views on the use of assistive devices in fall prevention. *Public Health Nursing, 15*(4), 297-304.

Ball, J., & Bindler, R. (1999). *Pediatric nursing 2nd edition.* Stamford, CT: Appleton & Lange.

Bilkasley, M., & Ryder, T. (1997). The halo orthosis. *Journal of Emergency Medical Services, 22*(12), 52-54, 56-57.

Black, J., & Matassarin-Jacobs, E. (1997). *Medical-surgical nursing: Clinical management for continuum of care* (5th ed). Philadelphia: WB Saunders Company.

Bryant, G. (1998). Modalities for immobilization. In A. Maher, S. Salmond, & T. Pellino (Eds.), *Orthopaedic nursing, 2nd edition* (pp. 296-322). Philadelphia: WB Saunders Company.

Ceccio, C. (1999). Key concepts in the care of patients in traction. In An introduction to *Orthopaedic nursing, 2nd edition* (pp. 45-60). Pitman, NJ: National Association of Orthopaedic Nurses.

Eckhouse-Ekeberg, D. (1999). Care of the patient with an external ambulatory device. In *An introduction to orthopaedic nursing, 2nd edition* (pp. 31-43). Pitman, NJ: National Association of Orthopaedic Nurses.

Folik, M. (1998). Traction for lower extremity fractures. In V. Williamson (Ed.), *Management of lower extremity fractures* (pp. 69-74). Pitman: NJ: National Association of Orthopaedic Nurses.

Gross, J. (1997). The child with musculoskeletal alterations. In J. Ashwill & S. Droske (Eds.), *Nursing care of children, principles and practice* (pp. 1090-1137). Philadelphia: WB Saunders Company.

Gunta, K. (1998). Common nursing diagnoses for patients with lower extremity fracture. In V. Williamson (Ed.). *Management of lower extremity fractures* (pp. 41-46). Pitman: NJ: National Association of Orthopaedic Nurses.

Hart, K. (1998). Circular external fixation for the lower extremity. In V. Williamson (Ed.), *Management of lower extremity fractures* (pp. 75-83). Pitman: NJ: National Association of Orthopaedic Nurses.

Harvey, C. (1998). Challenges of traction in critical care: A case study. *Critical Care Nursing Quarterly, 21*(2), 1-13.

Kunkler, C. (1999). Neurovascular assessment. In *An introduction to orthopaedic nursing, 2nd edition.* (pp.17-25). Pitman, NJ: National Association of Orthopaedic Nurses.

Kunkler, C. (1998). Care of the casted lower extremity. In V. Williamson (Ed.). *Management of lower extremity fractures* (pp. 63-68). Pitman: NJ: National Association of Orthopaedic Nurses.

Mellett, S. (1998). Care of the orthopaedic patient with traction. *Nursing Times, 94*(22), 52-54.

McCarthy, L. (1998). Safe handling of patients on cervical traction. *Nursing Times, 94*(14), 57-59.

McConnell, E. (1997). Clinical do's & don'ts: Assisting with cast application. *Nursing, 27*(12), 28.

Patient notes: Canes and crutches. (1998). *Postgraduate Medicine, 104*(2), 187-188.

Prior, M., & Miles, S. (1999). Casting: Part one. *Nursing Standard, 13*(28), 49-53.

Prior, M., & Miles, S. (1999). Casting: Part two. *Nursing Standard, 13*(29), 42-50.

Rush, K., & Ouellet, L. (1997). Mobility aids and the elderly client. *Journal of Gerontological Nursing, 23*(1), 7-15.

Schoen, D.C. (2000). Musculoskeletal trauma, immobility, and ambulation. In D.C. Schoen, *Adult orthopaedic nursing* (pp. 103-113). Philadelphia: Lippincott.

Schoen, D.C. (2000). Care of patients with casts and splints. In D.C. Schoen, *Adult orthopaedic nursing* (pp. 113-152). Philadelphia: Lippincott.

Schoen, D.C. (2000). Care of a patient in traction. In D.C. Schoen, *Adult orthopaedic nursing* (pp. 155-194). Philadelphia: Lippincott.

Schoen, D.C. (2000). Care of the patient with an external fixation device. In D.C. Schoen, *Adult orthopaedic nursing* (pp. 155-194). Philadelphia: Lippincott.

Sprague, J. (1998). Cast syndrome: The superior mesenteric artery syndrome. *Orthopaedic Nursing, 17*(4), 12-17.

Stewart, K., & Murray, H. (1997). How to use crutches correctly. *Nursing, 27*(5), 32hn 20-22.

Swezey, R., Swezey, A., & Warner, K. (1999). Efficacy of home cervical traction therapy. *American Journal of Physical Medicine and Rehabilitation, 78*(1), 30-32.

Wainapel, S. Langer-Broas, B., & Patak, R. (1999). Alternate four-point sweep-through gait: A technique for patients with combined neuromuscular and visual impairments. *American Journal of Physical Medicine and Rehabilitation, 78*(2), 163-165.

Williamson, V. (1998). Physical rehabilitation strategies for patients with a lower extremity fracture. In V. Williamson (Ed.), *Management of lower extremity fractures* (pp.115-123). Pitman: NJ: National Association of Orthopaedic Nurses.

STUDY QUESTIONS

Jerry Walker, a 22-year-old man, presents to the clinic with a painful edematous right ankle following a fall. X-ray examination reveals a fracture. Jerry's fracture will be treated with a long leg fiberglass cast. (Questions 1-5)

1. Prior to cast application the nurse should cut stockinette long enough to extend several inches beyond the cast. The purpose of the extra length is to:
   a. Allow for finishing the rough edges of the cast.
   b. Allow for shrinkage during cast drying.
   c. Provide a "handle" to use when moving the casted extremity.
   d. Provide extra padding over surfaces with bony prominences.

2. Pre-medication may be ordered prior to casting. The types of drugs most commonly used are:
   a. Analgesics, NSAIDs, and muscle relaxants.
   b. Analgesics, NSAIDs, and steroids.
   c. Anticoagulants and muscle relaxants.
   d. Anticoagulants and steroids.

3. Jerry will be using crutches for ambulation. Which of the following indicates that Jerry's crutches fit properly?
   a. He must lean slightly forward while ambulating to use his crutches effectively.
   b. The handgrips are positioned so that his arms are straight when using the crutches.
   c. The length of his crutches equals the distance from axilla to heel plus 2 inches.
   d. The tops of the crutches rest comfortably in his axilla during ambulation.

4. Jerry has steps in his home. Which of the following is the correct procedure for going up and down steps?
   a. The affected leg and crutches lead going both up and down.
   b. The affected leg and crutches lead going up, unaffected leg and crutches lead going down.
   c. The unaffected leg leads going both up and down.
   d. The unaffected leg leads going up, the affected leg and crutches lead going down.

5. Prior to discharge from the clinic, the nurse teaches Jerry to watch for signs and symptoms of complications. The nurse tells Jerry to call the clinic if he experiences:
   a. Itching of the skin under the cast.
   b. Mild swelling of the lower extremity following long periods of ambulation.
   c. Muscle soreness in the arms following ambulation with crutches.
   d. Numbness and paralysis of the toes which is unrelieved by elevation.

Nancy Terry, a 35-year-old, was injured in a motor vehicle accident. She sustained multiple injuries including a severe open fracture of her left tibia and fibula with a great deal of soft tissue damage, a ruptured spleen, and a left pneumothorax. Following insertion of a chest tube and surgery to remove her spleen and debride her fracture site, Nancy is admitted to the orthopaedic unit with an external fixator on her left lower leg. (Questions 6-7)

6. An external fixator is indicated for Nancy's fracture because:
   a. External fixation is less costly than other methods of fixation.
   b. She has extensive soft tissue injury and damage associated with her fracture.
   c. She has no one to help her manage at home if she is treated in a cast.
   d. Surgery for internal fixation is contraindicated because of her multiple injuries.

7. The nurse should include which of the following when teaching Nancy to do pin care?
   a. Copious drainage from the pin sites is normal for the first 48 hours.
   b. Looseness or motion of the pins should be reported.
   c. Mild pain at the pin sites is normal.
   d. Redness and swelling often occur at the pin sites when the patient becomes mobile.

Janice Brewster, a 60-year-old female with severe degenerative joint disease, has been admitted following a total knee arthroplasty. Postoperatively her right leg is placed in a continuous passive motion (CPM) machine. (Questions 8-10)

8. Ms. Brewster will only be allowed out of the CPM machine for limited periods of time. This is because:
   a. Continuous use of CPM decreased bleeding from the surgical site.
   b. Multisystem problems related to immobility and bedrest decrease when CPM is used continuously.
   c. The joint tends to swell when out of the CPM machine.
   d. The overall effectiveness of CPM increases when it is used continuously.

9. To increase Ms. Brewster's sense of control and to ensure her safety, the nurse should:
   a. Give her a planned schedule of activities for the time she is allowed out of the CPM machine.
   b. Instruct her to request assistance with all activities of daily living.
   c. Run the machine through one complete cycle before leaving her alone.
   d. Tell her to call for help if the machine needs to be stopped for an emergency.

10. Potential problems associated with the use of CPM include:
    a. Coagulation abnormalities.
    b. Joint swelling and tenderness.
    c. Loosening of the joint prosthesis.
    d. Muscle soreness and tenderness.

Dylan Cooper, a 28-pound 2½-year-old, is being treated at home with Bryant's traction for developmental dysplasia of the hip (DDH). The home health nurse is reviewing Dylan's care needs with his parents. (Questions 11-12)

11. The nurse must understand the critical elements for Bryant's traction to be effective. Which of the following is not a critical element for the traction to be effective?
    a. Dylan's buttocks/sacrum must just clear the mattress, his hips should be flexed at a 90- degree angle, and his knees should be extended.
    b. 2-4 pounds of weight is recommended in home traction.
    c. Bryant's traction must never be removed or changed until ordered to be discontinued.
    d. Toddlers may need to be restrained to prevent "flipping over."

12. Bryant's traction is a form of which type of traction?
    a. Manual.
    b. Skin.
    c. Reconstructive.
    d. Skeletal.

Chapter 11 Pediatric/Congenital Disorders

Kimberly J. Mason, MSN, RN

Contents

OBJECTIVES

At the completion of this chapter, the learner will be able to:

- Describe common orthopaedic conditions in children.
- Describe diagnostic findings for each condition.
- Discuss therapeutic interventions.
- Plan the nursing care of children with orthopaedic conditions.
- Discuss outcome criteria based on patient needs and home care considerations.

KEY POINTS

- Treatment and care of children with orthopaedic disorders must include an understanding of developmental needs.
- In children with chronic conditions, the needs of the child and demands on the caregivers will change as the child grows.
- Encourage as much independence in children with orthopaedic disorders as the disease severity will allow.
- The involvement of family members is a crucial part of patient care management.

CHAPTER 11

Pediatric/Congenital Disorders

METATARSUS ADDUCTUS

I. OVERVIEW

A. Definition: metatarsus adductus (also called metatarsus varus) is a deformity of the forefoot in which the metatarsals deviate medially.

B. Etiology.

1. May be related to intrauterine positioning.
2. Tends to run in families.
3. Commonly associated with internal tibial torsion.

C. Pathophysiology.

1. Varus deviation at tarsometatarsal joints.
   a. Most prominent at first joint.
   b. Deviation decreases in severity moving from the great toe to the small toe.
   c. May have mild supination of forefoot.
2. Exaggerated convexity of lateral border of foot may lead to excessive weight-bearing forces on the fifth metatarsal.
3. Hindfoot usually remains in neutral position.
4. Associated with increased risk of developmental dysplasia of the hip (DDH).

D. Incidence.

1. Most common congenital foot deformity.
2. One per 1,000 births.
   a. Increases to about 5% with subsequent pregnancies.
   b. Affects boys and girls equally.

E. Considerations across the lifespan: flexible metatarsus adductus generally improves as the child grows and matures.

F. Complications.

1. Flatfoot deformity with overcorrection of a flexible foot.
2. Pain and improper shoe fit if a rigid deformity left untreated.

II. ASSESSMENT

A. History.

1. Developmental history.
2. Medical history.
3. Family history.
4. Normal activities/play.
5. Concerns about gait, function, cosmesis.

B. Physical examination.

1. Forefoot adducted, may be mildly supinated.
2. Hindfoot usually in neutral position.
3. Great toe in varus with a widened interval between first and second toes.
4. Ankle and foot dorsiflexion normal.
5. Forefoot can be corrected to neutral but returns to adduction when released.

C. Diagnostic tests: diagnosis based on clinical findings.

III. COMMON THERAPEUTIC MODALITIES

A. Observation: the majority of cases resolve once child starts to wear shoes.

B. Stretching for mild to moderate flexible deformities.

1. Heel is stabilized with one hand; the forefoot is abducted in relation to hindfoot with the other hand.
2. Done five times with each diaper change.

C. Serial casting.

1. For severe and/or rigid deformities, or those refractory to stretching.
2. Long leg cast to control tibial rotation.
3. Weekly or biweekly cast changes.

D. Surgical interventions.

1. For patients with severe, residual deformity.
2. Surgical release of the tarsometatarsal joints.
3. Metatarsal osteotomies may be done in the older child.

IV. NURSING DIAGNOSES, OUTCOMES, AND INTERVENTIONS

A. See Table 11.1.

B. Anxiety, potential.

1. Outcome: patient and/or family verbalize knowledge of usual progression of metatarsus adductus.
2. Interventions.
   a. Reinforce the treatment plan.
   b. Reinforce that metatarsus adductus will resolve as child grows.
   c. Support parents and child throughout process.

V. PRACTICE SETTING CONSIDERATIONS: Office/Outpatient

A. Encourage family to allow time for correction of metatarsus adductus by growth alone.

B. Allow family to express concerns over lack of active treatment.

CLUBFOOT (TALIPES EQUINOVARUS)

I. OVERVIEW

A. Definition.

1. Clubfoot is a congenital foot anomaly with the following characteristics:
   a. Heel is inverted (varus).
   b. Forefoot adduction (metatarsus adductus).
   c. Downward pointing of the foot (equinus).
2. All three components must be present, although to varying degrees.
3. Deformity is rigid and fixed.

B. Etiology.

1. Etiology is controversial.

Table 11.1
Common Nursing Diagnoses, Outcomes, and Interventions for Pediatric Patients

Diagnoses	Outcomes	Interventions
A. Anxiety	• Patient and family will express their fears and concerns related to diagnosis and treatment. • Patient and family will understand the following: 1. Underlying pathology. 2. Normal developmental progression. 3. Treatment plan. 4. Availability of community resources. • Parents will seek genetic counseling if appropriate.	• Develop a plan of care to minimize patient/parental anxiety. • Allow patient/family to express fears and concerns related to diagnosis and treatment plan. • Recognize that guilt is a common parental response to which counseling/education must be targeted. • Include patient/family in decision-making process. • Provide education regarding: 1. Underlying pathology. 2. Normal developmental progression. 3. Treatment. 4. Community resources. 5. Genetic counseling.
B. Physical mobility, impaired	• Patient maintains mobility within activity restrictions. • Diversional activities reduce boredom/stress/fatigue.	• Promote mobility within restrictions. 1. Discuss, provide equipment to assist with mobility. 2. Plan alternate methods for patient to achieve developmental tasks to compensate for physical restrictions. 3. Teach family how to hold and cuddle patients. 4. Promote use of unaffected extremities. • Provide for diversional activities to alleviate boredom/stress/fatigue.
C. Pain, acute	• Patient demonstrates maximal degree of comfort.	• Assess patient's pain using age-appropriate assessment tool: observe for nonverbal cues, especially in those who cannot communicate effectively. • Promote patient comfort. 1. Relieve pain with appropriate pharmacologic and nonpharmacologic techniques. a. Pharmacologic: muscle relaxants, antispasmodics, analgesics, etc. b. Nonpharmacologic: rocking, holding/cuddling, distraction, play activities, moist heat, ice, relaxation, etc. 2. Encourage diversional activities. 3. Control environmental factors that precipitate or increase the pain experience.

Table 11.1 (continued)
Common Nursing Diagnoses, Outcomes, and Interventions for Pediatric Patients

Diagnoses	Outcomes	Interventions
C. Pain, acute (continued)	• Patient demonstrates maximal degree of comfort. (continued)	4. Discuss coping methods with patient/family. 5. Promote family participation in providing comfort. • See Chapter 7, Pain.
D. Self-concept, disturbed	• Strengths and weaknesses of child are identified. • Developmental skills consistent with age are attained.	• Promote a positive self-concept. 1. Focus on the patient as a whole, not just on the affected part or dysfunction. 2. Reinforce personal strengths and skills. 3. Recognize the reaction of parents/significant others as influencing the child's response. 4. Encourage attainment of developmental skills consistent with age. 5. Provide consistent feedback. 6. Praise the mastery of each new skill. • Allow the child to regain as much control as possible over self and care. 1. Allow choices when possible: daily routine, food choices etc. 2. Encourage patient to visually explore and touch the affected part; slowly encourage the patient to care for the area and become more self-sufficient. 3. Help child learn self-help skills. 4. Provide opportunities for child to demonstrate independence in self-care.
E. Role performance, altered; growth and development, altered	• The child attains developmental milestones. • The child participates in activities appropriate for developmental and physical needs.	• Provide realistic expectations regarding growth and development. 1. Identify special needs of child and adaptations required. 2. Teach caregivers about normal developmental milestones and associated behaviors. 3. Demonstrate activities that promote development. 4. Encourage activities/hobbies that can be mastered. • Facilitate integration of child with peers. 1. Provide activities that encourage interaction among children. 2. Encourage child to interact with others by role modeling interaction skills.

Table 11.1 (continued)
Common Nursing Diagnoses, Outcomes, and Interventions for Pediatric Patients

Diagnoses	Outcomes	Interventions
E. Role performance, altered; growth and development, altered (continued)	• The child attains developmental milestones. • The child participates in activities appropriate for developmental and physical needs. (continued)	• Provide opportunities for and encourage exercise and gross motor activities. • Promote the child's independence and decision-making in order to foster attainment of developmental tasks.
F. Parenting, altered	• Parent demonstrates parenting activities.	• Explore parent's feelings and concerns related to parenting a child with a progressive illness. • Provide information to help adapt parenting roles to rearing a child with an orthopaedic/neuromuscular disorder. • Reinforce caregiver role behaviors. 1. Demonstrate ways to interact with child despite limitations related to treatment. 2. Help parent learn adaptations to normal child care activities necessitated by treatment modalities. 3. Provide parents with a place to stay at child's bedside in hospital. 4. Support parent's role in decision-making regarding treatment plan. • Promote family cohesion. 1. Identify typical family coping mechanisms. 2. Provide for family privacy. 3. Provide for family visitation. 4. Promote care of patient by family members. • Assist the patient/family in readjusting role expectations as necessary.
G. Self-care deficit syndrome; home maintenance management, impaired	• Patient performs ADL with maximum independence. • Necessary home maintenance activities are accomplished.	• Promote independence in self-care and assist as needed. 1. Set goals with patient and family for maximum independence. a. Assess functional abilities. b. Assess activity tolerance. c. Assist patient to accept and realize when activities are beyond self-care capacity. 2. Structure environment to maximize patient independence. 3. Allow sufficient time to complete self-care activities. 4. Provide a consistent program for improvement of ADL skills to be followed at home and school.

Table 11.1 (continued)
Common Nursing Diagnoses, Outcomes, and Interventions for Pediatric Patients

Diagnoses	Outcomes	Interventions
G. Self-care deficit syndrome; home maintenance management, impaired (continued)	• Patient performs ADL with maximum independence. • Necessary home maintenance activities are accomplished. (continued)	5. Augment self-care activities with assistive devices, if needed. a. Check assistive devices for fit and safety. b. Arrange for repairs and fittings as needed. c. Instruct patient and family on the use of adaptive devices and ADL skill programs. d. Provide clothing that uses Velcro® fasteners instead of buttons or snaps. 6. Provide sensory stimulation/play activities. • Home maintenance management activities are provided for. 1. Space daily and weekly activities to facilitate energy conservation. 2. Negotiate completion of tasks with family/resources. 3. Reevaluate tasks: differentiate between what must get done and what would be nice to get done. 4. Make referral for home health aides when warranted.
H. Coping, ineffective; family processes, altered	• Patient/family demonstrates adequate coping mechanisms to deal with stressors imposed by illness/therapeutic regime. • Patient can identify specific sources of stress.	• Promote adaptation/coping. 1. Assist patient/family in verbalizing concerns, feelings, fears. 2. Provide current information on condition and changes in condition: prepare patient for prolonged course of therapy and permanent disability, when appropriate. 3. Help patient and family establish realistic goals. 4. Involve patient/family in treatment decisions. 5. Reinforce adaptive mechanisms successfully used. 6. Acknowledge and facilitate family strengths and effective coping strategies. 7. Assist patient/family in identifying support systems and community resources. 8. Reinforce need for respite care. • Enhance management of disease process. 1. Teach patient/family about diagnosis/management.

Table 11.1 (continued)
Common Nursing Diagnoses, Outcomes, and Interventions for Pediatric Patients

Diagnoses	Outcomes	Interventions
H. Coping, ineffective; family processes, altered (continued)	• Patient/family demonstrates adequate coping mechanisms to deal with stressors imposed by illness/therapeutic regime. • Patient can identify specific sources of stress. (continued)	2. Assess level of understanding and compliance with treatment plan. 3. Teach patient/caregiver in home care needs/techniques.
I. Noncompliance, nonparticipatory	• The child and parents participate in the treatment plan.	• Promote adherence to the treatment plan. 1. Identify the level of compliance with the prescribed regimen. 2. Assess the level of understanding regarding the condition and treatment. 3. Identify the difficulties patient and family experience in carrying out the home regimen. • Collaborate with the patient and family to develop the treatment plan. • Assist patient/family in identifying sources of supports and available resources.

2. Possible genetic role, given high incidence in first- and second-degree relatives.
3. Possible prenatal influences.
   a. Intrauterine mechanical factors.
      (1) Intrauterine crowding.
      (2) Oligohydramnios with formation of amniotic bands.
   b. Chemical insults, for example, sodium aminopterin ingestion to induce abortion and tubocurarine chloride for treatment of tetanus during first trimester of pregnancy are known to cause clubfoot.
   c. Arrest of embryonic development.
   d. Abnormal neuromuscular development.

C. Pathophysiology.
1. Bone and soft tissue develop synergistically in utero: altered development in bone will result in soft tissue abnormalities and vice versa.
2. Talus is short and abnormally angulated.
   a. Navicular, calcaneus, and cuboid bones are displaced around talus.
   b. Articular surfaces are abnormal.
3. Associated soft tissue abnormalities.
   a. Shortened Achilles tendon.
   b. Tight joint capsule and ligaments on medial side.
   c. Thin, atrophic muscles.
4. Untreated deformity will progress.

D. Incidence.
1. 1.24 per 1,000 live births.
2. Increased incidence in first degree relatives (parents, siblings).
3. Males are affected two times more frequently than females.

E. Considerations across the lifespan.
1. Neonate may have "positional clubfoot" due to intrauterine positioning.
   a. Foot is flexible and can be easily manipulated.
   b. True clubfoot deformity is rigid and difficult to manipulate.
2. The foot and calf will always be smaller.
3. Sports participation is possible.
4. Follow-up care is required until child reaches skeletal maturity.
5. Recurrence is possible in treated foot, although it is not as severe as initial deformity.

F. Complications.
1. Progressive deformity.
2. Potential leg length inequality.
3. Rocker-bottom deformity caused by pushing up on metatarsals while correcting equinus during casting.
4. Neurovascular compromise.
   a. Stress on neurovascular structures from overzealous equinus correction.
   b. Incorrect cast application.
   c. Uncontrolled drainage from wound or edema postoperatively.

5. Postoperative infection.
6. Recurrent and/or residual deformity

II. ASSESSMENT

A. History.

1. Prenatal and birth history, to rule out neurologic problems.
2. Diagnosis of clubfoot and previous treatment.
3. Family history.
4. Developmental milestones: developmental delay warrants examination for underlying problem.
5. Concerns about appearance, future function.

B. Physical examination.

1. Fixed deformity with hindfoot in equinus, heel in varus, and forefoot is adducted.
   a. Distinguish between true clubfoot and positional clubfoot.
   b. Prominent crease in the arch of the foot indicates severe or rigid form that may be less responsive to conservative treatment.
2. On affected side:
   a. Foot is smaller.
   b. Calf is smaller (atrophy).
   c. Leg may be shorter.
3. Inspect the back for tufts of hair, dimples, discoloration, cysts or masses near the spine, which can indicate at possible underlying neurologic problem, especially in a baby with bilateral club feet.

C. Diagnostic tests.

1. Usually diagnosed by clinical exam in neonates.
2. Radiographs.
   a. Usefulness in routine management of clubfeet is controversial.
   b. Anteroposterior (AP) and lateral of feet, weight-bearing or forced dorsiflexion views.
   c. Talocalcaneal angles can be measured to assess severity of clubfoot and the results of treatment.
3. CT scan with 3-dimensional reconstruction for older child with recurrent deformity.
4. Usefulness of MRI not yet determined.

III. COMMON THERAPEUTIC MODALITIES

A. Nonsurgical treatment: serial manipulation with casting.

1. Realigns navicular with talus.
2. Progressively stretches medial and plantar ligaments.
3. Casting to maintain position.

B. Surgical interventions.

1. Surgery is planned when non-operative correction has plateaued.
   a. Timing of initial surgery is controversial.
   b. Recommendations range from 6 weeks to 1 year.
2. Complete soft tissue release and correction of deformity.
   a. Posterior medial, plantar, and lateral release.
   b. Talonavicular and calcaneo-cuboid joints realigned and fixed with pin across talonavicular joint.
      (1) Smooth pin exits skin between the great and second toes.
      (2) Pin is removed in office after 3-4 weeks if it hasn't fallen out beforehand.
   c. Postoperative casting for 3 months.
   d. Reverse-last shoe may be worn for several months to 1 year postoperatively.
3. Tendon transfers may be done in severely deformed foot.
4. Osteotomy can correct adduction and residual deformity of hindfoot.
5. Triple arthrodesis may be needed in the adolescent with residual deformity.

IV. NURSING DIAGNOSES, OUTCOMES, AND INTERVENTIONS

A. See Table 11.1.

B. Skin integrity, impaired.

1. Outcome: skin remains intact.
2. Interventions.
   a. Instruct parents on cast removal prior to visit, if applicable.
      (1) Parents remove casts 1 day prior to reapplication.
      (2) Soak casts in vinegar and water (1:10 solution).
      (3) Use blunt scissors to remove casts or unwind softened casts.
      (4) Time consuming: may take 20 minutes or more to soak casts; may require one or more persons.
   b. Check skin for areas of redness/breakdown after cast removal.
      (1) Treat areas of breakdown.
      (2) Apply additional layers of cast padding over bony prominences/areas of redness.
      (3) Petal cast edges as necessary to protect skin.
   c. Gently wash legs (no scrubbing) to remove flakes of dead skin.

C. Anxiety.
Grieving.

1. Outcome: acceptance of congenital deformity.
2. Interventions.
   a. Support parents/significant others throughout treatment.
   b. Counsel to facilitate movement through grief process.
   c. Grief related to loss of the child they expected.
   d. Grief related to child's possible limitations.
   e. Explore parents' concerns/answer questions about their child's future (sports participation, appearance).
   f. Help family plan/problem-solve around weekly appointments for cast changes.
   g. Explore feelings regarding residual deformity.

V. PRACTICE SETTING CONSIDERATIONS

A. Office/outpatient.

1. Promote parents' ability to cope and participate in

treatment plan.

2. Promote healthy parenting and normal growth and development.
3. Encourage family to develop a response to public inquiry about casts on infant.

B. Hospital.

1. Help family anticipate what foot will look like when casts are removed.
   a. Position of foot may appear unchanged.
   b. Redundant skin will form large, deep wrinkles on lateral aspect of foot.
   c. After surgery, foot may appear bruised.
2. Prepare family for removal of skeletal pin at 3-4 weeks, either in office or as ambulatory surgical procedure. Let them know:
   a. Smooth pin is easily removed with no discomfort for baby.
   b. What to do if pin falls out before office visit.

C. Home care considerations – teach family how to manage child at home:

1. No tub baths while casted.
2. Some types of infant clothing will not fit over the casts.
3. Safety concerns as child learns to stand and walk in casts.

DEVELOPMENTAL DYPSLASIA OF THE HIP (DDH)

I. OVERVIEW

A. Definition.

1. Broad term now used to describe spectrum of hip dysplasias.
   a. Dysplastic hip: acetabulum is shallow so that femoral head does not fit well.
   b. Subluxable hip: femoral head moves partly out of the acetabulum.
   c. Dislocatable hip: femoral head moves completely out of the acetabulum.
   d. Dislocated but reducible hip: femoral head is out of the acetabulum but can be reduced.
   e. Dislocated and not reducible hip: femoral head is out of the acetabulum and cannot be reduced.
2. Term "developmental dysplasia of the hip" (DDH) preferable to "congenital dislocated hip" (CDH) since hip dysplasia may be diagnosed at birth or during early development.

B. Etiology.

1. Genetic and ethnic factors.
   a. More common in female infants.
   b. Increased incidence if parent or sibling had DDH.
   c. Increased incidence in certain ethnic groups: Lapps and Native Americans.
   d. Low incidence in children of African descent.
2. Prenatal factors.
   a. Intrauterine mechanical factors.
      (1) Breech position.
      (2) Oligohydramnios, which can limit fetal mobility.
      (3) Unstretched abdominal muscles and uterus in primagravida, which can force the fetus against the mother's spine.
   b. Neuromuscular mechanisms: myelomeningocele, lower limb deformity.
   c. Delay in formation and development of acetabulum.
3. Postnatal factors.
   a. Cultural practices, such as swaddling or strapping of infants with hips extended.
   b. Laxity in hip capsule.

C. Pathophysiology.

1. In a newborn with a normal hip, the surface tension of the synovial fluid in the joint capsule holds the femoral head firmly within the acetabulum.
   a. The joint capsule inserts just above the labrum, the fibrocartilaginous edge of the acetabulum.
   b. The acetabulum is shallowest at birth.
   c. The combination of a shallow acetabulum and the normal joint laxity of a newborn makes the time around delivery high-risk for dislocation.
2. A hypertrophied ridge of acetabular cartilage prevents a tight fit between femoral head and acetabulum in newborn with DDH.
3. If femoral head is not reduced and stabilized, normal growth and development of both the femoral head and the acetabulum are affected.
4. If hip remains dislocated or subluxated, secondary changes can develop.
   a. Adductor longus and iliopsoas shortening.
   b. Anteromedial constriction of hip capsule.
   c. Thickening or enlargement of ligamentum teres.
   d. Inverted labrum.
   e. Development of false acetabulum.
5. Pathologic changes are reversible, particularly when treated early.
   a. 95% of newborns successfully treated with abduction devices.
   b. Outcome is harder to predict for late-diagnosed cases.

D. Incidence.

1. Most common disorder of the hips in children under 3 years of age.
   a. Estimated 1 in 100 newborns has some degree of hip instability.
   b. Dislocation occurs in 1 out of 1,000 births.
2. Occurs more frequently in girls than in boys (6:1 ratio).
3. Left hip more frequently affected than right hip.
4. Associated with congenital torticollis, metatarsus adductus, and other lower limb deformities.

E. Considerations across the lifespan.

1. Most cases of DDH are detectable at birth.
2. Any delay in treating DDH will affect normal growth and development of hip. Patient can develop limited abduction, apparent femoral shortening, limb length inequality, waddling gait and hyperlordosis.
3. In adulthood.
   a. Patients with residual acetabular dysplasia are likely to develop degenerative joint disease.

b. Patients with complete dislocations who do not develop a false acetabulum have little disability.
c. Patients with complete dislocations who do develop a false acetabulum are likely to develop degenerative joint disease.

F. Complications.
1. Residual femoral and acetabular dysplasia.
2. Growth disturbance of proximal femur.
3. Failed reduction.
4. Avascular necrosis of femoral head.
5. Neurovascular injury related to surgery.
6. Degenerative joint disease in adulthood.
7. Back pain in patients with bilateral dislocation of hips.
8. In patients with untreated unilateral dislocations:
   a. Unstable gait.
   b. Pain with ambulation.
   c. Functional scoliosis.
   d. Valgus deformity of ipsilateral knee.
   e. Low back pain.

II. ASSESSMENT

A. History.
1. Presenting symptoms (older child).
   a. Difficult diapering because one leg does not abduct enough.
   b. Awkward gait.
   c. Leg length discrepancy.
   d. Pain with ambulation.
2. Onset of symptoms, progression, previous treatment.
3. Prenatal history.
   a. Breech position in utero.
   b. Birth order.
4. Family history of DDH or ligamentous laxity.
5. Developmental milestones.

B. Physical examination.
1. DDH is not always easy to identify in early infancy.
   a. Physical findings vary widely, depending on whether hip is dysplastic, subluxated, or dislocated.
   b. Bilateral dislocated hips may be missed because physical findings are symmetric.
   c. Hip exam is repeated at every postnatal check-up during infancy (first year of life).
2. Physical findings.
   a. Asymmetric skin creases/gluteal folds.
   b. Persistent limitation of abduction of flexed thigh.
   c. Femoral head can be dislocated (Barlow's maneuver): see Chapter 3, Musculoskeletal Assessment.
   d. Femoral head can be reduced (Ortolani maneuver): see Chapter 3, Musculoskeletal Assessment.
   e. Apparent discrepancy in limb lengths appearing as shortening of the femur on the affected side (positive Galleazi's sign and Allis sign): see Chapter 3, Musculoskeletal Assessment.
   f. Unusual attitude of lower limbs.
   g. In a child who is walking.
      (1) Positive Trendelenburg sign or gait: see Chapter 3, Musculoskeletal Assessment.
      (2) Pain.
      (3) Limp.
      (4) Toe walking.

C. Diagnostic tests.
1. Ultrasound of hips.
   a. Allows visualization of cartilaginous components of acetabulum and femoral head.
   b. Can be used to assess anatomic characteristics or to assess motion.
   c. Recommended for high-risk infants and infants with abnormal clinical exam.
2. Radiographs.
   a. AP and lateral to include both hips and pelvis after newborn period.
   b. Used to evaluate
      (1) Position of femoral head in relation to acetabulum.
      (2) Size and appearance of ossific nuclei.
3. CT: may be done to verify position of hips after closed or open reduction.
4. Intraoperative arthrogram to outline cartilaginous components of acetabulum and femoral head.

III. COMMON THERAPEUTIC MODALITIES

A. Treatment should begin immediately on diagnosis since success is directly related to the age at which treatment is initiated.

B. Treatment goals.
1. To reduce femoral head.
2. To maintain reduction to allow normal growth and development.
3. To avoid proximal femoral growth disturbance.

C. Initial treatment.
1. 0-6 months: abduction device such as Pavlik harness.
   a. Position in Pavlik harness
      (1) Maintains flexion and abduction, which leads to reduction and stabilization.
      (2) Prevents hip extension and adduction, which leads to dislocation.
      (3) Avoids forced adduction to protect blood supply to femoral head.
   b. Well tolerated by infant.
   c. Most often, worn full-time for 6-12 weeks after achieving hip stability.
   d. Complications.
      (1) Inferior hip dislocation from hyperflexion at hip.
      (2) Femoral nerve compression from hyperflexion at hip.
      (3) Skin breakdown in groin creases and popliteal fossa.
      (4) Damages to femoral head and physeal plate.
2. 6 months-2 years
   a. Difficult to maintain child older than 6 months in Pavlik harness.

b. Closed reduction and spica cast immobilization.
   (1) May be preceded by period of traction.
      (a) Stretches soft tissues until hip can be reduced without force to prevent avascular necrosis during reduction.
      (b) Modified Bryant's traction (skin traction).
         i. Hips flexed 45 to 60 degrees rather than the 90 degrees of true Bryant's traction.
         ii. Can be done at home or hospital.
         iii. Usually in traction for 1-3 weeks.
         iv. Effectiveness has not been clearly demonstrated.
      (c) May use skeletal traction.
   (2) Closed reduction.
      (a) Arthrogram prior to closed reduction.
         i. Outline normal cartilaginous structures of hip, such as the labrum.
         ii. Can help identify any structures blocking reduction.
      (b) Cautious reduction under general anesthesia to avoid injuring blood supply to femoral head.
      (c) Reduced position maintained in spica cast for 12 weeks.

c. Open reduction.
   (1) May be necessary to remove tissues blocking the reduction (labrum, ligamentum teres, fat pad) or to release soft tissues.
   (2) Followed by 12 weeks of immobilization in spica cast.

d. Abduction brace after spica cast removed.
   (1) Initially worn full-time for 8 weeks.
   (2) Worn during nap time and at night until development is normal.

3. Older than 2 years.
   a. Open reduction.
   b. Pelvic or femoral osteotomy to correct bony deformity.
   c. Femoral shortening may be necessary to prevent excessive pressure on proximal femur.
   d. Both procedures followed by immobilization in a spica cast.

IV. NURSING DIAGNOSES, OUTCOMES, AND INTERVENTIONS

A. See Table 11.1.

B. Physical mobility, impaired.

1. Outcome: parents understand application and purpose of abduction devices.
2. Interventions.
   a. Promote mobility within restrictions.
      (1) Help parents plan alternative methods to help child achieve developmental tasks to compensate for physical restrictions.
      (2) Promote use of unaffected extremities.
   b. Teach parents how to manage Pavlik harness/postoperative abduction brace at home.
      (1) The Pavlik harness strap should be placed at nipple line to prevent pressure on abdomen.
      (2) Wearing schedule.
      (3) Neurovascular assessments.
      (4) Skin care.
         (a) T-shirt and diaper under Pavlik harness or abduction brace to prevent skin breakdown.
         (b) Areas where skin may become irritated:
            i. Pavlik harness: groin folds, under axilla, feet, behind knee.
            ii. Abduction brace: thighs, knees, lower back.
   c. See Chapter 6, Effects of Immobility.

C. Anxiety.
Grieving.

1. Outcome: parents accept diagnosis of DDH and comply with treatment plan.
2. Interventions.
   a. Support parents/significant others throughout treatment.
   b. Counsel to facilitate movement through grief process.
      (1) Grief related to loss of child they expected.
      (2) Grief related to possible future limitations.
   c. Explore parents' concerns/answer questions about child's future and need for further treatment.
   d. Help family develop concrete plans for managing course of treatment.
      (1) How to deal with response of family and friends.
      (2) How to manage family/work issues.
      (3) What to expect over course of treatment/anticipated future needs.

V. PRACTICE SETTING CONSIDERATIONS

A. Office/outpatient.

1. Consider ultrasound for baby with congenital torticollis, metatarsus adductus, and other lower limb deformities to rule out DDH.
2. Complete examination of hip for DDH at well-child visits for first year.
3. Coordinate immunizations with primary care provider when child is casted.
4. Promote healthy parenting and normal growth and development.
5. Facilitate long-term follow-up of children with DDH, since problems can develop with growth.

B. Hospital: coordinate rental/purchase of adapted car seat (Spelcast CRD) for safe transportation on discharge in hip spica cast.

C. Home care considerations.

1. Help family develop a response to public inquiry about Pavlik harness/spica cast/abduction brace.
2. Teach family home management of baby in Pavlik harness/child in abduction brace.
3. Teach family how to manage traction at home in

Table 11.2
Factors in Child Abuse

Caregiver Characteristics	Child Characteristics	Environmental Characteristics
• Past or present victim of abuse • Negative relationship with parents • Difficulty controlling aggressive impulses • Inadequate knowledge of normal child development • Expect learning to take place automatically • Expect child to have maturity and responsibility of an adult • Low self-esteem and distrust of others • Often live in social isolation with few support systems • May be substance abuser	• Temperament • Position in family • Additional physical needs due illness/disability • Activity level • Sensitivity to parental needs • May be illegitimate or unwanted • May have cognitive or physical disabilities • History of prematurity • Age less than 1 year • Step child • Usually only one child abused	• Chronic stress in family, including divorce, financial difficulties, unemployment, poor housing • Substance abuse in family • Inadequate social supports • Not related to one educational, social or economic group • Lower socioeconomic group may be predisposed due to stress levels. • Cases in lower socioeconomic groups more likely to be reported. • Upper classes more likely to conceal abuse/less likely to be reported.

preparation for surgery.
   a. Teach family how to manage child at home in spica cast.
   b. Diapering/urinary and bowel elimination.
   c. Nutritional requirements of growing infant/child with restricted mobility.
   d. Positioning.
   e. Play/developmental activities for child with restricted mobility.
   f. Safe transportation.

PHYSICAL ABUSE (Battered Child Syndrome)

I. OVERVIEW

A. Definitions.

1. Child abuse: physical or mental injury, sexual abuse, negligent treatment, or maltreatment of a child under the age of 18 by a person who is responsible for the child's welfare under circumstances which indicate that the child's health or welfare is harmed or threatened.
2. Battered child syndrome: a clinical condition in young children who have received serious physical abuse.
3. Related child maltreatment definitions.
   a. Physical abuse: intentional or unintentional non-accidental injury by caregiver.
   b. Sexual abuse: behaviors and activities that involve sexual physical contact with the child.
   c. Physical neglect: acts of omission, including failure to provide adequate food, shelter, clothing, medical treatment, and a safe environment.
   d. Emotional abuse: use by caregiver of verbal expressions that are meant to dominate, belittle, reject, or instill fear in the child.
   e. Emotional neglect: failure of caregiver to provide nurturing, caring, affectionate, and developmental stimulation for the child.

B. Abuse is not a diagnosis but a symptom of severe family dysfunction.

1. No single behavior or combination of behaviors defines a parent/caregiver as abusive.
2. Diagnosis based on:
   a. History: often vague, changes over time, inconsistent with pattern of injury.
   b. Age of child.
   c. Behavior of parent/caregiver: self contradictory, over-reactive, under-reactive.
   d. Clinical findings.

C. Etiology.

1. No single cause of physical abuse or neglect has been identified.
2. Child abuse is the result of an interaction between the child and caregiver, a specific event, and the environment.
   a. Personality or physical characteristics can predispose a child to abuse or neglect: most often prematurity or disability.
   b. Caregiver stress and frustration have an impact on the situation.
      (1) Socioeconomic factors.
      (2) Significant life events.
      (3) Caregiver-child interaction patterns.
      (4) Caregiver role conflicts.
   c. Overall family functioning also has a role: inadequacy or excess.
3. See Table 11.2.

Table 11.3
Common Injuries in Child Abuse

Injuries	Description/Location
Bruises, welts, lacerations, abrasions	• Particularly on buttocks, perineum, trunk, back of legs, back of head or neck. • Found on several body surfaces • Bruises on young infant • Multiple injuries at different stages of healing • Geometric shapes • Shape of object that caused injury: electric cord, belt buckle, hand • Bite marks • Severe bruising that cannot be explained by history
Burns	• Circular burns (cigarettes), especially on soles of feet, palms, back or buttocks • Immersion burns • Sock- or glove-like • Symmetrical, regular, "water-mark" edge • On perineum, upper thighs, lower torso • Splash/spill burns • Rope burns on arms, legs, neck or torso • Burn in shape/pattern of object used: iron, radiator, stove burner • Infected burn indicating delay in treatment
Fractures, dislocations	• Metaphyseal "corner" fractures • Lower extremity fractures in non-ambulatory child • Bilateral acute fractures • Spine or rib fractures • Physeal fractures in young children • Multiple fractures in various stages of healing • Fractures of hands and feet in infants and young toddlers
Abdominal injuries	• External bruises • Ruptured pancreas • Laceration of liver and/or spleen • Intramural hematoma of bowel • Retroperitoneal hemorrhage • Kidney contusion • Rupture of ureter or bladder
Head injuries	• Subdural or subarachnoid hemorrhage • Skull fracture • Scalp swelling • Bald patches on scalp • Retinal hemorrhage • Black eye(s)

D. **Pathology: characteristics of physical abuse injuries.**
1. Injuries often related to abuse.
   a. Some physical injuries, depending on age of child and presentation (see Table 11.3).
   b. Unexplained repeat poisoning, drug overdose, alcohol ingestion, or other unusual substance.
   c. Growth retardation or failure to thrive.
2. Child often has multiple injuries.
3. Abused child most commonly injured by battering (53%) and shaking (10.3%).
4. Long-term impact of abuse is difficult to determine: can impair psychomotor, cognitive, psychosocial, and emotional development.

E. **Incidence.**
1. 30 per 1,000 children.
2. Increasing 15%-20% a year.
3. 68% of all cases may not be reported, particularly in older children.
4. Average age is 7 years.
5. Reporting.
   a. Required by law in suspicious cases.
   b. No penalty for reporting unsubstantiated cases.
   c. May be related to child custody conflicts.
   d. Over-reporting may overburden child protective services.
   e. Private pay cases may be under-reported.

F. **Considerations across the lifespan.**
1. Child younger than 18 months at highest risk, but physical abuse can occur at any age.
2. Skeletal injury in any child less than 2 years should be considered suspicious.
3. Physical abuse tends to be recurrent and can result in permanent sequelae.
4.. Accurate assessment and complete physical exam and x-rays are extremely important in children who are mentally/learning impaired and in children who are unable to communicate verbally. (Also important in frail elderly groups).

G. **Complications.**
1. Disfigurement.
2. Deformity.
3. Neurologic impairment.
4. Loss of mobility.
5. Hemorrhage.
6. Intestinal perforation.
7. Development delays.
8. Fear/withdrawal.
9. Sexual dysfunction.
10. Death.

II. ASSESSMENT

A. **Conduct separate interviews with parents, witnesses, or other significant persons, including verbal quotations.**

B. **Interview child, when appropriate, including verbal quotations and information from drawing or other play activities.**

C. **History.**
1. Presenting symptoms.
2. Onset, progression, and previous treatment.
   a. Date, time, and place of occurrence.
   b. Sequence of events and times.
   c. Time lapse between occurrence of injury and initiation of treatment.
   d. Presence of witnesses.
3. Developmental history.
4. Medical history to rule out other possible causes, such as OI, osteomyelitis, rickets.
5. Historic clues supporting suspicion of battered child.
   a. History of trauma that is incongruous, inconsistent, or not plausible in relation to physical findings.
   b. History of minor trauma with extensive physical injury.
   c. History of no trauma with evidence of injuries ("magical" injuries).
   d. History of self-inflicted trauma that is incompatible with child's development.
   e. History of injury that changes with time.
   f. Delay in seeking treatment.
   g. Caregiver ascribes blame for serious injury to young sibling or playmate.

B. **Physical examination.**
1. Height, weight, and head circumference.
2. General state of health and hygiene.
3. Location, size, shape, and color of injuries.
   a. Indicate location, size, and shape on drawing of body outline.
   b. Note distinguishing characteristics, such as a bruise in the shape of a hand; round burn (possibly caused by a cigarette).
4. Symmetry or asymmetry of injuries.
5. Degree of pain or bone tenderness.
6. Evidence of old injuries.
7. Psychosocial development.

C. **Observations.**
1. Caregiver behavior.
   a. Seems unaware of seriousness of injury.
   b. Seems indifferent to child's needs.
   c. Appears unsupportive of child.
   d. Belittles child.
   e. Is overly directive in his/her communication.
   f. Is inattentive to child's requests.
2. Child behavior.
   a. Interacts with caregiver in unusual manner.
   b. Does not look to caregiver for emotional support.
3. Caregiver-child interaction.

D. **Diagnostic tests.**
1. Skeletal survey to identify treated or untreated fractures in child with signs of physical abuse.
2. Radionuclide bone scan.
   a. Identify rib fractures.
   b. Determine presence of acute, non-displaced long bone fractures.
   c. Evaluate subperiosteal hemorrhage.
3. Ultrasound to identify metaphyseal "corner" fractures.
4. CT scan of head, abdomen.
5. Neurologic, ophthalmologic, or gynecologic examinations as indicated by injuries.
6. Diagnostic tests to rule out systemic cause of physical findings.
   a. CBC, PT/PTT, platelet count, bleeding time to rule out coagulopathy.
   b. Serologic testing for congenital syphilis.
   c. Rickets.
   d. Bone densitometry to rule out osteopenia, ostegenesis imperfecta.

III. COMMON THERAPEUTIC MODALITIES

A. **Protection of the child is the principal goal of treatment.**

B. **See Chapter 14, Trauma.**

IV. NURSING DIAGNOSES, OUTCOMES, AND INTERVENTIONS

A. **See Table 11.1.**

B. **Injury, risk for.**
1. Outcomes.
   a. Signs of abuse will be detected early and the child referred for appropriate intervention.
   b. Child abuse victim will be removed from abusive environment or returned to a healthy environment.

2. Interventions.
   a. Protect child from further injury.
      (1) Monitor caregiver/child interactions.
      (2) Monitor visits of family and friends.
   b. Provide therapeutic environment.
      (1) Ensure consistency in professional caregivers.
      (2) Use play to relieve tension and investigate relationships.
      (3) Establish daily routine.
      (4) Provide support during interactions, tests, treatments.
   c. Provide interventions for soft tissue and bone injuries.
   d. Objectively document physical condition and behavioral responses.
   e. Referral to Child Abuse/Protective team.

C. Self-concept, disturbed.

1. Outcomes.
   a. Caregiver will exhibit evidence of positive relationships with child.
   b. Caregiver verbalizes/demonstrates increased sense of self-worth.
2. Interventions.
   a. Promote a sense of caregiver adequacy.
   b. Help caregiver feel welcome and a part of child's care and recovery.
   c. Teach and reinforce competent child-care activities.
   d. Focus on abuse as a problem that requires therapeutic intervention, not as a deficiency of the caregiver.
   e. Foster healthy aspects of parent-child relationship.

D. Parenting, altered.

1. Outcomes.
   a. Caregiver will demonstrate appropriate parenting skills.
   b. Caregiver will provide for family's basic needs.
      (1) The child will be returned to a healthy environment.
      (2) There will be no further incidents of child physical abuse in the family.
   c. Family exhibits functional relationships.
2. Interventions.
   a. Teach caregivers parenting skills.
      (1) Age-appropriate behaviors of child.
      (2) Temperament pattern of child.
      (3) Methods of handling developmental problems, such as toilet training, independence.
      (4) Methods of discipline.
      (5) Person or agency to contact in crisis.
      (6) Appropriate babysitters/caregivers.
      (7) Home safety hazards and how to correct them.
      (8) Regular health care for child.
   b. Facilitate change in caregiver behavior.
      (1) Establish mutually agreed-upon goals.
      (2) Encourage caregiver to take personal responsibility and not project blame onto others.
      (3) Assist caregiver in identifying and using resources.
         (a) Telephone hotlines.
         (b) Homemaker services.
         (c) Day care programs.
         (d) Counseling.
         (e) Family or individual therapy.
         (f) Food or assistance programs.
   c. Assist caregiver(s) to develop insights into the emotional climate of the family.
      (1) Address caregiver's emotional needs first.
      (2) Identify factors that contribute to abusive behavior.
      (3) Find ways of coping with stressors.
      (4) Express feelings toward self and children.

E. Nutrition, imbalanced: less than body requirements.

1. Outcome: child will exhibit weight within expected range for age.
2. Interventions.
   a. Provide diet to promote weight gain.
   b. Provide information about good nutrition and diet to caregivers.
   c. Observe interaction between caregiver and child during feeding/meals.
   d. Assist caregivers in developing positive interactions during feeding/meals.

F. Social interactions, impaired: social isolation.

1. Outcome: caregiver will seek group and individual support.
2. Interventions.
   a. Assist caregivers in establishing a positive support system.
      (1) Identify family members and friends available for support.
      (2) Identify ways family, friends, and community can be helpful.
      (3) Identify ways the health care system can be helpful.
      (4) Encourage participation in groups, such as Parents Anonymous or Parents United.
   b. Refer caregivers to agencies that can help them.
      (1) Obtain adequate employment.
      (2) Manage public assistance optimally.
      (3) Manage budget to purchase basic needs.
      (4) Remain at the same residence without frequent moves.

V. PRACTICE SETTING CONSIDERATIONS. Office/outpatient or hospital: Protection of the child is the primary goal, in conjunction with developing a family-oriented service plan.

1. Report suspected child abuse as per state law.
2. Evidence preservation since all suspected inflicted injuries are possible forensic cases.
   a. Photographs to preserve evidence of physical findings; injuries disappear as healing occurs.
   b. Documentation includes complete, accurate written and diagramed description of injuries.

c. Maintain chain of possession for evidence as per legal counsel.

B. Teach caregivers skills necessary to care for child.

1. Home management of casts or braces.
2. Wound care/dressing changes.
3. Age-appropriate diet.

C. Social work referral to facilitate referral to community agencies.

1. Parenting classes.
2. Substance abuse treatment.
3. Financial assistance.

TORSIONAL PROBLEMS

I. OVERVIEW

A. Definitions.

1. Tibial torsion describes the rotation of the tibia along the long axis.
2. Internal tibial torsion.
   a. Distal end of the tibia is rotated medially in relation to proximal end.
   b. Also called medial tibial torsion.
3. External tibial torsion.
   a. Distal end of the tibia is rotated laterally in relation to proximal end.
   b. Also called lateral tibial torsion.
4. Femoral anteversion describes the rotation of the femur along its long axis.
   a. Caused by the anterior rotation of the femoral neck in relation to the femoral shaft.
   b. Also called medial femoral torsion.
5. Clinically, "torsion," "rotation," and "version" are used interchangeably.

B. Etiology.

1. Torsional changes in lower extremities occur as normal part of development in utero.
2. Prenatal influences.
   a. Genetic factors.
   b. Intrauterine positioning.
3. Postnatal influences.
   a. Prematurity: prone positioning can result in increased external tibial torsion.
   b. Comorbid conditions such as developmental dysplasia of the hip (DDH) or cerebral palsy.

C. Pathophysiology.

1. Tibial torsion.
   a. 0-20 degrees of internal tibial torsion normal at birth.
   b. Growth alone produces correction in over 90% of cases.
   c. May aggravate or compensate for rotational variations in the femur.
   d. 20 degrees external tibial torsion normal in adulthood.
   e. External tibial torsion is less common than internal tibial torsion.
      (1) Rare in pure form.
      (2) Compensatory mechanism for femoral anteversion.
      (3) Secondary to neuromuscular disease.
2. Femoral anteversion.
   a. 30-40 degrees of femoral anteversion normal at birth.
   b. Nearly all children exhibit some femoral anteversion.
   c. Gradually decreases to 10-15 degrees by skeletal maturity.
   d. Considered excessive when greater than 50 degrees or if it creates a functional disability.

D. Incidence.

1. In-toeing is the most common orthopaedic complaint in children.
2. May be caused by rotational problems: internal tibial torsion or femoral anteversion.
3. May be caused by angular problems: metatarsus adductus.
   a. Tibial torsion: persistent, disabling tibial torsion is rare.
   b. Femoral anteversion: excessive femoral anteversion is rare.

E. Considerations across the lifespan.

1. Most mild to moderate torsional problems will improve with growth during childhood, usually by age 8-10.
2. Severe torsional problems may persist into adulthood.
3. Early osteoarthritis in hip may be associated with femoral anteversion.
4. See Table 11.4.

F. Complications.

1. Torsional malalignment syndrome: excessive femoral anteversion with excessive tibial torsion.
   a. Significant in-toeing with internal rotation of entire lower extremity.
   b. Associated with ligamentous laxity.
      (1) Flatfoot deformity.
      (2) Genu recurvatum.
      (3) Lumbar lordosis.
   c. Usually presents in adolescence.
   d. Patellofemoral rotational malalignment can occur in severe cases.
      (1) Patellofemoral instability.
      (2) Early degeneration of patellofemoral joint.
2. Asymmetric growth stimulation and lower limb length discrepancy after surgery.

II. ASSESSMENT

A. History.

1. Presenting symptoms.
   a. Type of torsional problem.
   b. Knee pain.
   c. Difficulty with ambulation or physical activity.
2. Onset, progression, and prior treatment.
3. Birth history: risk factors for neurologic problems, such as cerebral palsy.
4. Family history: one or both parents often has same rotational problem.
5. Concerns about gait, function, cosmesis.

B. Physical examination.

Table 11.4
Torsional Problems Related to Pediatric Age Groups

Age	Torsional Problem	
	In-toeing	Out-toeing
1st year of life	Metatarsus adductus	Generally normal
Toddler	Internal tibial torsion	Generally continues to be normal
Preschool/early school-age	Femoral anteversion	Begin to see external tibial torsion
Late school-age	Internal tibial torsion and femoral anteversion usually resolve	External tibial torsion may increase
Adolescence	Malalignment syndrome – combination of femoral anteversion and external tibial torsion	Malalignment syndrome – combination of femoral anteversion and external tibial torsion

1. See Table 11.4.
2. See Table 11.5.
3. Spine and neurologic exam to rule out neuromuscular disorder.
4. Examination of entire lower extremity, including hip rotation, tibial rotation, and position of foot.
5. Evaluate gait.
   a. Tibial torsion.
      (1) Abnormal gait.
         (a) In-toeing: internal tibial torsion (more common).
         (b) Out-toeing: external tibial torsion.
         (c) In-toeing and out-toeing become less noticeable when running and barefoot.
      (2) Thigh-foot angle
         (a) Angular difference between the axis of the thigh and the foot as viewed from above with knee flexed at 90 degrees.
         (b) Normal range: 0-30 degrees of external rotation.
      (3) Foot progression angle (or angle of gait).
         (a) Angle child's foot makes in relation to forward progression.
         (b) Normal alignment is 10 degrees external rotation.
         (c) Internal rotation denoted with negative numbers to differentiate from external rotation.
   b. Femoral anteversion.
      (1) In-toeing gait.
      (2) Abnormal rotation of the hips.
         (a) Up to 90 degrees of internal rotation.
         (b) 30 degrees or less of external rotation.
      (3) Internal rotation of entire lower extremity.
      (4) Ligamentous laxity.

C. Diagnostic tests.
1. Tibial torsion.
   a. Can be adequately estimated by indirect physical measurements (see Physical Examination).
   b. Radiographs: standing anteroposterior (AP) view of entire leg on one cassette.
   c. Paper test assists in evaluation of foot progression angle. (Ink placed on bottom of child's foot, child walks on paper, gait pattern analyzed).
2. Femoral anteversion.
   a. Radiographs: standing AP of entire leg on one cassette.
   b. Standing AP pelvis to rule out hip dysplasia for symmetric femoral anteversion.
3. AP and lateral radiographs of hips for child with asymmetrical limitation of hip abduction to rule out DDH.
4. CT and MRI may be useful in assessing transverse plane deformity in severe cases.

III. COMMON THERAPEUTIC MODALITIES

A. Observational management is indicated for most children with torsional problems.
1. 90%-95% torsional problems remodel with growth, usually by 8-10 years.
2. Disability due to torsional problems is rare.

B. Tibial torsion.
1. Non-operative treatment is not felt to alter natural progression.
   a. Daytime bracing with twister cables or shoe modifications has been shown to be ineffective.
   b. Night splints, such as Denis Browne bar, are not harmful but have no proven value.
2. Tibial derotational osteotomy for persistent, severe tibial torsion.
   a. Indications.
      (1) Child over 8 years of age.
      (2) Significant functional deformity.
      (3) Greater than 15 degrees internal tibial torsion or 35 degrees external tibial torsion.

Table 11.5
Torsional Problems: Assessment Areas

Tibial Torsion	Femoral Anteversion
In-toeing gait (internal tibial torsion) or out-toeing gait (external tibial torsion)	In-toeing gait Abnormal rotation of hips Ligamentous laxity Internal rotation of entire lower extremity

b. Supramalleolar osteotomy reduces risk of compartment syndrome.

c. Non-weight-bearing long leg cast for 4 weeks postoperatively followed by 4 weeks in a weight-bearing cast.

D. Femoral anteversion.

1. Non-operative treatment (braces or splinting) is not effective.
2. Corrective derotational femoral osteotomy for persistent, severe femoral anteversion.
   a. Indications.
      (1) Child at least 8 years of age.
      (2) Significant functional deformity.
      (3) Greater than 50 degrees femoral anteversion.
      (4) 80 degrees or more of internal hip rotation, and less than 10-15 degrees of external hip rotation.
   b. Osteotomy may be performed at any level.
   c. Patient usually immobilized in a spica cast for 6 weeks postoperatively.
   d. Older patient may have osteotomy stabilized with femoral rod or external fixator.

IV. NURSING DIAGNOSES, OUTCOMES, AND INTERVENTIONS

A. See Table 11.1.

B. Anxiety, potential.

1. Outcome: patient and/or family verbalize knowledge of usual progression of torsional problem.
2. Interventions.
   a. Reinforce treatment plan.
   b. Stress the fact that torsional problems gradually resolve as a result of growth and neurologic development; treatment decisions may be deferred until school-age years.

V. PRACTICE SETTING CONSIDERATIONS

A. Office/outpatient.

1. Encourage family to allow time for correction of deformity by growth alone.
2. Encourage parents to focus on the child, not his/her deformity.
3. Allow patient/parent to express concern over lack of treatment during observation.
4. Assist family with symptom management (knee pain) as necessary.

B. Home care considerations: encourage parents to allow child to participate in normal activities as much as he/she is able.

GENU VARUS/GENU VALGUS

I. OVERVIEW

A. Definitions.

1. Genu varus.
   a. Characterized by increased distance between the knees.
   b. Clinically present when the distance between the knees is greater than 2.5 centimeters when child stands with ankles together.
   c. Often accompanied by internal tibial torsion.
2. Genu valgus.
   a. Characterized by an increased distance between the ankles (medial malleoli).
   b. Clinically present when the distance between the medial malleoli is greater than 2.5 centimeters when child stands with knees together.

B. Etiology.

1. Physiologic genu varus and genu valgus: normal developmental variations.
2. Pathologic genu varus.
   a. Partial physeal arrest on medial aspect of the proximal tibial or distal femoral physis, caused by bony bar, trauma, osteomyelitis.
   b. Rickets: vitamin D resistant rickets.
   c. Obesity.
3. Pathologic genu valgus.
   a. Partial physeal arrest on lateral aspect of the proximal tibial or distal femoral physis, caused by bony bar, trauma, osteomyelitis.
   b. Overgrowth of the tibia in relation to the fibula due to proximal tibial metaphyseal fracture.
   c. Overgrowth due to chronic synovitis of juvenile arthritis.
   d. Severely pronated feet.

C. Pathophysiology.

1. Angular variations are a normal part of growth and development.
   a. All infants born with genu varus.
   b. Genu varus will improve by 18 months to 2 years of age.

c. Genu valgus develops between 2-3 years of age, increasing until age 3-4 years.
d. Genu valgus improves by age 7.
e. Normal adult alignment is slight valgus.

2. Pathologic genu varus and genu valgus.
   a. Severe angular malalignment.
   b. Outside of normal developmental sequence.
   c. Deformity progresses rapidly.
   d. Family history of pathologic condition.
   e. A symmetric malalignment.
   f. Height less than 5th percentile.
3. Growth disturbance is a result of stress and growth.
   a. Heuter Volkman's law of epiphyseal growth states that compression inhibits growth and distraction stimulates growth.
   b. Compression on one side of the physis will slow growth and lead to continuing deformity as the opposite side grows normally.

D. Incidence.

1. More common in some families.
2. Higher incidence of pathologic genu varus and genu valgus in African Americans and Japanese.

E. Considerations across the lifespan.

1. Physiologic genu varus and genu valgus part of the normal developmental sequence.
2. Some genu varus or genu valgus may persist throughout life.
3. Osteoarthritis may develop in adulthood if pathologic genu varus or genu valgus is uncorrected.

F. Complications.

1. Pathologic genu varus or genu valgus.
   a. Gait awkwardness which increases the risk of sprains and fractures.
   b. Knee pain may limit physical activity.
2. Pathologic genu valgus.
   a. Subluxing/recurrent dislocation of patella.
   b. Predisposition to chondromalacia of patella.
   c. Easy fatigue.
   d. Joint pains.
3. Post-surgical.
   a. Vascular compromise due to entrapment of anterior tibial artery.
   b. Valgus deformity due to surgical trauma of osteotomy which stimulates overgrowth of tibia.
   c. Delayed healing of osteotomy if underlying problem is systemic.
   d. Upper tibial osteotomies may be associated with compartment syndromes or injury to peroneal nerve.
   e. Neurovascular injury from angular correction with Garch clamp and external fixator.
4. Lack of treatment may lead to degenerative joint disease in adulthood.

II. ASSESSMENT

A. History.

1. Present symptoms.
   a. Type of angular malalignment, onset, progression, and prior treatment.
   b. Pain with activity.
2. Developmental history.
3. Medical history.
4. Family history.
5. Normal activities/play.
   a. Difficulty walking, especially distances.
   b. Fatigue with activity.
6. Concerns about gait, function, cosmesis.

B. Physical examination.

1. Height and weight.
2. Medial or lateral thrust at knee, indicating joint instability or ligamentous laxity.
3. Rotational abnormalities of lower extremity.
4. Femoral – tibial angle measured with goniometer.
5. Symmetry/asymmetry of angular malalignment.
6. Genu varus: distance between medial femoral condyles when medial malleoli are touching.
7. Genu valgus: distance between the medial malleoli when medial femoral condyles are touching.
8. Foot abnormalities: valgus flat foot associated with genu valgus.

C. Diagnostic tests.

1. Radiographs if pathologic form suspected.
   a. Standing AP of entire leg with patellae forward.
      (1) Entire leg on a long cassette (one film) to measure hip-knee-ankle angle.
      (2) Pathologic genu varus.
         (a) Femoral-tibial angle 25 degrees of varus.
         (b) Medial tilting of transverse plane of knee and ankle joints and obvious angulation with normal epiphyseal appearance and development.
         (c) Pathologic genu valgus: femoral-tibial angle 15 degrees of valgus.
   b. Lateral radiograph if sagittal deformity is suspected.
   c. Skeletal survey if bone dysplasia is suspected.
   d. Teleroentgenograms and bone age if considering hemiepiphysiodesis.
2. See Table 11.6.

III. COMMON THERAPEUTIC MODALITIES

A. Physiologic genu varus and genu valgus usually correct over time without any intervention.

B. Pathologic genu varus and genu valgus.

1. Nonsurgical treatment.
   a. Bracing has not been shown to change the natural history, except in some cases of tibia vara (Blount's disease).
   b. Medical treatment of systemic disease, such as rickets.
2. Surgical interventions.
   a. Osteotomy.
      (1) Genu varus: opening- or closing-wedge osteotomy of proximal tibia.
      (2) Genu valgus: opening- or closing-wedge osteotomy of distal femur.
      (3) Both followed by long leg casting for 6-8 weeks.

Table 11.6
Genu Varus versus Blount's Disease

Physiologic Genu Varus	Pathologic Genu Varus	Blount's Disease
Genu varus is characterized by: • 2.5 cm or greater between medial femoral condyles when medial malleoli are together when child is standing and patellae are facing forward. • Normal in infants and toddlers. • Usually bilateral • No lateral thrust at knee with ambulation • X-rays normal • No treatment required	Pathologic genu varus is characterized by: • Severe malalignment • Occurs outside of normal developmental sequence • Asymmetry • Rapid progression • Positive family history • Height less than 5th percentile • Usually bilateral • Lateral thrust at knee evident with ambulation X-rays • Tibiofemoral angle 3/4 25 degrees of varus • Medial tilting of transverse plane of knee and ankle joints • Obvious angulation but epiphysis appears normal Treatment depends on age and severity Surgery	Blount's disease is characterized by: • A sharp, localized genu varum associated with growth suppression of posteromedial area of proximal tibial physis • Asymmetry • 50% unilateral • Lateral thrust at knee evident with ambulation X-rays • Changes in medial metaphyseal contour evidenced by "beaking" • Medial height of proximal tibial epiphysis is decreased Prominent localized tibial bowing Always requires treatment • Bracing • Surgery

b. Hemi-epiphysiodesis or hemi-stapling.
   (1) Hemi-epiphysiodesis stops growth on one side of physis so that deficient side can catch up.
   (2) Hemi-stapling slows growth on one side of physis: staples removed when deformity corrected.
   (3) Done after age 10 while physes are still open.
   (4) Timing is critical so that remaining growth can correct deformity.
c. Genu varus: gradual angular correction using Garch clamp and external fixator.
   (1) Garch clamp and external fixator applied after proximal tibial osteotomy.
      (a) Garch clamp provides angular correction.
      (b) External fixator stabilizes bone fragments, provides lengthening if necessary.
   (2) Patient/family do daily adjustment to external fixator similar to bone lengthening for limb length discrepancies.
   (3) When desired correction is obtained, Garch clamp and external fixator used to stabilize bone until healing is complete.

IV. NURSING DIAGNOSES, OUTCOMES, AND INTERVENTIONS

A. See Table 11.1.

B. Anxiety.
1. Outcome: patient and/or family verbalize knowledge of usual progression of genu varus/genu valgus.
2. Interventions.
   a. Reinforce the treatment plan.
   b. Reinforce that physiologic genu varus and genu valgus will resolve as child grows.
   c. Support parents and child throughout process as angular correction with Garch clamp and external fixator can last 3-6 months.

C. Peripheral neurovascular dysfunction, risk for.
1. Outcome: neurovascular status intact.
2. Interventions.
   a. Assess dorsiflexion and plantar flexion of foot.
   b. Use resting splint to prevent heel cord contracture.
   c. See Compartment Syndrome in Chapter 8, Complications.

V. PRACTICE SETTING CONSIDERATIONS

A. Office/outpatient.
1. Encourage family to allow time for correction of angular malalignment by growth alone.
2. Allow family to express concerns over lack of active treatment during growth.
3. Facilitate regular follow-up for child with pathologic genu varus or genu valgus.
   a. Regular follow-up important to monitor progression and/or improvement.
   b. If hemi-epiphyseodesis or hemi-stapling is rec-

ommended, timing of procedure is important.

c. If angular correction with Garch clamp and external fixator is performed.
   (1) Weekly appointments are necessary during the correction phase (while correcting angular deformity).
   (2) Appointments are every 2-4 weeks during healing phase (after angular deformity is corrected).

4. Promote medical follow-up for treatment of systemic condition.
5. Assist patient/family with symptom management (knee pain) as necessary.

B. Hospital.
1. Teach home management related to surgery/casting or Garch clamp and external fixator.
2. Inpatient rehabilitation may be needed for safe mobility before discharge with crutches or wheelchair.

C. Home care considerations.
1. Encourage parents to allow child to participate in normal activities, as much as he/she is able.
2. Avoid sports/physical activities that cause pain and consider alternatives.
3. Limit gym/physical activities if child has pain.
4. Teach patient/family proper application and care of braces.
   a. Wearing schedule.
   b. Skin care.
   c. Restriction of activities.

LEGG-CALVÉ-PERTHES (LCP) DISEASE

I. OVERVIEW

A. Definition: self-limiting disease of the hip characterized by idiopathic avascular necrosis of the femoral head occurring in children.

B. Etiology.
1. The etiology of initial avascularity is unknown.
2. Theories include hereditary, metabolic, chemical, or mechanical pathology.
   a. Trauma.
   b. Transient synovitis.
   c. Excessive femoral neck anteversion.
   d. Growth-related systemic abnormalities.
   e. Vascular embarrassment caused by intraosseous venous hypertension and venous obstruction.

C. Pathophysiology.
1. Cellular changes in epiphyseal and physeal cartilage.
2. Disorganization of physeal plate along with minimal trauma may interrupt vessels to femoral head causing necrosis.
3. Femoral head becomes deformed due to asymmetric repair process and molding of acetabulum.
4. During healing phase, blood supply starts from periphery and moves centrally.
5. Irregular areas of bone deposition and resorption.
6. Blood supply always returns but duration of disease process is unpredictable.
7. Residual deformity will vary depending on effectiveness of treatment.
8. Flattening of femoral head.
   a. Acetabular enlargement.
   b. Subluxation.

D. Incidence.
1. Occurs 1 in 1,200 in the general population.
2. Predominantly seen in males 4:1.
3. Occurs most frequently in 4-8 year olds.
4. About 85% of cases are unilateral.
5. More common in urban areas.
6. Reported association with attention deficit hyperactivity disorder (ADHD).

E. Considerations across the lifespan.
1. LCP affects children.
2. Age at disease onset significantly related to outcome.
   a. Older child has less time to remodel residual deformity before skeletal maturity.
   b. Residual deformity and hip joint congruity are most important in long-term prognosis.
3. Limitations placed on child's physical mobility may affect socialization and participation in developmental activities.
4. Most patients are active and pain-free in adulthood.
5. Residual deformity can cause pain, decreased range of motion and loss of function.

F. Complications.
1. Subluxation.
2. Subchondral fracture.
3. Deformity of epiphysis.
4. Residual deformity: coxa magna, premature physeal plate closure, irregular femoral head.

II. ASSESSMENT

A. History.
1. Presenting symptoms.
   a. Pain.
      (1) Localized to groin or medial aspect of thigh or knee.
      (2) Aggravated by activity.
      (3) Relieved by rest.
   b. Limitation in motion.
2. Onset and progression of symptoms.
   a. Insidious onset.
   b. Antalgic gait of several months duration.
3. History of trauma.
4. Physical activities/play.

B. Physical examination.
1. Height, weight to rule out growth disorder, systemic problem.
2. Limited hip motion, especially internal rotation and abduction.
   a. May hold leg in slight flexion and abduction.
   b. May have hip adduction contracture.
3. Increased pain with abduction and internal rotation.
4. Muscle spasm.
5. Disuse atrophy in upper thigh, calf, buttock.
6. Limb length inequality.

C. **Diagnostic tests.**
1. Radiographs: AP and frog-leg lateral of hips.
2. Radiographic stages.
   a. First phase: initial.
      (1) Interruption of blood supply to femoral ossific nucleus.
      (2) Affected femoral head appears smaller than unaffected side.
      (3) Widening of medial joint space.
      (4) Subchondral radiolucent zone (crescent sign) visible: result of subchondral stress fracture.
      (5) Physeal plate is irregular.
   b. Second phase: fragmentation.
      (1) Bony epiphysis appears fragmented.
      (2) Areas of increased radiolucency and radio-density.
   c. Third phase: reossification.
      (1) Normal bone density returns.
      (2) Deformity of femoral head and neck become apparent.
   d. Fourth phase: healed.
      (1) Healing complete.
      (2) Residual deformity of proximal femur may persist.
3. Arthrogram to determine if femoral head can be contained in acetabulum.

III. COMMON THERAPEUTIC MODALITIES

A. **Most patients do not need treatment.**
1. No treatment other than symptom management is necessary for patients with good prognosis.
2. Treatment considered for patients with poor prognosis.
   a. Prognostic factors.
      (1) Deformity of femoral head.
      (2) Hip joint incongruity.
      (3) Age at disease onset.
      (4) Extent of epiphyseal involvement.
      (5) Growth disturbance secondary to premature physeal closure.
      (6) Protracted disease course.
      (7) Remodeling potential.
      (8) Type of treatment.
      (9) Stage at treatment initiation.
3. Treatment considered for patients whose prognosis is not determined.
4. Treatment recommended for patients with clinical or radiographic risk signs.
   a. Clinical risk signs include loss of motion, joint contracture, and pain.
   b. Radiographic assessment includes stage of disease and extent of epiphyseal involvement.

B. **Primary goals of treatment are to prevent deformity and alter growth disturbances.**

C. **Treatment.**
1. Restore joint motion to enhance synovial and cartilage nutrition.
   a. Bed rest with skin traction and progressive abduction to relieve muscle spasm.
   b. Surgical release of adductors.
   c. Repeated casting in increasing abduction.
2. Position (contain) femoral head in acetabulum.
   a. Must be initiated early in course of disease process to effect femoral head deformity.
   b. Abduction orthosis, such as Atlanta Scottish Rite orthosis.
      (1) Femoral head maintained in abducted internal rotation position.
      (2) Allows for weight bearing.
      (3) Maintains hip range of motion in the desired position.
   c. Varus osteotomy of the femur, with or without derotation, repositions head of femur in acetabulum.
   d. Innominate osteotomy of pelvis redirects acetabulum to provide better anterolateral coverage.

D. **Salvage procedures.**
1. Treatment options for patients:
   a. Who present in late stage of LCP.
   b. With hip deformity that cannot be contained using other methods.
   c. Who have lost containment.
2. Salvage procedures include shelf arthroplasty, Chiari osteotomy, and chielectomy.

IV. NURSING DIAGNOSES, OUTCOMES, AND INTERVENTIONS

A. **See Table 11.1.**

B. **Activity intolerance.**
1. Outcome: patient/family plans activities appropriate for mobility restrictions.
2. Interventions.
   a. Explain pathology and expected outcome.
   b. Teach prescribed exercise program.
   c. Plan activities appropriate for restriction.
   d. Plan methods to allow expression of normal developmental tasks.
   e. Support family's efforts to enforce prescribed activity restrictions.

V. PRACTICE SETTING CONSIDERATIONS

A. **Office/outpatient.**
1. Support family through long healing process (18-36 months), with erratic improvement and uncertain prognosis.
2. Help family develop strategies to manage activity restrictions when necessary.

B. **Hospital.**
1. Coordinate transportation for discharge.
2. Child may not fit in car/mini-van with legs widely abducted postoperatively.

C. **Home care considerations.**
1. Encourage parents to allow as much activity as possible within activity restrictions.
2. Encourage prescribed exercise program.
3. Encourage self-care, educational, and diversional activities.
4. Home tutoring or special school arrangements while on bed rest, or in brace or casts.

OSGOOD-SCHLATTER DISEASE

I. OVERVIEW

A. Definition: a traction apophysitis of the tibial tubercle causing painful swelling.

B. Etiology: overuse – chronic, repetitive knee flexion.

C. Pathophysiology.

1. The tibial tubercle develops as an extension of the epiphysis of the proximal tibia.
2. An ossification center (apophysis) is susceptible to repeated trauma at the patellar tendon insertion.
3. Apophysitis and tendonitis cause pain at tibial tubercle.
4. Partial or complete separation of the tubercle can occur, interrupting the blood supply, resulting in necrosis.
5. The apophysis fuses to the tibia at skeletal maturity.

D. Incidence.

1. Occurs most frequently during the rapid growth during puberty (11-14 years).
2. Males more frequently affected than females.
3. Often bilateral.
4. More common in children involved in sports activities.

E. Considerations across the lifespan.

1. Self-limiting disease of pre-adolescence: symptoms stop when apophysis is fully ossified.
2. Commonly seen in boys ages 13-15; girls ages 10-13.
3. Failure of union of the tubercle to the tibia can cause symptoms that persist into adult years.

F. Complications.

1. Enlargement of the tibial tubercle may persist, causing a bony prominence.
2. Tibial tubercle fractures.
3. Premature closure of tibial tubercle apophysis, causing a recurvatum deformity.
4. Ossicles may develop in the tendon, causing pain and tenderness.

II. ASSESSMENT

A. History.

1. Presenting symptoms.
   a. Pain.
      (1) Increases with activities, such as kneeling, running, bicycle riding, stair climbing.
      (2) Diminishes or disappears with rest.
   b. May report rapid growth spurt prior to onset.
2. Onset, progression, and prior treatment.
3. Physical activities/limitations.

B. Physical examination.

1. Local pain at anterior aspect of knee.
2. Tender, bony prominence over tibial tubercle.
3. Subcutaneous swelling of soft tissues over the tibial tubercle.
4. Pain with forced knee extension against resistance.
5. Pain when squatting with full knee flexion.

C. Diagnostic tests.

1. Diagnosis usually made based on history and clinical exam.
2. Radiographs.
   a. To rule out tumor or infection.
   b. AP, lateral, and 10-degree oblique views.
      (1) Proximal tibial tubercle shows irregular areas of bone deposition and resorption.
      (2) One or more areas of calcification of tibial tubercle.
      (3) Excessive enlargement of tibial tubercle.
      (4) Separate ossicle may be visible between patellar tendon and tibial tubercle in skeletally mature patient.
3. CT and MRI rarely indicated.

III. COMMON THERAPEUTIC MODALITIES

A. Objective of treatment: reduce stress on the apophysis.

B. Nonsurgical treatment.

1. Limit activities to control pain.
2. Symptom management.
   a. Stretching exercises before sports activities, especially hamstrings.
   b. Ice to tibial tubercle after sports activities.
   c. Knee immobilizer or cylinder cast for severe pain.
   d. Quadriceps strengthening exercises.

C. Surgical interventions.

1. Surgical treatment is rarely indicated.
2. Excision of ossicles between tibial tubercle and patellar tendon if painful.

IV. NURSING DIAGNOSES, OUTCOMES, AND INTERVENTIONS

A. See Table 11.1.

B. Alteration in activity.

1. Outcome: patient/family plans activities appropriate for activity restrictions.
2. Interventions.
   a. Discuss activity limitations and symptom management.
   b. Support family's efforts to balance symptoms and activity.

V. PRACTICE SETTING CONSIDERATIONS: Office/Outpatient

A. Discuss symptomatology, expected course of treatment, and expectations.

B. Encourage parents to allow as much activity as possible within activity restrictions: restricting all activities may be counterproductive.

LEG LENGTH DISCREPANCY (LLD)

I. OVERVIEW

A. Definitions.

1. Discrepancy in leg length due to differences in length of tibia and/or femur.
2. Length differences are most common in the lower extremities but can occur in any limb for similar reasons.

B. Etiology.

1. LLD results from some process that changes the length of leg directly or that alters growth.
2. Direct change in leg length.

a. Trauma: fractures, bone loss, unreduced dislocations.
b. Malunion: overriding or angular deformity.
c. Congenital limb shortening or deficiency.
d. Angular malalignment.

3. Inhibition of growth.
   a. Slower growth in congenital short bones, possibly due to faulty genetic programming.
   b. Injury to physis (growth plate) from trauma, infection, or tumor.
   c. Paralysis: lack of compression forces across the growth plate from muscles will slow growth of bone.
   d. Avascular necrosis.
4. Stimulation of growth.
   a. Tumor.
      (1) Vascular malformations produce growth stimulation involving all physes (hemangiomatosis).
      (2) Certain nonvascular tumors (neurofibromatosis, fibrous dysplasia, Wilm's tumor).
   b. Inflammation: overgrowth is thought to result from increased blood flow.
   c. Fracture: overgrowth thought to result from increased blood flow to bone as part of healing process.

C. Pathophysiology.

1. Growth in leg occurs at four epiphyseal growth plates.
   a. Proximal and distal femoral physes.
   b. Proximal and distal tibial physes.
   c. 70% of growth occurs at the growth plates around the knee.
2. Inhibition or stimulation of growth at any physis can result in LLD.
3. Congenital or acquired loss of bone can change the length of the leg directly.

D. Considerations across the lifespan.

1. The difference in leg lengths will increase proportionately as the child grows.
2. Increased knee pain in athletes with LLD.
3. Degenerative arthritis of the hip of the long leg from pelvic obliquity and uncovering of the hip.
4. Conflicting evidence about LLD as a cause of low back pain later in life.

E. Complications.

1. Leg length discrepancy.
   a. Abnormal gait.
   b. Difficult ambulation.
   c. Contractures in contralateral leg.
   d. Conflicting evidence about LLD as cause of back pain.
   e. Degenerative joint disease.
2. Post-surgical complications.
   a. Infection.
   b. Delayed union/premature union.
   c. Unyielding soft tissues.
   d. Neurovascular complications
      (1) Sciatic or peroneal nerve palsy.
      (2) Vascular insufficiency.
   e. Hypertension related to distraction during limb lengthening procedures.
   f. Contracture of hip, knee, or heel cord.
   g. Fracture.
   h. Muscle weakness.

II. ASSESSMENT

A. History.

1. Presenting symptoms.
   a. Limp/awkward gait.
   b. Pain.
   c. Difficulty with physical activity.
   d. Unhappy with appearance.
2. Onset of symptoms.
3. History of causative factors.
4. Progression of inequality.
5. Prior treatment.
   a. Use of lifts in shoes, orthoses.
   b. Prior surgery.
6. Birth and developmental history.
7. Concerns about gait, function, cosmesis.

B. Physical examination.

1. Height.
2. Spinal deformity/scoliosis.
3. Pelvic obliquity.
4. Apparent leg length.
   a. Measured from the umbilicus to the tip of the medial malleolus.
   b. Affected by pelvic obliquity, hip position, contractures of hip or knee.
5. Real leg length: measured from the anterior iliac spine to the tip of the medial malleolus.
6. Soft tissue contractures.
   a. Knee and hip flexion contractures tend to shorten the leg.
   b. Heel cord contractures tend to lengthen the leg (causes toe walking).
7. Joint stability if bone lengthening procedures are being considered.

C. Diagnostic tests.

1. Radiographs.
   a. Generally need series of radiographs over time to evaluate altered pattern of growth. (Measurements from radiographs plotted on Moseley graph to evaluate pattern of growth, help predict future discrepancy and timing of surgical procedures.)
   b. Teleroentgenogram: single exposure of both legs against a ruler on one long film.
      (1) Shows angular deformities as well as length discrepancies.
      (2) May be distorted due to parallax of x-ray beam.
   c. Orthoroentgenogram: separate exposures of hip, knee, and ankle against a ruler on one long film (multiple exposures increase the risk of distortion due to patient movement).
   d. Scanogram: separate exposures of hip, knee, and ankle against a ruler on a single cassette which is moved between shots (patient movement may distort measurement).

2. CT can be used to accurately measure distance between two points to measure bone length.
3. Standing AP of spine to evaluate scoliosis.
4. Standing AP of pelvis to evaluate pelvic obliquity.
5. Bone age to determine skeletal maturity and to assist with planning appropriate treatment.

III. COMMON THERAPEUTIC MODALITIES

A. Choice of treatment depends on expected size of discrepancy at maturity.

1. 0-2 cm: no treatment.
2. 2-6 cm: shoe lift, epiphysiodesis.
3. 6-15 cm: shortening of longer leg or lengthening of shorter leg.
4. Greater than 15 cm: multiple, staged lengthening procedures or prosthetic fitting.
   a. Bone can be lengthened 20%-25% with good results.
   b. Lengthening bone more than 25% has increased incidence of complications.
   c. For discrepancy of 40%, two staged lengthenings of 20%.

B. Shoe lifts.

1. Prescribed to improve gait.
2. Height of lift is somewhat smaller than actual discrepancy.
3. Lifts higher than 5 cm are poorly tolerated because muscles controlling subtalar joints are not strong enough to resist inversion.

C. Surgical interventions.

1. Goal of surgery is equal leg lengths at skeletal maturity.
2. Timing of surgical intervention is critical.
   a. Determination of anticipated bone growth: several measurements needed for accuracy.
   b. Relative length of legs to torso/total height.
   c. Expected height.
   d. Degree of skeletal maturity.
3. Permanent arrest of growth in longer limb: epiphysiodesis.
   a. Continued growth in shorter leg to catch up.
   b. Produces bony bridge so that epiphysis is fused to metaphysis.
   c. No postoperative immobilization is necessary.
   d. Recreational/sport activities are restricted for 6-8 weeks.
   e. Complications.
      (1) Undercorrection or overcorrection.
      (2) Genu valgus or genu varus.
      (3) Stiff knee joint.
4. Shorten longer limb: Resect portion of tibia or femur after skeletal maturity is reached.
   a. Maximum femoral shortening possible is 5 cm.
   b. Complications.
      (1) > 3 cm shortening in tibia, foot, and ankle may have weakness and decreased function.
      (2) High rate of neurovascular complications following tibial shortening.
      (3) Delayed union/nonunion.
      (4) Compartment syndrome.
5. Lengthen shorter limb: bone lengthening.
   a. Surgery.
      (1) Corticotomy at desired level preserves intramedullary contents and blood supply.
      (2) Circular or bar external fixator applied.
         (a) Circular fixators (Ilizarov, Monticelli, Spinelli) allow correction of complex deformities on more than one plane (longitudinal, rotational, angular).
         (b) Bar fixator (EBI, Orthofix) used to correct primarily longitudinal discrepancies.
   b. Distraction.
      (1) Delayed 5-7 days after surgery to allow osteogenesis (new bone formation) at corticotomy site.
      (2) Distraction rate 0.25 mm every 6 hours (total 1 mm per day).
      (3) Partial to full weight bearing.
      (4) Callotasis method: distraction of newly formed callus starts 7-10 postoperatively.
   c. Consolidation.
      (1) Bone formed at site becomes strong enough to remove fixator.
      (2) Consolidation phase takes about two times as long as distraction phase.
      (3) Weight bearing increased.
   d. External fixator removed when new bone bridges and new cortex appears at lengthened site.
   e. Period of rehabilitation necessary to regain strength and motion.

IV. NURSING DIAGNOSES, OUTCOMES, AND INTERVENTIONS

A. See Table 11.1.

B. Physical mobility, impaired.

1. Outcome: neurovascular status remains unchanged from preoperative baseline. No signs of compartment syndrome are present.
2. Interventions.
   a. Monitor neurovascular status of involved extremity frequently postoperatively.
   b. Monitor pain.
   c. Monitor for signs and symptoms of compartment syndrome. See Chapter 8, Complications (Compartment Syndrome).
   d. Notify physician of abnormalities.

V. PRACTICE SETTING CONSIDERATIONS

A. Office/outpatient.

1. Answer questions regarding radiographs and evaluation of progression of discrepancy.
2. Anticipatory teaching regarding surgical interventions, using models of external fixation devices when possible.
3. Postoperatively.
   a. Assess pin sites at each appointment.

b. Evaluate range of motion at each appointment.
c. Coordinate rehabilitation referrals as needed.

B. Hospital.

1. External fixator.
   a. Keep external fixator covered until patient is "ready" to see it: appearance can be overwhelming.
   b. Bloody drainage from pins expected for 24-48 hours.
   c. Intravenous pain medication round-the-clock for 24 hours post-op before transitioning to PO medications.
2. Physical therapy for crutch training and mobility.

C. Home care considerations.

1. Teach home management related to external fixator.
   a. Pin site care.
   b. How to adjust fixator for distraction.
   c. Schedule of adjustments: usually "1/4 turn" every 6 hours.
   d. Watch for certain signs and symptoms.
   e. Shoe/clothing adaptions.
   f. Bathing and hygiene.
2. Help family with any special transportation needs due to fixator.
3. Help family develop plan for school while external fixator in place.

BLOUNT'S DISEASE (TIBIA VARA)

I. OVERVIEW

A. Definitions.

1. Blount's disease (tibia vara) is characterized by a localized varus deformity.
2. Caused by distorted growth of proximal medial physis and metaphysis.
3. Occurs in both early onset (infantile) and late onset (juvenile/adolescent) forms.

B. Etiology.

1. Underlying cause of distorted growth is unclear.
2. No known genetic element, but family tendency.
3. May represent an epiphyseal injury caused by early or excessive weight bearing in a child with extreme physiologic bowing.

C. Pathophysiology.

1. Asymmetric local pressure on posteromedial aspect of the proximal tibial epiphysis and physis (growth plate) is followed by selective growth slowing.
2. Result.
   a. An intra-articular deformity in posteromedial area of tibial plateau.
   b. Progressive, localized tibial bowing.
   c. Premature closure of medial tibial physis.
3. Early onset (infantile).
   a. May begin as exaggerated physiologic genu varum.
   b. Early walking may exacerbate tibial bowing with increasing knee sag when combined with internal tibial torsion and ligamentous laxity at the knee.
4. Late onset (juvenile/adolescent).
   a. Obesity may be a factor.
   b. May be a history of trauma.

D. Incidence.

1. Early onset form.
   a. Occurs most commonly between ages 1-4.
   b. Usually bilateral.
   c. Slightly more common in females.
2. Late onset form.
   a. Juvenile Blount's disease occurs between ages 4-10.
   b. Adolescent Blount's disease occurs after age 11.
   c. Usually unilateral.
   d. Increased incidence in African American children.
   e. Increased incidence of obesity.
   f. Increased incidence in Finland and the Caribbean.

E. Considerations across the lifespan.

1. Pain may limit physical activity.
2. Associated with degenerative joint disease in adulthood.

F. Complications.

1. Gait awkwardness which increases the risk of sprains and fractures.
2. Knee pain may limit physical activity.
3. Post-surgical.
   a. Vascular compromise due to entrapment of anterior tibial artery.
   b. Valgus deformity due to surgical trauma of osteotomy which stimulates overgrowth of tibia.
   c. Delayed healing of osteotomy if underlying problem is systemic.
   d. Upper tibial osteotomies may be associated with compartment syndromes or injury to peroneal nerve.
   e. Neurovascular injury from angular correction with Garch clamp and external fixator.
4. Lack of treatment may lead to degenerative joint disease in adulthood.

II. ASSESSMENT

A. History.

1. Present symptoms.
   a. Type of angular malalignment, onset, progression and prior treatment.
   b. Pain.
      (1) Pain and tenderness over lateral prominence of proximal tibia.
      (2) Pain with activity.
2. Developmental history: often walk before 12 months.
3. Medical history.
4. Family history.
5. Normal activities/play.
   a. Difficulty walking, especially distances.
   b. Fatigue with activity.
   c. Concerns about gait, function, cosmesis.

B. Physical examination.

1. Height and weight.

2. Medial or lateral thrust at knee, indicating joint instability or ligamentous laxity.
3. Rotational abnormalities of lower extremity.
4. Femoral-tibial angle measured with goniometer.
5. Symmetry/asymmetry of angular malalignment.
   a. Unilateral, sharp lateral angulation of the proximal tibia.
   b. Varus usually measures more than 20 degrees.
   c. 2-3 cm leg length discrepancy.
6. Palpable bony prominence over medial aspect of the proximal tibial condyle.

C. Diagnostic tests.

1. Radiographs
   a. Standing (if possible, depending on age of patient) AP and lateral radiographs of entire leg on long cassette.
   b. Changes in medial metaphyseal contours over time.
      (1) Local prominence or "beaking."
      (2) Height of proximal tibial epiphysis decreases.
      (3) Middle part of medial half of epiphyseal plate is narrowed, with increased bone density on its other side.
   c. Tibiofemoral angle on radiograph (25 degrees of varus).
   d. Internal tibial torsion visible on radiograph.
2. Laboratory studies: to rule out rickets or other systemic disease.
3. See Table 11.6.

III. COMMON THERAPEUTIC MODALITIES

A. Non-operative management.

1. Observation: follow-up with radiographs at 3-month intervals to evaluate progressive deformity.
2. Bracing.
   a. To relieve excessive stress on medial metaphysis of the tibia.
   b. To provide lateral stability to knee joint and external rotation of the leg.
   c. Up to age 24 months, with progressive deformity: hip-knee-ankle-foot orthosis (HKAFO).
   d. After age 24 months, with progressive varus deformity greater than 25 degrees.
   e. Worn full-time.
   f. May be difficult to get adequate stabilization in an adolescent.

B. Surgical interventions.

1. Indications.
   a. Failure to respond to bracing after 6 months of treatment.
   b. Over age 30 months who have not been treated with bracing.
   c. Depression of the tibial plateau, impending closure of medial physis of the upper tibia, and ligamentous laxity of the knee.
2. Procedures.
   a. Corrective proximal tibial osteotomy.
   b. Opening- or closing-wedge osteotomy. (May require internal or external fixation.)
   c. Hemiepiphysiodesis of lateral side of tibia and proximal fibula.
   d. Gradual angular correction using Garch clamp and external fixator.
      (1) Technique similar to bone lengthening procedures for limb length discrepancy.
      (2) Garch clamp and external fixator applied after proximal tibial osteotomy.
      (3) Garch clamp provides angular correction.
      (4) External fixator stabilizes bone fragments, provides lengthening if necessary.
      (5) Patient/family do daily adjustment to external fixator to create open gap on medial aspect of proximal tibia.
      (6) When desired correction is obtained, Garch clamp and external fixator maintained to stabilize bone until healing is complete.

IV. NURSING DIAGNOSES, OUTCOMES, AND INTERVENTIONS

A. See Table 11.1.

B. Anxiety.

1. Outcome: patient and/or family verbalize knowledge of usual progression of angular malalignment.
2. Interventions.
   a. Reinforce the treatment plan.
   b. Support parents and child throughout process.
   c. Angular correction with Garch clamp and external fixator can last 3-6 months.

C. Peripheral neurovascular dysfunction, risk for.

1. Outcome: neurovascular status intact.
2. Interventions.
   a. Assess dorsiflexion and plantar flexion of foot.
   b. Use resting splint to prevent heel cord contracture.
   c. See Compartment Syndrome in Chapter 8, Complications.

V. PRACTICE SETTING CONSIDERATIONS

A. Office/outpatient.

1. Facilitate regular follow-up for child with Blount's disease.
   a. Regular follow-up important to monitor progression.
   b. If angular correction with Garch clamp and external fixator is performed:
      (1) Weekly appointments are necessary during the correction phase (while correcting angular deformity).
      (2) Appointments are every 2-4 weeks during healing phase (after angular deformity is corrected).
2. Promote medical follow-up for treatment of systemic condition.
3. Assist patient/family with symptom management (such as knee pain) as necessary.

B. Hospital.

1. Teach home management related to surgery/casting

or Garch clamp and external fixator.
2. Inpatient rehabilitation may be needed for safe mobility before discharge with crutches or wheelchair.

C. Home care considerations.

1. Encourage parents to allow child to participate in normal activities, as much as he/she is able.
2. Avoid sports/physical activities that cause pain and consider alternatives.
3. Limit gym/physical activities if child has pain.
4. Teach patient/family proper application and care of braces.
   a. Wearing schedule.
   b. Skin care.
   c. Restriction of activities.

SLIPPED CAPITAL FEMORAL EPIPHYSIS (SCFE)

I. OVERVIEW

A. Definition: characterized by posterior displacement of the proximal femoral epiphysis on the femoral neck due to disruption of the physis (growth plate); the head of the femur "slips" off of the neck at the physis.

1. Acute: abrupt displacement. Symptoms less than 3 weeks.
2. Chronic: gradual displacement. More than 3 weeks of symptoms.
3. Acute-on-chronic: chronic slip with an additional acute episode of slipping, and marked increase in pain.

B. Etiology.

1. Exact cause is unknown but is believed to be multifactorial.
2. Biomechanical factors.
   a. Proximal femur subjected to shear stress as a result of certain body weight and rapid growth.
   b. Predisposed to slippage due to decreased femoral anteversion.
3. Trauma.
4. Hormonal/endocrine factors.
   a. Imbalance of sex and growth hormones.
   b. Hypothyroidism.
   c. Hypogonadism.
5. Other systemic medical problems such as renal osteodystrophy.
6. Immunosuppressive therapy after organ transplantation, particularly kidney.
7. Irradiation therapy for malignancy.

C. Pathophysiology.

1. In most cases, the femoral head displaces posteriorly and inferiorly in relation to the femoral neck.
2. "Slip" occurs through what would normally be the zones of cartilage cell hypertrophy and provisional calcification of the physis.
   a. Physeal plate abnormality apparently precedes slippage.
   b. Superimposing acute trauma or the chronic stresses of weight bearing may initiate displacement.
3. Proposed sequence of events:
   a. Rapid growth may cause weakening of proximal femoral physis.
   b. Shear stress of incumbent body weight may cause displacement.
4. Force required is often minimal; falling from bed or jumping may initiate acute slip.
5. As the "slip" progresses.
   a. Bone resorption occurs at anterior superior border of the femoral neck.
   b. Bone deposition occurs in the posterior inferior corner.
6. Once slippage has begun, it will continue until the growth plate is stabilized by either natural or surgical closure.

D. Incidence.

1. Most common disorder of the hip in adolescents.
2. Approximately 3 of 100,000 adolescents between ages 8-17 are hospitalized yearly for treatment.
3. Boys are affected two to three times as often as girls.
   a. Boys age range 10-17 years, with a peak incidence at age 13-14.
   b. Girls age range 8-15 years, with a peak incidence at 11 years; rarely occurs after menarche.
4. Occurs more often in left hip.
5. Bilateral disease in 25%-70% of patients.

E. Considerations across the lifespan.

1. Higher than normal risk of developing degenerative arthritis.
2. Long-term prognosis depends upon the amount of displacement.
3. More severe slips have a greater likelihood of degenerating in later life.
4. Joint arthroplasty, or arthrodesis, may be necessary to improve function or position.

F. Complications.

1. Avascular necrosis.
2. Chondrolysis or acute hyaline cartilage necrosis
3. Limitation of motion
4. Shortening of affected extremity.
5. Early degenerative arthritis.
6. Malunion.
7. Problems with internal fixation.
   a. Protrusion of pins into the joint space.
   b. Soft tissue irritation.
   c. Infection.
   d. Breakage of fixation devices.
   e. Fracture at the pin insertion sites.
8. Missed SCFE: limp, knee pain.

II. ASSESSMENT

A. History.

1. Presenting symptoms.
   a. Pain: location, duration, intensity.
      (1) Pain in groin, may be referred to anteromedial aspect of thigh and knee.
      (2) Pain is dull and vague.
      (3) Pain may be intermittent or continuous,

exacerbated by physical activity.
(4) No pain at rest.
b. Limitation in range of motion.
2. Onset of symptoms, progression, and prior treatment.
a. Chronic SCFE: insidious onset.
b. Acute SCFE: sudden onset of severe pain and inability to bear weight.
c. Acute-on-chronic slip.
(1) Sudden onset of acute pain and inability to bear weight.
(2) Previous history of pain in hip, thigh, knee.
3. Medical history: endocrine problems.

B. Physical examination.
1. *When doing physical examination, do not ask patient to walk or force ROM.*
2. Antalgic limp, holding leg in laterally rotated position.
3. Range of motion may be limited, depending on severity of slip.
a. Internal rotation and abduction are restricted.
b. At rest, limb usually lies in a laterally rotated position.
c. Flexing the involved hip produces concomitant external rotation.
4. Shortening of affected limb may be present (see Chapter 3, Musculoskeletal Assessment).
5. Often positive Trendelenburg test (see Chapter 3, Musculoskeletal Assessment).
6. Chronic or acute-on-chronic SCFE: disuse atrophy of proximal thigh.

C. Diagnostic tests.
1. Radiographs
a. Views.
(1) AP view of pelvis including both hips.
(2) True lateral view of hips: frog-leg lateral may exacerbate instability.
(3) Cross table, true lateral if high suspicion of acute, unstable hip.
b. Acute SCFE: contours of the femoral neck and head are sharp and easily defined.
c. Chronic SCFE: remodeling has occurred, and outlines may be blunted.
d. Grading: assessment of displacement can be obtained from the lateral radiograph.
(1) May classify widening and irregularity of the growth plate with no actual displacement of the epiphysis as "preslip."
(2) Grade I: displacement of less than one-third the diameter of the femoral neck is termed minimal slip.
(3) Grade II: displacement between one-third and one-half is termed moderate slip.
(4) Grade III: displacement greater than one-half is termed severe slip.
2. CT scan: to diagnose early slip in patients with symptoms but normal radiographs.
3. Teleroentgenogram and bone age to determine leg length discrepancy as needed.
4. Blood test to rule out hypothyroidism.
a. Recommended for patient who is obese, age 10 years or younger, other clinical signs of hypothyroidism.
b. Screening for all patients with SCFE not recommended.

III. COMMON THERAPEUTIC MODALITIES

A. Treatment should be initiated immediately after diagnosis to prevent further slippage and to decrease possibility of complications.
1. No weight bearing permitted on affected side.
2. Patient is put on bed rest at home or in hospital to prevent further slippage prior to surgery.

B. Surgical intervention.
1. The goal is to cause physeal "closure."
a. Physeal "closure," when cartilage cells of physis convert to bone, is normal in adolescence.
b. Femoral head will be fused to neck of femur.
2. Surgical pinning is most common procedure.
a. Large threaded pin(s) through femoral neck into head of femur.
b. Pins stimulate cartilage cells to convert to bone.
c. Non-weight-bearing or toe-touch weight bearing with crutches for 6 weeks after surgery.
d. Pins usually not removed.
3. Prophylactic pinning of contralateral hip in some patients.
4. Bone graft epiphysiodesis.
a. Bone graft used to bridge femoral neck and head of femur.
b. Cartilage cells of physis convert to bone.
c. Requires spica cast postoperatively.
5. Osteotomies of femoral neck and intertrochanteric and subtrochanteric regions.
a. Indicated for some chronic slips to restore more normal anatomy and mechanics.
b. Generally considered salvage procedure.
c. Varying complication rates.
6. Reconstruction by arthroplasty or arthrodesis.
a. Distraction of the joint using an external fixator may be needed prior to arthroplasty to pull the femur down, stretch the soft tissues, and provide better alignment.
b. Joint replacement for this age group is not recommended.

IV. NURSING DIAGNOSES, OUTCOMES, AND INTERVENTIONS

A. See Table 11.1.

B. Physical mobility, impaired.
1. Outcome: patient/parents understand and adhere to mobility restrictions after surgery.
2. Interventions:
a. Instruct patient regarding mobility restrictions after surgery: non-weight-bearing or toe-touch gait and use of crutches, as ordered by physician.
b. Reinforce restriction of activities/sports.

c. Reinforce need to report sudden onset of severe pain in affected or contralateral hip.
d. Coordinate physical therapy, if needed to restore mobility.

V. PRACTICE SETTING CONSIDERATIONS

A. Office/outpatient: promote participation in the prescribed physical therapy.

B. Hospital.

1. Reinforce need for bed rest and activity restrictions prior to surgery.
2. Teach patient appropriate crutch gait prior to discharge.

C. Home care considerations.

1. Provide reinforcement of the need for protected ambulation and restriction in activities.
2. Explain to patient the signs and symptoms of a slip.
3. Encourage patient to report changes in pain in the affected hip, or a sudden onset of pain and inability to bear weight on the unaffected hip.

ACHONDROPLASIA

I. OVERVIEW

A. Definition: a short-limbed, disproportionate dwarfing syndrome.

B. Etiology.

1. Caused by single gene mapped to 4th chromosome (4p16.3).
   a. Excludes locus for type II collagen on chromosome 12.
   b. Results in abnormal endochondral ossification.
2. Autosomal dominant trait.
3. Spontaneous mutations in 80% of cases.
4. May be associated with paternal age over 36 years.

C. Pathophysiology.

1. Normal endochondral ossification of cartilage at the physis does not occur.
2. Longitudinal growth is most affected.
   a. Defect is most apparent in fast-growing bones such as femora and humeri.
   b. Proximal segments are more severely affected than middle or distal segments, resulting in rhizomelic extremities.
3. Normal diameter is achieved through normal periosteal ossification.

D. Incidence.

1. The most common dwarfing syndrome.
2. Occurs in 1 of every 20,000-50,000 live births.

E. Considerations across the lifespan.

1. Early motor development is often slow due to hypotonia.
2. Recurrent otitis media is common due to position on eustachian tubes.
3. Cranial enlargement with poor head control increases infant's risk for cervical extension injuries.
4. Obesity is a lifelong problem.
5. Pregnancy and delivery may be affected by abnormal pelvic shape.
6. An adult with achondroplasia who mates with a person of normal size will have a 50% chance of having a child with achondroplasia.
7. An adult with achondroplasia who mates with another person with achondroplasia:
   a. 50% chance that child with receive single mutated gene.
   b. 25% chance that child with receive mutated gene from both parent: lethal in infancy.
   c. 25% chance that child will be unaffected.
8. Maxillary hypoplasia leads to dental crowding and malocclusion.
9. Low back pain may develop in the third decade due to stenosis of the spinal canal and intervertebral foramen.
10. Difficulties in using public restroom facilities, getting on buses, etc.
11. Average standing height for adults: male, 132 centimeters; female, 125 centimeters.

F. Complications.

1. Neurologic deficits from stenosis of spinal canal.
   a. Progressive stenosis is caused by disc herniation, lumbar lordosis, and anterior wedging of vertebral bodies.
   b. Symptoms include:
      (1) Backache.
      (2) Sciatica.
      (3) Disturbances of bladder and bowel function.
      (4) Paraplegia.
      (5) Sexual dysfunction.
2. Small size of foramen magnum may cause:
   a. Cervicomedullary compression.
   b. Increased risk of cervical extension injuries in infants.
   c. Increased risk of apneic spells and sudden death.
3. Respiratory complications due to narrow chest diameter.
   a. Pneumonia.
   b. Cyanotic spells.
   c. Apnea.
4. Abnormal spinal curvatures, particularly thoracolumbar kyphosis and hyperlordosis.
5. Pain and limitation of motion in legs due to progressive genu varum.

II. ASSESSMENT

A. History.

1. Presenting symptoms.
2. Onset of current symptoms, progression, and previous treatment.
3. Pregnancy and birth history.
4. Neurologic involvement.
5. Developmental history.
   a. Delayed motor milestones: 3-6 months behind peers.
   b. Speech and language normal.
6. Functional limitations.

B. Physical examination.
1. Height and weight, head circumference – plotted on growth curve for children with achondroplasia.
2. Disproportionate dwarfing, apparent at birth.
   a. Normal trunk length.
   b. Rhizomelic short extremities: humeri and femora appear most disproportionate.
   c. Head is enlarged with a flattened appearance due to early closure of cranial ossification centers.
3. Upper extremities.
   a. Trident hands: second and third fingers spread to form a large V-shaped space.
   b. Fingertips reach only to hip joint rather than to mid-thigh.
   c. Child may not be able to reach top of head, middle of back, or intergluteal region.
   d. Arm length improves somewhat with growth.
   e. Child may have elbow flexion contractures of 15-30 degrees.
4. Lower extremities.
   a. Genu varum, genu recurvatum, lateral torsion at knee.
   b. Hip flexion contractures associated with lordosis.
   c. Ankle varus deformity may be present.
   d. Child may have marked ligamentous laxity.
   e. Leg may be externally rotated at the hip.
5. Overdeveloped musculature.
6. Waddling gait.
7. Spinal abnormalities.
   a. Kyphosis before walking age related to ligamentous laxity and hypotonia.
   b. After independent ambulation, exaggerated lumbar lordosis associated with prominent abdomen and buttocks.

B. Diagnostic tests.
1. Radiographs.
   a. All long bones are short; flat bones are less affected.
   b. Metaphyseal flare with "ball and socket" relationship of epiphysis to metaphysis.
   c. Spine.
      (1) Small cuboid vertebrae.
      (2) Progressive narrowing of lumbar interpedicular distance.
      (3) Anterior vertebral wedging.
   d. Horizontal distance in pelvic outlet is broad giving champagne glass appearance.
2. Computerized tomography (CT).
   a. To evaluate size of foramen magnum.
   b. To evaluate cross sectional anatomy of spinal canal.
3. MRI to evaluate discogenic changes.

III. COMMON THERAPEUTIC MODALITIES

A. Nonsurgical treatment.
1. No medical treatment for underlying defect.
2. Nutritional management to prevent/manage obesity.
3. Exercises.
   a. Pelvic tilt exercises to relieve hyperlordosis.
   b. Stretching of hip flexion contractures.
4. Bracing.
   a. In extension for hyperlordosis after independent ambulation begins.
      (1) For wedging of vertebrae on x-ray.
      (2) May compromise mobility and create problems with activities of daily living (ADL).
   b. Not effective for genu varus deformity of lower extremities.

B. Surgical interventions.
1. Spine.
   a. Laminectomy.
      (1) For cauda equina syndrome.
      (2) Extend to pedicles with foraminoectomies.
      (3) Remove herniated disc material.
      (4) Maintain facet joints to prevent instability.
   b. Arthrodesis.
      (1) For instability or unresolved kyphosis.
      (2) Anterior fusion recommended.
      (3) Posterior fusion difficult due to small size of transverse processes.
      (4) No instrumentation because it will further decrease size of spinal canal.
   c. Discectomy.
      (1) Most beneficial in patients with intermittent symptoms.
      (2) Progressive neurologic loss can occur after procedure.
2. Lower extremities.
   a. Proximal tibiofemoral osteotomies.
      (1) Symptomatic or rapidly progressive deformity.
      (2) No internal fixation necessary.
      (3) Immobilized in long leg cast for 6 weeks.
   b. Proximal and distal fibular epiphysiodesis.
      (1) Stop relative overgrowth of fibula.
      (2) Correction by growth of tibia over time.
      (3) Asymptomatic patient between ages 7-10.
3. Limb lengthening is very controversial.

IV. NURSING DIAGNOSES, OUTCOMES, AND INTERVENTIONS

A. See Table 11.1.

B. See Table 11.7.

C. Nutrition, imbalanced: potential for more than body requirement.
1. Outcome: patient maintains healthy body weight as per achondroplastic growth charts.
2. Interventions.
   a. Counseling about potential for obesity should begin in early infancy.
   b. Monitor patient's weight.
   c. Refer to dietician for accurate assessment of caloric needs and dietary recommendations.

D. Self-care deficit: bathing/hygiene, feeding, dressing/grooming, toileting.
1. Outcome: patient is able to achieve independence in self-care activities.
2. Interventions.
   a. Promote independence in self-care activities.

Table 11.7.
Common Nursing Diagnoses, Outcomes, and Interventions for Chronic Pediatric/Congenital Disorders

Diagnoses	Outcomes	Interventions
A. Activity intolerance	• Patient makes adaptations in physical environment and lifestyle.	• Promote mobility within limitations. 1. Exercise programs to strengthen unaffected muscles and prevent disuse weakness. a. Teach family to assist/implement exercise program. b. Provide padded play area for walking, crawling, or rolling without injury. c. Encourage bilateral hand movement through use of play when patient prone. 2. Utilize assistive and ambulatory devices as needed. 3. Assess ambulatory stability and plan for safe ambulation. 4. Assess movements during sleep for need for side rails, padded rails. 5. Encourage patient to seek assistance for difficult activities.
B. Social isolation	• Patient participates in diversional/social activities.	• Promote socialization. 1. Assess patient satisfaction with level of participation in social and diversional activities. a. Assess for diminished self-esteem as a source of decreased interest or desire to participate in activities. b. Assess if pain is a factor in decreased interest in activities. 2. Assess interest and skills as sources of diversional and social activities. 3. Provide age-appropriate diversional activities. 4. Facilitate participation in activities appropriate to patient's physical and mental capabilities. 5. Develop alternate communication techniques as needed. 6. Remove physical/structural barriers to participation whenever possible. 7. Investigate community resources that may be of assistance in achieving socialization and diversional activity goals.

Table 11.7. (continued)
Common Nursing Diagnoses, Outcomes, and Interventions for Chronic Pediatric/Congenital Disorders

Diagnoses	Outcomes	Interventions
C. Aspiration, risk for	• Patient does not aspirate.	• Promote safe intake of food and fluids. 1. Assess ability to chew and swallow. 2. Offer foods and fluids of appropriate consistency. 3. Assist with feeding and drinking as needed. a. Stroke from neck to chin to stimulate swallowing. b. Allow sufficient time for meal to avoid rushing. 4. Provide smaller more frequent meals if needed. 5. Allow rest periods during meals. 6. Have suction equipment at bedside, if indicated. 7. Suction secretions before patient takes food/fluid. 8. Monitor for signs and symptoms of aspiration pneumonia.
D. Disuse syndrome	• Optimal musculoskeletal functioning is maintained.	• Maintain musculoskeletal functioning. 1. Provide passive and active range of motion to prevent contractures. 2. Maintain functional body alignment. 3. Teach patient/family to assess body position and proper positioning. 4. Collaborate with physical therapy for additional exercises or corrective treatment. 5. Exercise program to strengthen unaffected muscles and prevent disuse weakness. • Maximize function with braces, splints and assistive devices, as needed. 1. Encourage patient/family to utilize such devices. 2. Check assistive devices for fit and safety. 3. Arrange for repairs and fittings as needed. • Assess occurrence of spasms in relation to activity/movement and control them, if possible.

Table 11.7. (continued)
Common Nursing Diagnoses, Outcomes, and Interventions for Chronic Pediatric/Congenital Disorders

Diagnoses	Outcomes	Interventions
E. Pain, chronic	• Patient achieves maximal degree of comfort.	• Promote patient comfort. 1. Handle patient gently. 2. Relieve pain with appropriate nonpharmacologic and pharmacologic techniques. 3. Nonpharmacologic: massage, stretching, moist heat, ice, relaxation, etc. 4. Pharmacologic: muscle relaxants, antispasmodics, analgesics, etc. 5. Position to prevent problems, such as muscle spasms. 6. Encourage diversional activities. 7. Discuss coping methods with patient/family. • See Chapter 7, Pain.
F. Skin integrity, impaired	• Skin integrity is maintained.	• Check skin integrity, with special attention when: 1. Patient is unable to reposition self independently. 2. Spasms are severe or uncontrolled. 3. Sensation is impaired. 4. Patient is adjusting to a new positioning or mobilizing device. 5. Patient is splinted or casted. a. Irritability in a nonverbal patient with long-leg casts may indicate skin breakdown at heels or ankles. b. Window casts if no other cause of irritability is found. • Maintain skin integrity. 1. Turn and reposition frequently. 2. Keep skin clean and dry. 3. Use pressure-reducing or pressure-relieving devices such as air mattresses or special beds. 4. Avoid thermal injuries in sensation-impaired patients: heating pads, cooling blankets, overly hot water. 5. Position in proper alignment. • See Chapter 6, Effects of Immobility.

Table 11.7. (continued)
Common Nursing Diagnoses, Outcomes, and Interventions for Chronic Pediatric/Congenital Disorders

Diagnoses	Outcomes	Interventions
G. Communication, verbally impaired	• Patient is able to communicate verbally or nonverbally.	• Maximize communication capabilities. 1. Allow patient as much time as necessary to express thoughts. 2. Learn the patient's communication system (symbol board, pad and pencil, blinking, eye movements related to "yes" and "no" answers). 3. Stand in front of patient when speaking. 4. Pronounce words slowly and distinctly. 5. Help patient to repeat words as accurately as he/she is able. 6. Encourage use of nonverbal communications (gestures) if appropriate. 7. Communicate with other disciplines so patient is not frustrated by inconsistencies in care.
H. Grieving	• Patient/family is supported through grieving process.	• Encourage verbalization of feelings/fears associated with perceived losses. • Support patient/family through diagnostic period. • Assist patient/family in identifying life-style modifications. • Help family identify sources of support. 1. Refer to appropriate disease-related support group. 2. Provide for spiritual counseling if desired. 3. Provide for psychologic support as needed. • Help family recognize child's strengths and skills while acknowledging limitations.

b. Explore use of assistive devices (hand extensions to reach lights, step stools, etc.).
c. Explore methods of facilitating ADL within patient's capabilities.
d. Encourage verbalization of concerns regarding activity limitations.

V. PRACTICE SETTING CONSIDERATIONS

A. Office/outpatient: provide information about achondroplasia and the management of associated problems.

1. Need for good dental hygiene and care.
2. Treatment for frequent ear infections.
3. Speech evaluation if problems are due to persistence of tongue thrust.
4. Expected growth patterns.
5. Psychosocial implications.
6. School attendance.
7. Sports and gym participation.

B. Home care considerations.

1. Protect infant from cervical extension injuries.
   a. Support head whenever infant is moved.
   b. No infant swings, tossing baby into the air.
2. Home modifications and assistive devices may be necessary.

ARTHROGRYPOSIS MULTIPLEX CONGENITA (AMC)

I. OVERVIEW

A. Definition.

1. AMC is the best known of a group of syndromes characterized by joint contractures in all four extremities. (Syndromes classified according to joints involved.)
   a. Arthrogryposis involving all four extremities.
   b. Arthrogryposis involving the hands and feet.
   c. Ptergygia syndromes with skin webs across knees, elbows, and other joints.
2. Contractures are due to fibrosis of affected muscles, with thickening and shortening of the periarticular capsular and ligamentous tissue of the joint.
3. AMC is not progressive.

B. Etiology.

1. The cause of AMC is unknown.
2. It is not presently considered a genetic disorder.
3. Teratogens have been suggested by animal studies but none proven.
4. Decreased number of anterior horn cells indicated that a central nervous system disorder may have some role.

C. Incidence.

1. 0.03% in the general population.
2. Statistics vary widely from one geographic area to another.
3. Britain, Australia, and United States showed a tenfold increase between early 1940s and 1960s (may be attributed to improved diagnostic measures) followed by an unexplained subsequent decline.

D. Pathophysiology.

1. Neuropathic arthrogryposis (most common type).
   a. Reduction, degeneration, or absence of anterior horn cells.
      (1) Feet are most susceptible because the extrinsic muscles of the feet have the shortest anterior horn of all the columns in the lumbar spine.
      (2) Distal segments of limbs (hands, feet, and ankles) are the most frequently affected joints.
   b. Muscles may be normal, but small, or absent and replaced by fat or fibrous tissue.
   c. De-enervation atrophy is seen on muscle biopsy.
   d. In affected joints, there may be destruction of articulating surfaces.
   e. Degenerative changes and capsular thickening occur later.
2. Myopathic arthrogryposis.
   a. Fibrous, fatty alterations in muscles.
   b. No central nervous system alterations.
   c. Destruction of muscle fibers in unborn infant.
   d. Clinically apparent changes.
      (1) Partial fixation of joints.
      (2) Development of shortened restrictive ligaments and periarticular tissues.
3. Mixed arthrogryposis: pathophysiologic findings of both the neuropathic and myopathic types.

E. Considerations across the lifespan.

1. Joint contractures present at birth.
2. Newborn may suffer fractures during delivery.
3. Generally nonprogressive, although some contracture may seem to worsen with age.
4. Most adults become independent and gainfully employed.
5. Dependency in adulthood is related to personality, education, and overall coping skills rather than degree of physical involvement.
6. Normal lifespan expected.

F. Complications.

1. Fractures, particularly of the feet.
2. Recurrent foot deformity after surgery.
3. Transient nerve palsies may occur following pectoralis major transfers. These appear to resolve spontaneously after several weeks.
4. Pressure necrosis of articular cartilage may result when forceful methods used to correct contractures.

II. ASSESSMENT

A. History.

1. Presenting symptoms.
2. Onset and progression of presenting symptoms and previous treatment.
3. Family history usually negative.
4. Developmental history: normal intelligence.
5. Functional limitations.
6. Feeding history – often have stiff jaw, immobile tongue.

B. Physical examination.

1. Featureless extremities.
   a. Normal skin creases absent.
   b. Deep dimples over joints.
   c. Reduced muscle mass.
2. Joint motion is restricted.
3. Upper extremities.
   a. Shoulder adducted, internally rotated.
   b. Elbows extended.
   c. Wrists severely flexed with ulnar deviation.
   d. Finger flexed over thumb.
4. Lower extremities.
   a. Hips flexed, abducted, externally rotated.
   b. Unilateral or bilateral hip dislocation.
   c. Knees extended.
   d. Clubfeet.
5. Inguinal hernia.
6. 1/3 patients have scoliosis.

B. Diagnostic tests.

1. Radiographs: AP and lateral of involved areas.
   a. Loss of subcutaneous fat and muscle.
   b. Normal joints.
2. EMG and muscle biopsy of questionable diagnostic value.

III. COMMON THERAPEUTIC MODALITIES

A. Prognosis is better than might be expected based on clinical findings at birth.

B. Primary goals in treatment include.

1. Alignment and stability of lower extremities to allow weight bearing and ambulation.
2. Positioning and motion of upper extremities to allow independent ADL.

C. Complex problems are best managed by a comprehensive multidisciplinary team: pediatrician, neurologist, orthopaedist, geneticist, nurse, social worker, physical therapist, occupational therapist.

D. Nonsurgical treatment of contractures.

1. Aggressive physical therapy and occupational therapy immediately after birth.
2. Frequent ROM to affected extremities.
3. Splint joint in position of function.
4. Avoid casting: utilize bracing and assistive devices.

E. Surgical interventions.

1. Important to consider how one contracture relates to another when planning surgical intervention.
2. Hip flexion contractures: early release of soft tissue contractures.
3. Knees.
   a. Flexion contracture.
      (1) Soft tissue releases, including posterior capsulotomy before age 2.
      (2) Supracondylar osteotomies toward end of growth.
   b. Hyperextension deformity treated before hip contractures.
4. Clubfeet usually severe, very rigid.
   a. Treated after knees and hips.
   b. May require extensive release with resection of tendon insertions.
   c. Triple arthodesis may be necessary.
5. Upper extremity.
   a. Tendon transfer for active flexion if 90 degrees passive motion present.
   b. Distal humeral osteotomy for elbow flexion and to correct internal rotation at the shoulder.

IV. NURSING DIAGNOSES, OUTCOMES, AND INTERVENTIONS

A. See Table 11.1.

B. See Table 11.7.

C. Growth and development, altered.
Social interaction, impaired.
Body image, disturbed.
Self-care, deficient.

1. Outcomes.
   a. Achieves appropriate developmental tasks.
   b. Establishes positive peer relationships
   c. Participates in age-related activities.
2. Interventions.
   a. Promote accomplishments of developmental tasks and peer interactions.
   b. Plan alternative methods of stimulation and attainment of developmental tasks to compensate for physical restrictions.
   c. Encourage independence in ADL.
   d. Praise accomplishments of age-related tasks.
   e. Encourage involvement in age-related activities.
   f. Encourage and support involvement and interactions with peer groups.
   g. Focus on positive aspects of appearance (hair, eyes, etc.).

D. Physical mobility, impaired.

1. Outcomes.
   a. Able to perform own ADL, including feeding and toileting.
   b. Minimum limb atrophy as a result of disuse.
   c. Maximum use of upper extremities.
   d. Proper mobilization of limbs to inhibit growth of tissue webs (pterygium) across joints.
2. Interventions.
   a. Promote mobility within limitations.
   b. Teach significant others how to hold patient with immobilization devices.
   c. Plan methods of self-care, taking into consideration limitations of motion.
   d. Reinforce prescribed exercise program. For example, gait and balance training; stretching, strengthening, and range-of-motion exercises.
   e. Stress importance of aggressive program (beginning at birth and the relationship to outcome).

V. PRACTICE SETTING CONSIDERATIONS

A. Office/outpatient.

1. Collaborate with primary care provider to routine well-child and preventive health care.
2. Ongoing follow-up important to assess functional status and need for surgical intervention.
3. Child may require frequent surgeries to straighten

and maintain limbs. Give outline of surgical interventions and rationale for order and timing.

B. Home care considerations.

1. Reinforce importance of consistent and progressive implementation of physical/ occupational therapy regimens.
   a. Significant others will often need reassurance and encouragement as manipulation of limbs is often unpleasant.
   b. Contractures are worst at birth; with treatment, the condition improves.
   c. Although child will never have full range of motion, most can achieve normal lifestyle with adaptive equipment.
2. Provide support to parents as continuous caregivers.
   a. Parents are an important part in success/failure of treatment.
   b. Intelligence and life expectancy are usually not altered by AMC.
3. Encourage age-appropriate developmental behaviors and activities.
4. Offer information regarding community resources and support groups.
   a. National Arthrogryposis Foundation.
   b. Support groups.
   c. National Muscular Dystrophy Foundation.

OSTEOGENESIS IMPERFECTA (OI)

I. OVERVIEW

A. Definition.

1. An inherited connective tissue disorder that affects bone and soft tissues.
2. Clinical features and their severity are variable, depending on the type of OI (see Table 11.8).
3. Also called "brittle bone disease."

B. Etiology.

1. Mutations in one of two genes (COL1A1 or COL1A2) that encode the components of type I collagen.
2. Genetic defect results in abnormal structure or decreased amount of type I collagen.
3. Genetic defect usually transmitted as autosomal dominant.
4. High rate of spontaneous mutation.

C. Pathophysiology.

1. Basic defect is in type I collagen synthesis: decreased amount or quality.
   a. Normal epiphyseal and articular cartilage.
   b. Normal amounts of bone minerals.
   c. Skin thin, translucent, easily distensible.
   d. Increased vascular fragility but major aneurysms are rare.
2. Skeletal manifestations.
   a. Generalized osteopenia.
   b. Bone trabeculae are thin, frail, and sparsely distributed.
   c. Endochondral and intramembranous bone formation can be abnormal.
3. Fractures heal readily; callus is plastic and easily deformed.
4. Basilar impression may result from deformation of soft bone in skull.
   a. Elevation of the floor of the posterior cranial fossa, including occipital condyles and foramen magnum compresses the brain stem.
   b. Occurs most frequently in children with Type IV OI.
   c. May be prevented by delay upright posture in infants.
5. Cause of related metabolic abnormalities is unclear.
   a. Increased sweating.
   b. Heat intolerance.
   c. Increased body temperature.
   d. Resting tachycardia and tachypnea.

D. Incidence depends on type of OI (see Table 11.8).

E. Considerations across the lifespan.

1. Onset of fracture varies with the type of OI (see Table 11.8).
2. In general, frequency of fractures will decrease after puberty but increase again in later years.
3. Life expectancy ranges from neonatal death (Type II) to normal life expectancy (Type I).
4. Early death related to pulmonary insufficiency, cardiac decompensation, or brain stem compression.

F. Complications.

1. Progressive deformity.
2. Severe growth failure.
3. Pulmonary in sufficiency related to small thorax and/or kyphoscoliosis.
4. Cardiac decompensation related to aortic insufficiency or mitral regurgitation.
5. Brain stem compression from basilar impression.

II. ASSESSMENT

A. History: signs and symptoms will vary depending on type and severity.

1. Present symptoms.
   a. Signs of basilar impression/brain stem compression include:
      (1) Facial spasm and nerve paresis.
      (2) Pyramidal signs.
      (3) Proprioceptive defects.
      (4) Papilloedema.
      (5) Weakness in extremities.
      (6) Bladder dysfunction.
   b. Hearing loss.
   c. Abdominal pain/chronic constipation.
2. Pregnancy and birth history.
3. Developmental history.
   a. Delay in developmental milestones in some types of OI.
   b. Independent sitting by 10 months is important indicator of potential for independent ambulation.
4. Normal activities/play.
5. Onset and frequency of fractures
6. Past and current treatment.

Table 11.8
Types of Osteogenesis Imperfecta

	Type I	Type II	Type III	Type IV
Inheritance	Autosomal dominant	• Autosomal dominant (new mutations) • Autosomal recessive (rare)	• Autosomal dominant (new mutations) • Autosomal recessive (uncommon)	Autosomal dominant
Incidence	1/15-20,000	1/20-60,000	1/70,000	1/200,000
Onset of fractures	• Fractures usually begin when child starts to walk • Frequency of fracture decreases after puberty • Increase in frequency in women after menopause, in men, 60-80 years.	Multiple fractures in utero	Fractures at birth or within first year of life	• Fracture in utero, during labor and delivery or in newborn period • Fracture frequency increases when child starts to walk • Fractures decrease after puberty • Increase in frequency in post-menopausal women
Physical manifestations	• Mildest form • Mild to moderate bone fragility without deformity • Easy bruising • Mild joint hypermobility • Mild short stature	• Most severe form • Extreme fragility of connective tissue • Intrauterine growth retardation • Soft, large cranium • Extremities short • Legs bowed • Small thoracic cavity	• Severe fragility of bone • Fractures heal with deformity and bowing • Long bone deformity noted within first 2 years of life • Relative macrocephaly with triangular facies • Extreme short stature • Severe kyphoscoliosis	• Skeletal fragility and osteoporosis more severe than Type I • Bowing of long bones • Moderate short stature • Moderate joint hypermobility • Basilar impression results in brain stem compression • Mild to severe scoliosis
Appearance on x-ray	Mild osteopenia with recurrent fractures	• "Crumpled" bones • Skull severely osteopenic • "Beaded" ribs	• Progressive bony deformities • Undermineralized skull • Wormian bones • Thin, gracile long bones • Short, deformed long boned • Severe scoliosis	• Osteopenia with recurrent fractures • Bowing of long bones
Color of sclera	Blue sclera	Dark blue sclera	• Pale blue at birth • Fade to white	Grayish to white sclera
Dentinogenesis imperfecta	• Type A: No • Type B: Yes (uncommon)	Not known	Yes	• Type A: No • Type B: Yes
Other clinical findings	• Early onset hearing loss • Most achieve developmental milestones on time	• Associated with prematurity and low birth weight • Poor feeding	• Hearing loss common • Abdominal pain and chronic constipation or bowel obstruction due to protrusio acetabuli • Motor development severely delayed • Muscle weakness and joint contractures from immobility	Hearing loss in some families

Table 11.8 (continued)
Types of Osteogenesis Imperfecta

	Type I	Type II	Type III	Type IV
Life expectancy	Normal life expectancy	Lethal in perinatal period – 80% mortality in 1st month • Pulmonary insufficiency • Congestive heart failure • Infection	Shortened life expectancy • Cardiac decompensation • Pulmonary insufficiency • Brain stem compression from basilar impression	Near normal life expectancy

7. Family history.

B. Physical examination.
1. Height and weight.
   a. Short stature.
   b. Failure to thrive.
2. Musculoskeletal.
   a. Ligamentous laxity.
   b. Hypotonic muscles.
   c. Joint contractures.
   d. Deformity of skull, facial bones, and extremities.
   e. Scoliosis and/or kyphosis.
   f. Blue or gray sclera.
3. Neurologic exam for signs of basilar impression.
4. Cardiorespiratory exam for signs of respiratory insufficiency and cardiac decompensation.
5. Dentinogenesis imperfecta.
6. Hearing loss.

C. Diagnostic tests.
1. Radiographs to evaluate fractures, bony deformity, and scoliosis.
2. Skin biopsy for analysis of collagen defect.
3. Blood chemistry usually within normal limits. Serum alkaline phosphatase may be elevated.
4. Bone densitometry to measure bone strength.
5. Audiometry to evaluate hearing loss.

III. COMMON THERAPEUTIC MODALITIES

A. No established medical therapy to treat collagen defect.

B. Fracture prevention.
1. Physical therapy to strengthen soft tissues and prevent joint contractures.
2. Standing with bracing to prevent disuse osteopenia.
3. Develop ambulatory potential with orthotics and assistive devices as necessary.

C. Management of fractures.
1. Closed reduction best, if possible.
2. Precise fracture alignment to prevent deformities.
3. Lightweight immobilization and early return to weight bearing (standing frame or tilt-table as needed) to prevent disuse osteopenia.
4. In some small children, deformity will be accepted, pending corrective osteotomies when child is older.

D. Surgical interventions.
1. Open reduction of fractures: intramedullary (IM) fixation better than plates and screws.
2. Multiple corrective osteotomies with intramedullary fixation to correct deformities.
   a. Solid rod provides good stabilization but needs to be replaced as child grows.
   b. Elongating Bailey-Dubow rod "grows" with child but can break.
3. In situ spinal fusions for scoliosis (usually without instrumentation).
   a. Bracing ineffective for controlling progression.
   b. Poor quality of bone makes internal fixation difficult.

IV. NURSING DIAGNOSES, OUTCOMES, AND INTERVENTIONS

A. See Table 11.1.

B. See Table 11.7.

C. Injury, risk for.
1. Outcome: fractures are recognized and treated.
2. Interventions.
   a. Teach patient/family how to prevent fractures/recognize injuries.
   b. Handle patient gently, supporting patient's body when moving, positioning, and lifting.
   c. Plan with patient and family methods to achieve developmental tasks that lessen chance of fracture.
   d. Teach patient and family signs and symptoms of fracture.
   e. See Chapter 14, Trauma (Fractures).

D. Physical mobility, impaired.
1. Outcome: patient attains independent mobility.
2. Interventions.
   a. Promote mobility.
   b. Provide gentle, consistent exercise to extremities to avoid disuse atrophy.
   c. Assist with early weight bearing. May need to use tilt-table or standing frame.
   d. Lightweight orthoses are used whenever possible.

V. PRACTICE SETTING CONSIDERATIONS

A. Office/outpatient.

1. Child should receive routine pediatric and preventive health care.
2. Orthopaedist needs to share information regarding type of OI, clinical issues and prognosis with primary care provider.
3. Patient should have routine hearing evaluation to evaluate and treat hearing loss.
4. Family should be referred for genetic counseling.

B. Hospital.

1. Respiratory complications are common after surgery due to pulmonary insufficiency.
2. Risk of malignant hyperthermia now discounted. Elevated body temperature related to increased metabolic rate during surgery.
3. Friability and weakness of tissues makes suture lines weak.
4. Poor wound healing results in weak, wide scar.
5. May have increased risk of bleeding complications.

C. Home care considerations.

1. Teach parents appropriate handling techniques for baby or child.
   a. Support body when moving or lifting.
   b. Do not pull on limbs.
   c. Do not lift under arms.
   d. Use caution when bathing child.
2. Teach parents to recognize fractures and to follow physician's directions for fracture care.
3. Adapt clothing for comfort.
   a. Lightweight cotton clothing cooler and more absorbent will allow excessive perspiration to evaporate.
   b. Clothing must be easy to put on and take off.
4. Maintain gentle consistent exercise to prevent muscle atrophy.
5. Teach parents to make home as risk-free as possible to reduce likelihood of falls or other injuries.
6. Avoid "risky" physical activities, such as contact sports, heavy lifting, jumping, or falling.
7. Encourage as much independence as disease severity will allow.
   a. Motorized scooters or electric wheelchairs useful for severely involved patients.
   b. Adaptive aids to assist with ADL.
8. Encourage parents to restrict child's environment as little as possible.
   a. Avoid home tutoring.
      (1) Mainstream into public school.
      (2) Special school for physically (not mentally) handicapped.
   b. Participation in activities which are not physically contraindicated.
9. Offer family information about Osteogenesis Imperfecta Foundation.

MYELOMENINGOCELE

I. OVERVIEW

A. Definition: myelomeningocele is a neural tube defect (NTD) that involves the spinal cord, meninges, and vertebral bodies.

1. Neural tube eventually develops into brain and spinal cord.
2. Neural tube defects include.
   a. Spina bifida.
      (1) Spina bifida occulta: lack of fusion of spinous process of lower lumbar and sacral spine without neurologic abnormalities.
         (a) Usually has no visible or palpable malformations.
         (b) Occasionally, a cutaneous dimple or hair tuft is present.
         (c) Neurologic abnormalities and musculoskeletal changes in small percentage of patients.
      (2) Spina bifida cystica: term applied to all midline fusion defects in the spine in which there is external evidence of herniation of meninges.
         (a) Meningocele: unfused vertebral arches with a visible meningeal sac along the spinal axis.
            i. Less than one-third of all cases of spina bifida cystica.
            ii. Sac contains CSF, composed of dura or dura and arachnoid but no nerve tissue.
            iii. Usually no neurologic deficits.
         (b) Myelomeningocele: characterized by a failure of fusion between vertebral arches with dysplasia of the spinal cord and its membranes.
            i. Neural elements are abnormal and part of the sac.
            ii. Neurologic deficit at and caudal to the level of the lesion.
            iii. May have central nervous system abnormalities, such as Arnold-Chiari malformation.
   b. Encephalocele: a congenital gap in the skull, often with herniation of the brain or meninges.
   c. Anencephaly: absence of development above the brain stem.

B. Etiology.

1. The cause of myelomeningocele unclear, probably multifactorial.
2. Genetic factors.
   a. PAX3: gene involved in anterior-posterior closure of body axis.
   b. 5,19-methylene tetrahydrofolate reductase: enzyme involved in conversion of amino acid homocysteine to methionine.
   c. Chromosomal disorders: trisomy 13 and 18.

3. Nutritional and chemical factors.
   a. Low folic acid intake by the mother prior to conception.
   b. Maternal exposure to valproic acid or carbamazepine (seizure medications) or istotretinoin (acne medication).
   c. Maternal diabetes.
   d. Excessive maternal use of alcohol or hyperthermia (sauna) during pregnancy.

C. Pathophysiology.

1. Development of neural tube during days 21-29 of embryonic life is disrupted.
2. Two theories of abnormal development.
   a. Partial or complete failure of the neural tube to close.
   b. Rupture of a neural tube that is over-distended with ventricular fluid.
3. Partial or complete paralysis and sensory loss below affected neurosegmental area.
   a. Lesion occurs at any level of the spine but most frequently in the lumbosacral region.
   b. Most lesions are posterior, with rare instances of anterior or lateral lesions.
   c. Cause of neurologic deficits unclear.
      (1) Malformed spinal cord.
      (2) Combination of malformation and inflammatory effect of chronic expose of open cord to amniotic fluid.
      (3) Direct abrasion of cord against uterine wall as fetus grows.
      (4) Secondary trauma during delivery.
4. Associated brain abnormalities.
   a. Hydrocephalus in 85% of patients.
      (1) Obstruction of the flow of CSF at the fourth ventricle once lesion is surgically repaired
      (2) Obstruction of flow from Arnold Chiari malformation.
   b. Arnold-Chiari malformation: brain stem displaced through small foramen magnum.
      (1) Chiari Type II deformity most common: displacement of cerebellum.
      (2) Chiari Type III deformity: displacement of the entire cerebellum and lower brain stem.
   c. Cognitive impairments associated with diffuse changes in cerebral cortex.
5. Abnormal spinal curves.
   a. Result from bony malformations of spinal column and lack of muscle tone in trunk.
   b. Bony abnormalities can include hemivertebrae, unsegmented bars or diastematomyelia.
   c. Incidence of scoliosis increases as level of defect moves upward (toward chest).
   d. Lordosis may develop in relation to hip flexion contractures.
6. Lower extremity deformities.
   a. Result from abnormal neurologic development and muscle imbalance.
   b. Risk of hip dislocation in high lumbar (L1, L2, L3) myelomenigocele due to muscle imbalance.
   c. Foot deformities most common.
7. Some dysfunction of bowel and bladder in virtually all cases.
   a. Bladder, urinary outlet, and rectum all controlled by nerves that leave spinal cord in sacrum.
   b. Difficulty storing urine and emptying bladder.
   c. Uncoordinated propulsive action of intestines and ineffectual anal sphincter and lack of anal sensation.

D. Incidence.

1. 4.5 per 10,000 live births.
2. Incidence of myelomeningocele in the United States.
   a. 0.15% in Caucasian population.
   b. 0.04% in African American population.
3. Spina bifida is more common in females than males.
4. Families with one child with neural tube defect have 30 times greater risk of having second child with neural tube defect.
5. Adults with spina bifida have 1:23 risk of bearing child with neural tube defect.

E. Considerations across the lifespan.

1. Folic acid 0.4 mg per day at or before time of conception and continuing for first 3 months of pregnancy is recommended for prevention of neural tube defects.
2. Antenatal diagnosis is possible (see D. Diagnostic tests, to follow).
3. Myelomenigocele is being treated with fetal surgery.
   a. Defect repaired while fetus in still in the uterus.
   b. Surgery done between 22-30 weeks gestation.
   c. Early results.
      (1) Less neurologic damage, relative to level of defect.
      (2) Decreased incidence of Arnold-Chiari malformation.
   d. Long-term results are unknown.
4. Planned delivery by cesarean section before onset of labor or rupture of fetal membranes is recommended to prevent trauma to exposed nervous tissue.
5. Deterioration in neurologic function is not progressive.
   a. Neurologic function should remain steady throughout growth.
   b. Deterioration in neurologic function indicates a complication, which requires prompt evaluation and treatment.
6. As child reaches adolescence, changing relative strength and shift in center of gravity may decrease ability to ambulate.
7. Sexual dysfunction in adolescents and adults is common.
   a. Males.
      (1) 75% capable of erections, although not controlled.
      (2) Prone to retrograde ejaculation.
   b. Females.
      (1) Normal fertility.
      (2) Decreased genital sensation but can have orgasm.
      (3) Increased incidence of precocious puberty due to hypothalamus disorder.

Table 11.9
Functional Level in Myelomeningocele

Spinal Level	Motor Function/Sensation	Orthopaedic Problems	Mobility
Thoracic	• No motion in legs • Extremities lie in abduction, external rotation, and flexion • Variable weakness and sensory loss in abdomen and LE	• Flexion-abduction-external rotation contracture	• Requires extensive orthotics 1. Parapodium 2. Reciprocal gait orthosis 3. HKAFO
Upper lumbar L1-L2	• Hip flexion and adduction • Sensation in anterior hip joint and thigh	• Flexion contracture at hip • Hip dislocation	
Mid to lower lumbar L3-L5	• Hip flexion and adduction • Knee extension • Weak knee flexion • Foot dorsiflexion and eversion • Sensation to below the knee	• Flexion contracture at hip • Decreased hip abduction • Predisposed to progressive hip subluxation • Clubfeet	• Less extensive orthotics • Able to use crutches
Sacral	• Mild weakness of ankles and toes	• Cavus foot	• Minimal or no bracing • Ambulates with or without crutches

F. **Complications.**
1. Latex hypersensitivity.
   a. Increased incidence in patients with myelomeningocele.
   b. Cause unknown.
   c. Allergy characterized by swelling or itching of lips after blowing up balloons or dental exams, swelling or itching of skin after contact with rubber products, hand eczema, wheezing, bronchospasm.
   d. High-risk patients report oral itching after eating bananas, chestnuts, or avocados or report multiple surgical procedures in infancy.
2. Ventriculoperitoneal (VP) shunt infection or shunt malfunction.
3. Hydrosyringomyelia.
   a. From increased fluid pressure in spinal canal when shunt malfunctions.
   b. Characterized by increasing paralysis and/or spasticity of the lower extremities, weakness of hands and upper extremities, and occasional back pain.
4. Tethered spinal cord.
   a. Normal cephalad migration of cord impeded by ectodermal attachment of cord as part of initial defect or by adhesions after surgery.
   b. Characterized by increasing paralysis and/or spasticity in lower extremities, pain in lower back and along sacral nerve roots.
5. Infection.
   a. Chronic urinary tract infections due to urinary stasis.
   b. Postoperative, due to poor quality of soft tissues.
6. Urologic complications.
   a. Frequent urinary tract infections.
   b. Vesicoureteral reflux.
   c. Hydronephrosis.
7. Bowel complications.
   a. Impaction.
   b. Rectal prolapse.
8. Fractures of femur and tibia: peak at 3-7 years.
9. Pressure ulcers and skin breakdown on insensate areas.
10. Knee arthropathy in early 20s due to valgus-external rotation thrust during ambulation.
11. Charcot arthropathy.
    a. Progressive degeneration of metatarsal-phalangeal joint of great toe in insensate foot.
    b. Minor trauma causes swelling and redness around joint resembling cellulitis.
    c. Trauma progresses as patient continues to walk on injured foot.

II. ASSESSMENT
A. See Table 11.9.
B. History.
1. Presenting symptoms.
2. Onset and progression of presenting symptoms and

previous treatment.

a. Deterioration in neurologic status warrants careful evaluation.
b. Urinary tract infection.
c. Increased intracranial pressure/shunt malfunction.
   (1) Hydrocephalus.
      (a) High-pitched, shrill cry.
      (b) Malaise: vague symptoms of not feeling well.
      (c) Nausea, vomiting.
      (d) Severe headaches and/or neck pain.
      (e) Decreased upper extremity strength.
      (f) Increased paralysis or spasticity of lower extremities.
   (2) Shunt malfunction.
      (a) Symptoms of hydrocephalus.
      (b) Blurred vision.
      (c) Increased irritability.
      (d) Decreased perceptual motor function.
      (e) Short attention span.
      (f) Coma.

3. Pregnancy and birth history.
4. History of latex allergy or sensitivity.
5. Developmental history.
6. Neurologic status.
7. Functional limitations.
8. Bowel and bladder patterns.
9. Social interactions/relationships with peers.

C. Physical examination.

1. At birth, location, size, contents, and intactness of sac.
2. Height and weight.
3. Skin.
   a. Pressure ulcers from braces, sitting in wheelchair.
   b. Abrasion on insensate areas.
4. Eye: stabismus.
5. Musculoskeletal.
   a. Contractures.
   b. Foot deformities.
   c. Level of motor deficit.
   d. Strength in upper extremities.
   e. Scoliosis/kyphoscoliosis.
   f. Mobility/gait.
6. Neurologic.
   a. Signs and symptoms of increased intracranial pressure.
   b. Signs of Arnold-Chiari malformation.
      (1) Abnormal gag reflex.
      (2) Staring spells.
      (3) Nystagmus.
      (4) Apneic spells.
   c. Level of sensory deficit.
   d. Reflex activity of upper and lower extremities.
7. Genitourinary.
   a. Bladder size and tone, sphincter tone.
   b. Location and size of kidneys.
   c. Signs of precocious puberty.
8. GI: impaction or rectal prolapse.
9. Functional status.

D. Diagnostic tests.

1. Antenatal testing.
   a. Serum alphafetoprotein (AFP) at 16-18 weeks gestation.
   b. High-resolution ultrasound to detect abnormalities of head and back consistent with NTD.
   c. Amniocentesis for acetylcholinesterase (ACH) level in amniotic fluid: enzyme specific for NTD.
2. Radiographs.
   a. To evaluate bony abnormalities in involved areas (hips, knees, feet, spine, etc.).
   b. To evaluate function of ventriculoperitoneal (VP) shunt: shunt series.
3. MRI or CT: Head, spine, or hips.
4. Ultrasound of kidneys.
5. Cystometrogram.
6. Urodynamics.
7. Voiding cystourethrogram.
8. Intravenous pyelogram.

III. COMMON TREATMENT MODALITIES

A. Objectives of treatment.

1. Before surgical repair on myelomeningocele.
   a. Prevent infection of the sac.
   b. Protect exposed spinal cord and nerves from injury.
2. After surgical repair of myelomeningocele.
   a. Prevent development of complications.
   b. Maximize independence in ADL.
3. Care requires coordinated effort of interdisciplinary team.

B. Neurosurgical interventions.

1. Surgical closure of defect within the first 24-48 hours.
2. Placement of ventriculoperitoneal (VP) shunt to treat hydrocephalus.
   a. Cerebrospinal fluid drains into peritoneal cavity.
   b. Can become blocked, kinked, or infected.
3. Shunt revision for kinked, blocked, or infection VP shunt.
4. Release of tethered cord if necessary.

C. Orthopaedic interventions.

1. Orthotics.
   a. Stabilize weight-bearing joints.
   b. Support trunk in sitting and stance.
   c. Abduction brace for hip dysplasia.
   d. Cannot control fixed deformities.
   e. Use to maintain corrected position after surgery.
2. Parapodiums, standing tables, and other devices.
   a. Maintain an upright position.
   b. Teach ambulation.
   c. Place weight on the lower extremities.
3. Serial casting for clubfeet, in preparation for surgery.
4. Surgery.
   a. Stabilize and prevent progression of scoliosis or kyphoscoliosis.

b. Correct foot, ankle, and knee deformities.
c. Release soft tissue contractures

D. Urologic interventions.

1. Nonsurgical.
   a. Timed voiding with or without pharmacologic adjuncts.
   b. Clean intermittent catheterization.
   c. Anticholinergic therapy to decrease bladder wall contractions – oxybutynin chloride (Ditropan®).
   d. Pseudephedrine (Sudafed®) or imipramine chloride (Tofranil®) to increase storage of urine.
2. Surgery.
   a. Bladder augmentation.
      (1) A piece of colon or gastric tissue used to enlarge the bladder.
      (2) Appendico-vesicostomy – appendix used as conduit to catheterization.
   b. Artificial urinary sphincters control continence in a very select group of patients.

E. Pediatric care.

1. Routine pediatric care essential.
2. Monitor neurologic status.
3. Monitor development and refer to early intervention programs.
4. Oversee development and academic needs.
   a. Learning disabilities are prevalent in children with spina bifida.
   b. High incidence of visual/spacial and perceptual problems as well as attention deficit disorders.
5. Monitor weight.
   a. Obesity is a common problem.
   b. Early education regarding nutritional needs and physical activity.
   c. Gagging with delay in accepting textures is common.

IV. NURSING DIAGNOSES, OUTCOMES, AND INTERVENTIONS

A. See Table 11.1.

B. See Table 11.7.

C. Tissue perfusion, altered: cerebral.
Injury, risk for.

1. Outcome: no signs/symptoms of increased intracranial pressure.
2. Interventions.
   a. Instruct patient/significant others on signs and symptoms of increased intracranial pressure and shunt malfunction during childhood.
   b. Stress the importance of regular neurosurgical follow-up to check the functioning of the shunt and monitor child's status.
   c. Evaluate neurologic status on each visit.

D. Physical mobility, impaired.

1. Outcome: optimal mobility achieved.
2. Interventions.
   a. Encourage patient to work toward maximum mobility.
      (1) Benefits of ambulation.
         (a) Strengthening of upper extremities.
         (b) Protection against obesity.
         (c) Improved bone density.
         (d) Prevention of lower extremity contractures.
         (e) Increased independence.
         (f) Wider range of experiences.
      (2) When ambulation is not a realistic goal, help significant others secure mobility devices, such as wheelchair, cart, and parapodium.
      (3) Encourage patient/significant others to maximize mobility by using prescribed orthotic devices, such as the parapodium during the toddler stage and leg braces when patient grows older.
   b. Emphasize how bracing promotes ambulation and normalizes patient's life.
   c. Emphasize a program of active/passive range of motion to prevent contractures and promote mobility.

E. Skin integrity, impaired.

1. Outcome: intact skin evidenced by lack of sores or ulcers.
2. Interventions.
   a. Teach patient/family the importance of daily hygiene and skin checks for cuts, sores.
   b. Teach older child to check soles of feet with hand mirror and protect soles of feet from rough surfaces.
   c. Stress importance of protecting the skin from temperature extremes.
      (1) Test bath water to prevent burning of insensate skin.
      (2) Warm clothing to prevent frostbite.
   d. Instruct patient to "wean into" new braces and shoes to prevent pressure sores.
   e. Assess wheelchair needs and provide proper seating.
   f. Instruct wheelchair-bound patients to shift weight and do "wheelchair push-ups."

F. Urinary elimination, altered patterns.

1. Outcome: successful bladder training achieved.
   a. Social continence achieved.
   b. No signs/symptoms of urinary tract infections.
2. Interventions.
   a. Emphasize the importance of adequate fluid intake.
   b. Discuss importance of good perineal skin care.
   c. Counsel patient/family regarding long-term urologic management.
   d. Assist/instruct family in a bladder continence regime as needed.
   e. When required, provide teaching and demonstration of clean, intermittent catheterization technique.
      (1) Assess patient/family's success and compliance with catheterization program.
      (2) Educate patient/family on medications prescribed for catheterization program.
      (3) Support patient in developing social conti-

nence.

(4) When necessary, facilitate patient's catheterization program by contacting school nurse, teacher.

f. Teach patient/family signs and symptoms of urinary tract infections.

G. Incontinence, bowel.

1. Outcomes.
   a. Regular bowel elimination.
   b. Social continence.
2. Interventions.
   a. Interview significant others to obtain patient's bowel movement pattern.
   b. Teach family bowel regimen.
      (1) Initiate bowel regimen at age 2-3.
      (2) Establish morning or evening routine for patient's bowel program.
      (3) Educate patient/significant others on use of digital stimulation, suppository, enema, or oral adjuncts.
   c. Emphasize importance of adequate fluid intake.
   d. Emphasize diet which includes food high in bulk.
   e. Encourage physical activity, mobility.

H. Nutrition, imbalanced: more than body requirement.

1. Outcome: healthy body weight evidenced by weight for height on pediatric growth charts which does not exceed 80th percentile.
2. Interventions.
   a. Monitor patient's height and weight
   b. Begin counseling significant others when patient is an infant that patient will be prone to excessive weight gain.
   c. Give information and support to caretakers regarding gagging and introduction of textures.
   d. Counsel patient/significant others that obesity may interfere with ambulatory potential/function and self-care skills.

I. See Chapter 6, Effects of Immobility.

VI. PRACTICE SETTING CONSIDERATIONS

A. Office/outpatient.

1. Counsel patient and family about long-term health care needs.
   a. Multidisciplinary care to meet the multisystem needs of myelomeningocele patients.
   b. Ophthalmologist to monitor and treat strabismus.
   c. Neurosurgery to monitor shunt functioning and neurologic status.
   d. Endocrinology to evaluate precocious puberty.
   e. Orthopaedics to evaluate and treat musculoskeletal problems.
2. Neurologic exam on each visits: deterioration indicates development of tethered cord or shunt malfunction.
3. Collaborate with primary care provider regarding sexuality teaching and birth control education.

B. Hospital.

1. Latex allergy.
   a. Assess patient for latex allergy or risk factors.
   b. Administer premedication every 6 hours X 3 before surgery as ordered.
      (1) Corticosteroid IV or PO.
      (2) H1-Blocker IV or PO.
      (3) H2-blocker IV or PO.
   c. Administer intraoperative medications every 6 hours as ordered.
   d. Document allergy status.
   e. Use latex-free products whenever possible.
      (1) Latex products should not come in contact with patient's skin.
      (2) Powder-free gloves to prevent airborne particles.
   f. Be alert for new reactions in high-risk patients.
2. Maintain normal bladder and bowel regimen.
3. Increased risk of postoperative infection due to low-grade urinary tract infections and poor quality of soft tissues.

C. Home care considerations.

1. Stress importance of good hygiene and skin care, particularly in perineal and insensate areas.
2. Teach patient and family importance of at least daily skin checks to all insensate areas.
3. Well-balanced diet is important for good nutrition and prevention of obesity.
4. Modify home environment for handicapped accessibility.
5. Encourage independence in ADL. Stress to parents the importance of allowing child as much independence as his/her condition permits.
6. Maintain a consistent therapy program to prevent contractures and promote mobility.
7. Mobility aids as needed to maximize patient's function mobility.
8. Teach parents care of child in braces, when appropriate.
9. Offer family information about Spina Bifida Association.

CEREBRAL PALSY (CP)

I. OVERVIEW

A. Definition: a term used for a group of chronic neurologic disorders characterized by abnormal muscle control, movement, and posture.

1. Physiologic classification: three main types of motor abnormalities.
   a. Spastic type (80% of cases).
      (1) Lesion in cortical motor area or pyramidal tract.
      (2) Abnormally strong tonus of certain muscle groups.
      (3) Can affect any number of limbs.
   b. Dyskinetic (dystonic, athetoid) type.
      (1) Lesions of extrapyramidal tract and basal ganglia.
      (2) Involuntary, uncoordinated, uncontrollable

movements.
   c. Ataxic type (uncommon).
      (1) Lesion in cerebellum.
      (2) Disturbances of balance.
2. Anatomic classification.
   a. Hemiplegia.
      (1) One side of body involved.
      (2) Upper extremity more involved than lower extremity.
      (3) Most common type.
      (4) Seizure disorders common, possible due to focal brain lesion.
   b. Diplegia.
      (1) Both lower extremities involved.
      (2) Upper extremities involved to a lesser degree.
      (3) Spastic diplegia commonly associated with prematurity.
   c. Quadriplegia.
      (1) Involvement of all four limbs.
      (2) Many have global involvement.
   d. Anatomic patterns not always clear-cut.

B. Etiology.

1. Cerebral palsy (CP) is the result of hypoxia to the brain.
   a. Original insult results in a fixed static lesion affecting motor performance.
   b. Insult usually occurs during early CNS development.
2. Etiology is unknown in approximately one-third of cases.
3. Maternal factors.
   a. Multiple gestation pregnancy.
   b. Preterm labor/threatened abortion.
   c. Premature placental separation.
   d. History of fetal loss.
4. Prenatal factors.
   a. Intrauterine growth retardation.
   b. Congenital malformations.
   c. Twin gestation.
5. Perinatal factors.
   a. Prolonged, precipitous, or traumatic delivery.
   b. Apgar score less than 3 at 15 minutes.
   c. Venous cord blood pH less than 6.9.
   d. Premature or postmature birth.
   e. Abnormal fetal presentation.
6. Postnatal factors.
   a. Hypoxic-ischemic encephalopathy with multiorgan failure.
   b. Periventricular leukomalacia.
   c. Intracranial or intraventricular hemorrhage.
   d. Hyperbilirubinemia.

C. Pathophysiology.

1. Insult to developing brain in prenatal, perinatal, or postnatal period.
2. Clinical findings related to area of brain that is injured.
3. Brain lesion is permanent and nonprogressive.
   a. As the brain matures, the neuromotor signs of cerebral palsy change.
   b. Effects of growth of nervous system and growth and development of child can exacerbate characteristics.
4. Associated deficits due to CNS damage.
   a. Mental retardation (60% of cases) or some lesser degree of cognitive impairment.
   b. Hearing impairment.
   c. Visual impairments.
      (1) Strabismus.
      (2) Perceptual problems.
      (3) Nystagmus.
      (4) Cortical blindness.
   d. Speech-language disorders.
   e. Sensory impairment.
   f. Seizures (20%-30% of cases).
   g. Feeding and growth abnormalities
   h. Drooling, difficulty swallowing.
   i. Gait abnormalities due to loss of selective muscle control.
5. Gastrointestinal and genitourinary involvement.

D. Incidence.

1. 1.4-2.5 per 1,000 births overall.
2. 12 times more common in twin pregnancies.
3. More common in males.
4. More common in African American population.

E. Considerations across the lifespan.

1. Achievement of normal developmental milestones is delayed or absent.
2. Early intervention stimulates social, cognitive, and language development in infants.
3. Initial neurologic deficit is nonprogressive; however, physical deformities and functional impairments may progress due to abnormal tone or postural reflexes.
4. Scoliosis or hip dislocations may develop during childhood.
5. Thorough academic and psychologic evaluations should be done to develop a comprehensive program for preschool and school-age children.
6. As child grows in size, family may experience difficulty managing daily care.
7. Vocational counseling should be provided to assist adolescents in setting realistic career goals.

F. Complications.

1. Malnutrition.
2. Increased incidence of urinary tract infections.
3. Respiratory compromise.
4. Fractures due to disuse osteopenia.

II. ASSESSMENT

A. See Table 11.10.

B. History.

1. Presenting symptoms.
   a. Newborn/young infant.
      (1) Hypotonia ("floppy baby").
      (2) Asymmetry in motion or contour.
      (3) Listlessness, irritability, twitching, or stiffness.
      (4) Vomiting/reflux.
      (5) Difficulty feeding, sucking, keeping nipple

Table 11.10
Clinical Findings in Cerebral Palsy

	Spastic Diplegia	Hemiplegia	Quadriplegia	Dyskinetic (Dystonic, Athetoid)
	• LE more affected than UE or face	• Unilateral spastic motor weakness	• Involvement of head, neck and all four limbs	• Motor restlessness; intermittent movement of head, neck, limbs, hands and/or feet
Commonly related to	• Prematurity	• Congenital or acquired	• Full-term infant with cortical injury from hypoxemia-ischemia • Prematurity	• Kernicterus • Cardiac by-pass surgery
Early signs Later signs	• Hypotonia • Episodes of increased general tone caused by change in posture • Increasing spasticity	• Rarely suspected in newborn • "Hand preference" at 4-5 months • Delayed or absent pincer grasp		• Variable hypotonia or postural instability • Insidious development of adventitious movements at 6-12 months
Head/UE involvement	• Functional use of hands	• Held in abduction with flexion at wrist and hyperextension of fingers • Slower growth on affected side	• Weakness of facial and pharyngeal musculature: dysphagia, GE reflux • Cranial nerve palsies	• Tongue thrusting • Chewing movement • Orofacial grimacing • Hypotonia of neck and trunk
LE involvement	• Sitting: flexion of hips and knees • Standing: "scissoring of legs	• Ambulates within normative time	• Paucity of lower extremity movement	• Extensor posturing of foot
Speech/swallowing	• Minimally affected	• Language impairments with injury to either hemisphere	• Fail to acquire complex speech or language	• Marked impairment in language
Seizures	• Uncommon		• Common	
Sensory impairment	• Visual-spatial deficits • Strabismus		• Cortical blindness • Sensorineural hearing loss	• Hearing loss • Visual disturbances
Cognitive development	• Normal/near normal intelligence • Mild to moderate learning disabilities	• Intelligence variable: correlated with severity of seizures	• Variable: influence by underlying pattern of brain injury • Generally some degree of mental retardation exacerbated by seizures • Constipation/fecal impaction	• Receptive language and intelligence near normal
Treatment goals	• Independent ambulation		• Maximal functional independence and social adaptation	• Good positioning to support trunk and head • Language and communication

in mouth, or swallowing.
(6) Excessive irritability, high pitched, weak cerebral cry.
(7) Long, thin infants who are slow to gain weight.
b. Older infant/child.
(1) Abnormal tone, posture, and quality of movement.
(a) Difficulty separating legs when changing diapers.
(b) Tremors in arms or legs after sudden movement or crying.
(c) Hyperextension of neck when head is unsupported.
(d) Scissoring of legs when lifted (at any age).
(e) Any variation in quality of muscle tone or stiffness when handling.
(f) Thumb clenched tightly in palm after 4 months of age.
(g) Kicking legs in unison.
(2) Continuous tongue movement in and out of mouth.
(3) Weakness or apparent preference for one hand before 11-15 months.
(4) Excessive sleeping difficulties, overreaction to stimuli.
(5) Delayed or impaired speech.
(6) Visual or hearing impairments.
2. Onset and progression of presenting symptoms and previous treatment.
3. General health.
4. Pregnancy and birth history.
5. Developmental history.
a. Delayed developmental milestones.
b. Failure to follow normal pattern of gross and fine motor development.
c. Persistence of primitive reflexes.
6. Functional limitations.
7. History of seizures.
8. Nutrition and growth history.
9. Bowel and bladder patterns.
10. Social interactions/relationships with peers.

C. Physical examination.
1. Height and weight.
2. Skin.
a. Pressure ulcers from braces, sitting in wheelchair.
b. Abrasion due to uncontrolled movements/efforts to be mobile.
3. Musculoskeletal.
a. Muscle tone.
b. Strength and selective control.
c. Joint range of motion/contractures.
d. Hip subluxation/dislocation.
e. Angular or rotational deformities of extremities.
f. Scoliosis.
g. Gait, balance, standing, and walking postures.
4. Neurologic.
a. Cranial nerves.
b. Posture.
c. Trunk and neck (head control).
d. Deep tendon reflexes.
e. Primitive reflexes.
(1) Asymmetric tonic neck reflex.
(2) Truncal incurvations (Galant) reflex.
(3) Plantar grasp.
(4) Crossed extension.
(5) Truncal support.
f. Perceptual impairments.
g. Choking and difficulty in swallowing.
5. Dental anomalies.
6. Functional status.
7. Emotional and social problems.

D. Diagnostic tests.
1. Diagnosis is made on basis of clinical findings.
2. Radiographs.
a. Routine views of hips to evaluate hip subluxation/dislocation.
b. Weight-bearing films of feet and ankles prior to surgery.
c. Routine views of spine to evaluate scoliosis.
3. Barium swallow or pH probe to evaluate gastroesophageal reflux.
4. Electroencephalogram (EEG) to evaluate seizure disorder.
5. Blood tests to evaluate nutritional status.
a. Total serum protein and albumin.
b. Iron, iron-binding capacity, and transferrin levels.
c. Hemoglobin, erythrocyte mean corpuscular volume.
d. Total lymphocyte count.
6. Gait analysis for preoperative evaluation before tendon transfers.
7. MRI, PET, CT – may be used to evaluate intracranial pathology.

III. COMMON THERAPEUTIC MODALITIES

A. Goal is to treat the symptoms and prevent complications.
1. Early intervention for the child with CP is important because of the great adaptability and plasticity of the infantile brain.
2. Child with CP best managed by interdisciplinary team.
3. Functional priorities.
a. Communication.
b. ADLs.
c. Mobility in environment.
d. Walking.

B. Nonsurgical interventions.
1. Positioning to address tone and movement abnormalities.
a. Purpose is to:
(1) Promote skeletal alignment.
(2) Compensate for abnormal posture.
(3) Prepare child for independent mobility.
b. Includes side-liers, prone wedges, standers, specially-designed seating systems.

2. Physical therapy.
   a. Different modalities attempt to modify CNS by externally applied stimuli.
      (1) Modalities include.
         (a) Neurodevelopmental treatment (Bobath approach).
         (b) Sensory integration therapy.
         (c) Patterning.
         (d) Conducive-education.
         (e) Pressure-point stimulation.
         (f) Bracing and stretching.
         (g) Recreational therapies.
      (2) Results are controversial.
   b. Home program with parental involvement to maintain strength and range of motion.
   c. Postoperative rehabilitation to maximize benefits of surgery/regain preoperative strength.
   d. Assistance with adaptive and therapeutic equipment.
3. Braces and splints.
   a. Purpose is to:
      (1) Prevent deformity.
      (2) Provide support to joint by substituting for weakened muscle.
      (3) Protect weakened part.
   b. Lower extremity: (molded) ankle-foot-orthosis common to prevent plantar flexion.
   c. Upper extremity: resting hand splint to keep thumb adducted and wrist in neutral.
4. Manipulation and serial casting.
5. Medications (see Table 11.11).
   a. Seizure management.
   b. Management of gastroesophageal reflux.
   c. Nerve block and motor point blocks
      (1) Nerve block: direct injection of agent into motor nerve.
      (2) Motor-point block: injection interrupts nerve supply at entry site without compromising sensation.
      (3) Goal is to weaken muscle and balance forces across a joint.
         (a) May allow stretching and strengthening PT program.
         (b) Repeated injections may be necessary.
         (c) Can be painful.
   d. Botulinum-A injection.
      (1) Potent neurotoxin.
      (2) Injected directly into spastic muscles.
      (3) Causes weakening of muscle and reduction of spasticity for 3-6 months.
      (4) Little evidence regarding long-term effects.
6. Occupational therapy.
7. Speech therapy/hearing aid.

C. Surgical interventions.

1. To prevent or correct serious structural changes and decreased function in adult life.
2. Osteotomies to correct fixed bony deformities and stabilize joints.
3. Tendon lengthenings.
   a. Heel cords.
   b. Adductor tenotomy or myotomy.
   c. Hamstring releases or lengthening for knee flexion deformity.
4. Tendon transfers to restore muscle balance.
5. Anterior release and posterior spinal fusion with instrumentation to treat scoliosis.
6. Selective posterior rhizotomy.
   a. To reduce tone and facilitate normal movement by balancing muscle tone.
   b. Surgically divide dorsal roolets supplying spastic muscles.
   c. Intensive PT required after surgery.
   d. Results variable.
      (1) Have been best in 3-8 year olds with spastic diplegia.
      (2) Dramatic improvement in LE function.
      (3) Some improvement in UE, bladder control, swallowing/speech.
      (4) Does not affect joint contractures.
      (5) Can rapidly develop hip subluxation.

IV. NURSING DIAGNOSES, OUTCOMES, AND INTERVENTIONS

A. See Table 11.1.

B. See Table 11.7.

C. Aspiration, risk for.

1. Outcome: patient does not aspirate.
2. Interventions.
   a. If tongue thrust present, place food or medications to one side or back of tongue to facilitate swallowing.
   b. Stroke from neck to chin to stimulate swallowing.

D. Physical mobility, impaired.

1. Outcome: parent understands exercise/activity program.
2. Interventions.
   a. Assist with active/passive range of motion to joints to maintain and promote mobility.
   b. Lift patient in a flexed, sitting position.
   c. Encourage bilateral hand movement through use of play when patient is prone.
   d. Adapt wheelchair to maintain proper body alignment.

E. Pain, chronic.

1. Outcome: patient achieves maximal level of comfort.
2. Interventions.
   a. Assess for signs of discomfort related to spasticity.
      (1) Alternates between crying and calm.
      (2) Sudden, jerking movement of extremity, followed by crying.
      (3) Wakes from sleep.
      (4) Is relieved by change in position, especially to prone position.
      (5) Improves when treated with administration of muscle relaxants, not with analgesics alone.
   b. Assess for muscle spasms after surgery.

Table 11.11
Medications Used in Cerebral Palsy

	Drug	Medication Classification	Side Effects	Nursing Implications
Muscle spasms	Diazepam (Valium®) Baclofen (Lioresal®)	• Skeletal muscle relaxant; antianxiety agent • Skeletal muscle relaxant; antispasmodic	• Drowsiness; hypotension; fatigue • Drowsiness; dizziness; weakness	• Used primarily in the postoperative period to reduce muscle spasms and tone. • Taper dose when discontinued: withdrawal side effect includes seizures. • When teaching patient/family about medication, set realistic expectations of what drug can do: does not cause dramatic reduction in muscle spasms/tone. • May be injected intrathecally.
	Local anesthetic		• Sensory loss along nerve pathway	• Injected in immediate vicinity of specific nerve as nerve block. • Short acting, reversible conduction block.
	Alcohol		• Local pain at injection site	• Inject into muscle fibers in region distribution. • Inhibits nerve transmission and muscle contractions.
	Phenol		• Local pain at injection site	• Permanent nerve effect.
	Botulinum-A toxin	Neurotoxin		• Injected into sites of nerve branching in muscles • Blocks release of acetylcholine from synapses at myoneuronal junction • Effect begins in 12-72 hours, lasts 3-6 months • Contraindicated for fixed joint contractures
Seizures	Phenytoin sodium (Dilantin®)	Anticonvulsant	• Slurred speech • Confusion • Nystagmus • Gingival hyperplasia	• Therapeutic levels should be checked to achieve optimal dosage adjustments.

Table 11.11 (continued)
Medications Used in Cerebral Palsy

	Drug	Medication Classification	Side Effects	Nursing Implications
Seizures (continued)				• Give drug with or after meals to reduce gastric distress. • Instruct patient/family on importance of not missing doses. • Instruct patient/family on importance of meticulous oral hygiene.
	Carbamazepine (Tegretol®)	Anticonvulsant	• Dizziness; drowsiness; hematologic changes; nausea, vomiting	• Pre-treatment blood studies to identify any abnormalities. • Periodic evaluations necessary, especially with symptoms of potential hematologic problem. • Effective in partial seizures and tonic/clonic seizures.
	Valproic acid (Depakene®)	Anticonvulsant	• Nausea, vomiting; sedation; hepatotoxicity	• Liver function tests prior to initiation of therapy and at regular intervals. • Take with meals to prevent GI distress. • Effective in myoclonic seizures and absence(petit mal) seizures.
	Phenobarbital (Luminal®)	Anticonvulsant (barbiturate)	• Excitement and hyperactivity in children; drowsiness; GI upset	• Withdraw drug gradually to prevent convulsions, tremors.
GE Reflux	Metoclopramide (Reglan®)	Antiemetic	• Restlessness; agitation; seizures	• Contraindicated in patients with seizures. • Administer 30 minutes before meals.

c. Differentiate between soft-tissue/bony pain and muscle spasms.
d. Avoid startling patient.
(1) Approach slowly and speak softly.
(2) Initiate physical contact with firm but gentle pressure.
e. Explain occurrence of muscle spasms after surgery.
f. Assess degree of muscle spasms preoperatively: muscles involved, usual patterns, usual management.
g. Discuss postoperative management of muscle spasms.
(1) Comfort measures often impeded by postoperative immobilization.
(2) Muscle relaxant (commonly diazepam) is used.
(3) Opiates do not manage pain related to muscle spasms.
h. Administer muscle relaxant (commonly diazepam) round-the-clock for 48-72 hours.

F. Nutrition, imbalanced: less than body requirements.
1. Outcome: patient receives adequate nutrition as evidenced by stable growth curve.
2. Interventions.
a. Complete diet assessment, including calorie and nutrition intake and feeding history.
b. Assess for gastroesophageal reflux.
c. Identify high-calorie foods.
d. Teach enteric feeding regimens: nasogastric, gastric, or jejunal feedings

V. PRACTICE SETTING CONSIDERATIONS

A. Office/outpatient.
1. Orthopaedic findings indicative of CP.
a. Unexplained abnormal posturing.
b. Limp.
c. Toe walking.
d. Limb asymmetry.
e. Joint tightness.
f. Developmental delay.
g. Persistent primitive reflexes.
2. Single evaluation not as useful as series of exams over time.
3. Facilitate routine pediatric well-child care and preventive health follow-up.
4. Collaborate with primary care provider regarding orthopaedic issues.
5. Refer for Early Intervention services.
6. Facilitate follow-up with specialists.
a. Neurology for seizure management.
b. Gastroenterology for gastroesophageal reflux.
c. Speech therapy for language and communication.
d. Physical therapy for mobility and seating.
7. Facilitate communication between caregivers and members of the health care team.

B. Hospital.
1. Assess nutritional status prior to surgery.
2. Prepare carefully for major surgical procedures: patients with CP often have little reserves and frequently develop postoperative complications, such as respiratory compromise.
3. Utilize child's regular mode of communication: sound signals, communication board.
4. Reinforce that child may have normal intelligence despite communication barriers.

C. Home care considerations.
1. Help family develop a home care routine.
a. Managing ADL.
b. Opportunities for interactive play, visual, and tactile exploration.
c. Use of adaptive devices for mobility.
d. Home therapy program that includes positioning, range of motion, and sensory stimulation.
e. Time and resources for pleasurable activities and social interaction.
2. Provide patient and family with information on technologic advances, such as computer communication and mobility devices. (Assist patient/family in locating funding agencies to provide adaptive equipment.)
3. Refer to dietitian or teach family about high-calorie foods and foods to promote bowel elimination.
4. Teach patient and family about medications.
a. Purpose of drug.
b. Side effects.
c. Dosage.
d. Potential food and drug interactions.
e. When to report problems, dosage.
f. Importance of not missing doses.
5. Help family work with school system to provide appropriate learning environment.
a. Testing for appropriate school placement.
b. Teaching school personnel about CP and child's needs.
6. Offer family information about United Cerebral Palsy Association.

DUCHENNE'S MUSCULAR DYSTROPHY

I. OVERVIEW

A. Definition: Duchenne's muscular dystrophy is hereditary myopathy characterized by progressive weakness in proximal muscle groups and pseudohypertrophy.
1. The muscular dystrophies are a group of genetic myopathies characterized by progressive muscle degeneration and weakness (see Table 11.12).
a. Myopathies primarily involve striate (skeletal) muscle.
b. Myopathies are not caused by impairment of the central nervous system, anterior horn cells, peripheral nerves, or neuromuscular junctions.
2. Duchenne's muscular dystrophy is the most common type of muscular dystrophy.

B. Etiology.
1. Defect at Xp21 region on the short arm of the X-

Table 11.12.
Clinical Features of Major Types of Muscular Dystrophy

	Duchenne's	Becker's	Limb-Girdle	Congenital Muscular Dystrophy	Fascio-scapulohumeral	Distal
Incidence	Most common type	Less common than Duchenne's	Less common than Duchenne's and Becker's	Rare	Rare	Rare
Age at onset	Generally before age 3	Most between 5-15 years	Usually by second decade	At birth or soon after	Anytime from childhood until adulthood, usually in second decade	20-77 years; mean is 47 years
Sex distribution	Males; rare cases in females with Turner's syndrome	Males	Both sexes	Both sexes	More common in females	Both sexes
Inheritance	Sex-linked recessive gene; 33% due to mutations	Sex-linked recessive gene	Usually autosomal recessive; may occur as autosomal dominant	Not known	Usually autosomal dominant	Autosomal dominant
Pattern of muscle involvement onset	Proximal pelvis muscles; shoulder girdle muscles become involved 3-5 years later	Similar to Duchenne's	Proximal shoulder and pelvic girdle	Generalized muscle weakness, including respiratory and facial muscles	Face, shoulder girdle, upper arm	Distal: Intrinsic muscles of hand, anterior tibiali, and calf
Late muscle involvement	All muscles, including facial, oculo-pharyngeal, and respiratory	Face is spared	More distal muscles: brachioradialis, hand, calf		Lower limbs	Proximal
Pseudohypertrophy	Calf muscles	Calf muscles	Occurs in fewer than 1/3 of cases	No	Rare	No
Contractural deformities	Common	Less common	Late, milder than Duchenne's	Severe	Mild, late	Mild, late
Scoliosis/kyphoscoliosis	Common late	Not severe	Mild, late	Yes	Mild, late	No
Cardiac involvement	Yes	Late, uncommon	Very rare	Not known	Very rare	Very rare
IQ	Decreased	Normal	Normal	Not known	Normal	Normal
Course	Steadily progressive	Slowly progressive	Variable: generally slowly progressive	Variable: rapidly progressive or can stabilize	Insidious with prolonged periods of apparent arrest	Slow progression

chromosome.

2. X-linked recessive trait.
   a. Females are the carriers of the single gene defect.
   b. Trait expressed primarily in boys.
   c. Rare cases in females with Turner's syndrome.

C. Pathophysiology.

1. Because of genetic defect, body does not produce dystrophin, a component of the surface membrane of striated muscle cell.
   a. Necrosis caused by influx of Ca2+ into muscle fiber through defective surface membrane.
   b. Enzymes are lost from sarcoplasm of muscle into circulation.
2. Eventual decrease in number of muscle fibers due to necrosis of fibers accompanied by phagocytosis.
3. Regenerating fibers are structurally abnormal.
4. Hip contractures develop to help maintain standing posture as weakness in hip girdle increases.
5. Pseudohypertrophy of muscles as normal muscle is replaced with adipose and collagen.
6. Cardiac involvement includes tachycardia and right ventricular hypertrophy.
7. Patients have low-normal intelligence.
8. Progressive scoliosis develops after ambulation is lost.
9. Obesity may be related to limited physical activity, depression, and boredom.
10. Gastrointestinal (GI) tract involvement (megacolon, volvulus, cramping pain, malabsorption) is rare.

D. Incidence.

1. Occurs in 1 in approximately 3,500 live male births.
2. Primarily sex-linked inheritance, but 1/3 cases result from new mutations.

E. Considerations across the lifespan.

1. First trimester chorionic villous sampling can determine fetal gender and whether the deletion exists on the X chromosome.
2. Duchenne's muscular dystrophy is clinically evident at 3-6 years.
3. Most patient are wheelchair-bound by the end of the first decade.
4. Adolescents are usually unable to perform routine daily tasks with their arms, hands, and fingers.
5. Only 25% of patients survive beyond age 21.

F. Complications.

1. Low back pain with hip flexion contractures.
2. Fractures in wheelchair-bound.
3. Rapid deterioration in strength after being immobilized in bed.
4. Respiratory insufficiency.
5. Sudden cardiac failure.
6. Pulmonary infection.
7. Malignant hyperthermia with anesthesia.

II. ASSESSMENT

A. History.

1. Presenting symptoms.
   a. Muscle weakness.
      (1) Weakness begins in proximal muscle groups.
      (2) Weakness descends symmetrically in lower extremities.
         (a) Pelvic girdle affected first: gluteus maximus, gluteus medius, quadriceps.
         (b) Tibialis anterior and abdominal muscles affected.
      (3) Progresses to shoulder girdle (trapezius, deltoid, pectoralis major).
      (4) Lower facial muscles affected later.
   b. Frequently trips and/or falls.
   c. Difficulty running or climbing stairs (reciprocal motion).
   d. Unable to hop or jump normally.
2. Onset of presenting symptoms, progression, previous treatment.
3. Birth history.
4. Developmental history: independent ambulation often delayed.
5. Family history.
6. Functional status.

B. Physical examination.

1. Abnormal gait due to weakness of hip girdle muscles (gluteus maximus, gluteus medius, quadriceps).
   a. Rocks from side to side when walking.
   b. Waddling gait with lumbar lordosis.
2. Standing posture: wide-based stance, marked lumbar lordosis.
3. Uses maneuver known as Gower's sign to get up from the floor.
   a. Walks hands up thighs to push trunk erect.
   b. Compensates for quadriceps and gluteus maximus weakness.
   c. Usually seen by age 5 or 6.
4. Meyeron sign: child slips through truncal hold once shoulder girdle is involved.
5. Pseudohypertrophy of muscles.
   a. Typically in calf muscles.
   b. Also in vastus lateralis, infraspinous, deltoid.
6. Deep tendon reflexes.
   a. Absent in upper extremity and knee.
   b. Present in ankle until late stage of disease.
7. Presence of contractures.

C. Diagnostic tests.

1. Blood tests.
   a. Marked elevation in serum creatine phosphokinase (CPK): 200-300 times normal in early stages.
   b. Elevation in other serum enzymes: aldolase, serum glutamic oxaloacetic transaminase (SGOT)
2. Muscle biopsy from involved muscle.
3. EMG used to differentiate between myopathy and neuropathy.
4. Electrocardiogram to evaluate cardiac involvement.
5. Pulmonary function tests.

III. COMMON THERAPEUTIC MODALITIES

A. No treatment, surgery, or medication will halt disease progression: treatment with prednisone has been associated with short-term improvement and may prolong ambulation.

B. Orthopaedic problems.
1. Loss of independent ambulation.
2. Soft tissue contractures.
3. Spinal deformity.

C. Physical therapy.
1. Aimed at prolonged functional muscle strength and preventing contractures.
2. Active range of motion exercises.
3. Gait training and transfer techniques.
   a. Regular daily walking will enhance strength and prevent contractures.
   b. Ambulation may be achieved with crutches or walkers.
4. Wheelchair fitting and equipment recommendations when ambulation is lost.

D. Orthotics.
1. May have a role in preventing contractures.
2. In early stages, HKAFO with crutches for ambulation.

E. Surgery.
1. Tendon releases: soft tissue release of contractures when painful, interfere with ADL.
   a. Lower extremity.
      (1) Equinus and equinovarus contractures of feet.
      (2) Hip flexion and abduction contractures.
      (3) Knee flexion contractures in wheelchair bound.
   b. Upper extremity contractures common in adolescents, don't usually require treatment.
2. Spinal fusion with Unit rod for neuromuscular scoliosis (see Chapter 18, Spine).

IV. NURSING DIAGNOSES, OUTCOMES, AND INTERVENTIONS

A. See Table 11.1.

B. See Table 11.7.

V. PRACTICE SETTING CONSIDERATIONS

A. Office/outpatient.
1. Refer family for genetic counseling.
   a. Complete discussion of X-linked inheritance patterns.
   b. Methods of detecting carrier state in female siblings.
   c. Options for prenatal testing with subsequent pregnancies.
2. Reinforce information regarding signs, symptoms, expected clinical course.
   a. Child will become wheelchair dependent.
   b. Child is capable of continuing regular schooling and most daily activities.
3. Facilitate outpatient physical therapy.

B. Hospital.
1. Include a cardiac evaluation and pulmonary function tests as part of preoperative evaluation.
2. Implement measures to prevent malignant hyperthermia during anesthesia.
3. Consult with patient regarding positioning.
   a. Sensation is normal, though motion is not.
   b. Patient can get frustrated trying to explain what to do.
   c. Use calm, patient tone; try not to seem rushed.
   d. Assess for continued comfort or need to adjust position.
4. Mobilize the patient as soon as possible after surgery.

C. Home care considerations.
1. Reevaluate home care needs as child grows.
   a. Wheelchair adaptations as disease progresses.
   b. Hoyer lift/assistive devices to prevent injury to caregivers.
2. Offer family information about Muscular Dystrophy Association.

FREIDRICH'S ATAXIA

I. OVERVIEW

A. Definition: Freidrich's ataxia is a spinocerebellar degenerative disease, characterized by ataxia and corticospinal tract impingement. (Ataxia is the impaired ability to coordinate muscular movement, usually associated with staggering gait and postural imbalance).

B. Etiology.
1. Autosomal recessive trait.
2. Genetic mutation on chromosome 9 (9q13-21.1).
3. Defect causes abnormality in the protein frataxin: part of amino acid chain in repeated 700-800 times instead of the normal 7-22 times.

C. Pathophysiology.
1. Slowly progressive degeneration of cerebellar cortex and pathways in the spinal cord.
   a. Degeneration in cervical dorsal columns and lumbar pyramidal tracts of spinal cord.
      (1) Spinocerebellar tracts also involved.
      (2) Varying degrees of fiber loss, demyelination, and gliosis.
   b. Lesions in cerebellum and cerebrum more variable.
   c. Large myelinated axons in peripheral nerves affected.
2. As degeneration progresses, normal functions are lost.
   a. Progressive ataxia.
   b. Cerebellar dysarthria.
   c. Pyramidal weakness.
   d. Impaired vibration and joint position sense.
3. Ataxia may affect one side of the body before the other or both sides simultaneously.
4. Pathologic changes in heart include of cardiomyopathy and involvement of blood vessels, nerves, and ganglia.

D. **Incidence.**
   1. Most common hereditary ataxia.
   2. Affects 1 to 2 per 100,000 in the general population.
   3. Males and females and all races are equally affected.

E. **Considerations across the lifespan.**
   1. Onset before age 25 with a mean age of 7-15 years.
   2. Ability to walk may lost by early 20s.
   3. Remissions and stable periods are common.
   4. Existing symptoms may be aggravated or new deficiencies may appear in conjunction with concurrent infections.
   5. Patients survive into adult life and can have children.
   6. Death may occur in the 50s but some patients will live much longer.

F. **Complications.**
   1. Painful muscle spasms in hip adductors and knee extensors.
   2. Cardiac failure.
   3. Respiratory failure.
   4. Diabetes.
   5. Deterioration in mental status.

II. ASSESSMENT

A. **History.**
   1. Presenting symptoms.
      a. Progressive gait difficulty is usually first indication of disease.
         (1) Widening of base and wavering to either side.
         (2) May appear reeling or lurching.
      b. Difficulty walking.
      c. Difficulty making sudden turns.
   2. Onset and progression of presenting symptoms.
      a. Becomes increasingly "clumsy."
      b. Foot and ankle problems as foot deformity gradually develops.
         (1) Frequent episodes of ankles twisting.
         (2) Complaints of foot fatigue.
         (3) Difficulty finding comfortable shoes.
         (4) Often needs new shoes: wear out quickly or become misshapen.
   3. Developmental history: Ataxia of upper limbs may cause complaints of difficulty in learning to write or problems manipulating eating utensils.
   4. Family history.
   5. Trouble speaking or swallowing.
   6. Functional status.

B. **Physical examination.**
   1. Neurologic status.
      a. Ataxia.
         (1) Impaired balance (positive Romberg test).
         (2) Unsteady gait with wide base.
         (3) May present unilaterally but soon becomes bilateral.
      b. Loss of reflexes in lower extremities.
         (1) Absent knee and ankle deep tendon reflexes.
         (2) Extensor plantar response (Babinski reflex).
         (3) Abdominal and cremasteric reflexes usually preserved.
         (4) Reflexes in arms are usually retained longer.
      c. Dysarthria.
         (1) Quality of speech impaired early.
         (2) Decreased pace, slurring.
         (3) Uncontrolled outbursts of staccato volume changes.
      d. Swallowing difficulties delayed until terminal phases.
      e. Pyramidal weakness.
      f. Impaired vibration sense.
      g. Impaired proprioception.
   2. Musculoskeletal.
      a. Scoliosis.
      b. Pes cavovarus.
      c. Distal wasting.
      d. Muscle spasms.
         (1) Sudden onset, short duration.
         (2) Commonly hip adductors and knee extensors.
   3. Cardiac function.
   4. Optic atrophy.
   5. Higher cortical functioning appears to remain intact.
   6. Terminal stages.
      a. Personality changes.
      b. Bulbar disturbances.
      c. Loss of sphincter control.

C. **Diagnostic tests.**
   1. Diagnosis is based on physical exam.
   2. Nerve conduction studies show slight decrease in motor fiber conduction velocity but marked decrease in sensory action potential.
   3. ECG to evaluate cardiomyopathy.

III. COMMON THERAPEUTIC MODALITIES

A. **Scoliosis.**
   1. Bracing usually not well tolerated.
   2. Posterior spinal fusion.

B. **Pes cavovarus.**
   1. Orthotics usually not effective.
   2. Surgery.
      a. Tendo-Achilles lengthening with tibialis posterior tenotomy or transfer.
      b. Triple arthrodesis.

C. **Muscle spasms.**
   1. Initially treated with massage, heat.
   2. Muscle relaxants may be used: diazepam, baclofen.
   3. Tenotomy for spasms that interfere with sitting.

IV. NURSING DIAGNOSES, OUTCOMES, AND INTERVENTIONS

A. **See Table 11.1.**

B. **See Table 11.7.**

C. **Injury, risk for.**
   1. Outcome: patient remains free from injury.
   2. Interventions.

Table 11.13.
Clinical Features of Neurofibromatosis Types 1 and 2

	NF1	NF2
Diagnostic Criteria	Two or more of the following: • At least 6 café-au-lait spots 1. Larger than 5 mm in children 2. Larger than 15 mm in adults. • Two neurofibromas or a single plexiform neurofibroma. • Freckling in the axillae or inguinal region. • An optical glioma. • At least two Lisch nodules (white bumps on the iris). • A distinctive osseous lesion, such as vertebral scalloping or cortical thinning. • A first-degree relative with NF1.	Confirmed NF2: • Bilateral vestibular schwannomas (VS) or • Family history of NF2 plus: 1. Unilateral VS 2. Any two of the following: a. Meningioma b. Glioma c. Neurofibroma d. Schwannoma e. Posterior capsular lenticular opacities (SLO) Presumptive NF2 • Unilateral VS diagnosed before age 30 plus any two of the following: 1. Meningioma 2. Glioma 3. Neurofibroma 4. Schwannoma 5. SLO • Two or more Meningiomas plus: 1. Unilateral VS diagnosed before age 30 or 2. Any 2 of the following: a. Glioma b. Neurofibroma c. Schwannoma d. Cataract e. Cerebral calcification
Genetics	• Autosomal dominant • Defect on chromosome 17 (17q11.2) • Lack of protein neurofibrinomin	• Autosomal dominant • Defect on long arm of chromosome 22 (22q12.2) • Lack of gene product merlin or schwanomin
Incidence	1/3,000	1/40,000

a. Assess for sensory deficit routinely.
b. Instruct patient/significant other regarding need to assess body position and joint position.
c. Remind patient of need to compensate for sensory deficit (visual or tactile) as appropriate.
d. Assess body parts for unseen or unfelt injuries.

V. PRACTICE SETTING CONSIDERATIONS

A. Hospital.

1. Obtain cardiac consult to evaluate cardiomyopathy prior to surgery.
2. Complete careful neurologic exam preoperatively as baseline for postoperative assessments.

B. Home care considerations.

1. As care requirements become progressively greater, primary caregiver will require assistance.
2. Home remodeling may be necessary to accommodate required care equipment.

NEUROFIBROMATOSIS TYPE 1 (NF1)

I. OVERVIEW

A. Definition: Neurofibromatosis Type I (NF1) is a progressive disorder characterized by multiple tumors within the nervous system (central and peripheral) and is associated with variable abnormalities of the skin, skeleton, and soft tissues.

1. The most common types are neurofibromatosis Type 1(NF1) and neurofibromatosis Type 2 (NF2).
   a. NF1 (von Recklinhausen disease).
      (1) Peripheral form, characterized by café-au-lait spots and fibromas.
      (2) Orthopaedic involvement is common.
      (3) See Table 11.13.
   b. Neurofibromatosis Type 2 (NF2).
      (1) Central form, characterized by bilateral acoustic neuromas and few peripheral findings.

(2) See Table 11.13.

2. Numerous other types have been identified, including:
   a. Familiar spinal neurofibromatosis: extensive multiple spinal neurofibromas.
   b. "Neurofibromas alone": multiple subcutaneous and deep peripheral nerve tumors.
   c. Schwannomatosis: multiple peripheral and spinal schwannomas, CNS tumors and neurologic deficits.
3. The focus of this section will be NF1.
4. Mr. Merrick (the Elephant Man) probably had Proteus Syndrome, not neurofibromatosis.

B. Etiology.

1. Gene has been mapped to long arm of chromosome 17(17q11.2).
2. Autosomal dominant inheritance with variable penetrance.
3. Approximately 50% cases from spontaneous new mutations.

C. Pathophysiology.

1. Protein neurofibromin is decreased or absent.
   a. Neurofibromin has role in tumor suppression.
   b. Decreased amount/absence results in uncontrolled cell proliferation and tumor growth.
2. Growth disturbance apparent in neural crest cell growth and function.
   a. Cells of the neural crest become skin, brain, spinal cord, peripheral nerves, and adrenals.
   b. Cutaneous manifestations.
      (1) Café-au-lait spots.
         (a) Discrete tan spots, the color of "coffee with milk."
         (b) Wide variation in number, shape, size.
         (c) Found in areas of the skin not exposed to sun.
         (d) Primarily a cosmetic problem.
      (2) Freckling in axillae, groin, other skin folds.
   c. Cutaneous neurofibroma.
      (1) Composed of benign Schwann cells and fibrous connective tissue.
      (2) Occur anywhere, usually just under the skin.
      (3) Generally evident by age 10.
      (4) Usually no neurologic impact.
   d. Plexiform neurofibromas.
      (1) Proliferation of cells in nerve sheath extending along length of nerve.
      (2) Infiltrate into surrounding tissue.
      (3) May be visible or internal with no external evidence.
      (4) Soft tissue overgrowth results in hemihypertrophy.
      (5) Usually present at birth.
      (6) Tend to grow in early childhood and during periods of hormonal changes (adolescence, pregnancy).
      (7) Can undergo malignant transformation.
   e. Cerebral tumors.
      (1) Glioma, particularly optic pathway glioma.
         (a) Can block flow of cerebrospinal fluid.
         (b) Majority asymptomatic.
         (c) Can cause loss of vision.
      (2) Medulloblastoma and ependymoma of brain stem.
         (a) More indolent course than rest of oncology population.
         (b) 50% patients show clinical or radiological progression.
   f. Intraspinal and intermedullary tumors.
      (1) May be symptomatic: pain, loss of sensation, loss of reflexes at level of tumor.
      (2) Slowly progressive.
      (3) Difficult to treat.
   g. Spinal root neurofibromas.
3. Musculoskeletal manifestations.
   a. Scoliosis: idiopathic or dystrophic.
   b. Vertebral abnormalities.
      (1) Scalloping of posterior body, enlargement of neural formina, defective pedicles.
      (2) Dural ectasia may erode and thin posterior vertebral elements.
   c. Dysplasia of long bones.
      (1) Angular deformity.
         (a) Ranging from bowing to pseudoarthrosis.
         (b) Most common in tibia, but also ulna, radius, clavicle, femur.
      (2) Lytic areas resembling fibrous cortical defects.
      (3) Scalloping of cortex.

D. Incidence.

1. Most common single gene disorder in humans.
2. Affects 1 in 3,000 newborns.
3. No preference for either sex, any racial or ethnic group.

E. Considerations across the lifespan.

1. Disease cannot be diagnosed in many infants and children using standard criteria.
2. Anterolateral bowing of tibia warrants referral to orthopaedic surgeon.
3. Peak incidence of optic glioma is from 4-6 years.
4. Clinical manifestations develop during childhood: apparent in almost all affected individuals by age 8-10 years.
5. Learning disabilities common (30%-60% of children).
6. People with NF1 have fewer children than those who are unaffected.
7. Shortened life expectancy (early 60s) due to malignancies.

F. Complications.

1. Cutaneous or plexiform neurofibromas can affect appearance, depending on size and location.
2. Fractures characterized by poor healing, progressive pseudoarthrosis.
3. Seizures may signal existence of unrecognized tumor, hydrocephalus, or cerebrovascular disease.
4. Hydrocephalus may result from aqueductal stenosis.
5. Cerebrovascular disease is related to intrinsic abnor-

malities of intracranial vasculature.

6. Spinal meningoceles can cause headaches, minor neurologic symptoms, paraparesis.
7. Neurofibromatosis neuropathy due to accumulation of multiple peripheral neurofibromas.
8. Increased incidence of multiple sclerosis.
9. Increased incidence of childhood leukemia.
10. Malignant changes in peripheral cell tumors or plexiform neurofibroma.
11. Hypertension due to renal artery stenosis.

II. ASSESSMENT

A. History.

1. Present symptoms.
   a. Pain.
   b. Visual complaints.
   c. Neurologic symptoms.
      (1) Progressive neurologic deficits.
      (2) Changes in bowel or bladder function.
      (3) Weakness.
      (4) Seizures.
      (5) Headache
   d. Change in cutaneous findings.
2. History of development of clinical manifestations of NF1.
3. Present/past treatments.
4. Family history: tumors and skin lesions in 1st and 2nd degree relatives.
5. Neurologic deficits.
6. Musculoskeletal findings.
7. Cognitive or psychomotor deficits.
8. Exercise and play activities.

B. Physical examination.

1. Size and number of café-au-lait spots.
2. Freckling in axillae, groin, or other skin folds.
3. Cutaneous neurofibromas.
   a. Discrete nodules palpable just below the skin.
   b. Any body area.
   c. Rarely painful.
   d. May be itchy.
4. Plexiform neurofibroma.
   a. May be visible or internal.
   b. Skin may be hyperpigmented.
   c. May be tender or painful upon palpation.
   d. Hemihypertrophy from overgrowth of soft tissues.
   e. May affect cranial nerves.
5. Lisch nodules of the iris.
   a. Gelatinous elevations from the iris surface.
   b. Range from clear to yellow to brown in color.
   c. Usually bilateral.
6. Scoliosis.
   a. Idiopathic scoliosis: physical signs the same as idiopathic scoliosis in other populations.
   b. Dystrophic scoliosis.
      (1) Short curve with sharp angulation.
      (2) Onset at early age.
7. Tibial bowing.
   a. Apex usually anterolateral.
   b. Evident by age 2 years.
8. Pseudarthrosis of long bones.

C. Diagnostic tests.

1. Prenatal diagnosis is possible with chorionic villi sampling.
   a. Diagnosis through genetic linkage or by mutation, if family mutation is known.
   b. Cannot predict severity of clinical manifestations.
2. Radiographs.
   a. To monitor scoliosis.
   b. To evaluate intraspinal or paraspinal fibromas.
   c. To evaluate abnormalities of long bones.
3. MRI.
   a. To delineate extent of plexiform neurofibromas.
   b. To evaluate central nervous system tumors.
   c. "Unidentified bright spots" (UBOs) are incidental findings.
      (1) Areas of spongiform myelinopathy in basal ganglia, cerebellum, brain stem, pons.
      (2) Common in children, rare in adults.
      (3) Do not cause overt neurologic symptoms.
      (4) May be related to cognitive impairment.
4. Slit lamp eye exam to evaluate Lisch nodules or optic glioma.

III. COMMON THERAPEUTIC MODALITIES

A. Treatment is based on symptoms and complications of the illness.

B. Nonsurgical interventions.

1. Medical management of symptoms
2. Bracing.
   a. To protect long bone with pseudoarthosis.
   b. Does not prevent curve progression in dystrophic scoliosis.

C. Surgical interventions.

1. Spinal fusion for scoliosis.
   a. Idiopathic scoliosis managed with protocol similar to other populations.
   b. Dystrophic scoliosis.
      (1) Goal is stabilization, not correction.
      (2) 20-40 degree curves treated with posterior spinal fusion with instrumentation.
      (3) Curves greater than 40 degrees treated with combined anterior and posterior spinal fusion with instrumentation.
      (4) Postoperative bracing recommended.
2. Surgical removal of neurofibromas.
3. Pseudoarthrosis of the tibia.
   a. Resection of dysplastic bone with grafting.
   b. Transplant of vascularized fibula.
   c. Bone transport with external fixator.

IV. NURSING DIAGNOSES, OUTCOMES, AND INTERVENTIONS

A. See Table 11.1.

B. See Table 11.7.

C. Pain.

1. Outcome: patient has decreased pain or relief of pain.

2. Interventions: assist to minimize back pain.
   a. Teach relaxation techniques.
   b. Administer analgesics.
   c. Teach and encourage use of back brace.

V. PRACTICE SETTING CONSIDERATIONS: Office/outpatient

A. Referred family for genetic counseling.

B. Provide information on prognosis and anticipatory guidance.

1. Physical manifestations will develop and/or increase during first decade of life.
   a. Café-au-lait spots may be present at birth and may increase in number and size during first years of life.
   b. Skin fold freckling appears between 3-5 years.
2. Plexiform neurofibromas are usually congenital and may present as soft tissue enlargement.
3. Children with tibial dysplasia need to be followed for evaluation and/or treatment.
4. Annual ophthalmology exam to monitor development of optic glioma during first decade of life.
5. Children may need testing to evaluate learning disabilities.
6. Provide preliminary information about surgical options/possible surgical interventions.

C. Monitor blood pressure to assess development of hypertension.

D. Provide information to school to help plan for physical and psychosocial adjustment and proper academic placement.

E. Reinforce need for follow up to monitor nonmalignant and malignant tumors.

F. Offer family information about Neurofibromatosis Foundation.

Bibliography

Batshaw, M.L. (Ed.). (1997). *Children with disabilities (4th Ed).* Baltimore: Paul H. Brookes Publishing.

Bruce, R.W. (1996). Torsional and angular deformities. *Pediatric Clinics of North America, 43,* 867-881.

Byers, P.H. (1993). Osteogenesis imperfecta. In P.M. Royce & B. Steinmann (Eds). *Connective tissue and its heritable disorders: Molecular, genetic, and medical aspects* (pp. 317-350). New York: Wiley-Liss.

Davids, J.R., Foti, T., Dabelstein, J., Blackhurst, D.W., & Bagley, A. (1999). Objective assessment of dyskinesia in children with cerebral palsy. *Journal of Pediatric Orthopaedics, 19,* 211-214.

DiScala, C. (2000). Child abuse and unintentional injuries: A 10-year retrospective. *Archives of Pediatric and Adolescent Medicine, 154,* 16-22.

Drennan, J.C. (1999). Current concepts in myelomeningocele. *Instructional Course Lectures, 48,* 543-550.

Englebert, R.H.H., Pruijs, H.E.H., Beemer, F.A., & Helders, P.J.M. (1998). Osteogenesis imperfecta in childhood: Treatment strategies. *Archives of Physical Medicine and Rehabilitation, 79,* 1590-1594.

Giardino, A.P., Christian, C.W., & Giardino, E.R. (1997). *A practical guide to the evaluation of child physical abuse and neglect.* Thousand Oaks, CA: Sage Publications.

Green, M., Haggerty, R.J., & Weitzman, M. (Eds.) (1999). *Ambulatory pediatrics* (5th ed.). Philadelphia: Saunders.

Gutmann, D.H., Aylsworth, A., Carey, J.C., Korf, B., Marks, J., Pyeritz, R.E., Rubenstein, A., & Viskochil, D. (1997). The diagnostic evaluation and multidisciplinary management of neurofibromatosis I and neurofibromatosis 2. *JAMA, 278,* 51-57.

Hamdy, R.C., Fassier, F., Lachapelle, D., Gibis, J., Gervais, N., & Duhaime, M. (1998). The use of the Ilizarov method in children for limb lengthening. Medscape *Orthopaedics and Sports Medicine, 2,* 6.

Hecht, J.T., et al. (1985). Computerized tomography of the foramen magnum: Achondroplastic values compared to normal standards. *American Journal of Medical Genetics, 20*(2), 355-360.

Karol, L.A. (1997). Rotational deformities in the lower extremities. *Current Opinion in Pediatrics, 9,* 77-80.

Koeppen, A.H. (1998). The hereditary ataxias. *Journal of Neuropathology and Experimental Neurology, 57,* 531-543.

Liptak, G.S., (1999). Myelodysplasia. In M. Green, R.J. Haggerty, & M. Weitzman (Eds.), *Ambulatory pediatrics* (5th ed., pp. 251-258). Philadelphia: Saunders.

Marsden, C.D., & Fowler, T.J. (1998). *Clinical neurology* (2nd ed.). NewYork: Oxford University Press.

Morrissy, R.T., & Weinstein, S.L. (1996). *Lovell and Winter's pediatric orthopaedics* (4th ed.). Philadelphia: Lippincott-Raven.

Morton, R. (1999). New surgical interventions for cerebral palsy and the place of gait analysis. *Developmental Medicine and Child Neurology, 41,* 424-428.

Olutoye, O.O., & Adzick, N.S. (1999). Fetal surgery for myelomenigocele. *Seminars in Perinatology, 23,* 462-473.

Pellegrino, L. (1997). Cerebral palsy. In M.L. Batshaw (Ed.), *Children with disabilities* (4th ed., pp. 499-529). Baltimore: Paul H. Brookes Publishing.

Rose, R., Fuentes, A., Hamel, B.J., & Dzialo C.J. (1999). Pediatric leg length discrepancy: Causes and treatments. *Orthopaedic Nursing, 18*(2), 21-30.

Ruggieri, M. (1999). The different forms of neurofibromatosis. *Child's Nervous System, 15,* 295-308.

Staheli, L.T. (1989). Torsion-treatment indications. *Clinical Orthopaedics and Related Research, 247,* 61-66.

Tosi, L.L. (1997). Osteogenesis imperfecta. *Current Concepts in Pediatrics, 9,* 94-99.

STUDY QUESTIONS

1. Bobby, a 16-month-old, is brought in by his mother because she is concerned about his bowed legs. Bowed legs are normal (physiologic):
   a. Only in a neonate.
   b. Until 18-24 months.
   c. After age 18 months until approximately age 8.
   d. In adults.

David, a 3-day-old, is referred for evaluation of a bilateral foot deformity. He is the first baby born to healthy parents, and the pregnancy was uncomplicated. On examination, both of David's feet are in equinus, inversion, and adduction. After examining David, the orthopaedic surgeon makes the diagnosis of clubfeet. (Questions 2-3)

2. For a baby David's age, the treatment for clubfeet is:
   a. Manual stretching exercises.
   b. Serial casting and manipulation.
   c. Outflare shoes.
   d. Surgical correction.

3. David's father was an all-American football player. Both of David's parents are concerned about his ability to participate in sports when he is older. Your response to this concern would be:
   a. "It is too early to tell what David will be able to do."
   b. "David will not be able to participate in any sports activities."
   c. "David will be able to participate in adapted/handicapped sports only."
   d. "David may find some sports difficult but should be encouraged to try whatever interest him."

Melissa, a 2-month-old, is referred from the pediatrician's office for a right hip click. She was a breech presentation, but the pregnancy was otherwise uncomplicated. Physical findings include asymmetric skin folds on her thighs, a positive Galleazi's sign (right leg appears shorter than the left), and positive Barlow's and Ortolani maneuvers on the right. (Questions 4-5)

4. Given her diagnosis, the **first** treatment will be:
   a. Pavlik harness.
   b. Bryant's skin traction.
   c. Arthrogram.
   d. Closed reduction and casting.

5. Melissa could require further treatment for her hip dysplasia. The next course of treatment could be:
   a. Abduction brace followed by spica cast.
   b. Traction in preparation for arthrogram and closed reduction.
   c. Open reduction and immobilization in spica cast.
   d. Pelvic/femoral osteotomy to correct bony deformity.

Brian is a 14-year-old with myelomeningocele at level L1. (Questions 6-7)

6. Which of the following is **not** a problem associated with myelomeningocele?
   a. Hydrocephalus due to obstructed flow in the fourth ventricle.
   b. Talipes equinovarus and risk of hip dislocation.
   c. Vesicoureteral reflux and rectal prolapse.
   d. Chronic respiratory infection and extremity pain.

7. Orthotics are prescribed for Brian to:
   a. Help foot fit comfortably in shoes.
   b. Prevent contractures.
   c. Maximize ambulatory potential.
   d. Maintain alignment.

Molly, an 8-year-old, presents to the clinic with a 2-month history of pain with activity and an occasional limp. On physical examination, she has limited abduction and internal rotation of her left hip. Molly is diagnosed with Legg-Calvé-Perthes disease. (Questions 8-9)

8. Legg-Calvé-Perthes disease is:
   a. One of the developmental hip dysplasias.
   b. A condition where the epiphysis of the femur shifts position.
   c. The result of trauma before the age of six.
   d. Idiopathic avascular necrosis of the femoral head.

9. The orthopaedic surgeon tells the family that the first priority is to regain the lost motion in the hip. The most likely treatment will be:
   a. Bed rest with traction.
   b. Spica casting.
   c. Adductor release.
   d. Femoral osteotomy.

Jake, a 13-year-old, presents with a 1-month history of pain in his knee. He denies any trauma to the knee. Physical exam reveals limited internal rotation and abduction. (Questions 10-13)

10. Given Jake's age and history, the most likely diagnosis is:
    a. Legg-Calvé-Perthes disease.
    b. Slipped capital femoral epiphysis.
    c. Torn meniscus.
    d. Degenerative joint disease.

11. The initial treatment for this problem is:
    a. Bed rest at home or in the hospital.
    b. Casting in abduction to secure immobilization.
    c. Placement of pins across the physeal plate.
    d. Femoral osteotomy and bony grafting.

12. Osgood Schlatter disease is a(n):
    a. Inflammation of the tibial tubercle at the insertion of the quadriceps tendon.
    b. Recurrent dislocation of patella due to weakness of the quadriceps tendon.
    c. Meniscal injury due to quadriceps malalignment.
    d. Inflammation of the tibial tubercle at the insertion of the patellar tendon.

13. Patient teaching for Osgood Schlatter disease should include:
    a. There is a potential for long-term damage to the knee if inflammation persists.
    b. The symptoms will stop by the end of skeletal growth.
    c. Pain may be relieved by flexion exercises.
    d. All physical activity must be restricted for 3 months.

Erika, an 18-month-old, presents with a swollen left elbow. Her mother reports that she noticed the swelling yesterday when she returned from a shopping trip but waited to bring her in to see if it would get better. The mother's boyfriend was watching Erika while she was out. The mother denies knowledge of any injury or trauma, fever, and any recent ear or respiratory infections. When you remove Erika's shirt, you notice seven small circular scabs in the shape of a question mark on the left side of her back. On examination, Erika's left elbow is swollen and tender. Erika whimpers quietly during the examination, but does not cry. (Questions 14-15)

14. X-rays reveal a corner fracture of the left distal humeral epiphysis. What is your responsibility in a case of suspected child abuse?
    a. Reporting any suspected case of child abuse.
    b. Getting the mother to admit that the child was abused.
    c. Reporting only substantiated cases of child abuse.
    d. A nurse has no responsibility in a case of suspected child abuse.

15. An important nursing intervention for an abused child is to:
    a. Foster healthy aspects of parent-child relationship.
    b. Protect the child by prohibiting family visitors.
    c. Limit the amount of contact between the child and caregiver.
    d. Encourage the child to testify against the abusing caregiver.

Chapter 12 Arthritis and Connective Tissue Disorders

Dottie Roberts, MSN, MACI, RN,C, CNS, ONC

Contents

OBJECTIVES

At the completion of this chapter, the learner will be able to:

- Differentiate the three types of juvenile rheumatoid arthritis (JRA).
- Compare and contrast rheumatoid arthritis (RA) and osteoarthritis (OA).
- Discuss implications of the use of corticosteroids in the treatment of polymyalgia rheumatica (PMR), systemic lupus erythematosus (SLE), and other disorders.
- Describe three multifactorial features of fibromyalgia syndrome (FS).
- Review typical history and physical findings for patients with rheumatic fever.
- Identify appropriate treatments for both acute and chronic gout.
- Relate patient symptoms to each of the three stages of Lyme disease.
- Discuss differences in clinical presentation among three spondyloarthropathies.
- Describe complications of systemic sclerosis (SS).
- Review tests used to diagnose polymyositis/dermatomyositis (PM/DM).
- Identify nursing diagnoses, outcomes, and interventions appropriate for each of the arthritic or connective tissue disorders.

KEY POINTS

- Juvenile rheumatoid arthritis (JRA) is not a childhood version of rheumatoid arthritis but a heterogeneous group of diseases that includes three major subtypes: systemic onset, polyarticular onset, pauciarticular onset.
- Joint destruction begins early with rheumatoid arthritis, often in the first year of the disease, so correct diagnosis is critical to allow expedient use of disease modifying antirheumatic drugs (DMARDs).
- Osteoarthritis (OA) is no longer considered a degenerative disease but is instead recognized as a process in which all joint structures produce new tissue in response to joint insults and cartilage destruction.
- Polymyalgia rheumatica (PMR) occurs only in people over the age of 50 and is characterized by pain rather than weakness, swelling, or limitation of motion.
- Rheumatic fever remains the leading cause of heart disease among children and young adults in many developing countries.
- Gout results from either excessive uric acid production or underexcretion of uric acid.
- Lyme disease is now the most common vector-borne illness in the United States.
- The spondyloarthropathies share clinical and laboratory characteristics that make it difficult to distinguish among them in early stages.
- Treatment experience with burns may provide a logical approach to the care of patients with systemic sclerosis (SS).
- Patients with polymyositis/dermatomyositis (PM/DM) frequently experience respiratory muscle weakness that can lead to dysphagia and aspiration pneumonia.
- Sun exposure and burns may be the most significant environmental trigger for systemic lupus erythematosus (SLE), and sun protection is critical to disease management.
- Fibromyalgia can coexist with SLE and should be considered when developing a treatment regimen.

CHAPTER 12

ARTHRITIS AND CONNECTIVE TISSUE DISORDERS

JUVENILE RHEUMATOID ARTHRITIC CONDITIONS

I. OVERVIEW

A. Definition: systemic multisystem inflammatory disease that affects the body's connective tissue. Arthritis in children is most often termed juvenile rheumatoid arthritis (JRA), but the name is misleading in its implication of a positive (+) rheumatoid factor (RF) that is not always present in affected children. JRA is not a childhood version of rheumatoid arthritis but a heterogeneous group of diseases that includes three major types with two peak ages of onset (2-5 years of age, 9-12 years of age). It is one of the more common chronic diseases in children.

B. Etiology.

1. Exact cause unknown despite extensive research.
2. Autoimmune response considered most likely cause.
3. Triggers for possible autoimmune response include infection, trauma, emotional stress.
4. Recent belief that genetic factors called human leukocyte antigens (HLAs) may create predisposition to JRA.

C. Pathophysiology.

1. Chronic inflammation of synovium and joint effusion characterizes rheumatic process.
2. Eventual erosion, destruction, and fibrosis of articular cartilage occur.
3. Joint ankylosis, adhesions between articular surfaces follow if process persists.
4. General manifestations result from joint erosion, synovial thickening.
   a. Stiffness, especially after inactivity.
   b. Loss of motion due to muscle spasm, inflammation (early disease); or ankylosis, soft tissue contracture (later disease).

D-F. (See Systemic Juvenile Rheumatoid Arthritis, Polyarticular Juvenile Rheumatoid Arthritis, and Pauciarticular Juvenile Rheumatoid Arthritis.)

II. ASSESSMENT

A. History and physical examination.

1. Objective signs of inflammation in one or more joints.
2. Inflammation lasting at least 6 weeks.
3. Onset before patient's 17th birthday.
4. Exclusion of other underlying causes of joint problems, such as infection or malignancy.

B. Diagnostic tests: see Systemic Juvenile Rheumatoid Arthritis, Polyarticular Juvenile Rheumatoid Arthritis, and Pauicarticular Juvenile Rheumatoid Arthritis.

III. COMMON THERAPEUTIC MODALITIES

A. Management goals.

1. Accept lack of specific cure for JRA.
2. Preserve joint function.
3. Prevent physical deformities.
4. Relieve symptoms without iatrogenic harm.
5. Partner with patient, family in disease management.

B. Medications.

1. Given alone or in combination to suppress inflammation, relieve pain.
2. FDA-approved anti-inflammatory drugs used for rapid action require step-wise dose increase over 4-6 weeks.
   a. Naproxen sodium.
      (1) Dose 10 mg/kg/day divided into two oral doses.
      (2) Cannot monitor serum level.
      (3) Common side effects: nausea/vomiting, prolonged bleeding time/ inhibited platelet action, epigastric pain/GI bleeding, altered liver enzymes.
      (4) Toxicity/intolerance: hypersensitivity, nausea unrelieved by antacids or H^2 blockers; safety/efficacy in children under 2 years has not been demonstrated.
      (5) Precautions: administer with food; monitor BUN, creatinine, serum potassium in those with hepatic or renal dysfunction; regularly guiac stool.
   b. Tolmetin sodium.
      (1) Dose 10 mg/kg/day divided into three oral doses.
      (2) Cannot monitor serum level.
      (3) Common side effects: same as naproxen sodium.
      (4) Toxicity/intolerance: same as naproxen sodium.
      (5) Precautions: same as naproxen sodium.
   c. Ibuprofen.
      (1) Dose 20-30 mg/kg/day divided into three or four doses; not to exceed 40 mg/kg/day.
      (2) Cannot monitor serum level.
      (3) Common side effects: same as naproxen sodium.
      (4) Toxicity/intolerance: same as naproxen sodium.
      (5) Precautions: same as naproxen sodium.
   d. Aspirin (ASA).
      (1) Dose for child 25 kg or less, 60-100 mg/kg/day divided into 3 or 4 oral doses; for child over 25 kg, 2.4-3.6 g/day in divided doses.
      (2) Therapeutic serum level of 20-30 mg/dl monitored closely.

(3) Common side effects: nausea/vomiting, prolonged bleeding time, epigastric pain/GI bleeding.
(4) Toxicity/intolerance: tinnitus, hepatotoxicity with chronic high doses, vision changes, hypoglycemia with chronic dosing.
(5) Precautions: administer with food; monitor hematocrit, renal function, liver function, serum glucose.
(6) Salicylates no longer drug of first choice due to increased risk for gastric/hepatic toxicity and Reyes syndrome when compared to nonsteroidal anti-inflammatory drugs.

3. Disease modifying antirheumatic drugs (DMARDs) taken singly or in combination to slow, stop disease progression when one or two anti-inflammatory drugs ineffective.
   a. Methotrexate.
      (1) Dose 5-20 mg/m^2/wk in 1 dose, or 3 doses given 12 hours apart; low doses associated with fewer side effects.
      (2) Common side effects: nausea/vomiting, GI lesions, thrombocytopenia, anemia.
      (3) Toxicity/intolerance: osteoporosis in children on long-term therapy, hepatic fibrosis if on prolonged therapy, pulmonary toxicity.
      (4) Precautions: stomatitis usually resolves with continued administration but should be reported promptly; monitor liver function, renal function, WBC, platelets; I & O; watch for signs of uricemia.
      (5) Has replaced injectable gold salt therapy as second-line medication.
      (6) Symptomatic response usually occurs in 3-4 weeks.
   b. Cyclophosphamide.
      (1) Dose 10 mg/kg IV every 2 weeks.
      (2) Common side effects: faintness, flushing after IV especially if administered too quickly, nausea/vomiting, anorexia, leukopenia.
      (3) Toxicity/intolerance: thrombocytopenia; gonadal suppression in both sexes may occur; hemorrhagic cystitis in children may lead to dose limitation.
      (4) Precautions: monitor CBC, uric acid, serum electrolytes, liver function; regular weights.
   c. Aurothioglucose (injectable gold)
      (1) Dose 0.5-1.0 mg/kg weekly intramuscular injection.
      (2) Common side effects: burning at injection site, metallic taste in mouth, GI bleeding.
      (3) Toxicity/intolerance: stomatitis, pruritis, hematuria, proteinuria, anemia, leukopenia, thrombocytopenia, eosinophilia.
      (4) Precautions: administer intragluteally, observe for 10 minutes after injection; monitor CBC, UA before each injection; assess for mouth ulcers before each injection.
      (5) Injectable gold used in refractory cases after methotrexate has been tried.
4. Corticosteroids.
   a. Very limited role in treating childhood arthritis, used mainly for severe systemic manifestations such as pericarditis, pleuritis, severe anemia.
      (1) Diagnosis of JRA should be definite because use of corticosteroids may make it difficult to diagnose a malignancy.
      (2) Side effects with long-term use seldom warranted because corticosteroids make the patient feel better but do not prevent joint destruction.
      (3) Effectiveness may in fact decrease over time.
   b. Dosage determined by severity of condition, child's response.
   c. Topical corticosteroids combined with mydriatics valuable in controlling eye disease.
   d. Occasional intra-articular corticosteroids used, usually in conjunction with physical therapy.
5. Biologic agents.
   a. May be available in the future for treatment of arthritis in selected children.
   b. Synthesized proteins (monoclonal antibodies) may be directed at specific molecular targets in arthritic joints.

C. Physical management.

1. Individualized programs designed to preserve function, prevent deformity.
   a. Joint rest.
   b. Joint protection.
      (1) Splint to maintain neutral position, minimize pain.
      (2) Rest on firm mattress with no pillow/very low pillow, no support under knee to maintain extension and avoid flexion contractures.
   c. Exercise.
      (1) Pool exercise beneficial due to warmth, mild resistance.
      (2) Isometric/tensing exercises used during peak inflammation to avoid joint motion that may aggravate pain.
      (3) Continued ROM exercises after disease remission allows easy detection of JRA recurrence.
   d. Nutritional support.
      (1) Avoid growth retardation.
      (2) Decrease likelihood of obesity.
2. Physical therapy directed toward joints that are most limited.
   a. Strengthen muscles to provide joint support.
   b. Mobilize restricted joints to avoid deformity.
   c. Prevent/correct deformities to decrease mobility impairment.
3. Occupational therapy builds on child's natural tendency to be active.

a. Generalized mobility.
b. Performance of activities of daily living (ADLs).
4. Other modalities proven to be effective adjuncts.
a. Warm baths, hot packs to reduce joint stiffness, muscle spasm.
b. Cold to decrease acute inflammation.
c. Ultrasound, electrical stimulation to decrease pain, increase joint mobility.
5. Surgery considered for joint contractures, unequal growth of extremities.
a. Soft tissue release (tenotomy) for contractures.
b. Leg length correction.
c. Arthroplasty.

VI. NURSING DIAGNOSES, OUTCOMES, AND INTERVENTIONS (See Table 12.1)

VII. HOME CARE CONSIDERATIONS

A. Because majority of child's care occurs in home, nurse in clinic or hospital must help parent and child cope with/adapt to limitations of disease.

1. Question parents sensitively to determine if they have stopped giving medication due to fears about side effects, doubts concerning efficacy.
2. Encourage parents to avoid overprotecting child, especially if under misconception that inactivity will spare child pain.
3. Encourage parents to contact local chapters of the Arthritis Foundation for information, ongoing emotional support.
4. Link parents with social workers for help in locating resources to cope with financial demands of chronic illness.

B. Follow-up for individual exercise program essential to encourage consistent participation.

C. Provide age-appropriate care to meet developmental needs.

1. Toddlers – choose play that encourages small and large muscle exercise.
a. Blocks.
b. Puzzles.
c. Art projects.
2. School-age children – participate in less strenuous activities to keep involved with peer group, conserve energy, preserve joint/muscle movement.
a. Board games.
b. Collections.

D. Offer strategies for child's success in school.

1. Inform teacher of child's illness and its impact on school performance.
2. Have child use a backpack to eliminate strain on small joints.
3. If possible, obtain two sets of books so child does not have to carry them between school and home.
4. Encourage child to wear high-quality running shoes to decrease ankle pain exacerbated by walking at school.
5. Prevent pain, stiffness, fatigue in hands.
a. Use felt-tip pen, pen covered with foam or wedge.
b. Schedule oral rather than written tests.
c. Use electric typewriter, computer for long reports.
d. Use chalk holder for blackboard work.
e. Use flip chart, felt-tip pen instead of blackboard.

SYSTEMIC JUVENILE RHEUMATOID ARTHRITIS

I. OVERVIEW

A. Definition: (see Juvenile Rheumatoid Arthritic Conditions). Formerly known as Still's Disease; the title is rarely used now due to its lack of precision.

B. Etiology (see Juvenile Rheumatoid Arthritic Conditions.)

C. Pathophysiology.

1. Often begins with daily intermittent fever (up to 105 degrees), chills that continue for weeks.
2. May be accompanied by maculopapular rash on thighs, chest.
3. Inflammation present in variable number of joints.
4. Enlarged spleen, lymph nodes likely.
5. Inflammation of liver, heart, and surrounding tissues possible.

D. Incidence.

1. 10%-15% of JRA.
2. More common in males.

E. Considerations across the lifespan.

1. Systemic involvement requires consistent management.
2. Residual joint destruction affects function in adulthood.

F. Complications.

1. 25%-35% progress to severe crippling arthritis.
2. High mortality rate due to systemic involvement (pericarditis, myocarditis).
3. Growth retardation during periods of active disease, possibly due to corticosteroid use.

II. ASSESSMENT

A. History.

1. Acute onset.
2. Fever spikes, return to baseline without antipyretics.
3. Transient rashes.
4. Fatigue, anemia common.
5. Anorexia, possible weight loss.
6. Joint stiffness after periods of immobility, especially upon awakening.

B. Physical examination.

1. Intermittent high fever.
2. Transient rash, often occurring with fever.
3. Swelling, warmth, painful motion in affected joints.
4. Possible hepatosplenomegaly.

C. Diagnostic tests.

1. No definitive serologic tests; possible abnormal values include:
a. Elevated erythrocyte sedimentation rate (ESR),

Table 12.1
Common Nursing Diagnoses, Outcomes, and Interventions

Diagnoses	Outcomes	Interventions
A. Pain, acute; pain, chronic	Pain is managed adequately to allow patient participation in routine activities, ADLs.	• Define pain experience with patient. 1. Identify location, type, duration of pain. 2. Assess level of pain using pain intensity scale. 3. Determine factors that alleviate or aggravate pain. • Collaborate with patient, other health team members in choosing appropriate pain management strategies. 1. Discuss use of pharmacologic and nonpharmacologic pain management options. 2. Recommend a preemptive approach to use of analgesics for pain management (e.g., ATC rather than PRN dosing). 3. Assess effectiveness of chosen therapies and modify as needed. • Review principles of joint protection. 1. Instruct patient in use of assistive devices. 2. Assist patient to determine alternate ways to perform tasks in order to decrease stress on joints, tissues. 3. Advocate a balance of rest, activity.
B. Physical mobility, impaired	Patient's joint mobility and muscle strength will be maintained and/or improved, with deformities and contractures minimized.	• Review history of mobility impairment with patient. • Assess effect of mobility impairment on functional ability. • Promote optimal mobility and joint movement. 1. Collaborate with therapist in initiating exercise regimen to target affected joints. 2. Encourage use of analgesics prior to activity. 3. Instruct patient in use of heat or cold to reduce pain, inflammation that restrict movement. 4. Encourage weight loss if indicated to facilitate movement.
C. Activity intolerance	Patient will tolerate activity with minimal fatigue.	• Assess patient's response to activity. • Instruct patient in principles of energy conservation, joint protection, alternative methods of task performance. • Assist patient in reorganizing daily schedule to optimize rest, avoid excesses in activity that can increase pain. • Encourage gradual progression of activity.

Table 12.1 (continued)
Common Nursing Diagnoses, Outcomes, and Interventions

Diagnoses	Outcomes	Interventions
C. Activity intolerance (continued)	Patient will tolerate activity with minimal fatigue. (continued)	• Encourage participation in an exercise/conditioning program to maximize endurance.
D. Sleep pattern, disturbed	Patient will report an optimal balance of rest and activity.	• Identify factors that contribute to sleep disturbance. • Encourage use of sleep aids. 1. Warm bath. 2. Snack, milk. 3. Relaxation/breathing exercise. 4. Reading material. 5. Soft music, audiotaped story. • Encourage use of analgesics prior to bedtime. • Limit amount, length of daytime sleeping if necessary.
E. Self-care deficit syndrome **• Bathing/hygiene** **• Dressing/grooming**	Patient will demonstrate optimal level of independence in performance of ADLs.	• Assist patient to identify barriers to mobility/activity in home environment. • Assist patient to modify activities and environment to accommodate limitations. 1. Hand rails. 2. Ramp. 3. Safety treads, nonslip mats. • Instruct patient in use of appropriate assistive devices to meet hygiene, dressing, grooming needs. 1. Shower chair, raised toilet seat. 2. Dressing aids (sock donner, long-handled shoe horn, reacher). 3. Adapted toothbrush. • Encourage use of analgesics to relieve pain that may affect patient's ability to provide self-care.
F. Skin integrity, impaired	Patient will demonstrate minimal skin impairment.	• Assess for patient risk factors that contribute to the development of skin impairment. • Attempt to modify contributing factors that increase patient risk for skin impairment. 1. Immobility. 2. Impaired circulation. 3. Malnourishment. 4. Sensory deficit. • Educate patient and family about preventive strategies. • Discuss psychosocial impact of skin impairment, disfigurement.

Table 12.1 (continued)
Common Nursing Diagnoses, Outcomes, and Interventions

Diagnoses	Outcomes	Interventions
G. Body image, disturbed	Patient will verbalize/demonstrate acceptance of appearance.	• Encourage verbalization regarding effects of disease on patient's appearance. • Emphasize patient's life/attributes apart from disease. • Encourage use of clothing, make-up to enhance feelings of attractiveness. • Encourage patient to avoid isolation due to changes in physical appearance. • Suggest professional counseling for patient with poor ego strengths, inadequate coping resources.
H. Sexuality pattern, altered	Patient will report optimal sexual role functioning.	• Discuss impact of disease on patient's sexuality. • Encourage patient's attention to details which reinforce sense of personal sexuality. 1. Grooming. 2. Hygiene. 3. Communication with partner. • Encourage use of pain management modalities (e.g., analgesics, warm bath) prior to sexual activity. • Encourage patient to plan sexual activities when not fatigued. • Provide information on alternative positions that may be less stressful on joints, tissues. • Suggest professional counseling for continued sexual problems.
I. Nutrition, imbalanced • **More than body requirements** • **Less than body requirements**	Patient will consume daily nutritional requirements in accordance with activity level, metabolic needs.	• Assess patient's nutritional needs related to weight loss or gain. • Assess for underlying depression/grief that may contribute to dietary imbalances. • Assist in development of appropriate diet plan that integrates patient's personal, cultural, age-related food preferences. • Assist in development of exercise program for overweight patient.
J. Role performance, ineffective	Patient will manage home/work roles.	• Assess for functional deficits which may require vocational/lifestyle adaptations. 1. Refer for vocational retraining if indicated. 2. Assist in determining needed adaptations for current employment. 3. Assist in obtaining resources for necessary lifestyle changes. 4. Discuss appropriate changes that can be made to enable patient to meet home role responsibilities.

Table 12.1 (continued)
Common Nursing Diagnoses, Outcomes, and Interventions

Diagnoses	Outcomes	Interventions
J. Role performance, ineffective (continued)	Patient will manage home/work roles. (continued)	• Encourage verbalization regarding role changes, their impact on self-concept.
K. Individual coping, ineffective Family coping, compromised	Patient and family will cope effectively with changes imposed by chronic illness and treatment regimen.	• Educate patient and family regarding disease process, possible complications, appropriate therapies. • Identify stresses that contribute to disease exacerbation and methods of stress reduction. • Discuss role of alternative therapies in patient treatment plan and provide current information on strategies of interest to patient. • Assist with problem-solving strategies for dealing with perceived difficulties. • Create a supportive environment that encourages verbalization of patient concerns related to chronic disease. • Assist patient and family to identify support networks within the community.

depending on degree of inflammation.

b. Low hemoglobin, hematocrit related more to anorexia than to disease progression.
c. Leukocytosis in early stages.
d. Elevated C-reactive protein (CRP).
e. Negative antinuclear antibody (ANA), rheumatoid factor (RF) in systemic disease.
f. Latex fixation test negative in 90% of JRA cases.

2. Radiographic findings variable.
   a. Early widening of joint space.
   b. Gradual evidence of fusion, articular destruction.

III-V. (See Juvenile Rheumatoid Arthritic Conditions.)

POLYARTICULAR JUVENILE RHEUMATOID ARTHRITIS

I. OVERVIEW

A. Definition (see Juvenile Rheumatoid Arthritic Conditions).

B. Etiology (see Juvenile Rheumatoid Arthritic Conditions).

C. Pathophysiology.

1. Arthritis in five or more joints.
   a. Commonly affects knees, ankles, hips, feet, small joints of hands.
   b. Usually symmetric joint involvement.
2. Unlikely extra-articular manifestations.

D. Incidence.

1. 35%-40% of JRA.
2. More common in females.
3. Two subtypes:
   a. Subtype I (10% occurrence).
      (1) More common at 8-10 years of age.
      (2) Positive RF.
      (3) Potential for severe joint damage.
   b. Subtype II (25% occurrence).
      (1) Negative RF.
      (2) Less crippling deformities.

E. Considerations across the lifespan.

1. Most negative RF cases go into remission by adulthood but leave residual joint damage.
2. Permanent disability occurs with chronic disease.
3. Small percentage with effects of systemic involvement if not managed appropriately.

F. Complications.

1. Joint subluxations.
2. Soft tissue contractures.

II. ASSESSMENT

A. History.

1. Insidious onset.
2. Joint stiffness after periods of immobility, especially in the morning.

B. Physical examination.

1. Edema, warmth, painful motion/decreased ROM in

affected joints.
2. Possible limp or obvious favoring of one lower extremity.

C. Diagnostic tests.
1. No definitive serologic tests.
    a. Elevated ESR possible.
    b. Positive RF in subtype I.
2. Radiologic findings similar to systemic onset JRA.

III-V. (See Juvenile Rheumatoid Arthritic Conditions.)

PAUCIARTICULAR JUVENILE RHEUMATOID ARTHRITIS

I. OVERVIEW

A. Definition: see Juvenile Rheumatoid Arthritic Conditions.

B. Etiology: see Juvenile Rheumatoid Arthritic Conditions.

C. Pathophysiology.
1. Asymmetric joint involvement.
2. Commonly affects knees, elbows, wrists, ankles.
3. Possible iridocyclitis (uveitis), potentially dangerous eye inflammation.
    a. Annual ophthalmic screening recommended.
    b. Annual slit lamp examination recommended.

D. Incidence.
1. 50% of all JRA.
2. More common in females.
3. Three subtypes:
    a. Subtype I (early onset)
        (1) 5%-10% occurrence in females less than 6 years of age.
        (2) Positive ANA.
        (3) High risk of eye inflammation.
    b. Subtype II (late onset).
        (1) 5%-10% occurrence in males over 8 years of age.
        (2) Arthritis in spine, although involvement may not occur until adolescence.
        (3) Possible positive test for HLA-B27 gene.
    c. Subtype III (late onset).
        (1) 10%-15% occurrence.
        (2) Best prognosis.
        (3) Joint involvement the extent of disease.
        (4) May evolve into polyarticular arthritis.
4. Also classified based on patient function.
    a. Class I – patient can perform all activities.
    b. Class II – patient performs activities adequately but with some limitations.
    c. Class III – patient's activities very limited, can perform self-care only.
    d. Class IV – patient wheelchair-bound or bedridden.

E. Considerations across the lifespan.
1. Growth retardation.
2. Disability.

F. Complications.
1. Blindness from iridocyclitis.
2. Leg-length discrepancies.
3. Muscle atrophy.
4. Spondyloarthritis.

II. ASSESSMENT

A. History. Same as polyarticular disease.

B. Physical examination. Same as polyarticular disease.

C. Diagnostic tests.
1. No definitive serologic tests.
    a. Mild leukocytosis.
    b. Elevated ESR.
    c. Possible positive ANA.
    d. Positive HLA-DR5, HLA-B27.
    e. Positive RF in later onset disease.
2. Radiologic findings similar to systemic onset JRA.

III-V. (See Juvenile Rheumatoid Arthritic Conditions.)

RHEUMATOID ARTHRITIS (RA)

I. OVERVIEW

A. Definition: chronic systemic progressive disease characterized by inflammation of connective tissue, primarily in diarthrodial joints, with unexplained periods of remission and exacerbation.

B. Etiology.
1. No known single cause.
2. Theory suggests RA is generated by intermeshed pathogenic pathways in a susceptible host who experiences an initial immune response to an antigen.
    a. Probably not the same antigen in all patients.
    b. Multifactorial, complex genetic factors involved.
3. Possible triggering stimuli would be integrated with immunogenetic factors.
    a. No infectious agent has been cultured from synovial tissue, synovial fluid, blood with enough reproducibility to suggest causation.
    b. Autoimmunity suggested as cause of RA due to association with rheumatoid factor (RF), the antibody against gamma globulin.
4. No known risk factors exist.

C. Pathophysiology.
1. Changes first seen in synovial tissue where immune response appears to localize.
    a. RF antibodies develop against immunoglobulin IgG, form immune complexes.
    b. Formation of complexes leads to activation of complement system, release of lysosomal enzymes from leukocytes.
    c. Synovitis develops as immune complexes are formed.
2. Immune complexes are deposited onto synovial membrane or superficial articular cartilage.
    a. Phagocytosis of complexes occurs by polymor-

phonuclear leukocytes, monocytes, lymphocytes.

b. Phagocytosis simultaneously deactivates complex, produces additional enzymes that cause hyperemia, edema, thickening of synovial lining.

3. Hypertrophied synovium invades surrounding tissue (cartilage, ligaments, joint capsule, tendons).
   a. Granulation tissue eventually forms, covering entire articular cartilage.
   b. Formation of characteristic pannus (highly vascularized fibrous scar tissue) results.
4. Destructive pannus erodes, destroys articular cartilage.
   a. Subchondral bone erosions, bone cysts, fissures, bone spurs result.
   b. Production of tumor necrosis factor (TNF) by cells at cartilage-pannus junction may lead to cartilage destruction.
   c. Pannus also scars, shortens tendons and ligaments to create laxity, subluxation, contractures.
5. Systemic involvement characteristic of RA.
   a. Tendon sheaths; bursae; connective tissue in heart, lungs, arteries affected.
   b. Rheumatoid nodules appear as subcutaneous masses over pressure points.

D. Incidence.

1. Exact prevalence unknown, generally due to past use of two different diagnostic classification systems for disease activity.
2. After age 55, estimated prevalence rates for men and women are 2% and 5% respectively.
3. Genetic predisposition seen, with higher rate of concordant disease among identical twins (32%) than fraternal twins (9%).
4. Higher prevalence in North American Indians, Eskimos also supports theory of genetic predisposition.

E. Considerations across the lifespan.

1. In younger people, disease tends to have a slow, insidious onset.
2. With disease onset after age 60, symptoms tend to be acute, explosive, and widespread but have shorter duration, better prognosis.
3. Genetic differences between mother, fetus may alter disease activity during pregnancy.
   a. Most women report improvement in joint pain and/or swelling.
   b. Up to 1/3 report no change in symptoms during pregnancy.
4. 10% of patients with RA typically experience remission, 15% develop severe progressive destructive disease, 75% experience a slowly progressive and worsening course.

F. Complications.

1. Direct cause of death, severe morbidity more often than has been appreciated.
   a. Life expectancy shortened by 7 years in males, 3 years in females.
   b. About 50% of patients with RA cannot function in their jobs within 10 years of disease onset.
2. Joint destruction begins early, often within first year of disease.
3. Flexion contractures, deformity in hand result in diminished grasp strength.
   a. Ulnar deviation ("zigzag" deformity) of wrist.
   b. Swan-neck deformity (flexion of distal interphalangeal [DIP], metacarpophalangeal [MCP] joints with hyperextension of proximal interphalangeal [PIP] joint).
   c. Boutonnière deformity (avulsion of extensors, producing flexion of PIP joint).
   d. Resorptive arthropathy with appearance of shortened digits in hands.
      (1) Excess skin folds present.
      (2) Phalanges can be retracted (telescoped) into each other, then pulled out into abnormally long extension.
      (3) Associated with aggressive synovitis of longer duration.
4. Popliteal cysts may cause various complications.
   a. Intact cysts compress venous flow, producing vessel dilation and/or edema.
   b. Cyst rupture may resemble acute thrombophlebitis with swelling, tenderness.
5. Pronation deformities, eversion of foot occur due to stretching, erosion of ligaments.
6. Nodular myositis, muscle fiber degeneration lead to severe pain similar to that of vascular insufficiency.
7. Effects of vasculitis range from occasional nail fold infarcts to deep, erosive, scarring pyoderma gangrenosa.
8. Episcleritis can lead to keratitis, cataract development that result in vision loss.
9. Complications may result from rheumatoid nodules.
   a. Ulceration, with appearance similar to pressure sores.
   b. Progressive hoarseness from nodules on vocal cords.
   c. Bone destruction from nodules within vertebral bodies.
   d. Valvular deformities from nodules in heart.
10. Later disease may have cardiopulmonary effects.
    a. Pleurisy, pleural effusion, pleural and parenchymal nodules.
    b. Pericarditis, pericardial effusion, nodules, cardiomyopathy.
11. Neuromuscular involvement may include carpal tunnel syndrome.
12. Rotator cuff insufficiency commonly leads to loss of motion.

II. ASSESSMENT

A. History (see Table 12.2 for comparison of RA, OA).

1. Fatigue, lethargy, weight loss.
2. Joint pain, swelling particularly in hands, wrists.
3. Morning stiffness lasting at least 1 hour, up to 4 hours.
4. Hoarseness.

Table 12.2
Comparison of Rheumatoid Arthritis (RA) and Osteoarthritis (OA)

Characteristic	RA	OA
Age at onset	2nd - 5th decade	4th - 5th decade
Gender	Females 2 or 3:1 Differences less marked after age 60	Females 2:1 over age 55
Disease course	Exacerbations, remissions	Variable, progressive
Symptomatology	Systemic	Local
Commonly affected joints	Small joints first (PIPs, MCPs, MTPs), wrists, knees	Weight-bearing joints (knees, hips), MCPs, DIPs, PIPs, cervical and lumbar spine
Morning stiffness	1 hour to all day	10-30 minutes after rising
Joint involvement	Symmetric	Asymmetric
Effusions	Common	Uncommon
Synovial fluid	Decreased viscosity; 3000 - 25,000 WBCs	Usually normal viscosity, few cells
Synovium	Thickened, may be severely inflamed	Possible localized synovitis with point tenderness
Nodules	Rheumatic nodules over bony prominences, extensor surfaces, juxtarticular regions	Heberden's nodes (DIPs); Bouchard's nodes (PIPs)
X-rays in advancing disease	Global narrowing of joint space, erosions, subluxations; osteoporosis RT corticosteroid use	Asymmetric narrowing of joint space; osteophytes, subchondral cysts & sclerosis

5. Difficulty with mobility, self-care.

B. **Physical examination.**
1. Deformities.
   a. Spindle-shaped fingers (early disease).
   b. Swan-neck, boutonnière deformities.
   c. Clawed toes.
2. Swollen, red, warm, tender joints.
3. Muscle weakness, atrophy.
4. Subcutaneous nodules.
5. Spongy synovium, decreased ROM in affected joints.
6. Tenderness in paravertebral muscles, around spinous processes.
7. Guarded movement, gait abnormalities, posture changes.
8. Joint effusion, especially in knee or elbow.

C. **Diagnostic tests.**
1. Diagnosis based predominantly on history, physical findings.
2. Laboratory results typically used to confirm diagnosis, monitor disease progression.
   a. ANA titers seen in 5%-20% of patients.
   b. Positive RF in approximately 80% of patients, with higher titers in active disease.
   c. Elevated ESR, CRP indicative of active inflammation.
   d. Slight anemia.
   e. Genetic markers not a practical screening test.
3. Radiographs not commonly needed to make diagnosis.
   a. May be inconclusive in early disease.
   b. Baseline films, especially of hands, may be useful in monitoring disease progress, determining prognosis if erosions present.
   c. Soft tissue swelling in early disease indicated by increased shadowing around affected joint.
   d. Loss of articular cartilage leads to narrowed joint space with advanced disease.
   e. Joint subluxation, malalignment seen on x-ray, reflect destructive changes noted on physical examination.
   f. Osteopenia/osteoporosis may be evident due to corticosteroid use.
4. Bone scans detect early joint changes, confirm diagnosis.
5. Synovial fluid in early disease straw-colored, slight-

ly cloudy with many flecks of fibrin, WBCs (3,500-25,000/mm³).
6. Arthroscopy typically reveals pale, thick, edematous (hypertrophic) synovium with cartilage destruction, fibrous scar formation.

III. COMMON THERAPEUTIC MODALITIES

A. Management goals.

1. Reduce inflammation.
2. Alleviate pain.
3. Preserve function.
4. Prevent deformity.

B. Medications. Drug therapy remains the most important part of interdisciplinary care approach.

1. Correct diagnosis critical to allow expedient use of DMARDs.
   a. Consistent use shown to impede erosive course of RA.
   b. Recommended initiation within 3 months of diagnosis.
   c. Choice of drug based on disease activity, patient's functional status, relevant lifestyle considerations (affected female of childbearing age).
      (1) Methotrexate 7.5-25 mg weekly (orally or intramuscularly) most frequently prescribed by rheumatologists in United States.
      (2) Sulfasalazine 2000-3000 mg daily.
      (3) Hydroxychloroquine 200-400 mg daily.
      (4) Gold 25-50 mg intramuscularly every 1-4 weeks, 3-6 mg orally daily has been standard therapy for more than 60 years.
      (5) Penicillamine 250-1000 mg daily.
      (6) Azathioprine 1.5-2.5 mg/kg/day.
      (7) Cyclosporin 2.5-5 mg/kg/day.
      (8) Cyclophosphamide 1-2 mg/kg/day.
   d. New DMARD leflunomide approved in 1998 for treatment of RA in adults.
      (1) Shown to reduce signs and symptoms; retard joint space narrowing, structural damage, erosions.
      (2) Improvement typically occurs within 4-6 weeks; no benefit likely from drug if no positive response by that time.
      (3) No known pulmonary effects, less destructive to bone marrow than methotrexate.
   e. Laboratory monitoring (renal, liver function) required with all DMARDs.
2. Biological response modifiers (BRMs) interfere with cell surface antigens of modulating cytokines.
   a. Etanercept approved for symptom management in patients with moderate/severe RA who have not responded to DMARDs.
      (1) Narrow indication because effects of long-term use unknown.
      (2) Has produced rapid, dramatic results.
      (3) Regimen calls for self-injection, which may be problematic for patients with poor muscle strength, severe disease.
   b. Infliximab recently approved for treatment of Crohn's disease, under investigation for treatment of RA.
3. Various NSAIDs have fairly equal analgesic, anti-inflammatory effects on RA.
   a. NSAIDs do not affect disease progression.
   b. The ability of NSAIDs to alleviate symptoms may delay initiation of DMARD therapy or referral to rheumatologist.
   c. Choice should be based on side-effect profile, cost, duration of action, patient preference.
   d. Approval of cyclooxygenase-2 (COX-2) inhibitors (celecoxib, rofecoxib) offers alternative to traditional NSAIDs.
      (1) Patients with history of MI, TIA, or stroke can safely use COX-2 inhibitors without foregoing antiplatelet therapy because they have no effect on bleeding time, platelet aggregation.
      (2) Drugs offer less GI toxicity than traditional NSAIDs.
         (a) Specifically inhibit prostaglandin synthesis by acting on COX-2 enzyme.
         (b) Do not inhibit COX-1 enzyme, which is believed to protect the gastroduodenal mucosa.
4. Corticosteroids can help in symptom relief.
   a. Direct injection into affected joints can temporarily alleviate pain, inflammation associated with flare ups.
   b. Long-term use of oral corticosteroids is associated with development of osteoporosis, avascular necrosis.
      (1) Should not be mainstay of RA treatment.
      (2) Low-dose prednisone may be used with caution in selected patients to minimize disease activity for limited time until DMARD effect is seen.
5. Use of antibiotics to treat RA has seen resurgence of interest in recent years.
   a. Multiple studies have validated usefulness of minocycline in RA treatment but many rheumatologists remain unconvinced of its value.
   b. Minocycline's antirheumatic effect could be related to immunomodulatory/anti-inflammatory properties.
   c. Preliminary data suggest drug's efficacy sustained over 3 years.
   d. May be reasonable alternative for patients with benign prognosis but probably would not be tried in severe, potentially destructive disease.
6. Future drug therapies may stem from continued research on underlying causes of RA-associated inflammation.
   a. Calcitonin may down-regulate monocyte function.
   b. Anecdotal reports have noted patient improvement with rifampin (antitubercular drug), which acts on pathways of RNA synthesis.
   c. Retinoid compounds have multiple effects on

biologic systems.

   d. Anti-CD4 monoclonal antibodies target subpopulations of T lymphocytes to interfere in the immune system's attack on joint disease.
   e. Anti-tumor necrosis factor (TNF) monoclonal antibodies may delay abnormal growth of cartilage, bone.
   f. Collagenase inhibitor showed safety at 2-year mark in phase II/III trial but clinical efficacy was undetermined.

C. Therapeutic exercise and other modalities.

1. Range of motion (ROM), strengthening, endurance exercises typically prescribed.
   a. Passive, active, assisted ROM exercises done to improve joint mobility.
   b. Isometric, isotonic exercises build muscles surrounding, connecting joints.
      (1) Provide support.
      (2) Minimize further joint injury.
   c. Appropriate low-resistance exercises include bike riding, swimming, golfing, dancing.
   d. Progressive muscle contraction, relaxation should be used cautiously due to tendency to exacerbate pain.
   e. Exercise programs should be done step-wise to achieve optimal long-term benefits.
2. Heat, cold are important adjuncts to exercise.
   a. Superficial heat provided with hot packs, hydrotherapy, paraffin baths.
   b. Deep heat achieved with ultrasound.
   c. Cold packs may provide greater relief of pain and stiffness than heat but should not be used in patients with Raynaud's phenomenon.
3. Use of splints appears to resolve inflammation more quickly than leaving joint unsplinted.

D. Medicinal oils.

1. Some patients resist proven prescriptive medicine preferred in severe disease due to concerns about side effects.
2. Oil supplements (fish oils, evening primrose oil, flaxseed oil, borrage seed oil) are not a cure, appear to give relief similar to NSAIDs.
3. Researchers have been unable to determine optimal dose or combination of oils that might work best.
4. Recommendations include taking oil supplements while lowering overall fat intake, changing oils in diet, eating oil-rich cold water fish at least twice weekly.

E. Alternative therapies.

1. Patient must be aware that use of alternative may delay care/access to care and lead to exclusion of proven remedies.
2. Acupuncture has been confirmed in randomized clinical trials to have safe effects in pain modulation.
3. Use of bee venom is a controversial unconventional therapy that carries potential for anaphylaxis, unknown long-term side effects.

IV. NURSING DIAGNOSES, OUTCOMES, AND INTERVENTIONS (See Table 12.1)

V. HOME CARE CONSIDERATIONS

A. Patient should receive information about purpose, dose, frequency, anticipated side effects of all medications.

1. When to report adverse symptoms to health care providers.
2. What to do if missed dose.

B. Patient should receive assistance in meeting self-care needs at home.

1. Assistive devices such as easy-to-grip combs and long-handled brushes may help with grooming.
2. Use of long-handled bath brush creates less stress on joints.
3. Clothing can be selected, adapted to allow self-dressing (zipper pulls, buttoners, velcro closures, pull-on pants).
4. Equipment needs for hygiene care should be identified (shower chair, elevated toilet seat).
5. Mobility aids such as platform cane, walker may be helpful.

C. Reinforce pain management strategies.

1. Analgesic use.
2. Positioning, joint protection.
3. Use of heat, cold.
4. Relaxation techniques (imagery, rhythmic breathing, music).

D. Enlist support of family members.

1. Instruction on disease process, treatments should be provided to family.
2. Family should be encouraged to allow patient to function independently when able but be available for assistance (for example, severe morning stiffness).
3. Family should be encouraged to collaborate with patient in developing nutritionally sound diet.

E. Strategies to maximize sleep and rest.

1. Reinforce good sleep habits.
   a. Follow regular sleep schedule.
   b. Avoid caffeine, alcohol before bed.
   c. Participate in soothing activities before bed.
2. Ease painful joints by taking a bath, warming bed.
3. Take analgesic with light snack 30 minutes before retiring.
4. Use relaxation exercises if difficulty in falling asleep.

F. Developing coping mechanisms.

1. Encourage patient to actively participate in decision making related to disease treatment, lifestyle changes.
2. Discuss effects of disease on patient's sexuality, suggest strategies to allow sexual expression.
3. Discuss adaptive strategies for workplace.
4. Encourage involvement in support groups through agencies such as the Arthritis Foundation.

OSTEOARTHRITIS

I. OVERVIEW

A. Definition: osteoarthritis (OA) is a slowly progressive, non-inflammatory disorder of movable (diarthrodial) joints. Previous term degenerative joint disease (DJD) not as commonly used due to view of OA as process in which all joint structures produce new tissue in response to joint insults, cartilage destruction. OA ischaracterized by deterioration of articular cartilage, subsequent formation of new bone at joint margins with synovial hyperplasia, capsular thickening. No systemic involvement.

B. Etiology.

1. Idiopathic (formerly primary) OA cause obscure or unknown.
   a. Aging an important factor associated with decreased quality, quantity of proteoglycans in cartilage.
   b. Evidence suggests idiopathic OA may be inherited as autosomal recessive trait with gene defects causing premature cartilage destruction.
2. Secondary OA caused by any condition that damages cartilage directly; subjects joint surfaces/underlying bone to chronic, excessive, or abnormal forces; or causes joint instability.
   a. Trauma: sprains, strains, dislocations, fractures (possibly leading to avascular necrosis, osteonecrosis).
   b. Mechanical stress: long-term involvement in repetitive physical tasks or activities such as athletics or ballet.
   c. Inflammation in joint structures: inflammatory cells release enzymes that can digest cartilage.
   d. Joint instability: damage to supporting structures such as ligaments, tendons, joint capsule.
   e. Neurologic disorders: pain, proprioceptive reflexes diminished or lost, leading to increased tendency for abnormal movement, positioning, weight bearing (diabetic neuropathy, Charcot arthropathy).
   f. Congenital/acquired skeletal deformities: varus leg deformity, dislocated hip, joint laxity, Legg-Calvé-Perthes disease.
   g. Hematologic/endocrine disorders: hemophilia with chronic bleeding into joints; hyperparathyroidism with calcium loss from bone.
   h. Selected drug use: activity of collagen-digesting enzymes stimulated in synovial membrane (colchicine, indomethacin, steroids).
3. Sex hormones, other hormonal factors seem to influence disease development, progression.
   a. Excessive growth hormone produces progressive overgrowth of bone.
   b. Excessive parathyroid hormone results in hypercalcemia, produces skeletal changes.

C. Pathophysiology.

1. Smooth, glistening, white articular cartilage normally covers synovial joint surfaces.
   a. Characterized by extremely low friction with movement, shock-absorbing capacity due to compressibility, elasticity.
   b. Composed of chondrocytes and matrix made of type II collagen, proteoglycans.
2. OA results from articular cartilage damage, tremendous metabolic response at level of chondrocytes.
   a. Enzymatic breakdown results in decreased proteoglycan content in matrix and softening, loss of elasticity in cartilage.
   b. Compensatory increase in synthesis of proteoglycans, collagen cannot keep pace with progressive cartilage destruction by lysosomal enzymes.
   c. Decreased proteoglycan content also leads to loss of support for collagen fibrils, makes cartilage more susceptible to joint friction.
3. Decreased cushioning, permeability of matrix results as some hydrophilic properties of proteoglycans lost and type I collagen replaced with more fibrous form.
   a. Cartilage loses ability to resist wear with heavy use.
   b. Nutrients from synovial fluid have increased difficulty reaching deeper layers of cartilage.
4. Loss of collagen support, changes in collagen structure cause fibers to rupture.
   a. Fissuring, fibrillation, erosion of articular cartilage result.
   b. Joint surface becomes yellowish, dull, granular.
5. Softened, fibrillated cartilage is gradually abraded to subchondral bone in center of joint surface.
   a. Cartilage in peripheral joint area responds with proliferation of fibroblasts, new bone formation.
   b. Bone outgrowth, spurs develop on joint margins.
6. Loss of central cartilage, build up of peripheral cartilage and bone create incongruity in joint surfaces.
   a. Change occurs in normal distribution of stress.
   b. Joint motion restricted.
7. Small pieces of articular cartilage (osteophytes) may shear from joint surface, attract phagocytic cells that will try to cleanse joint of loose debris.
   a. Secondary synovitis can result, leading to enlarged joint capsule.
   b. Inflammatory response also leads to increased synovial fluid production, further swelling in joint.
8. Early pain, stiffness of OA result from inflammatory changes in synovium, joint capsule.
   a. Possible causes include prostaglandin release, microfractures of subchondral trabeculae, joint effusion, irritation of periosteal nerve endings by osteophytes, compromise of circulation to bone, effects on tendons or fascia, muscle spasm.
   b. Because cartilage has no nerve supply, joint surfaces do not become painful until subchondral bone exposed in later stages of OA.

9. Classification based on joint involvement.
   a. Localized – one or two joints affected.
   b. Generalized – three or more joints affected.

D. Incidence.
1. Most common form of articular disease in the United States.
2. Leading cause of disability among the elderly.
3. Cartilage destruction begins from ages 20 to 30.
4. More than 90% of population affected by age 40, but few experience symptoms until after age 60.
5. 30%-60% of people older than 65 years are symptomatic.
6. 25%-65% of people ages 45-64 have radiographic changes consistent with OA in at least one diarthrodial joint.
7. Incidence over age 55 twice as great in women (11.7 million).
8. OA demonstrates site specificity – only certain synovial joints show high prevalence.
   a. Weight-bearing joints (hips, knees).
   b. Cervical and lumbar spine.
   c. DIP, PIP, MCP joints in hands.
   d. Metatarsophalangeal (MTP) joints in feet.
9. Hands more affected in women, especially after menopause.
10. Hips more affected in men.

E. Considerations across the lifespan.
1. OA in younger people secondary to trauma, joint bleeds, infection may cause lifelong disability.
2. Resulting limitations in physical activities increase with age.
   a. 78% of elderly with arthritis describe limitations in physical activity.
   b. More than 1/3 report limitation in at least one ADL.
3. Arthritic involvement of feet, knees may cause unstable gait, increased risk for falling.
4. Emotional, social problems result from coping with chronicity, pain, limitations of arthritis.

F. Complications.
1. Chronic pain.
2. Decreased joint ROM, loss of function.
3. Synergistic action with other chronic diseases.
4. Decreased independence due to altered ability to perform ADLs.

II. ASSESSMENT

A. History (see Table 12.2 for comparison of RA, OA).
1. Joint pain.
   a. Dominant symptom, usual reason for seeking medical opinion.
   b. Typically mechanical ("aching") in nature, differentiating OA from inflammatory arthropathies.
   c. Increased with joint use, relieved by rest in early disease; night pain, pain at rest possible with disease progression.
   d. Possibly increased with falling barometric pressure before inclement weather.
   e. Hip OA may cause complaint of referred pain around groin, inner thigh radiating to buttocks, knee, outer thigh that can cause limp.
   f. Localized, asymmetric complaint with insidious onset; patient may not be able to remember exactly when pain started.
2. Joint stiffness.
   a. Varies in meaning from slowness of movement to pain on initial movement.
   b. Early morning stiffness after inactivity (articular gelling) or with prolonged static posture later in the day.
   c. Overactivity of joint often causes swelling due to a moderate effusion.
   d. Usually short-lived compared to generalized stiffness of inflammatory arthropathies.
3. Functional impairment.
   a. Difficulty in performance of ADLs.
   b. Limited joint movement, possibly with creaking or grating noise.
   c. Loss of work opportunities, with subsequent financial concerns.

B. Physical examination.
1. Symptoms localized, not systemic.
2. Tenderness to palpation.
   a. Capsular/joint line tenderness suggests capsular/intracapsular origin of pain.
   b. Point tenderness away from joint line suggests accompanying periarticular lesions (bursitis) often readily amenable to local treatment.
3. Reduced ROM as principal feature or contributor to overall disability.
   a. Extremely common in OA joints.
   b. Crepitation may be felt during joint movement, indicating loss of smooth cartilaginous joint surface.
   c. Accompanying loss of function more important than precise loss of movement.
   d. Mainly results from osteophyte encroachment, remodeling, capsular thickening but may be accentuated by mild effusion, soft tissue swelling.
4. Deformity/instability.
   a. Heberden's nodes on DIP joints.
      (1) Indicate osteophyte formation, loss of joint space.
      (2) Appear most often in women with OA.
      (3) Occur as early as age 40.
      (4) Tend to be seen in families.
   b. Bouchard's nodes on PIP joints indicate similar involvement to Heberden's nodes.
   c. Varus or valgus deformities possible in advanced knee OA.
   d. Leg length discrepancy resulting from loss of joint space in advanced hip OA.
   e. Large effusions uncommon, but slight to moderate effusion possible due to mild synovitis.
   f. Muscular atrophy in advanced disease secondary to joint splinting for pain relief.
   g. Weakness, numbness in arms or legs possible

from nerve root impingement by osteophytes in spine involvement.

5. Joint warmth.
   a. Can indicate varying degrees of synovitis.
   b. May accompany or precede signs of joint damage.
   c. Most evident at the knee or during early development of OA in fingers.
   d. Large warm effusion uncommon, should suggest alternative pathology.

C. Diagnostic tests.

1. Accurate diagnosis of type of arthritis allows prompt initiation of appropriate treatment, prevention of unnecessary suffering, disability, cost.
2. Laboratory findings.
   a. No observable changes in peripheral blood to confirm diagnosis of OA.
   b. Testing done to rule out autoimmune disorders, assess general function before initiating treatment.
   c. ESR may be minimally elevated with acute synovitis.
3. Radiographic findings.
   a. Help to confirm disease activity, monitor treatment effectiveness.
   b. Findings do not always correlate well with severity of clinical symptoms.
   c. Plain films may display typical changes.
      (1) Joint space narrowing due to loss of cartilage.
      (2) Cyst formation.
      (3) Subchondral sclerosis.
      (4) Enlarged, deformed asymmetric joints in severe OA.
   d. Bone scan used to determine skeletal distribution of OA.
      (1) Detects early changes.
      (2) Used to monitor complications of total joint arthroplasty (infection, loosening of prosthesis).
   e. Magnetic resonance imaging (MRI) used to determine extent of joint destruction.
      (1) Thinning of articular cartilage.
      (2) Capsular edema.
      (3) Subchondral cysts, inflammation.
      (4) Extent of collapse with avascular necrosis.
      (5) Possible effusion.
4. Synovial fluid analysis differentiates between OA, other forms of arthritis.
   a. Clear yellow joint fluid in OA.
   b. High viscosity due to normal amount of hyaluronic acid.
   c. Low WBC.
   d. Serum and fluid glucose equal.

III. COMMON THERAPEUTIC MODALITIES

A. Management goals. Conservative management with physical therapy, drug therapy, and/or self-care modifications.

1. Manage pain, inflammation.
2. Maintain joint function, mobility.
3. Prevent, correct deformity.
4. Accept chronic illness, individualized therapeutic regimen.
5. Use positive coping strategies.
6. Achieve maximal role function, independence in self-care.

B. Pharmacologic management.

1. Because no drug can reverse structural, biochemical abnormalities of OA, therapy aimed at pain management.
2. OA frequently occurs in elderly patients who may have other chronic diseases, take multiple medications.
   a. May take over-the-counter (OTC) medications that adversely interact with recommended OA regimen.
   b. Often receive health care from multiple providers, possibly leading to drug duplication or polypharmacy.
3. Nurses in all practice settings must be aware of factors that may affect drug therapy in elderly.
   a. Normal changes in body composition.
   b. Normal functional decline in body systems.
   c. Presence of other chronic diseases.
   d. Need to "start low and go slow."
4. Nonopioid analgesics.
   a. Acetaminophen now recommended as initial drug of choice for treating pain associated with OA.
      (1) Dose up to 1,000 mg 4 times daily.
      (2) Supplemented in short-term with opioid analgesics (propoxyphene, codeine, oxycodone) for acute exacerbations of pain.
   b. Nonsteroidal anti-inflammatory drugs (NSAIDs).
      (1) If acetaminophen proves inadequate for pain control, low dose of NSAIDs (OTC) or nonacetylated salicylate recommended for patients with normal renal function, no prior history of GI problems.
      (2) If pain persists, prescription dosages of NSAIDs may be ordered.
      (3) Analgesic effect exerted by inhibition of prostaglandin synthesis via inactivation of cyclooxygenase (COX) enzymes.
         (a) Reduction of prostaglandin levels in stomach, kidney due to COX-1 inhibition can result in gastric ulceration,renal impairment.
         (b) Elderly patients at higher risk for these side effects due to multiple comorbidities, diminished physiologic reserve.
         (c) Less GI, renal toxicity with newer NSAIDs with COX-2 selectivity (celecoxib, rofecoxib).
      (4) Careful monitoring should always accompany treatment with NSAIDs.
         (a) Renal function.

(b) Hemoglobin, hematocrit.
(5) Prophylactic treatment to reduce risk of GI ulceration, perforation, bleeding recommended in patients over 60 years of age with prior history of peptic ulcer disease, anticipated therapy of more than 3 months, moderate to high doses of NSAIDs, concurrent corticosteroids.
(a) Significant protective effect with misoprostol 200 mg four times daily but poorly tolerated due to diarrhea.
(b) Cytotec 100 mcg better tolerated, with increase to 200 mcg two to three times daily.
(c) Histamine[2] blocker or omeprazole can be substituted but efficacy limited to prevention of duodenal ulcers.

5. Biologic products.
a. Chondroitin sulfate acts as connecting matrix between protein filaments in cartilage.
(1) Idea of cartilage regeneration has become popularized in consumer literature.
(2) Chondroitin sulfate availability suggested to stimulate matrix synthesis, accelerate healing process.
(3) Research ongoing with some controversial outcomes regarding role of chondroitin sulfate in arthritis treatment.
b. Glucosamine sulfate perceived as "building block" for regeneration of cartilage glycosaminoglycans.
(1) Several studies indicate glucosamine sulfate may be better than some NSAIDs, placebos in relieving both pain, inflammation of OA.
(2) Intramuscular, intra-articular treatment appears to be well-tolerated.
(3) Further studies warranted on various dosage regimens, potential long-term effects.
c. Studies suggest dietary supplement S-adenosylmethionine (SAM-e) may help OA symptoms.
(1) No gastrointestinal side effects similar to NSAIDs.
(2) No sexual dysfunction, dry mouth, nausea as with antidepressants.
(3) Patient education must be initiated.
(a) Take stabilized SAM-e product.
(b) Easily loses potency, needs to be carefully packaged in airtight, light-proof container.
(c) Dose not to exceed 1600 mg daily.
(d) Take B vitamins (folic acid, B_{12}) with SAM-e to facilitate body's utilization.

6. Local therapies.
a. Capsaicin, methyl salicylate creams used as adjunctive agents.
b. Intra-articular corticosteroid injections appropriate for elderly OA patients with effusions, local inflammation but four or more injections suggest need for additional intervention.
c. Periarticular injections possibly effective in treating bursitis, tendinitis that may accompany OA.

C. Physical management.

1. American College of Rheumatology (ACR) guidelines highlight importance of nonpharmacologic therapies to relieve pain, improve joint biomechanics and function in patient with OA.
a. Local heat or ice to reduce pain, stiffness.
b. Ultrasound to increase collagen elasticity, flexibility.
c. Stimulation with electrical devices (TENS) to strengthen muscles.
d. Use of orthotic devices, shock-absorbing shoes to reduce discomfort with movement.
2. Weight reduction in obese patients reduces biomechanical stress on weight-bearing joints, may significantly relieve pain.
a. Cartilage, subchondral bone particularly vulnerable to effects of obesity in middle age, elderly patients.
b. OA progresses more rapidly in overweight individuals.
3. ACR guidelines also acknowledge importance of exercise as integral part of OA management.
a. Evidence suggests joint loading, mobilization are essential for articular integrity.
b. Quadriceps weakness develops in early disease, may contribute to progressive articular damage.
c. Exercise prescription should focus on cardiovascular conditioning, improvements in strength and flexibility, increased joint mobility.
(1) Aerobic or resistance exercises have led to improvements in physical performance, painful symptoms, reports of disability.
(2) Strengthening and weight bearing ROM exercises have improved gait, strength, overall function.
(3) Low-impact, gravity-limiting activities (bicycle training) increase muscle tone/strength, neuromuscular function, cardiovascular endurance without excessive force across joints.
d. Appropriate timing of analgesics helps patient participate more comfortably in exercise sessions.
4. Physical therapy may be ordered to facilitate exercise, help control joint symptoms.
a. Therapist can educate, motivate patient and monitor progress.
b. Therapy should be a transition strategy in almost all cases, with patient ultimately exercising independently.
5. Alternative therapies may be sought for symptom relief.
a. Some therapies (use of copper bracelets) are harmless, probably worthless.
b. Some therapies may have severe toxicities.
c. A few therapies (acupuncture) may have modest beneficial effects.

d. The nurse should consider asking about patient's interest in this area.
   (1) Maintain nonjudgmental attitude.
   (2) Recommend continuation of conventional therapies.
   (3) Request information to determine safety of other medications, nutritional supplements being taken by patient.
   (4) Support patient if relief is obtained from an alternative substance, treatment poses no medical risks and does not interfere with conventional treatments.

6. Surgical intervention may be considered for patients whose function, mobility remain compromised despite maximal medical therapy.
   a. Arthroscopy for removal of loose bodies, resection of torn tissue when joint space is sufficiently wide.
   b. Tibial osteotomy for patient with knee OA who has relatively small varus angulation, stable ligamentous support.
   c. Arthroplasty for patient with severe varus/valgus deformity (with related ligamentous instability), advanced hip OA, ineffective pain relief with other modalities.

IV. NURSING DIAGNOSES, OUTCOMES, AND INTERVENTIONS (See Table 12.1; see Chapter 19 (Hip), Chapter 20 (Knee) for surgical care considerations.)

V. HOME CARE CONSIDERATIONS

A. Education, counseling are nurse's primary role in assisting patients with chronic, potentially disabling OA.

1. Help families to become partners with patient in effective disease management.
   a. Schedule educational sessions when key family members can attend.
   b. Focus content on concerns of all family members to facilitate care.
2. Provide education about disease process, treatment, probable impact.
   a. Highlight nonsystemic nature of OA.
   b. Discuss unpredictable course of OA.
   c. Stress importance of exercise.
   d. Describe use of proper body mechanics, joint protection.
   e. Discuss importance of weight reduction in obese patient.
   f. Review pharmacologic therapies for OA, other medications taken by patient.

B. Advancing disease may lead to self-care deficits, threat to independent functioning.

1. Collaborate with occupational therapist to obtain assistive devices that facilitate patient's independence in self-care.
2. Discuss impact on self-esteem of arthritic deformities, decreased independence.
3. Review effects of disease on sexual relationship.
   a. Suggest alternative positions.
   b. Discuss strategies to relieve pain, stiffness before intercourse (analgesics, warm bath).
4 Retraining if needed by working patient.

POLYMYALGIA RHEUMATICA (PMR)

I. OVERVIEW

A. Definition: clinical syndrome characterized by pain, stiffness in shoulder girdle, pelvic girdle, neck occurring in people over 50 years of age. Primarily a pain syndrome rather than one of weakness, swelling, limitation of motion. Often associated with giant cell arteritis (GCA).

B. Etiology.

1. Unknown.
2. Possible causes include genetic factors, immune system abnormalities.
3. Reason for association with GCA unknown.

C. Pathophysiology.

1. Infiltrating mononuclear cells lead to mild synovitis.
2. Bilateral symmetric proximal myalgia develops in shoulders, hips, with prominent morning stiffness.
   a. Onset often acute, may be insidious.
   b. Due in part to synovitis.
3. Strong expression of HLA class II antigens appears on synovial, inflammatory cells.
4. Musculoskeletal symptoms may occur before, after, or simultaneously with GCA.

D. Incidence.

1. Mean age of occurrence 70 years.
2. Varies by geographic location possibly due to differing genetic, environmental factors.
3. Affects women more than men.
4. 70%-95% of patients present with shoulder pain, 50%-70% with hip or neck pain.

E. Considerations across the lifespan.

1. Extremely rare in anyone under age of 50.
2. PMR generally self-limiting unless associated with GCA.
3. Spontaneous disease exacerbations can occur, more frequently in first 2 years.

F. Complications.

1. PMR generally benign.
2. Associated GCA may have severe vascular complications.
   a. Blindness.
   b. Stroke.
   c. Ischemia to limbs or bowel.
   d. Aortic dissection (rare).
3. Corticosteroid-related side effects (a dangerous complication of therapy).

II. ASSESSMENT

A. History.

1. Morning stiffness, bilateral pain in shoulders, hips.
2. Discomfort may extend to proximal arms and thighs, axial muscles.

3. Pain may be severe, limiting activity and aggravated by joint movement.
4. Fever, malaise, anorexia, weight loss in about 1/3 of patients.
5. Headache, scalp tenderness, vision changes associated with GCA.

B. Physical examination.

1. Pain at rest in affected joints, increased with joint movement.
2. Tenderness over affected joints.
3. If associated with GCA, findings may include:
   a. Impaired visual acuity.
   b. Swollen, tender temporal and scalp arteries in 25% of patients.
   c. Bruits over large arteries.
   d. Low-grade fever.

C. Diagnostic tests.

1. Diagnosis based on clinical presentation rather than laboratory findings.
2. Elevated ESR may assist in diagnosis, but 20%-25% of affected patients have normal ESR.
3. Synovial fluid shows evidence of mild synovitis (1,000-8,000 WBCs).
4. Bone scan may demonstrate more uptake in presence of synovitis.
5. Temporal artery biopsy done to confirm GCA.

III. COMMON THERAPEUTIC MODALITIES

A. Corticosteroids are drug of choice for treatment.

1. Initial dose of prednisone 10-20 mg/day adequate in absence of cranial signs, symptoms.
2. Dose must be raised to 40-60 mg/day if GCA also present.
3. Rapid response to corticosteroids common, with resolution of symptoms within a few days.
4. Dose generally reduced after 1 month if symptoms subside and ESR normal.
5. Long-term therapy (> 2 years) may be required.

B. Short course of NSAIDs may be tried with patients with mild disease.

C. Methotrexate proposed as corticosteroid-sparing drug, but data are conflicting.

IV. NURSING DIAGNOSES, OUTCOMES, AND INTERVENTIONS (See Table 12.1)

V. HOME CARE CONSIDERATIONS

A. Educate patient on use, side effects of corticosteroids.

1. Recommend consistent calcium, vitamin D supplementation.
2. Recommend bone densitometry studies.

B. Patient should go immediately to ophthalmologist or emergency department in event of any alterations in vision.

RHEUMATIC FEVER

I. OVERVIEW

A. Definition: an acute multisystem inflammatory disease that occurs within weeks after an episode of group A (beta-hemolytic) streptococcal pharyngitis.

B. Etiology.

1. Caused only by group A (beta-hemolytic) streptococcal pharyngitis.
   a. Does not follow infection by other strains at other sites (soft tissue infection).
   b. Not all pharyngeal infections lead to rheumatic fever.
2. Strongly suspected to be hypersensitivity reaction induced by the bacterium.
   a. Proposed that antibodies to certain strains of streptococci cross-react with tissue glycoproteins in heart, joints, other tissues.
   b. Also suggested that streptococcal infection evokes autoimmune response against self-antigens.

C. Pathophysiology.

1. Acute presentation.
   a. Widely disseminated inflammatory lesions found in various sites, most notably in the heart (Aschoff bodies).
   b. Diffuse inflammation may be found in all three layers of the heart, leading to pancarditis with characteristic clinical features.
   c. Migratory polyarthritis leaves successive large joints painful, swollen.
      (1) Subsides spontaneously.
      (2) Leaves no residual disability.
   d. Sydenham's chorea.
      (1) Erratic, jerky movements.
      (2) Transitory local muscle weakness.
      (3) Emotional lability, personality changes.
      (4) Usually after earlier signs of fever, polyarthritis, carditis.
      (5) Commonly overlooked in children, attributed to restlessness, clumsiness if first, only major sign of rheumatic fever.
      (6) Self-limiting disease with no significant effects.
   e. Subcutaneous nodules, erythema marginatum.
      (1) Characteristic signs of rheumatic fever that actually occur rarely, are easily overlooked.
      (2) Small, painless nodules located over bony prominences, in tendon sheaths.
      (3) Rash obvious only in fair-skinned patients, generally hidden by clothing.
   f. Minor signs include fever, systemic inflammation.
2. Recurrent attacks.
   a. Increased vulnerability to reactivation of disease with subsequent pharyngeal infections.
   b. Same manifestations likely to reappear.
      (1) Chorea frequently reactivated.
      (2) Carditis probably worse with each recurrence.
      (3) Cardiac damage cumulative.

3. Chronic rheumatic heart disease.
    a. Characterized by acute inflammation, subsequent deforming fibrosis.
    b. Mitral valve usually affected in chronic disease.
    c. Involvement of another valve (aortic) may be more clinically significant in some patients.

D. Incidence.

1. Prevalence reflects adequacy of preventive medical care.
    a. Rare in developed countries (0.2-0.5 per 100,000).
    b. Remains leading cause of heart disease among children, young adults in many developing countries (from 1.25 to 24 per 1,000).
    c. Inadequate prevention among populations may lead to striking disparity within same country.
2. Most common among schoolchildren.
3. Affects both genders, all races.

E. Considerations across the lifespan.

1. Valve replacement may become necessary, particularly with profound mitral regurgitation.
2. No group known to be free of risk of rheumatic fever if exposed to pharyngeal infection with causative organism.

F. Complications.

1. Infective endocarditis leading to formation of bulky vegetations on heart valves.
2. Embolic events (cerebral or myocardial infarct).
3. Cardiac hypertrophy, heart failure due to myocarditis.
4. Atrial fibrillation, especially with mitral stenosis.

II. ASSESSMENT

A. History.

1. Recent group A streptococcal pharyngitis.
2. Previous rheumatic fever.
3. Complaints of joint pain, fever, rash.
4. Personality changes, emotional lability.
5. Muscle weakness.

B. Physical examination.

1. Evidence of chorea.
    a. Local muscle weakness.
    b. Jerky, purposeless movements.
2. Rash over trunk.
    a. Pink borders not indurated.
    b. Blanches on pressure.
    c. Changes shape before provider's eyes.
3. Subcutaneous nodules.
    a. Found with careful palpation of bony prominence such as vertebral spines.
    b. Also found with palpation of back of scalp.
4. Change in heart sounds.
    a. New murmur, change in previous murmur.
    b. Weak heart sounds.
    c. Pericardial friction rub.
    d. Tachycardia, arrhythmias.

C. Diagnostic tests.

1. No specific laboratory test is diagnostic, though throat cultures provide useful negative predictive test.
2. Diagnosis may be quite subtle unless indicated by presentation.
    a. Requires clinical skills and experience to diagnose.
    b. With diagnosis of rheumatic heart disease in later life, patient often does not recall previous attack.

III. COMMON THERAPEUTIC MODALITIES

A. Spontaneous healing may be present in about 80% of patients.

B. Detection should lead to prompt treatment to avoid introducing strains of disease-causing bacteria into community.

C. Medical management.

1. Current debate on effectiveness of cephalosporins versus penicillin in treatment of rheumatic fever.
    a. Low doses of penicillin may do little harm for treatment after false-positive tests due to non-*group A streptococci.*
    b. Use of broad-spectrum antibiotics may contribute to emergence of resistant pharyngeal strains.
2. Salicylates indicated for routine treatment of inflammation.
3. Corticosteroids indicated for a small minority of patients needing powerful suppression of inflammation.
4. Chronic disease management appropriate to specific manifestations.
5. Follow-up throat cultures not advised when treatment has been adequate, compliance good.

IV. NURSING DIAGNOSES, OUTCOMES, AND INTERVENTIONS (See Table 12.1)

V. HOME CARE CONSIDERATIONS

A. Primary prevention.

1. About 6%-29% of treated patients continue to carry *group A streptococci* after clinical recovery but bacteria pose no threat to family, other contacts in populations with low incidence of rheumatic fever.
2. Penicillin prophylaxis depends on eradication of strains that cause post-infection complications.
3. In populations where rheumatic fever remains a problem, causative strains need to be identified, studied.

B. Secondary prevention.

1. Patients at greatest risk for rheumatic recurrences should receive weekly intramuscular or daily oral penicillin, or daily sulphadiazine.
2. Duration of prophylaxis also risk-dependent, safely stopped if rheumatogenic strains disappear from community.
3. Several studies point to potential of an oral vaccine for rheumatic fever.

GOUT

I. OVERVIEW

A. Definition: disorder in purine metabolism characterized by monosodium urate crystal deposits in articular, periarticular, subcutaneous tissues that lead to acute attacks of arthritis. Umbrella term for multiple disorders characterized by elevated serum uric acid concentration (hyperuricemia).

B. Etiology.

1. Excess production of uric acid due to either accelerated purine synthesis, accelerated nucleotide breakdown, or increased nucleic acid turnover.
2. Primary gout (90% of cases) results from inborn error in either production or excretion of uric acid.
3. Secondary gout (10% of cases) results from known cause.
   a. Various acquired diseases (hyperuricemia or other clinical dysfunction such as hemolytic anemia, psoriasis, renal insufficiency).
   b. Obesity or starvation.
   c. Lead toxicity.
   d. Use of certain common drugs (salicylates, diuretics, nicotinic acid, alcohol).
   e. Organ transplant recipients (especially with renal/cardiac allografts) who take cyclosporin, diuretics.

C. Pathophysiology.

1. Uric acid is end product of purine metabolism, has no physiologic role.
   a. Humans may accumulate uric acid due to lack of uricase, enzyme that breaks down uric acid into more water-soluble products.
   b. 90% of patients with gout have underexcretion of uric acid.
   c. Hyperuricemia is a risk factor in development of gout, but gouty arthritis can occur in presence of normal serum uric acid concentrations.
2. Synovial fluid serves as poor solvent for monosodium urate.
   a. Urates become supersaturated in joint fluid, especially in peripheral joints.
   b. Prolonged hyperuricemia leads to crystal development in synovial lining cells, joint cartilage.
3. Unknown event (such as trauma) initiates crystal release into synovial fluid.
   a. Released crystals attract leukocytes, activate complement.
   b. Neutrophils, macrophages accumulate in joints, synovial membrane.
   c. Phagocytosis of crystals induces release of toxic free radicals, leukotrienes.
4. Activated neutrophils release destructive lysosomal enzymes.
   a. Inflammatory reaction intensified.
   b. Injury to articular structures augmented.
5. Four stages of clinical progression for gout.
   a. Asymptomatic stage marked by elevation of serum uric acid levels.
   b. About 5% of patients progress to second stage, acute gouty arthritis.
      (1) Rapid onset.
      (2) Exquisite pain usually involving one joint (especially great toe, joints in foot and leg).
      (3) Often precipitated by surgery, trauma, drugs, alcohol, emotional stress.
   c. Patient is essentially symptom-free during intercritical period (third stage), which may last months to years.
   d. Chronic tophaceous gout (fourth stage) marked by persistent pain after multiple episodes of acute disease.
      (1) Results from chronic inability to eliminate uric acid.
      (2) Sodium urate crystal deposits (tophi) now observed in earlobes, fingers, hands, knees, feet, ulnar sides of forearms.
      (3) Narrowed joint space with cartilage destruction seen on x-ray.
      (4) Gouty nephropathy possible from crystal deposits in renal medullary interstitium.

D. Incidence.

1. More than 10% of population of Western hemisphere have hyperuricemia, but only 0.5% develop gout.
2. Prevalence of gout equal in men and women, but men are six times more likely to have serum uric acid elevations.
3. Typically occurs during middle age, uncommon before 30 years of age.
4. Gout in great toe (podagra) accounts for over 50% of acute attacks.

E. Considerations across the lifespan.

1. Incidence raises with age, with first attack typically occurring between ages 40 and 60.
2. Patients with recurrent attacks have longer duration of illness, are more likely to have polyarthritic disease.
3. Average of 12 years passes between initial acute attack, development of chronic disease.
4. Elderly patients who have diminished renal function, use a diuretic, are particularly susceptible to development of polyarticular tophaceous gout.
5. Estrogen generally protects women against hyperuricemia until menopause.

F. Complications.

1. Soft tissue damage, deformity.
2. Joint destruction, crippling deformity.
3. Nerve compression syndromes.
4. Nephrolithiasis, gouty nephropathy.

II. ASSESSMENT

A. History.

1. Development of pain, swelling.
   a. Gout attack occurs within hours.
   b. If time frame is weeks to months, gout is less likely.
2. Number of involved joints.
   a. Early gout usually monoarticular or oligoarticular.

b. Initially not uncommon to have two joints involved, especially adjacent joints.
3. Any contributing factors.
a. Trauma, from major surgery to a long walk without physical conditioning.
b. Use of alcohol with high guanosine content that catabolizes to uric acid.
c. Use of thiazide diuretics, low dose aspirin, cyclosporin that raise serum urate level.
d. Physiologic disruption from acute illness that triggers attack.
e. Family history of gout that increases patient risk, especially in early onset disease.

B. Physical examination.
1. Swelling, pain, decreased ROM of affected joints (classically MTP joint in great toe; also fingers, knees, ankles, wrists, elbows).
2. Other possible findings.
a. Fever.
b. Headache.
c. Hypertension.

C. Diagnostic tests.
1. Laboratory findings.
a. Hyperuricemia (7-10mg/dl).
b. Albuminuria (>100 mg/24 hours).
c. Increased urinary uric acid.
d. Leukocytosis.
e. Elevated ESR.
2. Radiologic findings.
a. Normal films in early gout but may reveal intraosseus tophi that are not visible above the skin.
b. Asymmetric swelling seen within joint on x-ray, should also be found on physical examination.
c. Bony abnormalities on x-ray indicate presence of chronic disease.
(1) Tophi.
(2) Overhanging edge of cortex.
(3) "Punched out" erosion of bone with sclerotic borders.
d. Foot films in early disease serve as baseline, help in recognition of unsuspected destructive disease.
e. MRI necessary if gouty tophus mimics infection, neoplasm.
3. Synovial fluid aspiration potentially controversial aspect of patient work-up.
a. Accurate diagnosis possible without aspiration 80% of the time if patient has classic acute, painful swelling in MTP joint.
b. Aspiration may have therapeutic as well as diagnostic value, providing relief by decompressing swollen joint capsule.
c. Only reliable way to distinguish septic arthritis, pseudogout from gout.
d. Affected fluid generally reveals distinctive needle-like intracellular crystals of sodium urate.
4. Evaluation of renal, cardiac vascular systems essential due to typical occurrence of hypertension, renal impairment with gout.
a. CBC.
b. Serum creatinine.
c. Serum uric acid.
d. Blood urea nitrogen.
e. Urinalysis.

III. COMMON THERAPEUTIC MODALITIES

A. Nonpharmacologic therapy may reduce serum uric acid concentrations.
1. Weight reduction.
2. Decreased alcohol ingestion.
3. Decreased consumption of foods with high purine content.
4. Control of hypertension, hyperlipidemia.
5. Maintenance of high liquid intake (>2 liters/day).

B. Symptomatic hyperuricemia requires medication in addition to diet and lifestyle changes.
1. Acute gouty arthritis treatment.
a. NSAIDs currently most favored treatment.
(1) Indomethacin generally drug of choice.
(2) Other NSAIDs (naproxen sodium, sulindac, ketorolac) have achieved pain relief in affected patients.
(3) Used with caution in patients with history of peptic ulcer disease, congestive heart failure, chronic renal failure.
(4) Discretionary use in patients who are allergic to aspirin, have asthma or nasal polyps.
b. Colchicine is effective alternative to NSAIDs.
(1) Most beneficial when given in first 12-36 hours after attack.
(2) Appears to inhibit phagocytosis of uric acid, block release of chemotactic factor.
(3) Has anti-inflammatory effects but no analgesic activity.
(4) Oral administration started with two 0.5-0.6 mg tabs, followed by one tab hourly until joint symptoms relieved, GI side effects develop, or total of 5-7 mg given.
(5) Intravenous administration in 1 mg doses (not to exceed 4 mg/day) if oral route not available or GI side effects must be avoided.
c. Intra-articular injection of corticosteroids effective against monoarthric gout.
d. Systemic steroids (e.g., prednisone 20-30 mg/day) used only when NSAIDs, colchicine ineffective or contraindicated.
2. Prevention of recurrent attacks.
a. Hyperuricemic therapy initiated after acute attack has ended in patients with frequent attacks, tophi, or urate nephropathy.
(1) Uricosuric drugs decrease serum uric acid level by increasing renal excretion (probenecid, sulfinpyrazone).
(2) Contraindicated in patients with urine output <1 ml/minute, creatinine clearance <50 ml/minute.
(3) Frequently limited use in elderly due to physiologic decline in renal function that occurs with aging.

(4) Probenecid also blocks tubular secretion of other organic acids, may result in increased plasma concentrations of penicillin, cephalosporins, sulfonamides, indomethacin.
(5) Sulfinpyrazone can act as antiplatelet drug, requires cautious use in patients who are anticoagulated, have bleeding disorders.

b. Allopurinol impairs conversion of xanthine to uric acid.
   (1) Drug of choice in patients with severe tophaceous deposits, history of impaired renal function, uric acid nephropathy or nephrolithiasis.
   (2) Initial treatment with 100 mg/day, increasing by 100 mg/day at weekly intervals until maximum of 800 mg/day attained.
   (3) Initiation of allopurinol therapy can precipitate acute gouty attack.
   (4) Dosage must be adjusted in patients with renal impairment.

c. If mechanical problems result from tophi despite adequate control of arthritis, joint replacement or surgical excision of tophi may be necessary.

IV. NURSING DIAGNOSES, OUTCOMES, AND INTERVENTIONS (See Table 12.1)

V. HOME CARE CONSIDERATIONS

A. Patient, family must understand dietary guidelines for appropriate food selections at home, in restaurants if restrictions are recommended.
1. Decreased intake of red and organ meats.
2. Decreased alcohol intake.
3. Avoidance of sudden, severe dietary modifications.

B. Patient may use heat, ice, elevation to alleviate pain in affected extremity.

C. Patient should receive information on all gout medications, potential interactions with other drugs.

D. Focus should be on prevention, decrease of future attacks through consistent health care.

LYME DISEASE (LD)

I. OVERVIEW

A. Definition: tick-borne multisystem infectious syndrome. Often called the "great imitator" because symptoms can mimic those of mononucleosis, meningitis, multiple sclerosis, other diseases.

B. Etiology.
1. Caused by spirochete *Borrelia burgdorferi* transmitted by tick bite.
2. Infected ticks most commonly of Ixodes species (deer tick in United States, sheep tick in Europe).
3. Person-to-person transmission does not occur.

C. Pathophysiology.
1. Tick must obtain blood meal in order to molt, lay eggs.
   a. Leads to obligatory parasitism on mammals, reptiles, amphibians, birds in various locales.
   b. Humans become suitable alternative hosts when participating in activities in wooded areas where ixodid ticks are prevalent.
2. When tick in nymphal stage attaches to mammalian host, spirochetes begin to migrate to salivary glands, are regurgitated into host.
3. Organism may travel rapidly via blood to any area of body, with special affinity for skin, nerve tissue, synovium, heart's conduction system.
4. Bite by infected tick does not automatically result in infection but likelihood increases with longer duration of tick attachment to host.
5. Disease frequently appears as localized skin lesion but in its disseminated form may affect joints, cardiovascular and nervous systems.
6. *Early localized disease* (stage 1) characterized by appearance of typical LD rash (erythema migrans).
   a. Expanding erythematous rash (sometimes in shape of bull's eye) often occurs at site of tick bite 2-30 days after exposure (most commonly 7-10 days).
   b. Early symptoms appear to be related to live organism.
   c. Early localized disease usually cured with 3-4 weeks of antibiotic therapy.
7. *Early disseminated disease* (stage 2) associated with hematogenous spread to other body sites.
   a. Occurs after infection of several weeks or months.
   b. Neurologic, cardiac manifestations possible.
      (1) Bell's palsy, radicular neuronitis, lymphocytic meningitis possible.
      (2) AV nodal block most common manifestation of cardiac involvement.
   c. Malaise, myalgia, arthralgia likely in very ill patient at this stage.
8. *Late disease* can occur months to years after initial infection.
   a. May be immune-mediated but precise mechanism for tissue damage unknown.
   b. Approximately 10% of people affected with disease develop chronic Lyme arthritis if untreated.
   c. Late neurologic involvement possible.

D. Incidence.
1. Named after Lyme, CT, site of initial identification in mid-1970s.
2. Now most common vector-borne illness in United States.
3. Annual average of 11,000 cases reported between 1990 and 1996, represents significant increase over previous decade.
4. Both sexes, all ages susceptible but attack rate is highest in children younger than age 15, adults older than age 29.

5. Although disease has been reported in nearly every state, more than 80% of cases originate in eight states (New York, New Jersey, Connecticut, Rhode Island, Maryland, Pennsylvania, and Wisconsin).
6. Clusters of patients with rashes identical to erythema migrans also reported in North Carolina and Missouri but symptoms appear to be caused by unrelated borrelial species.

E. Considerations across the lifespan.

1. Because of similarities between Lyme disease and syphilis, there was initially great concern related to possible fetal transmission in pregnancy, teratogenicity.
   a. Recent studies suggest that antepartum Lyme disease is uncommon, even in endemic areas.
   b. Even with reported transplacental transmission of spirochete, fetal immunologic response is lacking.
   c. Suspected or early disease treated with oral amoxicillin or penicillin for 3 weeks.
   d. More aggressive treatment not warranted except for severe acute/ chronic disease, neurologic complications.
2. Patients with history of treatment for Lyme disease may have higher incidence of persistent impairment in overall health.
3. Studies under way to define clinical spectrum, pathogenesis of chronic disease in order to design better treatment regimens for persistent symptoms.

F. Complications.

1. Persistent soft tissue pain, fatigue even after otherwise successful treatment (post-Lyme syndrome).
2. Arthritic attacks resolve in a few days to weeks but may be recurrent, mimicking reactive arthritis.
3. Neurologic complications include triad of cranial neuropathy, meningitis, radiculoneuropathy unique to *B. burgdorferi* infection.
4. Variable AV block usually transient but sometimes high grade, requiring temporary cardiac pacing.
5. Pericarditis, impaired cardiac contractility can occur but are unusual.

II. ASSESSMENT

A. History.

1. Early localized skin infection at site of tick bite.
2. Disseminated disease causes systemic complaints 1-4 months after infected tick bite, requires clinical acumen for accurate diagnosis.
   a. Flat rash generally found on thorax, in body creases, or areas where tick experienced an obstacle (hair line, panty line).
   b. Complaints of fever, neck stiffness, joint pain, fluctuating headache, malaise possible.
3. Patient may not remember recent tick bite but reports activities in endemic areas.
4. Memory, mood, sleep disturbances possible from late neurologic involvement.

B. Physical examination.

1. Flat rash (erythema migrans).
   a. Previously emphasized "bull's eye" rash actually occurs in minority of cases.
   b. Lesion can also present with central necrosis, induration, vesiculation.
   c. Treatment with topical steroids leads to pale lesion.
2. Regional or generalized lymphadenopathy.
3. Acute joint effusions, especially in knee, leading to gait changes.
4. Dizziness, palpitations related to variable AV block in disseminated disease.

C. Diagnostic tests.

1. Routine laboratory tests have only minor role in diagnosis.
   a. CBC, ESR usually normal.
   b. Lyme serology test results not readily available as basis for rapid initiation of treatment.
   c. False-positive enzyme-linked immunosorbent assay (ELISA) result occurs in 5% of normal population.
   d. Serologic testing has no impact on treatment choices.
2. To optimize predictive value of positive finding, serologic testing should be performed only in patients who have clinical features truly suggestive of disseminated disease and are considered to be at risk.
3. Cerebrospinal fluid should be examined in cases of possible neurologic involvement.
4. ECG indicated in patients with cardiovascular symptoms.
5. Synovial fluid can be tested to exclude other causes of arthritis.

III. COMMON THERAPEUTIC MODALITIES

A. Treated with antibiotics in all stages.

1. Amoxicillin, doxycycline are drugs of choice.
   a. Amoxicillin safe in pediatric, pregnant patients.
   b. 2-3 week treatment recommended for solitary erythema migrans.
   c. Lyme arthritis typically slow to respond to antibiotic therapy.
2. Disseminated disease treatment based on severity of disease, may include parenteral antibiotic therapy.

B. Patients with carditis, any symptom more severe than mild PR prolongation should be admitted for cardiac monitoring, possible insertion of temporary pacemaker.

C. Arthritic symptoms treated with NSAIDs.

IV. NURSING DIAGNOSES, OUTCOMES, AND INTERVENTIONS (See Table 12.1)

V. HOME CARE CONSIDERATIONS

A. Education must focus on disease prevention, prompt evaluation of suspicious symptoms.

1. Counter public sources (Internet, call-in help lines from advocacy groups) that may provide misinformation.
2. Outdoor safety.
   a. Walk in center of path.
   b. Tuck long pants into socks.
   c. Wear white clothing to make ticks more visible.
   d. Check for ticks daily, remove attached ticks

before they are likely to transmit disease.
   e. Use tick repellent.
3. Vaccine for persons whose occupations, recreational activities place them at risk for *B. burgdorferi* exposure.
   a. Approved for people 15-70 years of age.
   b. Limited safety data for pregnant women, people with RA or certain heart conditions.
   c. Given in three doses spread over a year.
   d. Use of usual protective measures against Lyme disease recommended even after vaccination.
   e. Produces positive blood tests that might make diagnosis more difficult.

B. Provide rationale for decision not to perform serologic testing.

C. Ensure patient understanding of treatment plan.

SPONDYLOARTHROPATHIES

I. OVERVIEW

A. Definition: an interrelated group of multisystem inflammatory disorders that affect spine, peripheral joints, periarticular structures (Ankylosing Spondylitis, Reiter's Syndrome, and Psoriatic Arthritis).

B. Etiology.
1. Inheritance of HLA-B27 gene strongly associated with susceptibility to all forms of spondyloarthropathy, but gene is neither necessary nor sufficient for disease development.
2. Both genetic, environmental factors likely to play a role in pathogenesis.

C. Pathophysiology. (European Spondyloarthropathy Study Group criteria.)
1. Inflammatory spinal pain.
2. Asymmetric synovitis primarily affecting joints of lower extremities.
3. May be accompanied by one or more of following:
   a. Episodes of alternating buttock pain.
   b. Radiographic evidence of sacroiliitis.
   c. Heel enthesopathy at plantar fascia, insertion of Achilles tendon.
   d. Positive family history of spondyloarthopathy in first-degree relative.
   e. Current psoriasis or documented history of psoriasis.
   f. Current chronic inflammatory bowel disease or documented history of bowel disease.
   g. Urethritis, cervicitis, or acute diarrhea that occurred within month before onset of arthritic symptoms.
4. Spondyloarthropathies share clinical, laboratory characteristics that make it difficult to distinguish among them in early stages.

D-F. See Ankylosing Spondylitis, Reiter's Syndrome, and Psoriatic Arthritis.

II. - V. (See Ankylosing Spondylitis, Reiter's Syndrome, and Psoriatic Arthritis.)

ANKYLOSING SPONDYLITIS (AS)

I. OVERVIEW

A. Definition: systemic inflammatory disease of axial skeleton, including sacroiliac joints, intervertebral disc spaces, costovertebral articulations.

B. Etiology.
1. Unknown.
2. Tendency toward familial aggregation in disease development.
   a. HLA-B27 gene found in 90% of whites, 50% of African Americans with AS.
   b. Other genes may play a role.
3. Sex-linked hormone may be significant.

C. Pathophysiology.
1. Aseptic synovial inflammation with lymphoid infiltration, pannus formation occur in spine, affected peripheral joints (hip, shoulder).
2. Proliferative fibroblastic response leads to development of dense fibrous scars that tend to calcify/ossify in creating fusion of articular tissues.
3. Extra-articular inflammation can affect eyes, lungs, heart, peripheral nervous system, kidneys.

D. Incidence.
1. Overall prevalence estimated to be 1%-2% of population.
   a. Higher prevalence rates (27-62 per 1,000 males) in some high-risk North American Indian groups.
   b. Comparable to rheumatoid arthritis.
2. Usual age of onset 15-35 years of age, but highest incidence occurs at 25-34 years of age.
3. Males 3-4 times more likely to get disease than females.
   a. Generally seen in men in third decade of life.
   b. May go undetected in women due to milder course, caution regarding pelvic x-rays during childbearing years.

E. Considerations across the lifespan.
1. Usually manifests with onset of chronic low back pain, stiffness during late adolescence, early adulthood.
2. Symptoms begin before age 16 in juvenile-onset AS.
3. May result in severe limitation of spinal motion in some patients that affects quality of life.
4. Course varies greatly with periodic remissions, exacerbations.
5. Severe disease may result in shortened lifespan.

F. Complications.
1. Aortic insufficiency.
2. Pulmonary fibrosis.
3. Uveitis.
4. Impaired spinal ROM, fixed kyphosis cause inability to move head/neck and lead to altered visual function.
5. Severe postural abnormalities, deformity with disability.
6. Increased risk for spinal fracture due to osteoporosis.
7. Cauda equina syndrome with lower extremity weakness, bladder dysfunction.

II. ASSESSMENT

A. History.

1. Insidious complaints of dull ache, stiffness in neck, back.
2. Gradually increasing pain and muscle spasms with motion restriction in back, ribs, neck.
3. Morning stiffness persisting 1 hour or more, generally relieved by exercise.

B. Physical examination.

1. Restricted back motion with reduced extension, lateral flexion, forward flexion.
2. Tenderness to palpation of sacroiliac joints while patient is in position of forward flexion.
3. Reduced chest expansion, diaphragmatic breathing with costovertebral involvement in thoracic spine.

C. Diagnostic tests.

1. Diagnosis based primarily on physical findings, radiologic evidence.
   a. Sacroiliac joint distortion due to inflammation in early disease.
   b. Later appearance of "bamboo spine" due to calcifications (syndesmophytes) that bridge from one vertebra to next.
2. Laboratory testing not specific but elevated ESR, mild anemia may be seen.
3. Pulmonary function tests not diagnostic of AS but may show deterioration with thoracic involvement.

III. COMMON THERAPEUTIC MODALITIES

A. Treatment goals include mobility maintenance, decrease in inflammation, pain management.

B. Physical therapy critical to patient's ability to manage disease.

1. Instruction provided on back, neck, chest stretching exercises.
2. Hydrotherapy shown to decrease pain, facilitate spinal extension.
3. Light exercise often more comfortable than bed rest or reclining position.
4. Appropriate exercise, involvement in ADLs essential to minimize spinal curvature.

C. Successful pain management depends on reducing inflammation, stiffness.

1. NSAIDs, salicylates commonly prescribed.
2. Phenylbutazone may be effective in acute flare-ups but use should be limited due to possible bone marrow suppression.
3. Intractable pain may respond to sulfasalazine, methotrexate.

D. Use heat application for local relief of symptoms.

E. Spinal osteotomy, total joint replacement may be necessary for severe deformity, mobility impairment.

1. Heterotrophic bone development possible after joint replacement.
2. Radiation therapy, treatment with indomethacin may be needed.

IV. NURSING DIAGNOSES, OUTCOMES, AND INTERVENTIONS (See Table 12.1)

V. HOME CARE CONSIDERATIONS

A. Continue prescribed exercises at home.

B. Sleep on back with flat pillow on firm surface to allow any back, neck fusion to occur in functional position.

C. Use office furniture, equipment that reduces spinal flexion (tilting artist's table rather than conventional desk, correct placement of computer work station).

D. Continue normal activities except in severe disease.

REITER'S SYNDROME (Reactive Arthritis)

I. OVERVIEW

A. Definition: typical form of reactive arthritis, now synonymous with that disease. A symptom complex of urethritis or cervicitis, conjunctivitis, and asymmetric arthritis is considered classic but fewer than 1/3 of diagnosed cases show all three clinical signs.

B. Etiology.

1. Acute inflammation following within 1-4 weeks of an infection of GI or GU tract in genetically predisposed persons.
2. Presence of HLA-B27 antigen correlates with severity, chronicity of Reiter's syndrome.
3. Environmental, geographic, social influences being investigated.

C. Pathophysiology.

1. Primary microbial trigger is *Chlamydia trachomatis* infection.
2. Other triggers include enteric pathogens Salmonella, Yersinia, Shigella, Campylobacter.
3. Unclear if HLA-B27 antigen itself is linked to pathogenesis of Reiter's syndrome or if it is an immune response-linked gene.

D. Incidence.

1. Postvenereal disease course affects more men than women.
2. Enteric disease found equally in men and women.
3. Almost all cases in elderly; children develop after enteric infection.
4. 80% of patients positive for HLA-B27.
5. Patients who exhibit classic triad of clinical symptoms likely to have intermittent disease course, while those with incomplete syndrome are prone to chronic course.

E. Considerations across the lifespan.

1. Approximately 20% of patients experience severe progressive degenerative disease in peripheral joints, axial spine that can create functional disability.
2. Ankylosing spondylitis develops in about 10% of Reiter's patients, possibly leading to additional disability.
3. Because considerable variation exists in individual manifestations of disease, nursing care must be based on each patient's physical, developmental needs.

F. Complications.

1. Some attacks are self-resolving, but about 50% of patients will have recurrence at intervals from 3 weeks to 18 years.
2. About 50% of patients develop some type of permanent disability.
3. Keratitis, iritis, uveitis may recur.
4. Cardiac conduction problems such as AV block may occur in early disease.
5. Cardiac fibrosis may occur in chronic disease, leading to prolonged PR interval and aortic regurgitation.

II. ASSESSMENT

A. History.

1. History of infection.
   a. Episode of dysentery, bacterial gastroenteritis may have been forgotten.
   b. Sexually transmitted disease may not be readily admitted or discussed, but questioning about sexual contacts essential to appropriate diagnosis.
2. Painful urination, urinary urgency, possible blood in urine.
3. Possible penile discharge, edema/erythema at urinary meatus, painless ulcers on glans penis.
4. Joint stiffness, muscle aches, low back pain.
5. Eye redness, discomfort, tearing.
6. Skin lesions identical to those of psoriasis.
7. Chest wall pain from inflamed tendons in sternum, vertebral attachments.

B. Physical examination.

1. Asymmetric polyarticular joint involvement with or without edema, effusions.
   a. Sausage-shaped fingers, toes found only in Reiter's syndrome, psoriatic arthritis.
   b. Knees, ankles also often affected.
   c. Muscle wasting possible near affected joints.
2. Evidence of urethritis.
   a. Edema, redness at urinary meatus.
   b. Muculopurulent drainage.
3. Psoriasis-like lesions on soles of feet, other body surfaces.
4. Red, irritated eyes.

C. Diagnostic tests.

1. Greatest problem comes in differentiating Reiter's syndrome from other spondyloarthropathies.
2. Diagnosis based largely on clinical signs, symptoms, and history of infection.
3. Laboratory testing (urethral swab) confirms presence of sexually transmitted disease (STD).
4. Debatable if HLA-B27 antigen is worthwhile as screening device despite high incidence in patients with disease.
5. Other laboratory findings common but not diagnostic.
   a. Anemia, mild thrombocytosis.
   b. Elevated ESR in about 50% of patients.
   c. Leukocytosis with shift to left.
   d. Joint fluid analysis with 500-50,000 leukocytes/ul.
   e. Pyuria, hematuria per urinalysis.

III. COMMON THERAPEUTIC MODALITIES

A. No cure, no treatment regimen shown to have lasting effect on disease course.

B. Treatment includes patient education, symptom management.

C. Pharmacologic interventions may be used.

1. Antibiotics used to treat confirmed STD.
2. Joint discomfort initially treated with NSAIDs, though response usually incomplete.
3. Local steroid injections may produce more rapid control of arthritis.
4. Immunosuppressive agents (methotrexate) may be recommended for cases that do not show improvement with NSAIDS.
5. Skin lesions treated with etretinate, local corticosteroids.
6. Steroid eye drops or subconjunctival preparations may be needed for eye symptoms.
7. Use of prophylactic antibiotics remains controversial.

D. Nonpharmacologic interventions supplement other therapies.

1. Splinting recommended for joint protection.
2. Managed exercise program indicated for joint mobility.
3. Orthotics may prevent foot contracture, decrease deformity.

E. Knee surgery may be indicated for persistent effusion, popliteal cysts.

IV. NURSING DIAGNOSES, OUTCOMES, AND INTERVENTIONS (See Table 12.1)

V. HOME CARE CONSIDERATIONS

A. Education imperative to help patient understand, manage chronic disease.

1. Skin, optical care.
2. Energy conservation, joint protection.
3. Home exercise program.
4. Use of assistive devices.
5. Use of medications.

B. Safe sexual practices must also be discussed.

1. Condom may protect from postvenereal exacerbation.
2. Patient advised to avoid multiple sexual partners.

PSORIATIC ARTHRITIS

I. OVERVIEW

A. Definition. Inflammatory arthritis associated with psoriasis, a common skin disorder.

B. Etiology.

1. Cause appears to be combination of immunologic, genetic, environmental factors.
   a. Elevated IgG, IgA titers and presence of immune complexes.
   b. Possible environmental factors such as *group A streptococci*, trauma.
2. Family history of psoriasis or arthritis is useful

pointer to correct diagnosis.
3. Certain clinical HLA markers may help identify early in course who will have progressive, disabling disease.

C. Pathophysiology.
1. Scaling of psoriasis occurs when cells in skin's outer layer reproduce faster than normal, piling up on skin surface as plaques.
   a. Common sites are knees, elbows, trunk.
   b. Lesions may also be seen in scalp/hairline, umbilical area.
2. Joint erosion, deformity may precede or follow development of psoriasis.
   a. Extent pattern, severity of arthritis generally do not correlate with extent of skin lesions.
   b. When arthritis develops before skin lesion, spondylitic pattern of arthritis appears to be more common.
   c. If psoriasis precedes arthritis, most prevalent patterns are spondylitis, polyarthritis, and mixture of two.

D. Incidence.
1. Occurs in about 0.1% of general population, 5%-7% of patients with psoriasis.
2. Affects men, women equally.
3. Peak age of onset is 30-55 years of age.
4. Incidence as low as 0.3% in African and American Blacks, Latin American Indians, Chinese.
5. Almost nonexistent among Eskimos.

E. Considerations across the lifespan.
1. Now recognized as progressive and destructive disease, capable of causing significant disability.
2. Considerable social, economic distress possible due to double disfigurement from psoriasis, arthritis.

F. Complications.
1. High prevalence of joint damage, loss of motion.
2. Chronic pain, sleep disturbances.
3. Joint laxity limiting fine movements needed for performance of ADLs.
4. Ankylosis in proximal joints (wrist, MCP) leading to disability.
5. Severe joint deformity (arthritis mutilans) relatively rare (approximately 1% of patients with disease).
6. Conjunctivitis or iritis.

II. ASSESSMENT

A. History.
1. Nail changes.
2. Swollen, painful digits.
3. Appearance of pruritic silver scales on patches of bright red skin.
4. Possible low-grade back pain, loss of motion, stiffness.
5. Family history of psoriasis, arthritis.
6. Fever, malaise uncommon.

B. Physical examination.
1. Asymmetric swelling ("sausage digit"), erythema in small peripheral joints.
2. Tendency toward "ray" involvement, with inflammation of several joints in one digit.
3. Scaly skin lesions on knees, elbows, trunk, scalp.
4. Pitted, ridged, partially discolored nails.
5. Evidence of sacroiliitis.
6. Inflammation at areas of tendon or ligament insertion into bone (enthesopathy).

C. Diagnostic tests.
1. Most rheumatologists agree that diagnosis cannot be made without evidence of skin, nail changes.
2. Radiologic findings help monitor disease progression.
   a. Early soft tissue swelling.
   b. Erosion of DIP joints in hands, feet.
   c. Evidence of sacroiliitis with spinal involvement.
3. Laboratory findings inconclusive.
   a. Mild hyperuricemia not uncommon, can lead initially to diagnosis of gout.
   b. RF positive in only about 25% of patients, many of whom have co-existing psoriasis and RA.
   c. Slightly elevated ESR not specifically diagnostic.

III. COMMON THERAPEUTIC MODALITIES

A. Goals include symptom relief, disease suppression, rehabilitation.

B. Severe or generalized skin disease requires systemic therapy.
1. 1,25-dihydroxyvitamin D3.
2. Etretinate.
3. Tar preparation for scalp lesions.

C. Most patients receive some symptomatic relief from NSAID therapy.
1. Indomethacin, naproxen, diclofenac, piroxicam commonly used.
2. Trial of at least 4-6 weeks needed to fully evaluate efficacy.

D. DMARDs indicated for persistent inflammatory joint disease in patients with evidence of erosive arthritis, significant joint deformities.
1. Choice of drug depends on toxicity ratio, potential effect on skin, cost of drug, monitoring requirements.
2. Methotrexate, azathioprine, sulfasalazine, gold compounds, cyclosporin most widely used agents.
3. Patient withdrawal rate is significant with DMARDs.

E. Intra-articular or topical corticosteroids may be effective when used sparingly.
1. Injection through psoriatic plaque must be avoided to minimize risk of septic arthritis.
2. Oral agents used cautiously due to risk of exacerbating psoriasis.

F. Control of psoriasis with methoxypsoralen and UV light treatments may lead to control of arthritis in some patients.

G. Physical therapy, occupational therapy referrals appropriate for orthoses, assessment of social support needs.
1. Spinal mobility exercises important to maintain normal upright stance.
2. Weight-bearing exercise encouraged to decrease risk of osteoporosis common to patients with inflammatory arthritis.

H. Synovectomy, joint replacement may be indicated as in any chronic inflammatory arthritis.

IV. NURSING DIAGNOSES, OUTCOMES, AND INTERVENTIONS (See Table 12.1)

V. HOME CARE CONSIDERATIONS

A. Engaging patient's partnership essential to continued participation in therapeutic regimen.

B. Balance of rest, activity recommended.

C. Education must be provided on key treatment strategies for both skin, arthritis.

D. Significant image disturbance may result, requiring emotional support from caregivers.

SYSTEMIC SCLEROSIS (SS)

I. OVERVIEW

A. Definition: a multisystem disease affecting the microvasculature and the connective tissue, causing alterations in the skin and in a variety of internal organs. Painful symmetric arthropathy may also develop. Previously called scleroderma due to skin induration; later termed progressive systemic sclerosis to reflect generalized multisystem course. Systemic sclerosis now preferred because of limited skin, organ involvement in many patients.

B. Etiology.

1. Cause unknown.
2. Multiple interacting factors lead to endothelial injury, production of a variety of fibroblast growth factors.
3. Both immunologic derangements, vascular abnormalities play a role in development of fibrosis.
4. Risk factors associated with skin thickening:
    a. Environmental factors such as working with coal, plastics, silica dust.
    b. Similar conditions resulting from genetic factors (phenylketonuria), metabolic disorders (Hashimoto's thyroiditis), malignancies, postinfection disorders, neurologic conditions.

C. Pathophysiology.

1. General consensus that fibrosis is secondary to abnormal activation of the immune system.
    a. CD4+ T cells responding to unidentified antigen accumulate in skin.
    b. Release of cytokine by T cells attracts inflammatory cells such as mast cells, macrophages.
2. Accumulated T cells, inflammatory cells release mediators.
    a. Transcriptional up-regulation results in genes that encode collagen, other extracellular matrix proteins.
    b. Hypothesis supported by presence of CD4+ T cells in skin of many patients with SS.
3. Damaged vascular endothelium releases vasoactive substances.
    a. Collagen, mucopolysaccharides overproduced.
    b. Subintimal tissue proliferates, leading to fibrous thickening and narrowing of lumina.
4. Two major types of SS based on degree of systemic involvement.
    a. Diffuse cutaneous scleroderma.
        (1) Begins with symmetric widespread thickening of skin on face, trunk, extremities.
        (2) Bilateral symmetric swelling of face, fingers, feet seen in early disease.
        (3) Skin becomes thicker, shiny, hidebound as disease progresses.
        (4) Face becomes mask-like with rigid mouth, immobile expression.
        (5) Early visceral changes tend to develop.
    b. Limited cutaneous scleroderma.
        (1) Skin changes usually confined to face, fingers, distal extremities.
        (2) Often accompanied by CREST syndrome.
            (a) Calcinosis – calcium deposits in tissues.
            (b) Raynaud's phenomenon – intermittent vasospasm of fingertips.
            (c) Esophageal hardening.
            (d) Sclerodactyly – scleroderma of digits.
            (e) Telangiectasias – capillary dilations leading to lesions on face, lips, fingers.

D. Incidence.

1. Seen worldwide.
2. Incidence for women more than three times that of men, especially between ages of 14 and 40.
3. Black women at higher risk than white women.
4. Overall incidence rises with age.

E. Considerations across the lifespan.

1. Rare in men under 35, children.
2. 10-year survival rate after diagnosis with CREST syndrome approximately 65%.

F. Complications.

1. Loss of hand grasp ability due to skin retraction, musculoskeletal problems leading to functional disability.
2. Reduced general joint mobility.
3. Chronic vascular insufficiency with CREST syndrome leading to painful ulcers at fingertips, in areas of calcinosis.
4. Malabsorption syndrome leading to severe diarrhea.
5. Colonic hypomotility leading to constipation.
6. Interstitial pulmonary fibrosis leading to cough, shortness of breath.
7. Renal involvement leading to malignant hypertension.
8. Esophageal fibrosis leading to dysphagia.
9. Severe skin induration leading to erectile dysfunction, loss of penile length in men; dyspareunia, vaginal dryness in women.

II. ASSESSMENT

A. History.

1. Blanching, cyanosis, erythema in fingertips (Raynaud's phenomenon).
2. Changes in texture, color, consistency, moisture of skin.
3. Difficulty opening mouth, swallowing.

4. Diarrhea or constipation.
5. Nausea, vomiting, abdominal distention.
6. Shortness of breath.
7. Joint pain, swelling.
8. Decreased endurance, muscle strength.

B. Physical examination.

1. Telangiectasias on face, lips, fingers, palms, fingernails.
2. Edematous hands with thickened or hardened skin, loss of skin folds or wrinkles.
3. Calcific nodules, dilated capillary loops in fingers.
4. Edema, thickening, or tightening over forearms, face, legs, trunk.
5. Reduced temporomandibular joint range of motion.
6. Reduced peripheral joint mobility, evidence of polyarthritis.
7. Decreased strength in proximal muscles.
8. Rhythm changes, hypertension, signs of heart failure.
9. Decreased thoracic excursion, dyspnea, adventitious breath sounds.

C. Diagnostic tests.

1. Relatively normal laboratory findings.
   a. Mild hemolytic anemia often present due to mechanical red cell damage from diseased small vessels.
   b. Slightly elevated ESR common.
2. Scleroderma ANA SCL-70 found in about 35% of patients with diffuse disease, rarely seen in patients with limited cutaneous involvement and CREST syndrome.
3. Serum RF found in 30% of affected patients.
4. Definite diagnosis of systemic sclerosis requires clinical presentation with one major or two minor criteria.
   a. Major criterion is proximal scleroderma marked by skin thickening, tightening proximal to MCP joints.
   b. Three minor criteria are:
      (1) Sclerodactyly, with skin changes limited to fingers.
      (2) Digital pitting scars with depressed areas at fingertips or loss of fingerpad tissue.
      (3) Bibasilar pulmonary fibrosis.

III. COMMON THERAPEUTIC MODALITIES

A. Currently no rehabilitative guidelines for treating skin problems, but treatment experience with burns may provide logical approach to care of patients with SS.

1. ROM exercises may prevent skin retraction, help skin vascularization.
   a. Mouth excursion (yawning with open mouth).
   b. Active, passive exercise with progressive loads for trunk, limbs.
2. Massage compliments ROM in stimulating vascular function.
3. Heat applications increase skin flexibility.
   a. Superficial moist heat application.
   b. Paraffin baths of hand, feet.
   c. Ultrasound.
   d. Spa therapy.
4. Acupuncture, transcutaneous electrical nerve stimulation (TENS) both reported to improve skin vascularization.

B. Joint, tendon, muscle involvement treated with variety of interventions.

1. Rest appropriate for short periods of time with severe myositis, prominent synovitis.
   a. Splints applied locally.
   b. Systemic rest not suggested.
2. Passive, active exercises used to decrease joint deformity, muscle shortening.
   a. Passive exercises benefit patients with joint retraction, severe muscle weakness but may worsen inflammation in patients with severe arthropathy.
   b. Isometric exercises best suited for patients with arthropathy because no joint movement occurs.
3. Heat beneficial in improving ROM.
   a. Ultrasound may improve temporomandibular function, hand flexion-extension.
   b. Local heat application increases collagen extensibility.

C. Pharmacologic management.

1. Treatment has historically included three therapeutic agents.
   a. Vasoactive agents often given in early disease.
      (1) Prazosin, nicotinic acid, dipyridamole commonly prescribed.
      (2) Calcium channel blockers now more widely used.
   b. Anti-inflammatory medications (low-dose corticosteroid therapy) used when patients have significant joint, muscle involvement or extensive skin disease with severe digital ulcers.
   c. Immunosuppressive drugs used with minimal effectiveness, can also produce skin disorder quite similar to SS.
2. Penicillamine not accepted as established therapy by all clinicians, requires considerable patient support and monitoring due to possible toxic side effects.
3. Topical treatments may offer some relief from joint pain.
   a. Blistering fluids rubbed onto skin as home remedy produce "hyperstimulation analgesia."
   b. Capsaicin may be considered not only as pain controller but also as vasodilating drug.
4. Other agents used to treat specific systemic problems.
   a. Tetracycline for diarrhea associated with malabsorption syndrome.
   b. H^2 blocker for esophageal dysphagia, esophagitis.
   c. Captopril reported effective for hypertension with renal involvement.

D. Ergonomic work interventions may be needed due to peak incidence of SS during highly productive decade of patient's work life (35-44 years of age).

1. No data on such interventions available for SS patients.

2. Usual treatment includes protocols for hand stiffening originally developed for burns, OA.

IV. NURSING DIAGNOSES, OUTCOMES, AND INTERVENTIONS (See Table 12.1)

V. HOME CARE CONSIDERATIONS

A. Treatment involves shared management of chronic disease.

B. General education needed regarding nature, course, treatment of disease.

1. Digit protection, avoidance of exposure to cold.
2. Exercises to minimize hand contractures, facial rigidity.
3. Smoking cessation to decrease risk for vasoconstriction.

C. Nutritional goals developed to maintain patient's weight, minimize elimination problems.

1. Assist in choice of easy-to-swallow, high-calorie foods.
2. Instruct on dental hygiene practices to prevent inflammation, ulceration of mucous membranes.
3. Encourage use of high-fiber foods, increased fluids with constipation.
4. Identify, eliminate foods known to promote diarrhea.

POLYMYOSITIS (PM) AND DERMATOMYOSITIS (DM)

I. OVERVIEW

A. Definition: PM is an inflammatory myopathy of symmetric proximal skeletal muscles. DM is an inflammatory myopathy of skeletal muscle that includes distinctive skin involvement.

B. Etiology.

1. Unknown.
2. Tissue injury seems to be mediated by immunologic mechanisms.
3. Severity of disease not correlated well with altered immune complexes, so it is unclear if complexes represent primary or secondary phenomena.
4. Other possible triggers include viral, bacterial, parasitic agents; neoplasms; drugs or vaccinations; stress.
5. Genetic predisposition proposed in juvenile dermatomyositis.

C. Pathophysiology.

1. PM appears to be caused by cell-mediated injury.
   a. Cytotoxic T cells, macrophages seen near damaged muscle fibers.
   b. Expression of HLA Class I molecules increased on normal muscle fibers.
2. Capillaries seem to be principal targets in DM.
   a. Microvasculature attacked by antibodies, complement.
   b. This deposition precedes inflammation, destruction of muscle fibers.
3. Fibers, skin show evidence of regeneration.

D. Incidence.

1. Overall annual incidence of PM/DM 5 per million.
2. Biomodal distribution of age of onset.
   a. Children ages 5-14 years.
   b. Adults ages 45-65 years.
3. Occurrence in females twice that of males.
4. Seasonal onset inconclusively linked to course of disease.

E. Considerations across the lifespan.

1. Increased mortality associated with DM.
2. Close monitoring of outpatients required to detect flare-up of muscle disease.
3. Cautious agreement that there appears to be increased incidence of malignancy in adult patients.

F. Complications.

1. Early contractures if muscle weakness severe.
2. Muscle atrophy later in disease.
3. Aspiration pneumonia due to ineffective swallowing, muscle weakness in advanced disease.
4. Calcium nodules on skin surface.
   a. Seen in long-standing DM, especially in children.
   b. Nodules may ulcerate, crust over, develop eschar in severe cases.

II. ASSESSMENT

A. History.

1. Increasing fatigue, weight loss, malaise often occurring over several months.
2. Difficulty performing tasks due to muscle weakness.
3. Muscle pain, tenderness not always present in early disease.
4. Tendency to fall that is unrelated to balance.
5. Nail or skin changes including rash, scaling, reddened area.
6. Weakened cough effort, difficulty swallowing.
7. Palpitations.

B. Physical examination.

1. Characteristic skin changes.
   a. Violet-colored or erythematous papules, small plaques at PIP joints (Gottron's papules).
   b. Reddened, smooth, scaly patches at PIP joints (Gottron's sign).
   c. Violet-colored, cyanotic, or erythematous symmetric rash with edema around eyelids (Heliotrope rash).
   d. Irregular, thickened, or fissured cuticles with dilated vessels (telangiectasias) in nailbeds.
   e. Calcium nodules of varying size throughout skin (calcinosis cutis).
   f. Erythematous, scaling, atrophic rash on extensor surfaces, back (poikiloderma).
2. Muscle weakness.
3. Joint erythema, pain, synovitis with limitations in ROM.
4. Poor chest expansion, dyspnea.
5. Arrythmias.

C. Diagnostic tests.

1. Diagnosis confirmed after excluding other neuromuscular diseases.

2. Most important laboratory finding is elevated creatine kinase (CK).
    a. Indicates muscle injury.
    b. Level changes according to disease activity.
3. Electromyography (EMG) often shows bizarre, high-frequency discharges with spontaneous fibrillation, positive spikes at rest.
4. Muscle biopsy shows necrosis, fibrosis, evidence of regeneration.
5. Complete pulmonary function testing determines nature of pulmonary disorder.
    a. More sensitive to clinical changes than chest films.
    b. Evidence of restrictive lung disease, diminished carbon monoxide (CO) diffusing capacity.
6. Five criteria used to diagnosis PM/DM.
    a. Proximal symmetric muscle weakness, with or without respiratory muscle weakness or dysphagia.
    b. Elevated serum muscle enzymes.
    c. Characteristic EMG changes.
    d. Muscle biopsy evidence of PM/DM.
    e. Typical skin rash of DM.

III. COMMON THERAPEUTIC MODALITIES

A. Initial drug treatment consists of high-dose corticosteroids.

B. If corticosteroids ineffective or side effects intolerable, alternative medications may be prescribed (unlabeled use).
1. Methotrexate.
2. Azathioprine.
3. Cyclophosphamide.

C. Bed rest often prescribed, with slow return to normal activity level when CK levels return to normal.

D. Active, passive ROM exercises used to prevent joint contracture.

IV. NURSING DIAGNOSES, OUTCOMES, AND INTERVENTIONS (See Table 12.1)

V. HOME CARE CONSIDERATIONS

A. Return for frequent monitoring of CK because elevations indicate muscles have been overworked.

B. Patient education focused on safety.
1. Fall prevention strategies.
    a. Muscle strengthening program.
    b. Use of assistive devices.
2. Aspiration prevention strategies.
    a. Rest before meals.
    b. Diet of easily swallowed foods.
    c. Upright posture during meals.

C. Patient education focused on corticosteroid use.
1. Report low-grade fevers, chills, joint pain due to increased risk of infection.
2. Develop awareness of long-term effects of drug.
    a. Facial edema.
    b. Increased appetite.
    c. Development of diabetes mellitus, osteoporosis, avascular necrosis.
3. Understand administration requirements.
    a. Never change dose.
    b. Never discontinue therapy suddenly.

SYSTEMIC LUPUS ERYTHEMATOSUS (SLE)

I. OVERVIEW

A. Definition: multisystem inflammatory connective tissue disorder associated with abnormalities of the immune system. Occurs in subsets: discoid lupus erythematosus, subacute cutaneous lupus erythematosus, antiphospholipid syndrome, neonatal lupus syndrome, drug-induced lupus.

B. Etiology.
1. Long suspected genetic influence in SLE.
    a. High prevalence of condition in identical twins.
    b. 5%-12% of relatives of patients also develop SLE.
    c. Multiple susceptibility genes (HLA complex), null complement play a role.
2. Environmental factors may contribute to disease development.
    a. Sun exposure, burns may be most significant environmental trigger.
    b. Infectious agents could serve as stimulus for immune hyperactivity.
    c. Drugs (sulfa antibiotics) may play role in SLE development.

C. Pathophysiology.
1. Results from abnormal reaction of body against its own tissues, cells, serum proteins.
2. Affected persons have both self and nonself antigens, indicating possible hyperactivity of B cells.
    a. Interleukin-6 may play role in B cell hyperactivity.
    b. Abnormal B cell response due in turn to defective T cell function.
3. Increased number of antigen-antibody complexes form.
    a. Complexes penetrate basement membranes of capillaries.
    b. Affected tissues include kidneys, heart, skin, brain, joints.
4. Immune complexes then trigger inflammatory response that leads to tissue destruction.
    a. Severity of clinical response, organ damage directly related to intensity of inflammation.
    b. Elevation in concentration of interleukin receptor antagonists also a good indicator of disease activity.
5. Along with inflammatory activity, lupus erythematosus (LE) cells develop in blood.
    a. LE cells are neutrophils resulting from ANAs.
    b. LE bodies develop in LE cells as result of another antibody (anti-DNA of IgG type).
    c. Relationship between serum LE factor and pathological changes of SLE unclear, but absence of LE factor is strong evidence against existence of disease.

6. One of underlying defects in SLE may center on programmed cells death (apoptosis), when exposed cellular antigens incite an immune response.

D. Incidence.

1. Recognized worldwide but prevalence varies from country to country.
2. More prevalent in women (90%-95% of cases), particularly those between puberty and menopause.
3. African Americans, Asian Americans, Native Americans approximately three times more likely to be diagnosed with SLE than white Americans.
4. Despite many published cases, true incidence of SLE in children, adolescents unknown.
5. Overall incidence in United States is 15-100 per 100,000.
6. Age, gender, race, socioeconomic status appear to affect disease progression.
   a. Blacks seem to have worse prognosis with increased prevalence of renal disease.
   b. Deprived groups seem to fare worse than those from affluent background.

E. Considerations across the lifespan.

1. Neonatal lupus erythematosus (NLE) may appear in children of women with SLE.
   a. Risk for congenital heart block correlated with high antibody titers.
   b. Cutaneous involvement noted in more than 1/3 cases of NLE.
2. Children, adolescents with SLE are extremely vulnerable to psychologic impact of both chronic illness and medication regimen.
   a. Although many cases of mild SLE may go unreported, early age of onset may be associated with worse prognosis due to significant renal, central nervous system (CNS) involvement.
   b. Delayed diagnosis due to physician failure to consider SLE is great risk to children, adolescents with disease.
3. Most common in women of childbearing age, may cause multiple peripartum complications.
   a. Infertility may occur due to renal involvement, high-dose corticosteroid therapy.
   b. 22%-49% incidence of spontaneous abortion, fetal death in women with SLE.
   c. Placenta affected by immune complex deposits, inflammatory responses in placental vessels leading to common problems.
      (1) Spontaneous abortion.
      (2) Stillbirth.
      (3) Intrauterine growth retardation.
   d. Renal, cardiovascular, pulmonary, central nervous systems may be affected significantly during pregnancy.
   e. 60% incidence of peripartum exacerbations requires treatment as high risk pregnancy.
   f. Many practitioners, investigators believe that pregnancy does not affect the long-term prognosis of SLE.
   g. Patient should plan pregnancy when disease state is in control, conceive during inactive phase.
4. Late-onset lupus (in patients over age of 50) often has insidious onset, may be difficult to distinguish from other autoimmune disorders.

F. Complications.

1. Severe maternal morbidity with permanent renal and/or CNS compromise complicating about 10% of pregnancies.
2. 10-year survival now 80% in children, adolescents but significant numbers continue to progress to chronic renal failure and/or death.
3. Fibromyalgia can co-exist with SLE, should be considered when developing treatment regimen.
4. Panniculitis, a rare but severe complication, affects middle or deep dermal layer and leaves a deep scar on resolution.
5. Permanent alopecia may result from scalp lesions.
6. "Shrinking lung syndrome" may result from myopathy of the diaphragm associated with pleural adhesion.
7. Peripheral neuropathy can result in sensory and/or motor deficits.
8. Diffuse proliferative nephritis associated with poor prognosis.
9. Rare gastrointestinal complications include mesenteric vasculitis, inflammatory bowel disease, pancreatitis, liver disease.
10. Risk for thromboembolism due to the hypercoagulable state of antiphospholipid antibody syndrome.
11. Premature atherosclerosis often associated with corticosteroid use.
12. Vasculitis, impaired circulation to distal extremities lead to ulcers, difficulty with healing.

II. ASSESSMENT

A. History.

1. Hair loss, rash, other skin lesions.
2. Muscle pain, weakness.
3. Joint pain, especially in hands, wrists, knees.
4. Pleuritic chest pain.
5. Headaches, possibly of classic migraine type.
6. Anxiety, mood swings, insomnia.
7. Visual disturbances, photosensitivity.

B. Physical examination.

1. Cutaneous, vascular lesions.
   a. Appear in any location, especially after exposure to sunlight.
   b. Classic butterfly rash over cheeks, bridge of nose affects less than 50% of patients with SLE.
   c. Atrophied scaling areas (discord lesions) can appear on face, neck, arms.
   d. Mild to moderate hair loss possible if disease is active.
2. Joint symptoms.
   a. Earliest features of disease, occur in more than 90% of patients with SLE.
   b. Diffuse swelling, joint and muscle pain, stiffness may be noted.
   c. Deformities usually result from soft tissue stresses rather than erosive joint changes.
3. Central nervous system involvement.

a. Evidence of cranial neuropathies include facial weakness, asymmetric expression, nystagmus, extraocular muscle weakness.
b. Psychosocial effects may include changes in mood/affect, cognition, emotional stability.

4. Cardiopulmonary involvement.
   a. Tachypnea, cough suggest restrictive lung disease.
   b. Adventitious breath sounds possibly related to pneumonia, pleural effusion.
   c. Arrhythmias due to fibrosis of SA, AV nodes.
5. Hematologic manifestations.
   a. Hemolytic anemia in up to 25% of patients with SLE, associated with autoimmune antibodies directed against RBC antigens.
   b. Leukopenia usually associated with active disease.
   c. Thrombocytopenia may follow course of disease (refractory) or occur as isolated finding.

C. Diagnostic tests.

1. No specific diagnostic test exists for SLE.
2. Like several other connective tissue diseases, SLE is characterized by ANA against various cell nucleus components.
3. Other antibodies include anti-DNA, antineuronal, anticoagulant, anti-WBC, anti-RBC, antiplatelet, anti-basement membrane.
   a. Most specific tests for SLE are anti-double-stranded DNA, anti-samarium (Sm).
   b. High levels of anti-DNA rarely found in any condition other than SLE.
   c. Anti-Sm nuclear antigen almost exclusively found in SLE.
4. LE cell test has been generally superseded by anti-DNA, anti-Sm tests.
5. ESR, CRP not diagnostic but may be useful to distinguish between lupus flare and infection.

III. COMMON THERAPEUTIC MODALITIES

A. Treatment for active disease depends on organ systems involved, disease severity.

B. Major challenge is to treat active phase of SLE without allowing treatment itself to cause long-term damage.

1. NSAIDs remain a mainstay of treatment, especially for patients with mild polyarthralgias or polyarthritis.
   a. Need to avoid more gastrotoxic NSAIDs due to likelihood of GI effects during long-term therapy.
   b. NSAIDs affect renal function, which must be monitored due to risk for nephritis with SLE.
2. Antimalarial agents (hydroxychloroquine) frequently used to treat polyarthritis.
   a. Generally very safe.
   b. Retinopathy may develop in 1% of patients, reverses when drug discontinued.
3. Physicians now less reluctant to use immunosuppressive drugs (azathioprine, cyclophosphamide).
4. Corticosteroid exposure limited if at all possible.
   a. Intravenous methylprednisolone may be indicated to control severe flare-up of polyarthritis, followed by low-maintenance dose of prednisone.
   b. Steroid-sparing drugs (methotrexate) can be added to regimen with folic acid to counter minor side effects.
5. D-Penicillamine, minocycline, sulfasalazine effective for RA, SS but may exacerbate SLE.

C. Cutaneous manifestations usually treated with strict use of sun block, careful use of topical steroids (not all indicated for use on face), antimalarial therapy.

1. If patient cannot tolerate antimalarials, antileprosy drugs (dapsone) or retinoids are additional therapeutic options.
   a. Glucose-6-phosphate dehydrogenase status must be checked in patients before initiating dapsone.
   b. Retinoids should not be used in pregnant patients.
2. Patients with very severe cutaneous LE may require high doses of corticosteroids or use of steroid-sparing drug.

D. Manifestation of antiphospholipid antibody syndrome is a common cause of hypercoagulability.

1. Patients with history of venous, arterial thrombosis appear to benefit from high-intensity warfarin sodium with International Normalized Ratio maintained at 3-4.
2. Women with recurrent pregnancy loss have a greater chance of successful pregnancy if given heparin and low-dose aspirin.
3. Heparin and warfarin may be inappropriate for patient with thrombocytopenia.

E. Therapeutic plasma exchange (plasmapheresis) is designed to relieve clinical manifestations of SLE by removing immune complexes from the affected patient.

1. Repeated treatments usually necessary.
2. Pheresis therapy does not provide cure for SLE.
3. Plasmapheresis must be given with corticosteroids, often cytoxan to avoid a disease flare.

F. Supportive therapies may be more important than drug therapy, experimental treatments.

1. Physical and emotional support.
   a. Avoid excessive bed rest.
   b. Manage fatigue by pacing activities.
   c. Develop positive coping skills.
   d. Use support groups (American Lupus Society, Arthritis Foundation).
2. Diet and supplements.
   a. Three well-balanced meals needed daily.
   b. Fish oil suggested as beneficial but various studies failed to show anti-inflammatory effects.
   c. Salt intake restricted if patient is taking corticosteroids, is hypertensive.
   d. No controlled studies demonstrate clear-cut benefits for vitamin use beyond normal supplementation.

3. Skin protection.
   a. Sunscreen protection (at least SPF 15) needed.
   b. Limit sun exposure from 11 a.m. to 3 p.m.
   c. Avoid drying soaps, powders, harsh household chemicals.
   d. Monitor for infection if steroid-dependent.

IV. NURSING DIAGNOSES, OUTCOMES, AND INTERVENTIONS (See Table 12.1)

V. HOME CARE CONSIDERATIONS

A. Consider referral to pain management center if patient unresponsive to conventional therapies.

B. Counsel patient to expect some increased stiffness, aching in relation to changes in barometric pressure.

C. Urge tobacco abstinence, avoidance of secondhand smoke because smoke contains potentially lupogenic hydrazines.

D. Encourage muscle strengthening exercises that improve endurance while avoiding undue stress to inflamed joints.

FIBROMYALGIA SYNDROME (FS)

I. OVERVIEW

A. Definition: syndrome of chronic nonarticular musculoskeletal pain that is nondegenerative, nonprogressive, noninflammatory. Currently second most commonly diagnosed musculoskeletal disorder, major cause of disability; diagnosis especially increased in geriatric population.

B. Etiology.
1. Multifactorial features contribute to unknown etiology.
2. Abnormalities of musculature have been implicated, but none remain fully reproducible/confirmatory.
3. May coexist with certain rheumatic diseases (RA, SLE) or overlap with myofascial pain syndrome.

C. Pathophysiology.
1. FS historically believed to be either an inflammatory or psychiatric condition, but no current evidence supports either theory.
   a. Light microscopy has not shown evidence of inflammation in either muscle or tendons.
   b. Electron microscopy has revealed severe damage, dissolution of myofilaments to support the reality of patient complaints.
2. Loss of stage 4 non-REM sleep believed to lead to ineffective tissue restoration, pain modulation.
3. Abnormality in serotonin metabolism can alter perception of pain in affected or damaged tissues.
4. Some preliminary work also suggests possible role for autoimmunity.

D. Incidence.
1. 80%-90% of affected patients are women.
2. Peak age is 30-50 years.
3. Prevalence reported to be 2%-5% overall, increasing with age.

E. Considerations across the lifespan.
1. Highest prevalence between ages 60 and 79.
2. Anecdotal reports indicate pregnancy may exacerbate symptoms.
   a. Trigger points may worsen.
   b. Joint pain during the night may increase.
   c. Temporary remission may be followed by later worsening of symptoms.
   d. Symptom monitoring critical during pregnancy.
3. Occurs in children (predominantly in girls) with age of onset ranging from 9 to 15 years.
4. May overlap with chronic fatigue syndrome, making differentiation especially difficult in children.

F. Complications.
1. Clinical depression, anxiety may develop related to uncertainty of disease.
   a. Average FS patient visits more than five medical practitioners, spends thousands of dollars, and has symptoms for 5 years before diagnosis is made.
   b. Suggestion is often made that symptoms are "all in the patient's head."
   c. Some relief of psychological symptoms occurs with confirmed diagnosis.
2. Headache, symptom of irritable bowel syndrome, excess sensitivity to cold reported in 50% of patients with FS.
3. Patient experiences decreased ability to remain at job due to pain, fatigue.

II. ASSESSMENT

A. History (see Table 12.3).
1. Diffuse burning pain that waxes and wanes during the day, difficult to tell if in muscles, joints, soft tissues.
2. Sleep deprivation.
3. Extreme fatigue, weakness.
4. Frequent absence from work due to pain, fatigue.

B. Physical examination.
1. Skin, soft tissue tenderness, especially in skin folds.
2. Positive for point tenderness at 11 or more points, existence of which are generally not known by patient.
3. Reactive hyperemia (localized erythema) may be seen after point palpation.
4. Weary look, flat or anxious affect.

C. Diagnostic tests.
1. Routine laboratory analysis, diagnostic studies reveal little or nothing about course, symptoms of FS.
2. Results of evaluation in most cases rule out differential diagnoses postulated from history, physical examination.
3. Occasionally a low ANA titer is seen but is not considered diagnostic.
4. Muscle biopsy may reveal nonspecific moth-eaten appearance in Type I fibers, fiber atrophy in Type II fibers.

Table 12.3
ACR 1990 Criteria for Classification of Fibromyalgia

1. **History of widespread pain for at least 3 months.**
   Definition: pain is considered widespread when all of the following are present: pain in left side of body, pain in right side of body, pain above waist, and pain below waist. In addition, axial skeleton pain (cervical spine, anterior chest, thoracic spine, or low back) must be present. In this definition, shoulder and buttock pain is considered as pain for each involved side. "Low back pain" is considered lower segment pain.

2. **Pain in 11 of 18 tender point sites on digital palpation.**
   Definition: pain on digital palpation must be present in at least 11 of the following 18 tender point sites:
   - *Occiput*: bilateral, at the suboccipital muscle insertions.
   - *Low cervical*: bilateral, at the anterior aspects of the intertransverse spaces at C5-C7.
   - *Trapezius*: bilateral, at the midpoint of the upper border.
   - *Supraspinatus*: bilateral, at origins, above the scapula spine near the medial border.
   - *Second rib*: bilateral, at the second costochondral junctions, just lateral to the junctions on the upper surfaces.
   - *Lateral epicondyle*: bilateral, 2 cm distal to the epicondyles.
   - *Gluteal*: bilateral, in upper outer quadrants of buttocks in anterior fold of muscle.
   - *Greater trochanter*: bilateral, posterior to the trochanteric prominence.
   - *Knee*: bilateral, at the medial fat pad proximal to the joint line.

Digital palpation should be performed with an approximate force of 4 kg. For a tender point to be considered "positive," the patient must state that the palpation was painful. "Tender" is not be considered "painful."

Patient will be said to have fibromyalgia if both criteria are satisfied. The presence of a different clinical disorder does not exclude the diagnosis of fibromyalgia.

Source: The American College of Rheumatology, 1990 Criteria for the Classification of Fibromyalgia. (1990). *Arthritis and Rheumatism*, *33*(2), 160-172.

III. COMMON THERAPEUTIC MODALITIES

A. Long-term follow-up suggests little symptom improvement over time, so coordinated collaborative approach to care required.

B. FS is not generally responsive to corticosteroids, only minimally responsive to NSAIDs.

C. Adjunctive medications may be prescribed before bedtime to decrease pain, improve sleep.

1. Low-dose tricyclic antidepressants.
2. Low-dose selective serotonin re-uptake inhibitors (SSRIs).
3. Benzodiazepines.
4. Muscle relaxants.

D. Localized pain can be treated with topical creams (capsaicin, EMLA) or by injection of tender points.

E. Other interventions often attempted.

1. Massage, reflexology may alleviate symptoms.
2. Local heat often beneficial.
3. Herbal therapies (St. John's wort) have apparently helped some patients but have not been tested to determine safety, efficacy.
4. Anecdotal reports of symptom management with a variety of health food nutrients.
   a. Side effects and bioequivalencies of health food nutrients have often not been studied.
   b. Patient may discuss use of varied products.
      (1) Chrominum picolinate to decrease "carbo craving" experienced by some patients with FS.
      (2) Melatonin or Calms Forte (mixture of herbs, calcium, magnesium phosphates) to assist with sleep problems.
      (3) Raw thymus to address possible immune impairment.
      (4) L-Threonine to help with "restless legs syndrome."
      (5) Peppermint oil to help with irritable bowel syndrome.
5. Studies suggest dietary supplement S-adenosylmethionine (SAM-e) may help FS symptoms (see Osteoarthritis section in this chapter for discussion of SAM-e).
6. Meditation allows escape from the burden of sensory overload that often accompanies FS.

IV. NURSING DIAGNOSES, OUTCOMES, AND INTERVENTIONS (See Table 12.1.)

V. HOME CARE CONSIDERATIONS

A. Educate patient, family regarding effects of chronic illness.

B. Review basics of sleep hygiene to try to maximize sleep behaviors.

C. Encourage regular exercise to promote restorative sleep.

D. Discuss possible nutritional triggers for symptom

exacerbation.

1. Cereals made of wheat or corn.
2. Dairy products.
3. Caffeine.
4. Yeast.
5. Citrus.

E. Promote use of pain management strategies.

F. Discuss ways to manage FS during travel, vacation.

1. Begin trip in the best possible shape.
2. Try to find easiest air routes with fewest possible connections.
3. Dress for expected weather.
4. Request rental car with automatic transmission, cruise control.
5. Change position often when traveling.
6. Maintain normal exercise regimen while traveling.

G. Assist with vocational retraining if FS causes significant functional disability.

Bibliography

Alarcon, G.S. (1999). Antibiotics for rheumatoid arthritis? Minocycline shows promise in some patients. *Postgraduate Medicine, 105 (4), 95-98.*

Altizer, L.L. (1998). Degenerative disorders. In A.B. Maher, S.W. Salmond, & T.A. Pellino (Eds.). *Orthopaedic nursing* (2nd ed., pp. 480-544). Philadelphia: W.B. Saunders Company.

American College of Rheumatology Ad Hoc Committee on Clinical Guidelines (1996). Guidelines for the initial evaluation of the adult patient with acute musculoskeletal symptoms. *Arthritis & Rheumatism, 39*(1), 1-8.

Ashwill, J.W., & Droske, S.D. (1997). *Nursing care of children: Principles and practice.* Philadelphia: W.B. Saunders Company.

Barrett, J.H., Brennan, P., Fiddler, M., & Silman, A.J. (1999). Does rheumatoid arthritis remit during pregnancy and relapse postpartum? Results from a nationwide study in the United Kingdom performed prospectively from late pregnancy. *Arthritis & Rheumatism, 42*(6), 1219-1227.

Bindler, R.M., & Howry, L.B. (1997). *Pediatric drugs and nursing implications* (2nd ed.). Stamford, CT: Appleton & Lange.

Briant, C., Roye, K., & Kutscher, A.H. (1997). Pericarditis as a manifestation of Lyme disease. *Journal of Emergency Nursing, 23*(6), 525-529.

Bryant, G.A. (1998). Reiter's syndrome. *Orthopaedic Nursing, 17*(1), 57-62.

Burrage, R.L., & Sutter, C.A. (1999). Arthritis. In J.T. Stone, J.F. Wyman, & S.A. Salisbury (Eds.). *Clinical gerontological nursing: A guide to advanced practice* (pp. 469-487). Philadelphia: W.B. Saunders Company.

Casale, R., Buonocore, M., & Matucci-Cerinic, M. (1997). Systemic sclerosis (scleroderma): An integrated challenge in rehabilitation. *Archives of Physical Medicine & Rehabilitation, 78*(7), 767-773.

Chondroitin. (1998, April). The Review of Natural Products, 1-2.

Classen, S.R., Paulson, P.R., & Zacharias, S.R. (1998). Systemic lupus erythematosus: Perinatal and neonatal complications. *JOGNN, 27*(5), 493-500.

Clough, J.D., Lambert, T., & Miller, D.R. (1996). The new thinking on osteoarthritis. *Patient Care, 30*(14), 110-137.

D'Cruz, D., Ross, E., & Morrow, J. (1998). Psoriatic arthritis: Identifying and controlling an insidious disease. *Journal of Musculoskeletal Medicine, 15*(2), 17-20, 26-28, 33-35.

DiNubile, N.A. (1997). Osteoarthritis: How to make exercise part of your treatment plan. *The Physician and Sportsmedicine, 25*(7), 47-56.

Dunkin, M.A. (2000). Juvenile rheumatoid arthritis. *Arthritis Today, 14*(1), 32-33.

Dwolatzky, T., Sonnenblick, M., & Nesher, G. (1997). Giant cell arteritis and polymyalgia rheumatica: Clues to early diagnosis. *Geriatrics, 51*(6), 38-40, 43-4.

Garry, E. (1999). Caring for the elderly client with rheumatic disease. In S. Zang, & J.A. Allender (Eds.), *Home care of the elderly* (pp. 279-299). Philadelphia: Lippincott.

Glaser, V. (1999). *Recognizing the spondyloarthropathies.* Patient Care [On-line]. Available: http://pc.pdr.net/pc/content/journals/p/data/1999/p4a/p4a183.html

Glucosamine sulfate. (1996, November). The Review of Natural Products, 1-2.

Gremillion, R. (1998). Fibromyalgia: Recognizing and treating an elusive syndrome. *The Physician and Sportsmedicine, 26*(4), 55-65.

Gremillion, R.B., & van Vollehoven, R.F. (1998). Rheumatoid arthritis: Designing and implementing a treatment plan. *Postgraduate Medicine, 103*(2), 103-123.

Halverson, P.B. (1997). The spondyloarthropathies. *Orthopaedic Nursing, 16*(4), 21-25.

Hasselbacher, P., Schumacher, H.R., Simkin, P.A., & Saunders. C.S. (1998). *Gout: Applying current knowledge.* Patient Care [On-line]. Available: http://pc.pdr.net/pc/content/journals/p/data/1998/p5b/p5b125.html.

Holmes, S.B. (1998). Autoimmune and inflammatory disorders. In A.B. Maher, S.W. Salmond, & T.A. Pellino (Eds.), *Orthopaedic nursing* (2nd ed., pp. 351-430). Philadelphia: W.B. Saunders Company.

Horstman, J. (1999). Medicinal oils. *Arthritis Today, 13*(4), 56-58.

Horstman, J. (2000). Sam-e. *Arthritis Today, 14*(1), 52-54.

Hunt, A.H. (1998). Metabolic conditions. In A.B. Maher, S.W. Salmond, & T.A. Pellino (Eds.), *Orthopaedic nursing* (2nd ed., pp. 431-479). Philadelphia: W.B. Saunders Company.

Kitridou, R.C.(1997). The neonatal lupus syndrome. In D.J. Wallace & B.H. Hahn (Eds.) *Dubois' lupus erythematosus* (5th ed., pp. 1023-1036). Baltimore: Williams & Wilkins.

Krug, B. (1997). Rheumatoid arthritis and osteoarthritis: A basic comparison. *Orthopaedic Nursing, 16*(5), 73-75.

Langenegger, T., & Michel, B.A. (1999). Drug treatment for rheumatoid arthritis. *Clinical Orthopaedics and Related Research, 366*, 22-30.

Lehman, T.J.A. (1997). Systemic lupus erythematosus in childhood and adolescence. In D.J. Wallace & B.H. Hahn (Eds.), *Dubois' lupus erythematosus* (5th ed., pp. 851-870). Baltimore: Williams & Wilkins.

Ling, S.M., & Bathon, J.M. (1998). Osteoarthritis in older adults. *Journal of the American Geriatrics Society, 46*, 216-225.

Luggen, A.S., & Luggen, M.E. (1998). Arthritis and musculoskeletal/immunological disorders: Osteoporosis, mobility issues, pain, and comfort. In A.S. Luggen, S.S. Travis, & S. Meiner (Eds.), *NGNA core curriculum for gerontological advanced practice nurses* (pp. 435-446). Thousand Oaks, CA: SAGE Publications.

Lyme disease vaccination: Who needs it? How effective? (1999). *The Physician and Sportsmedicine, 27*(4), 15-17.

Matteson, M.A. (1997). Age-related changes in the musculoskeletal system. In M.A. Matteson, E.S. McConnell, A.D. Linton (Eds.), *Gerontological nursing: Concepts and practice* (2nd ed., pp. 197-221). Philadelphia: W.B. Saunders Company.

Miller, M.L (1999). Arthritis in children. In R.A. Dershewitz (Ed.). *Ambulatory pediatric care* (3rd ed., pp. 700-708). Philadelphia: Lippincott-Williams & Wilkins.

Mourad, L.A. (1998). Alterations in musculoskeletal function. In K.L. McCane & S.E. Huether (Eds.). *Pathophysiology: The biologic basis for disease in adults and children* (3rd ed., pp. 1435-1485). St. Louis: Mosby.

O'Dell, J.R., Pischel, K.D., & Weinblatt, M. (1997). *Rheumatoid arthritis: What's new in treatment.* Patient Care (On-line). Available: http://pc.pdr.net/pc/content/journals/p/data/1997/p3a/03a081.html.

Opperman, C.S., & Cassandra, K.A. (1998). *Contemporary pediatric nusing.* St. Louis: Mosby.

Osteoarthritis: Old scourge, new hope (1996, January). *Consumer Reports on Health,* 3-5.

Ouslander, J.G., Osterweil, D., & Morley, J. (1997). *Medical care in the nursing home* (2nd ed.). New York: McGraw Hill.

Peschken, C.A., & Esdaile, J.M. (1999). Rheumatic disease in North America's indigenous peoples. *Seminars in Arthritis and Rheumatism, 26*(6), 368-391.

Petri, M. (1998). Treatment of systemic lupus erythematosus: An update. *American Family Physician, 57*(11) 2753-2760.

Pittman, J.R., & Bross, M.H. (1999). Diagnosis and management of gout. *American Family Physician, 59*(7), 1799-1806.

Rahn, D.W., & Felz, M.W. (1998). Lyme disease update: Current approach to early, disseminated, and late disease. *Postgraduate Medicine, 103*(5), 51-64, 70.

Rosenberg, A. (1999). Bones, joints, and soft tissue tumors. In R.S. Cotran, V. Kumar, & T. Colins (Eds.), *Robbins pathologic basis of disease* (6th ed., pp. 1215-1268). Philadelphia: W.B. Saunders Company.

Salvarani, C., Macchinio, P., & Boiardi, L. (1997). Polymyalgia rheumatica. *Lancet, 359*(9070), 43-47.

Schoen, F.J. (1999). The heart. In R.S. Cotran, V. Kumar, & T. Collins (Eds.). *Robbins pathologic basis of disease* (6th ed., pp. 543-599). Philadelphia: W.B. Saunders Company.

Silver, H.M. (1997). Lyme disease during pregnancy. *Infectious Disease Clinics of North America, 11*(1), 93-97.

Simon, L.S. (1999). Arthritis: New agents herald more effective symptom management. *Geriatrics, 54*(6), 37-44.

Smith, W.A. (1998). Fibromylagia syndrome. *Nursing Clinics of North America, 33*(4), 653-669.

Starlanyl, D., & Copeland, M.E. (1996). *Fibromyalgia & chronic myofascial pain syndrome: A survival manual.* Oakland, CA: New Harbinger Publications, Inc.

Stollerman, G.H. (1997). Rheumatic fever. *Lancet, 349*(9056), 935-942.

Taylor, M. (2000). Lyme disease. *Arthritis Today, 14*(2), 34-35.

Wallace, D.J. (1997). Occasional, innovative, and experimental therapies. In D.J. Wallace & B.H. Hahn (Eds.), *Dubois' lupus erythematosus* (5th ed., pp. 1191-1202). Baltimore: Williams & Wilkins.

Wong, D.L. (1997). *Whaley & Wong's essentials of pediatric nursing* (5th ed.). St. Louis: Mosby.

STUDY QUESTIONS

1. Which of the following is an effective alternative to NSAIDs in the treatment of acute gout?
   a. Ethotrexate.
   b. Allopurinol.
   c. Colchicine.
   d. Sulfasalazine.

2. Ultraviolet light treatments may be helpful in controlling:
   a. Polymyalgia rheumatica
   b. Psoriatic arthritis.
   c. Reiter's syndrome.
   d. Dermatomyositits.

3. To maximize sleep for the patient with rheumatoid arthritis, the nurse will suggest that the patient:
   a. Have a glass of wine before bed.
   b. Apply ice to painful joints before bed.
   c. Exercise to create fatigue before bed.
   d. Take an analgesic before bed.

4. When answering questions about alternative therapies for a patient who has osteoarthritis, it is important that the nurse:
   a. Share personal experiences with alternative therapies.
   b. Encourage the patient to consider alternative therapies.
   c. Maintain a nonjudgmental attitude about alternative therapies.
   d. Discuss the lack of medical risk associated with alternative therapies.

5. The treatment of choice for polymyalgia rheumatica is:
   a. Corticosteroids.
   b. Monocycline.
   c. Gold injections.
   d. Calcium supplements.

6. Syndenham's chorea is associated with
   a. Systemic lupus erythematosus.
   b. Fibromyalgia syndrome.
   c. Rheumatic fever.
   d. Ankylosing spondylitis.

7. Erythema migrans is a flat rash characteristic of:
   a. Lyme disease.
   b. Fibromyalgia syndrome.
   c. Polymyalgia rheumatica.
   d. Reiter's syndrome.

8. A patient needs assistance in choosing easy-to-swallow, high-calorie foods because of the risk of dysphagia. Dysphagia is associated with:
   a. Lyme disease.
   b. JRA.
   c. PMR.
   d. Systemic sclerosis.

9. The patient with systemic lupus erythematosus may complain of:
   a. Migraine headaches.
   b. Bladder dysfunction.
   c. Drowsiness.
   d. Hirsutism.

10. In discussing possible nutritional triggers for fibromyalgia syndrome with an affected patient, the nurse should mention:
    a. Rice cereals.
    b. Red meat.
    c. Dairy products.
    d. Graham crackers.

11. The most important laboratory finding in polymyositis to which the nurse should be alert is:
    a. Elevated ESR.
    b. Elevated CK.
    c. Positive RF.
    d. Positive ANA.

Chapter 13 Metabolic Bone Conditions

Kathleen A. Geier, MS, RN, ONC

Contents

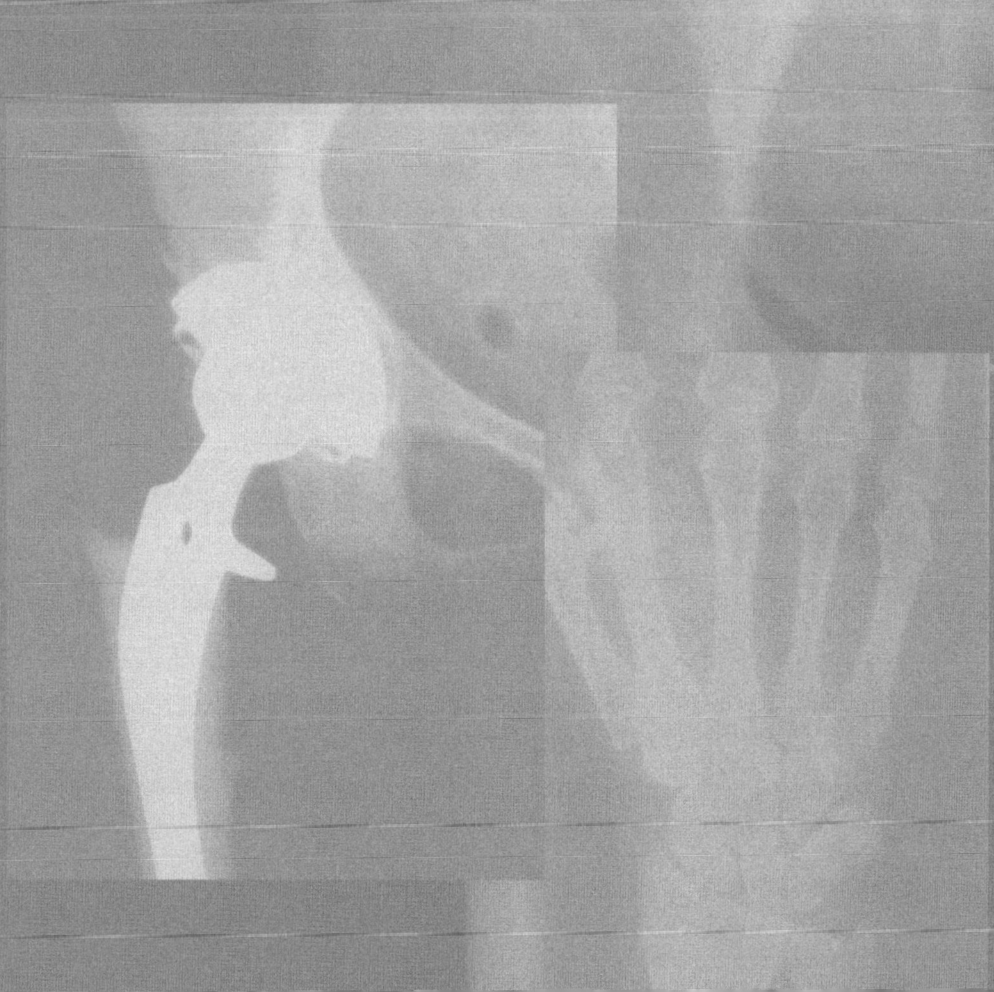

OBJECTIVES

At the completion of this chapter, the learner will be able to:

- Define metabolic bone disease.
- Describe the anatomy of the parathyroid glands.
- List the physiologic action of parathyroid hormone on the body.
- Define the disease process for hyperparathyroidism, hypoparathyroidism, rickets, osteomalacia, osteoporosis, and Paget's disease.
- Describe the clinical picture of each disorder by describing the pathophysiology, incidence, etiology, and diagnostic findings.
- List the treatment modalities used in the management of each disorder.
- Identify the nursing diagnoses for each disorder.
- Outline appropriate nursing interventions to assist in the management of each disorder.
- Define the expected outcome of each disorder.

KEY POINTS

- Hypoparathyroidism is a clinical condition that results when insufficient parathyroid hormone is produced to maintain serum calcium levels within the normal range. Treatment and care of the patient with hypoparathyroidism must include accurate assessment of the clinical signs of hypocalcemia.
- In the classification of osteoporosis proposed in 1993 by the World Health Organization, a bone mass measurement result of more than 2.5 standard deviations below peak bone mass (T-score below -2.5) was classified as osteoporosis. Although this definition helps identify patients requiring treatment, the real hope for eradication of osteoporosis lies in prevention.
- Most cases of osteomalacia are the result of vitamin D deficiency and can be classified as extrinsic or intrinsic. Extrinsic causes include reduced dietary intake and reduced production in skin; intrinsic causes are due to some combination of impaired intestinal absorption and increased catabolism, often initiated by malabsorption of calcium.

CHAPTER 13

METABOLIC BONE CONDITIONS

ANATOMY AND PHYSIOLOGY

I. OVERVIEW

A. Definition: metabolic bone disease may result from an inappropriate function of one or several metabolic processes and may be manifested by physical and chemical changes within the bone. Conditions that alter the normal equilibrium existing in bone remodeling – causing metabolic bone disease – include parathyroid malfunction, vitamin or dietary deficiency, estrogen deficiency, and malabsorption syndrome.

B. Anatomy.

1. Parathyroid glands.
   a. Description: four small round (about 6 mm by 3 mm by 2 mm in size) bodies that are attached to the posterior surfaces of the four lateral lobes of the thyroid gland.
   b. Function: produce parathyroid hormone (PTH) which exerts a potent influence on determining the functional effects of vitamin D in the body, specifically vitamin D's effect on calcium absorption in the intestine and bone.
2. Thyroid glands.
   a. Description: located immediately below the larynx on either side of and anterior to the trachea, connected by a band of tissue.
   b. Function: secrete thyroxine, triiodothyronine, and calcitonin.
3. Ovaries.
   a. Description: female sexual organs located in the abdomen, attached to the uterus via the fallopian tubes.
   b. Function: secrete the hormone estrogen which plays vital role in minimizing loss of bone in women.
4. Testes.
   a. Description: male sexual organs located in the scrotum.
   b. Function: secrete several male hormones (androgens), including testosterone which increases size and strength of bones.
5. Bone.
   a. Description: skeleton provides structure and support for the body, point of attachment for tendons, protection for vital organs, as well as a dynamic system that constantly remodels.
   b. Function: deposition (by oeteoblasts) and resorption (by osteoclasts) of bone.

C. Physiology.

1. Parathyroid hormone (PTH).
   a. PTH exerts potent influence on determining the functional effects of vitamin D in the body.
   b. Efficient feedback system accurately maintains proper concentrations of serum calcium; rate of secretion of PTH controlled almost entirely by plasma calcium concentration.
   c. Hypercalcemia leads to decreased PTH secretion and, therefore, decreased formation in the kidney of the active form of vitamin D, decreased intestinal absorption of calcium, and decreased resorption of bone at cellular level.
   d. Hypocalcemia leads to increased PTH secretion and, therefore, increased renal tubular reabsorption of calcium, increased intestinal absorption of calcium, and increased movement of calcium from bone into extracellular fluid.
2. Calcitonin.
   a. Calcitonin is manufactured by perifollicular cells (C cells) in the thyroid gland.
   b. Calcitonin effects are opposite to those of PTH; calcitonin is released when plasma calcium concentration is increased.
   c. Calcitonin is also released with ingestion of administration of glucagon and/or magnesium.
   d. Calcitonin's primary effect is on bone: calcitonin acts to lower plasma calcium concentration by inhibiting osteoclastic bone resorption, increasing osteoblastic activity, and inhibiting the formation of new osteoclasts.
   e. Calcitonin decreases formation of active vitamin D which is needed for absorption of calcium from the intestine.
   f. Calcitonin interacts with PTH which regulates urinary excretion of magnesium, calcium, phosphates, and other electrolytes.
3. Estrogen.
   a. Estrogen inhibits bone resorption directly by attaching to specific receptors in bone cells.
   b. Estrogen promotes osteoblastic activity.
   c. Estrogen promotes renal reabsorption of calcium.
   d. Estrogen helps promote intestinal absorption of calcium.
   e. Estrogen results in increased amounts of bone matrix with retention of both phosphate and calcium.
   f. Estrogen stimulates the thyroid gland to secrete calcitonin, thereby protecting bones at the cellular level.

II. METABOLIC DISEASES (See the following conditions.)

PRIMARY HYPERPARATHYROIDISM

I. OVERVIEW

A. Definition.

1. Excessive secretion of PTH.
2. Interrupts metabolism of calcium, phosphate, and bone.
3. Enlargement of one or more parathyroid gland(s), resulting in increased PTH secretion, rapid absorption of calcium salts from bones, and elevated serum calcium levels (hypercalcemia).

B. Etiology.

1. Most common cause: benign, solitary adenoma.
2. Other causes: genetic or multiple endocrine disorders.
3. Familial pattern of occurrence.

C. Pathophysiology: excessive PTH secretion.

1. Results from growth of a parathyroid mass with its own feedback mechanism.
2. Remains controlled by a negative feedback mechanism resulting in hypercalcemia, yet the level at which calcium exerts feedback control is altered.
3. Physical signs and symptoms.
   a. Bone.
      (1) Extreme osteoclastic activity occurs in presence of vitamin D, resulting in an osteodystrophy (defect in bone development).
      (2) Increased osteoblastic activity, in an attempt to form enough new bone to make up for the old bone absorbed by osteoclastic activity.
      (3) Increases subperiosteal bone resorption.
      (4) Decreases bone density.
      (5) Extensive decalcification can lead to large punched-out cystic areas of bone that are filled with giant cell tumors (osteitis fibrosa cystica).
      (6) Generalized bone weakness.
      (7) Anemia as a result of fibrous tissue replacing bone marrow.
   b. Kidneys.
      (1) Hypercalciuria results because high calcium levels overwhelm renal tubular resorptive mechanism.
      (2) Renal calculi are formed as a result of excretion of large amounts of phosphates and calcium in the urine.
      (3) Renal calculi (nephrolithiasis) result in obstruction, urinary tract infection, and renal failure.
      (4) Polyuria results because calcium loss impairs renal water conservation by interfering with action of antidiuretic hormone (ADH).
   c. Gastrointestinal system.
      (1) Hypercalcemia may result in anorexia, nausea, vomiting, and constipation due to diminished contractility of muscular walls of gastrointestinal tract.
      (2) Increased secretion of gastrin and pepsin results in increased incidence of peptic ulcers.
      (3) Increased incidence of pancreatitis.
   d. Heart.
      (1) Electrocardiograph changes:
         (a) Shortened QT interval.
         (b) Prolonged PR interval.
      (2) Other heart conditions:
         (a) Dysrhythmias.
         (b) Heart block.
         (c) Cardiac arrest may occur.
   e. Central nervous system (CNS).
      (1) Nervous system is depressed in presence of hypercalcemia.
      (2) Reflex activities of CNS become sluggish.
      (3) Muscles become weak and hypotonic due to effects of elevated calcium on muscle cell membranes.

D. Incidence.

1. Primary hyperparathyroidism occurs in 1 of every 1,000 individuals.
2. Affects women at least twice as frequently as men.
3. Effects seen in any bone.
4. Hypercalcemia ranges from asymptomatic to severe where patients deteriorate rapidly and become confused, dehydrated, and lethargic.

E. Considerations across the lifespan.

1. Can occur at all ages, even in children.
2. Frequently seen in patients over 70 years of age.

F. Complications.

1. Renal calculi.
2. Renal insufficiency due to nephrolithiasis.
3. Bones fracture easily due to osteoporosis.
4. Pancreatitis.
5. Peptic ulcers.
6. Central nervous system disorders, ranging from mild personality disturbances to severe psychiatric disorders.
7. Skin necrosis.
8. Cataracts.
9. Calcium thrombi to lungs and pancreas.

II. ASSESSMENT

A. History and physical examination.

1. Renal.
   a. Pain.
   b. Urinary output changes.
   c. Nephrolithiasis.
2. Skeletal.
   a. Chronic low back pain.
   b. Fractures.
   c. Bone tenderness.
   d. Traumatic synovitis.
   e. Pseudogout.
   f. Deformities.
   g. Shortening of body stature.
3. Gastrointestinal.
   a. Severe epigastric pain radiating to the back.
   b. Peptic ulcers.
   c. Pancreatitis.

d. Nausea and vomiting.
e. Constipation.

4. Neuromuscular: marked muscular atrophy and weakness, especially in the legs.
5. Central nervous system.
   a. Stupor.
   b. Coma.
   c. Overt psychosis.
   d. Depression.
   e. Psychomotor disturbances.
   f. Personality disturbances.
   g. Neurosis.
   h. Apathy.
   i. Emotional irritability.
6. Other.
   a. Cataracts.
   b. Skin necrosis.
   c. Subcutaneous calcification.
   d. Fatigue.
   e. Cardiac dysrhythmias.

B. Diagnostic tests.

1. Laboratory studies.
   a. Serum calcium: exceeds 10 mg/dl in 95% of patients.
   b. Serum phosphorus: usually falls below 1.8 mg/dl due to inverse relationship with calcium.
   c. Serum magnesium: directly affects PTH secretion; when it falls below 1 mEq/L, PTH secretion is impaired.
   d. Serum chloride: greater than 102 mEq/L because of high urinary bicarbonate losses and metabolic acidosis.
   e. Serum alkaline phosphatase: increased.
      (1) Mediates some complex reactions of bone formation.
      (2) Elevated levels in bone disease are nonspecific because any disease process that results in hypercalcemia can lead to elevated serum alkaline phosphatase levels.
   f. Urine cyclic AMP: increased in 97% of patients because it is controlled by PTH (used predominantly in research).
   g. PTH radioimmunoassy: increased in 80% of patients.
   h. Urine calcium levels elevated: levels usually less than 25 mEq/L.
   i. Creatinine clearance decreased.
   j. Urinary PO4 less than 1.8 mEq/L.
   k. Hydroxyproline (a serum and urinary marker of bone resorption) increased.
2. Radiographic studies:
   a. X-rays of hands, clavicle ends, and skull are taken when bone changes are suspected.
   b. X-rays show demineralization, decreased bone density, and cyst formation.
3. Bone mineral density measurements show decreased bone density; these studies are helpful in evaluating degree of bone resorption in hyperparathyroidism.
4. Localized studies.
   a. Cervical esophagography.
   b. Computerized tomography.
   c. Parathyroid ultrasound: may show enlargement of one or more of the parathyroid glands.
   d. Digital subtraction angiography.
   e. Magnetic resonance imaging (MRI) of parathyroid glands.
   f. Thallium scan.
   g. Fine-needle biopsy of thyroid and/or parathyroid.

III. COMMON THERAPEUTIC MODALITIES

A. Medical.

1. Force fluids up to 3,000 ml/day IV or PO.
2. Encourage salt intake of 8-10 grams/day.
3. Phosphorus supplements except in patient with renal calculi.
4. Annual physical examination and history.
5. Biannual serum calcium and creatinine clearance tests.
6. Annual x-rays of hands to check for subperiosteal bone resorption.
7. Annual x-rays of abdomen to check for renal calculi.
8. Treatment for hypercalcemia greater than 14 mg/dl.
   a. Normal saline infusions given concurrently with furosemide (Lasix®): 20-80 mg every 1-8 hours IV or PO.
   b. Magnesium and potassium supplements.
   c. Bisphosphonates: pamidronate or etidronate IV.
   d. Plicamycin (an antihypercalcemic agent) IV.
   e. Calcitonin 4-8 IU/kg of body weight, IM or subcutaneously every 6-8 hours.
   f. Inorganic phosphate decreases serum calcium by complexing it and depositing it in bone.
   g. Encourage ambulation.
   h. Dialysis may be used in emergency situations when calcium needs to be reduced quickly.

B. Surgical.

1. Removal of parathyroid glands, all but half of one gland.
2. Preferred for symptomatic hyperparathyroidism.
3. Removal of adenoma.
4. Autotransplantation of parathyroid remnant to forearm.

IV. NURSING DIAGNOSES, OUTCOMES, AND INTERVENTIONS

A. Fluid volume, deficient.
Fluid volume, excess.

1. Outcomes.
   a. Patient's serum calcium levels are within normal limits.
   b. Patient maintains normal hydration.
2. Interventions.
   a. Administer diuretics and antihypercalcemic agents as prescribed.
   b. Hydration per physician's order to promote excretion of calcium.
   c. Monitor strict intake and output.
   d. Monitor for signs of fluid overload.

(1) Respiratory assessment.
(2) CVP readings.
(3) Pedal edema.

e. Monitor for dehydration, which may occur with severe hypercalcemia.
   (1) Numbness or tingling of fingers and toes.
   (2) Muscle cramps.

B. Urinary elimination, impaired.

1. Outcome:
   a. Patient will not develop large residual urine volume.
   b. Patient does not develop renal calculi.
2. Interventions.
   a. Force fluids: at least 4 liters/day unless contraindicated.
   b. Ambulate patient as much as possible to prevent stasis.
   c. Strain all urine output.
   d. Keep strict record of intake and output.
   e. Assess patient for signs and symptoms of urinary tract infection, urinary stasis, and nephrolithiasis.

C. Constipation.

1. Outcome: patient maintains normal bowel patterns.
2. Interventions.
   a. Force fluids.
   b. Encourage diet high in fruit and fiber.
   c. Monitor bowel patterns.
   d. Administer stool softeners and laxatives as needed per physician's order.

D. Pain (see Table 13.1).

1. Outcomes: patient will remain in a state of relative comfort with decreased or absence of pain.
2. Interventions.
   a. Avoid extreme temperature changes.
   b. Assure a balance between rest and activity.
   c. Administer warmth to areas of pain.
   d. Handle patient gently.
   e. Reinforce good body alignment.

E. Decreased cardiac output.

1. Outcomes.
   a. Patient's blood pressure and pulse rate remain within normal ranges.
   b. Patient's urine output is maintained.
2. Interventions:
   a. Assess for signs of hypoperfusion (urine output, vital signs, mental status changes).
   b. Vital signs at least every 4 hours to include pulse check for bradycardia.
   c. Assess cardiac function via EKG.
   d. Monitor for secondary causes of anemia (check for blood in stools, emesis, urine, and sputum).
   e. Assess for bruising and petechiae.

V. PRACTICE SETTING CONSIDERATIONS

A. Office/outpatient.

1. Provide information regarding diagnosis and prescribed treatment or intervention.
2. Describe signs and symptoms of pathophysiology and identify which symptoms require intervention by health care provider.
3. Instruct patient and family regarding completion, interpretation, and potential intervention related to diagnostic tests and localized studies.
4. Pre/postoperative teaching and wound care.
5. Arrange follow-up care, including appropriate outpatient diagnostic tests, to manage hyperparathyroidism.

B. Home Care.

1. Patient teaching to include:
   a. Monitoring and maintaining fluid balance.
   b. How to check the urine for stones and blood.
   c. Good body alignment.
   d. Plan of progressive activities of daily living (ADL) to promote rapid mobilization.
   e. Plan for alternative pain management.
   f. Pulse checks for bradycardia.
   g. Signs and symptoms of hypocalcemia.
   h. Lifestyle modifications.

C. Long-term care.

1. Lifelong monitoring of serum calcium and kidney function.
2. Annual history and physical examination to monitor status of hyperparathyroidism.
   a. Serial x-rays and bone mineral density studies.
   b. Evaluation for renal calculi.

SECONDARY HYPERPARATHYROIDISM

I. OVERVIEW

A. Definition.

1. Excessive secretion of PTH.
2. Interrupts metabolism of calcium, phosphate, and bone.
3. Acquired metabolic disorder in which excessive PTH secretion is brought about by any factor that initiates hypocalcemia.
   a. There is a lack of response to the normal feedback regulation, and PTH continues to be secreted.
   b. It is encountered in various diseases that result in resistance to effects of PTH.

B. Etiology: abnormalities that result in resistance to the metabolic action of PTH.

1. Chronic renal failure.
2. Vitamin D deficiency.
3. Osteomalacia.
4. Intestinal malabsorption syndrome.
5. Rickets.

C. Pathophysiology.

1. Hypocalcemia stimulates PTH secretion.
2. PTH secretion continues despite rise in calcium level.
3. High PTH levels result in excess bone reabsorption.
4. Calcium and phosphorus resorption from the bone matrix causes bone demineralization.

D. Incidence: same as primary hyperparathyroidism once secondary hyperparathyroidism evolves into primary hyperparathyroidism.

E. Considerations across the lifespan: see primary hyperparathyroidism.

Table 13.1
Common Nursing Diagnoses, Outcomes, and Interventions

Diagnoses	Outcomes	Interventions
A. Injury, risk for	• Patient remains free of injury. • Patient and/or significant others promote a safe environment. • Patient adheres to an activity/exercise program to increase strength and endurance.	• Prevent injury. 1. Assist patient with transfers and ambulation as needed. 2. Emphasize that patient should avoid heavy lifting. 3. Demonstrate proper body mechanics for lifting. 4. Provide the patient with a safe environment. 5. Promote safety in home environment. a. Remove scatter rugs. b. Caution about door sills. c. Ambulatory devices should be properly fitted with rubber tips. d. Rubber strips in bathtub to prevent falls; handrails. 6. Promote increased strength and endurance. • Establish an individualized exercise and activity program for the patient. • Educate patient and family on potential for injury even with minor trauma.
B. Pain	• Patient knows own limitations for activity/pain and has decreased or no pain.	• Assess levels of pain. • Handle patient gently. • Reinforce good body alignment. • Use bracing as needed. • Assure a balance between rest and activity. • Use mild analgesics as needed. • Refer to Chapter 7, Pain.
C. Individual coping, ineffective	• Patient able to cope with a chronic illness by identifying and utilizing personal strengths.	• Assist patient and family to adjust to the realities of a chronic illness. • Assess anxiety and concern over diagnosis, limitation in activity, pain, and altered body image. • Identify personal strength that could be used in coping with chronic illness. • Identify and evaluate options relative to activity limitations and lifestyle alterations needed. • Promote independence in ADL.
D. Knowledge, deficient	• Patient will be familiar with disease process. • Patient will adhere to the specific treatment regime.	• Instruct patient on the disease process and specific factors contributing to the disease. • Patient teaching should at least contain: 1. Dietary requirement. 2. Behavior modification to assist with lifestyle changes.

F. **Complications.**
   1. Same as primary hyperparathyroidism.
   2. Skeletal deformities of the long bones (Rickets).

II. ASSESSMENT

A. **History and physical examination.**
   1. See primary hyperparathyroidism.
   2. Emphasis also is placed on identifying and evaluating signs and symptoms of underlying disease processes resulting in hypercalcemia.
   3. Determine patient's ability to carry out ADL.

B. **Diagnostic tests: see primary hyperparathyroidism.**

III. COMMON THERAPEUTIC MODALITIES

A. **Correct underlying cause of parathyroid hypertrophy.**
B. **Vitamin D therapy.**
C. **Aluminum hydroxide for hyperphosphatemia in patients with renal disease. (Limit duration in order to avoid aluminum intoxication.)**
D. **Peritoneal dialysis for patients with renal failure.**

IV. NURSING DIAGNOSES, OUTCOMES, AND INTERVENTIONS

A. **See Table 13.1.**
B. **See primary hyperparathyroidism.**

V. PRACTICE SETTING CONSIDERATIONS (See Primary Hyperparathyroidism)

HYPOPARATHYROIDISM

I. OVERVIEW

A. **Definition: deficiency of PTH because of disease, injury, or congenital malfunction of the parathyroid glands.**

B. **Pathophysiology – low PTH levels result in:**
   1. Neuromuscular excitability and tetany.
   2. Hypocalcemia.
   3. Decreased bone resorption.
   4. Decreased renal phosphate excretion.
   5. Activation of vitamin D.
   6. Decreased intestinal absorption of calcium.
   7. Mild metabolic alkalosis.
   8. Mental status changes.
   9. Dry skin.
   10. Parkinson-like symptoms.

C. **Etiology.**
   1. Hypoparthyroidism may be acute or chronic.
   2. Classified as idiopathic, acquired, and/or reversible.
      a. Idiopathic.
         (1) May result from idiopathic atrophy of parathyroid gland.
         (2) May be congenital.
      b. Acquired.
         (1) Accidental removal of or injury to one or more parathyroid glands during surgery or ischemic infarction.
         (2) Other causes: tuberculosis (TB), neoplasms, trauma.
      c. Acquired reversible.
         (1) Resulting from any condition that causes hypomagnesemia, such as alcoholism or malabsorption syndrome, and which therefore inhibits PTH secretion.
         (2) Resulting from any disorder that limits vitamin D availability such as:
            (a) Gastric or intestinal surgery.
            (b) Pancreatitis.
            (c) Small intestine malabsorption.
            (d) Hepatic or renal disease.

D. **Incidence.**
   1. Idiopathic and reversible forms occur most often in children.
   2. Irreversible, acquired forms occur in older patients who have undergone surgery for hyperparathyroidism.

E. **Considerations across the lifespan (see D. Incidence, above).**

F. **Complications.**
   1. Tetany.
   2. Carpopedal spasm.
   3. Seizure.
   4. Laryngospasms.
   5. Respiratory insufficiency.
   6. Psychosis (anxiety, irritability, depression, delirium).
   7. Neuromuscular irritability.
   8. Cardiac dysrhythmias.
   9. Congestive heart failure (CHF).
   10. Dementia.
   11. Dysphagia.
   12. Pain.
   13. Cataracts.
   14. Dental abnormalities:
      a. Caries.
      b. Hypoplasia of enamel.
      c. Pitting.
      d. Delayed eruption of teeth.
   15. Photophobia.

II. ASSESSMENT

A. **History.**
   1. Intestinal diseases.
   2. Alcohol abuse.
   3. Recent neck irradiation or surgery.
   4. Family history.

B. **Physical examination.**
   1. Neuromuscular.
      a. Irritable skeletal muscles: twitches, cramps, tetany.
      b. Paresthesias.
         (1) Tingling and numbness sensations.
         (2) Positive Chvostek's sign:
            (a) Ipsilateral contraction of the facial muscles elicited by tapping the facial nerve just anterior to the ear.
            (b) Since slightly positive Chvostek's sign occurs in 10%-30% of adults with normal serum calcium levels, this sign cannot be considered diagnostic

unless it was known to be previously absent.
(3) Positive Trousseau's phenomenon:
(a) Occurrence of carpal spasm after compression of the nerves in the upper arm.
(b) Typically elicited by inflating blood pressure cuff on upper arm to above systolic blood pressure for 3-5 minutes.
(4) Even in patients with definite hypocalcemia, both the Chvostek's sign and the Trousseau's phenomenon can be absent.
c. Hyperactive deep tendon reflexes.
d. Laryngospasms.
2. Central nervous system.
a. Mood disorders.
b. Syncopal spells.
c. Seizures.
d. Dementia or memory impairment.
3. Cardiovascular.
a. Electrocardiogram abnormalities.
(1) Prolonged QT interval.
(2) Prolonged ST interval.
(3) Tachycardia.
(4) Decreased cardiac output.
b. Congestive heart failure (rare).
4. Gastrointestinal.
a. Increased gastric motility.
b. Hyperactive bowel sounds.
c. Abdominal cramping and diarrhea.
5. Skin.
a. Dry, flaking skin.
b. Brittle nails and hair.
c. Thinning eyebrows.

C. Diagnostic tests.
1. Laboratory studies: see hyperparathyroidism.
2. Laboratory studies, finding of hyperparathyroidism are reversed.
a. Serum calcium:
(1) Decreased.
(2) Tetany occurs at 6-7 mg/dl.
b. Serum phosphorus: increased greater than 5.4 mg/100 ml.
c. Magnesium: increased.
d. Chloride: increased.
e. Uric acid: increased.
f. Alkaline phosphatase: decreased.
g. PTH radioimmunoassay: decreased; this test used as a chronic measure as well.
h. Creatinine: increased.
i. Vitamin D levels are low.
j. Urinary calcium is decreased in an attempt to balance the system by preserving calcium.
2. Radiographic studies: increased bone density is a late manifestation of chronic hypoparathyroidism.
3. EKG: Prolonged ST and QT intervals.

III. COMMON THERAPEUTIC MODALITIES

A. Acute hypoparathyroidism:
1. Is a medical emergency.
2. Treatment aim is to control tetany and prevent laryngeal spasms and seizures.

B. Medical management.
1. Treatment is lifelong except in patients with reversible disease.
2. Vitamin D with or without supplemental calcium.
3. If patient has renal disease and cannot tolerate pure form of vitamin D, alternatives such as dihydrotachysterol or calcitriol are used.
4. Acute life-threatening tetany calls for immediate IV administration of calcium gluconate.
5. Sedatives and anticonvulsants are administered to control spasm until calcium levels rise.
6. Maintenance of serum calcium levels with oral calcium supplements in chronic tetany.

IV. NURSING DIAGNOSES, OUTCOMES, AND INTERVENTIONS

A. Skin integumentary, impaired.
Oral mucous membrane, altered.
1. Outcomes.
a. Patient has increased knowledge of special skin, nail, and hair care needed because of hypocalcemia.
b. Patient understands need for strict dental hygiene and regular dental care visits.
2. Interventions.
a. Prevent alteration in skin integrity.
(1) Back and skin care to meet the patient's needs.
(2) Turn patient every 2 hours if on bed rest.
(3) Monitor skin integrity status daily.
(4) Use flotation and pressure relieving devices.
b. Increase patient's knowledge about skin and nail care.
(1) If skin is scaly, teach patient to use creams.
(2) Keep nails trimmed to prevent splitting.
(3) Special moisturizing shampoos may be indicated.
c. Increase patient's knowledge about dental care.
(1) Regular brushing and flossing to control increased decay.
(2) Avoid chewing hard foods (hard candy, taffy, etc.) because of dental fragility.

B. Fatigue.
1. Outcome: patient able to carry out ADL with increased tolerance.
2. Interventions.
a. Prevent muscle spasm with heat and gentle positioning.
b. Teach the patient to avoid positions that aggravate muscle spasms (leg crossing).
c. Assist the patient in establishing alternate periods of mild exercise and rest.
d. Assist patients when applicable.
e. Instruct patient to use assistive devices PRN.

C. Injury, risk for.
1. Outcomes.

a. Seizures are controlled.
b. Patient has no injury if seizures occur.
2. Interventions.
a. Maintain seizure precautions.
b. Pad patient's side rails for ongoing seizure.
c. Keep suction equipment at bedside for ongoing seizure activity.
d. Administer anticonvulsant drugs and sedatives as ordered.
e. Keep environment free of noise, sudden draft, bright lights, or sudden movement.

D. Nutrition, altered: less than daily body requirement.
1. Outcome: patient will meet calcium requirements by improving nutrition.
2. Interventions.
a. Assess dietary intake of calcium.
b. Patient teaching to include foods high in calcium (yogurt, milk, sardines, dark green vegetables).
c. Monitor for Chvostek's sign and Trousseau's phenomenon (see Chapter 3, Musculoskeletal Assessment).
d. Dietary plan to include meals/snacks that are high in calcium.
e. Calcium replacements per order.
f. Vitamin D preparations per order.

V. PRACTICE SETTING CONSIDERATIONS

A. Office/outpatient.
1. Provide information regarding diagnosis and prescribed treatment or intervention.
2. Describe signs and symptoms of pathophysiology and identify which symptoms require intervention by health care provider.
3. Instruct patient and family regarding completion, interpretation, and potential intervention related to diagnostic tests and localized studies.

B. Home care. Patient teaching to include:
1. Pulse checks for bradycardia.
2. Dietary or over-the-counter supplements of calcium and vitamin D.
3. Side effects of drug therapy.
4. Early assessment of signs and symptoms of hypocalcemia.
5. Seizure precautions.
6. Skin, nail, hair, and dental care.

C. Long-term care.
1. Lifelong monitoring of serum calcium and kidney function.
2. Annual history and physical examination to monitor status of hypoparathyroidism.
a. See complications.
b. EKG changes.
c. Radiographic incidence of increased bone density (late manifestation).

OSTEOMALACIA

I. OVERVIEW

A. Definition: a disease in which the bone becomes abnormally soft resulting in marked deformities of weight-bearing bone and pathologic fractures. Osteomalacia is characterized by inadequate concentration of calcium or phosphorus and inadequate mineralization of bone matrix after cessation of growth.

B. Etiology: osteomalacia is always due to an inadequate concentration of calcium or phosphorus in the body fluids and may be due to:
1. Vitamin D disturbances.
a. Inadequate production of vitamin D.
b. Inadequate sunlight exposure.
c. Dietary deficiency of vitamin D.
d. Abnormal metabolism of vitamin D, such as in hepatic or renal disease.
(1) Chronic renal failure.
(2) Tubular necrosis
(3) Hypophosphatemia
2. Inadequate absorption of vitamin D and calcium from gastrointestinal system.
a. Gastrectomy.
b. Gastric or intestinal bypass surgery.
c. Malabsorption syndromes.
d. Inflammatory bowel disease.
3. Drug therapy.
a. Phenytoin.
b. Fluoride.
c. Antacids containing aluminum.
d. Anticonvulsants.
e. Etidronate (Didronel®).
4. Increased urinary excretion of calcium.
5. Loss of calcium or phosphorus from body during pregnancy or lactation.

C. Pathophysiology.
1. Calcium is needed for bone formation and resorption.
2. Vitamin D is needed for intestinal absorption of dietary calcium and therefore affects bone strength, formation, and resorption.
3. Osteomalacia is an inadequate concentration of calcium or phosphorus and therefore affects the bone.
4. Absence of adequate calcium or phosphorus to promote mineralization of bone leads to softened skeletal structure.
5. Softening causes marked deformities of weight-bearing bones, distortion in bone shape, and pathologic fractures.

D. Incidence.
1. Adults, mainly women.
2. Endemic in the Orient and in individuals with no exposure to the sun (prisoners of war; residents of institutions).
3. Severe malnourishment and famine.
4. Occasionally in strict vegetarians.
5. Occasionally in postgastrectomy patients.

6. Women who have multiple, frequent pregnancies and who have breast-fed.
7. Patients on long-term anticonvulsants, phosphate-binding antacids, tranquilizers, sedatives, muscle relaxants, or antidiuretic.
8. Small intestinal diseases.
   a. Celiac disease (idiopathic steatorrhea).
   b. Regional enteritis.
   c. Small bowel resections.
9. Hepatobiliary diseases.
   a. Chronic biliary obstruction.
   b. Cirrhosis.
10. Pancreatic insufficiency.
11. Renal tubular disorders.
    a. Renal tubular acidosis.
    b. Fanconi's syndrome.
       (1) Rickets.
       (2) Polyuria.
       (3) Growth failure.
12. Primary hypoparathyroidism.

E. Considerations across the lifespan.

1. Occurs only in adults; often called the adult form of rickets.
2. Osteomalacia in adult causes less severe clinical features than does childhood rickets due to less turnover of bone at older ages.
3. Reversible with treatment.
4. Homebound or institutionalized elderly susceptible due to lack of exposure to sunlight and/or inadequate intake of vitamin D-fortified foods.

F. Complications.

1. Proximal myopathy.
2. Fractures.
3. Bone deformities.

II. ASSESSMENT

A. History.

1. Clinical manifestations are subtle.
2. Complaints of bone pain ranging from mild aching to extreme tenderness when weight or pressure is applied to affected bones.
3. Poorly localized muscle pains and weakness.
4. Pelvic region and dorsolumbar area usually affected.
5. Complaints of low back pain and difficulty walking or changing positions.
6. Muscle weakness contributes to waddling, unsteady gait and high risk for falls.
7. Loss of vertebral height causes kyphosis.
8. History of multiple fractures may be present.
9. Other symptoms are related to the causative dietary, gastrointestinal, or renal factors.
10. Decreased intake or absorption of vitamin D.

B. Physical examination.

1. Deformities, particularly of weight-bearing structures.
2. Kyphoscoliosis.
3. Coxa vara deformity of femoral neck due to pressure on femoral head.
4. Muscle weakness.
5. General malaise.

C. Diagnostic tests.

1. Radiographic findings.
   a. Significant osteomalacia can exist without radiographic manifestations.
   b. Pseudofractures (Looser's zones) which are radiolucent bands considered to be a type of stress fracture; may precede other radiographic changes in osteomalacia.
   c. Looser's zones most often found along the concave side of the femoral neck, the pubic rami, the ribs, the clavicles, and the lateral aspects of the scapulae.
   d. Generalized demineralization with loss of transverse trabeculae and severe osteopenia.
   e. Compression fractures of vertebrae.
   f. Bowing deformities of the long bone.
   g. Areas of spongy bone show decreased trabeculae with coarsened and unsharp appearance.
   h. Osteoid may be deposited in excessive amounts at various sites, particularly in vertebral bodies and pelvis.
2. Laboratory findings.
   a. Serum calcium low or low-normal.
   b. Serum phosphorus normal or low-normal.
   c. Alkaline phosphatase level moderately elevated.
   d. 24-hour urine calcium and creatinine excretion low (below 100 mg calcium per 24 hours).
3. Bone biopsy.
   a. May be necessary due to difficulty diagnosing osteomalacia.
   b. Rib or iliac crest often used or biopsy done during open reduction of fracture.
   c. Depressed appositional rate, increased mineralization lag time, and reduced calcification.

III. COMMON THERAPEUTIC MODALITIES

A. Intervention is related to etiology.

B. If nutritional vitamin D deficiency is cause:

1. Oral vitamin D in doses of 2,000-5,000 IU/d for several months.
2. Replacement oral vitamin D doses of 200-400 IU/d.

C. If malabsorption is cause:

1. Oral vitamin D in doses of 25,000-100,000 IU/d.
2. May require parenteral administration of vitamin D.
3. Possible surgical intervention for intestinal disease.

D. If altered renal function is primary cause:

1. Patient education regarding how kidneys increase urinary excretion.
2. Review with patient the physiology of calcium loss via kidneys.
3. Collaborative care of patient involves multispeciality focus.

IV. NURSING DIAGNOSES, OUTCOMES, AND INTERVENTIONS

A. See Table 13.1.

B. Nutrition, imbalanced: less than daily body requirement.

1. Outcome: patient meets RDA requirements for calcium and vitamin D.

2. Interventions.
   a. Adequate nutrition to meet needs.
   b. Assess intake of milk and products that contain vitamin D and calcium.
   c. Administer supplements per orders.
   d. See the next section in this chapter on osteoporosis.

C. **Knowledge, deficient.**
1. Outcome: patient is familiar with disease process and adheres to specific treatment regime.
2. Interventions.
   a. Instruct patient on disease process and specific factors contributing to the disease.
   b. Patient teaching should include:
      (1) Dietary requirements.
      (2) Exposure to sunlight.
      (3) Serum calcium levels monitored throughout therapy.
      (4) Importance of complying with medication regime.
      (5) Importance of keeping follow-up appointments.

V. PRACTICE SETTING CONSIDERATIONS

A. **Office/outpatient.**
1. Provide information regarding diagnosis and prescribed treatment or intervention.
2. Describe signs and symptoms of pathophysiology and identify which symptoms require intervention by health care provider.
3. Instruct patient and family regarding completion, interpretation, and potential intervention related to diagnostic tests and localized studies.
4. Review prescribed medication/supplement regime and reinforce specific protocols for taking prescribed medications.
5. Arrange follow-up, including appropriate outpatient diagnostic tests, to manage osteomalacia.

B. **Home care.**
1. Encourage adequate sunlight exposure.
2. Follow medication plan.
3. Follow dietary plan.
4. Encourage weight-bearing activities: 30-40 minutes three times a week.

C. **Long-term care (related to origin of osteomalacia).**
1. Appropriate, regular exposure to sunlight (if vitamin D deficiency is cause).
2. Lifelong treatment and therefore avoidance of malnourishment.
3. If vegetarian, appropriate vitamin D supplementation to prevent deficiency.
4. Lifelong monitoring/treatment of hepatic, renal, or gastrointestinal disease (if this is source of vitamin D deficiency).
5. Avoidance or substitution of drug that induced osteomalacia (avoid aluminum-containing antacids).
6. Appropriate vitamin D supplementation/replacement in mother throughout childbearing years and beyond.

OSTEOPOROSIS

I. OVERVIEW

A. **Definition:**
1. A common metabolic bone disease where the rate of bone resorption is more rapid than the rate of bone formation.
2. It occurs when there is severe general reduction in skeletal bone mass and susceptibility to fractures.
3. Definitions for low bone mass give diagnostic criteria to clinicians who make decisions about interventions.
4. The World Health Organization defines bone loss in terms of bone mineral density:
   a. Normal bone mass is categorized as a bone density value, a T-score that lies between +1 and -1 standard deviation of the mean for young adults.
   b. Osteopenia, low bone mass, is categorized as a T-score value for bone density that lies between -1 and -2.5 standard deviations below the mean value for young adults.
   c. Osteoporosis is categorized as a statistical value of bone mineral density or content that is -2.5 standard deviations or more below the standardized mean value for young adults.

B. **Etiology.**
1. The exact cause of osteoporosis is unknown.
   a. Peak bone mass is achieved by age 35 and influenced by genetic factors. It is enhanced by adequate calcium intake, weight-bearing exercise, and absence of risk factors.
   b. Rate of bone loss is strongly influenced by genetics, estrogen, and risk factors.
2. Factors contributing to bone mass (hardness or density of bone):
      (1) Peak bone mass achieved during young adulthood.
      (2) Rate of bone loss that occurs after menopause or during late adulthood.
3. Rate of bone loss strongly influenced by genetics, estrogen, and risk factors.
4. Contributing (risk) factors.
   a. Immobilization.
   b. Endocrine disorders.
   c. Increased age.
   d. Iatrogenic causes.
   e. Nutritional abnormalities.
   f. Genetic/sex factors.
   g. Chronic diseases, such as malignant tumors and collagen diseases.
   h. Certain drugs and substances.
      (1) Corticosteroids.
      (2) Heparin.
      (3) Anticonvulsants.
      (4) Immunosuppressants.
      (5) Alcohol.

C. **Pathophysiology.**
1. Disturbance of normal osteoblastic and osteoclastic

balance occurs, and mineral and protein matrix components are diminished.
2. Loss of trabecular bone, medullary widening, and decreased bone density occurs.

D. Incidence/risk factors.
1. Hereditary tendencies.
2. More prevalent in women over age 60.
3. More prevalent in Caucasians and Asians.
4. Individuals with small body structure are at greater risk than those with a larger frame.
5. Heavy cigarette smokers, caffeine users, and persons who use alcohol to excess are at greater risk.
6. Postmenopausal (estrogen-deficient) women are at high risk.
7. Inactive or bedridden people.
8. People on long-term steroid therapy.
9. Can occur in any or all bone; most common in spine, hip, ribs, wrist, or pelvis.
10. People with a northern European background at higher risk.
11. Higher risk in people with endocrine disorders, diabetes, scoliosis, and rheumatoid arthritis.
12. Onset may be insidious; diagnosis often not made until injury/fracture occurs.
13. Gonadal insufficiency in men (testosterone increases total quantity of bone matrix and causes calcium retention).
14. High protein diet.
15. Eating disorders (anorexia, bulimia) and resultant amenorrhea.
16. Excessive exercise resulting in amenorrhea.

E. Considerations across the lifespan.
1. Calcium intake.
   a. Adolescent girls and young adults should ingest 1,200 mg Ca daily (ages 12-24).
   b. Premenopausal women and men and postmenopausal women on estrogen should ingest 1,000 mg Ca daily.
   c. Postmenopausal women not on estrogen should ingest 1,500 mg of Ca daily.
   d. Adult men need 1,500 mg of Ca daily.
2. Establish appropriate and regular weight-bearing exercise regime daily.
3. Calcium intake in all age groups is generally found to be deficient.
4. Presence of fractures is greater in the aging population.

F. Complications.
1. Vertebral compression fractures.
2. Hip fractures.
3. Thoracic kyphosis.
4. Wrist (forearm or Colles) fractures.
5. Other fractures, depending on the severity of the condition.

II. ASSESSMENT

A. History.
1. Family history of osteoporosis.
2. Excessive height loss or fractures from minor trauma.
3. Onset of menarche and menopause.
4. Dietary calcium intake, over the lifespan.
5. History of steroid use.
6. Northern European heritage.
7. History of gum disease or tooth decay.
8. Excessive caffeine intake.
9. Cigarette smoking.
10. High alcohol intake.
11. Long-term immobilization; sedentary lifestyle.
12. Lactose intolerance; avoidance of dairy products.
13. History of thyroid problems, liver problems, diabetes, renal failure, and other endocrine disorders.
14. Medication history: corticosteroids, isoniazid, heparin, tetracycline, anticonvulsants, and thyroid supplements.

B. Physical examination.
1. May present with Colles' fracture, femoral fractures, or vertebral compression fractures.
2. Marked kyphosis of thoracic spine (dowager's hump).
3. Shortened stature.
4. Muscle wasting or muscle spasms of the back.
5. Difficulty bending over.
6. Occasional impaired breathing due to deformities of spine and rib cage.

C. Diagnostic tests.
1. Laboratory findings.
   a. Urinary calcium may be elevated.
   b. Serum calcium, phosphorus, and alkaline phosphatase are normal, because of body's efficient calcium/phosphorus balance system.
   c. Serum osteocalcin is elevated.
   d. Serum and urinary markers of pyridinoline crosslinks (markers of bone turnover) elevated.
2. Radiographic findings.
   a. Osteoporotic changes not seen until over 30% of bone mass lost.
   b. Diffuse radiolucency of bones.
   c. Transverse trabeculae are sparse, vertical trabeculae are normal.
   d. Articular cortices indistinct.
   e. Thoracic vertebrae may be wedge-shaped.
   f. Lumbar vertebral bodies may be biconcave.
   g. Old and/or recent compression fractures are noted.
3. Bone mineral density (BMD) evaluation.
   a. Dual energy x-ray absorptiometry (DEXA) indicates low bone density.
      (1) Precise, economical, and readily available.
      (2) Minimal radiation exposure, short procedure time and very precise.
   b. Quantitative ultrasound (QUS) indicates low bone density.
      (1) Low-cost, extremely fast (5 minutes), portable, and radiation-free.
      (2) Evaluates density, elasticity, and strength of the os calcis and patella.
   c. QUS correlates well with DEXA measurements and both predict fractures.
4. Bone biopsy.
   a. Invasive and reserved for gathering more pre-

cise information about metabolic bone activity.
   b. Performed when diagnosis by noninvasive measures has been unreliable or when patient has not responded to therapy.
   c. Iliac crest is preferred site of bone sampling.
   d. Tetracycline labeling (oral tetracycline) given pre-biopsy according to precise schedule.

III. COMMON THERAPEUTIC MODALITIES

A. Prevention and early detection strategies should be started before bone loss occurs.

B. Active treatment required if prevention fails.

1. Estrogen replacement therapy for women.
2. Antiresorptive therapy.
   a. Alendronate (Fosamax®) used for treating postmenopausal osteoporosis (10 mg), as well as for preventing osteoporosis (5 mg).
   b. Risedronate (Actonel®) 5 mg used for treating and preventing postmenopausal osteoporosis. Also used for treating and preventing glucocorticoid-induced osteoporosis in men and women on systemic glucocorticoid treatment (7.5 mg or more of prednisone or equivalent) for chronic disease.
   c. Calcitonin available to treat osteoporosis; either nasal spray or parenteral preparation.
3. Slow released sodium fluoride.
4. Selective estrogen receptor modulators (raloxifene [Evista®]) provide treatment option for women who cannot take estrogen.
5. Calcium supplementation and adequate vitamin D (either from sunlight exposure, or from diet and/or supplementation) necessary for optimum bone health.

C. Exercise for improving strength and flexibility.

1. Regular, weight-bearing exercise, at least 30 minutes three times a week.
2. Prevent risk of fractures:
   a. Avoid high impact.
   b. Avoid vertebral spine rotational activities.

D. Fall prevention strategies.

1. Safe home environment.
2. Hip pads to lower fracture risk with fall.

E. Pain management.

1. Rest and activity.
2. Lumbosacral brace for vertebral fractures; short-term use only.
3. Heat application.
4. Medications (anti-inflammatories; non-narcotic and/or narcotic analgesics).

F. Diet high in vitamins, calcium, and protein.

IV. NURSING DIAGNOSES, OUTCOMES, AND INTERVENTIONS

A. See Table 13.1.

B. Nutrition, imbalanced: less than body daily requirement.

1. Outcome: patient meets RDA requirement for calcium and vitamin D.
2. Interventions.
   a. Instruct on dietary and medical needs and calcium and vitamin D supplements.
   b. Provide education regarding the relationship between adequate calcium and vitamin D intake and strong bones.
   c. Provide current information regarding calcium and vitamin D supplements.
   d. Provide nutritional information on foods high in calcium and vitamin D.
   e. Instruct on dietary habits that diminish ability to maintain total body calcium stores.
      (1) High-protein diet.
      (2) High-fiber diet.
      (3) High-sodium or carbohydrate diet.

C. Knowledge, deficient.

1. Outcome: patient adheres to a regular weight-bearing activity program.
2. Interventions.
   a. Discuss with the patient the role of weight-bearing activities in developing and maintaining bone mass.
   b. Instruct patient on safe weight-bearing activities that are essential for maintaining strong, healthy bones.
      (1) Weight bearing exercise at least 30 minutes three times a week: walking.
      (2) Avoid high-impact aerobics.
      (3) Avoid vertebral spine rotational activities.
   c. Caution patient on risk-taking behaviors that could lead to falls or other injuries to the musculoskeletal system.

D. Body image, disturbed.

1. Outcome: patient has a positive self-image.
2. Interventions.
   a. Instruct on coping strategies for altered body shape and size.
   b. Provide resources for obtaining clothing that fits properly.
   c. Provide information regarding support groups/classes for people with osteoporosis.
   d. Provide information regarding the National Osteoporosis Foundation (1232 22nd Street N.W., Washington, D.C., 20037-1292; phone: (202) 223.2226; Web site: http://www.nof.org).

V. PRACTICE SETTING CONSIDERATIONS

A. Office/outpatient.

1. Provide information regarding diagnosis and prescribed treatment.
2. Describe signs and symptoms of pathophysiology and identify which symptoms require intervention by health care provider.
3. Instruct patient and family regarding completion, interpretation, and potential intervention related to diagnostic tests (DEXAs; laboratory tests) and localized studies (peripheral bone mineral density studies).
4. Monitor patient's height (measure annually).
5. Arrange follow-up, to include appropriate outpatient diagnostic tests (serial bone mineral densities

at appropriate intervals) to manage osteoporosis.

B. Home care.

1. Maintain a healthy diet.
2. Maintain an adequate calcium intake.
3. Engage in regular weight-bearing exercise.
4. Take estrogen or bisphosphanates when and how indicated, and under medical supervision.
5. Assure safe home environment, free of obstacles and other risks of falling.
6. Continue self-administration of calcitonin, when indicated, under medical supervision.
7. Encourage adequate sunlight exposure and adequate vitamin D intake.
8. Maintain normal bowel elimination.
9. Decrease risk factors such as smoking and excessive alcohol intake.

C. Long-term care.

1. Lifelong monitoring of bone mineral density.
2. Annual physical examination and bone mineral density to monitor response to therapy and/or progression of osteoporosis.
3. Lifelong intake of appropriate amount of calcium and vitamin D.
4. Promotion of healthy dietary habits that help maintain total body calcium stores.
5. Ongoing participation in regular weight-bearing exercise.
6. Treatment (possibly surgical) of any fractures that result from osteoporosis.
7. Lifelong intake of appropriate bone sparing medications (estrogen or other antiresorptive medications).
8. Safety and fall precautions.

PAGET'S DISEASE (OSTEITIS DEFORMANS)

I. OVERVIEW

A. Definition: slowly progressive metabolic bone disease characterized by an initial phase of excessive bone resorption, followed by a reactive phase of excessive abnormal bone formation.

B. Etiology.

1. Exact cause unknown.
2. Possibly early viral infection causes dormant skeletal infection that develops into Paget's disease several years later; possible genetic predisposition.
3. Familial tendency; 25%-40% of patients with Paget's disease have at least one relative with the disorder.

C. Pathophysiology.

1. Characterized by an osteoclastic phase of excessive bone resorption which is followed by an osteoblastic phase in which there is excessive abnormal bone formation.
2. New bone structure is fragile and weak resulting in painful deformities and susceptibility to fractures.
3. Bone marrow is frequently replaced by loose fibrous tissue increasing vascularity.
4. As bone formation continues, it forms a classic mosaic pattern of bone matrix.
5. Early stages may be asymptomatic, but when pain develops, it is severe and persistent.

D. Incidence.

1. Occurs worldwide but is extremely rare in Asia, the Middle East, Africa, and Scandinavia.
2. In the United States, Paget's disease affects approximately 3% of people over age 50.
3. Males are affected slightly more than females.
4. Usually localizes in one or several areas of the skeleton, most frequently in lower torso (femur, tibia, pelvic bones, and vertebrae).
5. Skeletal deformity can be widely distributed.

E. Considerations across the lifespan.

1. Patient and family members should be instructed about possible role changes necessitated by the progressive nature of this disease.
2. Patient and family members should be instructed about aid for continuity of care.

F. Complications.

1. Bone pressing on cranial nerves may result in:
   a. Vertigo.
   b. Hearing loss with or without tinnitus.
   c. Blindness.
2. Hypertension.
3. Congestive heart failure or calcific aortic disease.
4. Hypercalcemia/hypercalciuria.
5. Fractures.
6. Renal calculi.
7. Waddling gait due to softening of pelvic bones and bowing of femur and tibia.
8. Gout, pseudogout, and arthritis.
9. Calcific periarthritis.
10. Pain.

II. ASSESSMENT

A. History.

1. Complete with special emphasis on history of viral infections (mumps virus).
2. Chief complaints.

B. Physical examination.

1. Complete physical examination with special emphasis on:
   a. Areas of deformity.
   b. Pain.
   c. Impaired movement.
2. Signs to note:
   a. May be asymptomatic or vague and difficult to distinguish from other diseases.
   b. Persistent and severe bone pain.
   c. Pain intensified with weight bearing.
   d. Impaired movement as a result of abnormal bone formation impinging on the spinal cord or spinal nerve root.
   e. Skull involvement results in cranial enlargement.
   f. Kyphosis with barrel-shaped chest and asymmetric bowing of the tibia and femur which leads to reduced height.
   g. Pagetic sites that are warm and tender due to increased vascularity.

h. Pagetic fractures that heal slowly and often incompletely.
i. Hearing loss.
j. Signs of congestive heart failure as overworked heart attempts to pump blood through the increased mass of blood vessels in active pagetic bone.
k. Hypertrophy and bowing of long bones.
l. Irregular deformities of the long bones.
m. Joint destruction and arthritis because pagetic joint deformity can invade the joints and contribute to osteoarthritis.
n. Involvement of spine can lead to development of kyphosis and height loss from vertebral compression fractures.

C. Diagnostic tests.

1. Laboratory findings.
   a. Increased serum alkaline phosphatase due to excessive osteoblastic activity.
   b. Complete blood count (CBC) may show anemia.
   c. Serum calcium, phosphorus, and albumin levels are usually normal.
   d. Serum and urinary markers of bone resorption – hydroxyproline or pyridinoline crosslinks.
2. Radiographic findings.
   a. Primary means of confirming diagnosis of Paget's disease.
   b. Early phases: characteristic osteolytic lesions, most commonly in long bones and skull.
   c. Adjoining overgrowth of bone appears on x-ray, providing coarse irregular appearance and enlargement of bone contours.
   d. After symptoms present, weakened bone usually shows characteristic mosaic pattern.
   e. Long bones may have tiny cracks; surface of skull may appear irregular because of varying thickness of the bone and low-density lesions.
   f. Radioactive bone scan helps diagnose when x-ray is unreliable.
      (1) Areas of active pagetic bone absorb more radioisotopes and can be detected with scanner.
      (2) Radioactive bone scan is also used to determine activity vs. inactivity of existing pagetic lesion.
   g. Bone biopsy occasionally necessary to confirm an unusual clinical or radiologic finding, or in patients who do not respond to therapy.

III. COMMON THERAPEUTIC MODALITIES

A. Medical.

1. Symptomatic and supportive therapy for pain (aspirin, nonsteroidal anti-inflammatory drugs [NSAIDs]).
2. Calcitonin and etidronate (Didronel®), which retard bone resorption and decrease bone lesions.
3. Alendronate (Fosamax®), which decreases rate of bone resorption.
4. Pamidronate (Aredia®), which is given intravenously to suppress bone resorption by inhibiting osteoclasts, binding calcium phosphate crystals in bone, and blocking calcium reabsorption.
5. Tiludronate (Skelid®), which is a strong inhibitor of bone resorption.
6. Management of hypercalcemia (see Primary Hyperparathyroidism).
7. Reserved for patients who are unresponsive to other treatment, those requiring rapid treatment due to serious complications, or the occasional young patient.

B. Surgical.

1. Reduce pathologic fractures.
2. Correct secondary deformities.
3. Relieve neurologic impairment.
4. Drug therapy prior to surgery to decrease risk of excessive bleeding due to hypervascular bone.
5. Total joint replacement when arthritis reaches advanced stage.
6. Spinal decompression to alleviate severe pain and neurologic symptoms.

IV. NURSING DIAGNOSES, OUTCOMES, AND INTERVENTIONS

A. See Table 13.1.

B. Self care, deficient; instrumental.

1. Outcome: patient and/or significant other able to administer medications as prescribed.
2. Interventions: educate patient/significant others about drugs the patient will be on at home.
   a. When patient takes calcitonin:
      (1) Teach patient how to comply with scheduling.
      (2) Teach how to inject the medication and rotate the sites of administration.
      (3) Warn patient that side effects may occur, that they are mild and infrequent and usually diminish with continued use of calcitonin.
   b. When patient takes etidronate (Didronel®):
      (1) Teach patient to take medication with juice 2 hours before meals.
      (2) Daily dose should be divided to minimize side effects.
      (3) Tell patient to watch for and report stomach cramps, diarrhea, new bone pain, or fractures.
      (4) Due to high incidence of side effects, etidronate usually not taken for longer than 6 months at a time.
   c. When patient takes alendronate (Fosamax®):
      (1) Teach patient to take with 6-8 ounces of plain water, on empty stomach at least 30 minutes before first food or drink of the day and to remain in upright position after taking.
      (2) Tell patient to report any abdominal pain, esophagitis, gastritis, nausea, and vomiting.
   d. When patient takes tiludronate (Skelid®): teach patient to take with 6-8 ounces of plain water

and not within 2 hours of meals.

C. **Body image, disturbed.**
   1. Outcome: patient will cope with body image changes.
   2. Interventions.
      a. Assess effects of disease on the patient's body image.
      b. Encourage patient to vent his/her feelings.
      c. Physical therapy consult to maintain ADL and role performance.
      d. Instruct family of changes in role as disease progresses.

D. **Pain.**
   1. Outcome: patient will have adequate pain management.
   2. Interventions.
      a. Assess pain.
      b. Schedule medications appropriately.
      c. Encourage periods of rest and activity.
      d. Heat therapy and gentle massage for mild discomfort.

E. **Knowledge, deficient.**
   1. Outcome: patient is familiar with disease process and adheres to specific treatment regimen.
   2. Interventions.
      a. Instruct patient on disease process and the treatment he/she will undergo.
      b. Describe pagetic process and provide information about The Paget Foundation (120 Wall St., Suite 1602, New York, NY 10005; phone: (800) 23-PAGET; fax: (212) 509-8492; http://www.healthanswers.com/Sources/nhc/homepages/pf/pf1.html; e-mail: pagetfdn@aol.com).

V. PRACTICE SETTING CONSIDERATIONS

A. **Office/outpatient.**
   1. Provide information regarding diagnosis and prescribed treatment.
   2. Describe signs and symptoms of pathophysiology and identify which symptoms require intervention by health care provider.
   3. Instruct patient and family regarding completion, interpretation, and potential intervention related to diagnostic tests and localized studies.
   4. Arrange follow-up, to include appropriate outpatient diagnostic tests to manage Paget's disease (x-rays; bone scans; bone biopsies).
   5. Review fracture prevention and fall precautions.
   6. Treat hearing loss (referral to ENT as needed).
   7. Treat CHF (referral to cardiologist as needed).
   8. Perioperative education and management (related to fracture reduction; deformity correction; neurological impairment; total joint replacemene [TJR]; spinal decompression).

B. **Home care considerations.**
   1. Maintain a healthy diet.
   2. Take prescribed medications according to schedule, under medical supervision.
   3. Assure safe home environment, free of obstacles and other risks of falling.
   4. Continue pain management interventions and assess regularly for effectiveness.

C. **Long-term care.**
   1. Lifelong monitoring of skeletal deformity.
   2. Patient and family instruction and support related to role changes and continuity of care.
   3. Supportive medical care related to progressive complications.

RICKETS

I. OVERVIEW

A. **Definition:**
   1. A disturbance in formation of the bone in the growing skeleton. Is characterized by softened and deformed bones caused by a failure of the organic matrix osteoid of the growth plate (epiphysis) and newly formed, trabecular and cortical bone to calcify normally.
   2. Deficient mineralization due to inadequate calcium and/or phosphate deposition in the osteoid formed by the growth plate. This deficience leads to a defect in growing bone, specifically in the growth plates before closure.

B. **Etiology.**
   1. Nutritional rickets.
      a. Failure to ingest required amounts of vitamin D.
      b. Lack of sufficient absorption of minerals from gastrointestinal tract such as with celiac disease.
      c. Reflected in decreased levels of calcium and phosphorus in the tissue fluids that perfuse the organic matrix of the bone.
   2. Renal rickets.
      a. Abnormally high level of excretion of minerals through kidneys causes a continual negative balance.
      b. Two types:
         (1) Malfunction of tubercles.
         (2) Loss of glomerular function
   3. Vitamin D-resistant rickets: apparently due to a person's inability to satisfactorily use the amount of vitamin D which in a healthy person is sufficient to promote gastrointestinal absorption of adequate amounts of minerals.
   4. Congenital hypophosphatemia.
      a. Adequate ingestion of minerals and vitamin D.
      b. Inadequate synthesis of calcitriol (1,~, 25-dihydroxyvitamin D3).
      c. Vitamin D utilized normally and kidneys resorb minerals satisfactorily, but a failure by osteoblasts laying down the matrix to form alkaline phosphatase causes a failure of calcification.

C. **Pathophysiology.**
   1. Calcium is needed for bone formation and resorption.
   2. Vitamin D results in intestinal absorption of dietary calcium and therefore affects bone strength, formation, and resorption.
   3. Rickets is a vitamin D deficiency that results in failure of normal bone calcification.

D. Incidence.

1. Infancy and childhood, most often noted between 5 months and 3 years.
2. Can affect all bones, but most common deformities are noted in spine and lower extremities.
3. Family tendencies toward the disease.
4. Children of vegetarian parents who avoid milk products, and breast-fed children who are not weaned to vitamin D-supplemented milk.
5. Endemic in northern India; China, and Africa.
6. Occurs mainly in winter and nontropical areas.

E. Considerations across the lifespan.

1. Infancy and childhood to include adolescents.
2. Most often noted between the ages of 6 months to 3 years.

II. ASSESSMENT

A. History.

1. A history of dietary deficiency.
2. Infant displays increased restlessness at night, profuse diaphoresis, skin pallor, and lack of interest in play.

B. Physical examination.

1. Generalized inflammation of mucous membranes manifested by diarrhea and respiratory infections.
2. Occasional CNS irritability resulting in spasticity or convulsions.
3. Head often has enlarged, squared appearance, and fontanelles are late in closing.
4. Chest has a beading enlargement at the costochondral junction (rachitic rosary), a horizontal depression a few inches above the lower costal margin caused by a pull of the diaphragm on the softened ribs (Harrison's groove), and the chest cage is narrowed transversely and elongated anteroposteriorly (pigeon breast).
5. Compression fractures of vertebrae resulting in a twisted and bent spinal column.
6. Abdomen may be prominent.
7. Enlarged epiphyses especially at areas of most rapid growth, such as knee and wrist.
8. Delayed dentition.
9. Poor muscle tone resulting in delayed walking.
10. Deformities of extremities consequent to weight bearing (genu varum or genu valgus)
11. Occasionally shortened stature is observed.

C. Diagnostic tests.

1. Laboratory findings.
   a. Serum phosphorus is typically reduced.
   b. Serum alkaline phosphatase is elevated.
   c. Urinary calcium level is diminished.
   d. Serum calcium is decreased and serum phosphorus is elevated in renal rickets.
   e. Serum phosphorus is decreased, calcium is normal, and alkaline phosphorus is elevated in vitamin D-resistant rickets.
2. Radiographic findings.
   a. In acute stage, the epiphysis is poorly defined and frayed looking.
   b. Metaphyseal cortices flare outward (trumpeting).
   c. Trabeculae are reduced and less prominent except in vitamin D-resistant rickets where they are coarser and broader.
   d. Pelvis is compressed transversely and the inlet is narrowed.
   e. Long weight-bearing bones bend; cortices are thickened on the concave side.
   f. Intestinal dilation is noted in celiac disease.

III. COMMON THERAPEUTIC MODALITIES

A. Administration of vitamin D.

B. Exposure to sunlight, especially for premature infants and those on artificial milk feedings.

C. Braces for deformities are usually unnecessary if adequate amounts of vitamin D are given.

D. Gluten-free diet; high-protein diet; supplemental vitamin D for celiac disease.

E. Occasionally an osteotomy is necessary after growth is complete to correct deformities.

IV. NURSING DIAGNOSES, OUTCOMES, AND INTERVENTIONS

A. See Table 13.1.

B. Nutrition, imbalanced: less than daily body requirement.

1. Outcomes.
   a. Significant others able to identify dietary and medical needs.
   b. Patient has adequate dietary intake of vitamin D.
2. Interventions.
   a. Provide information regarding disease process and sources of vitamin D.
   b. Improved nutrition to meet individual's body requirements by:
      (1) Assessing fluid intake to include milk and other foods containing calcium and vitamin D.
      (2) Dietary supplements when indicated.

C. Injury, risk for.

1. Outcomes.
   a. Decreased anxiety demonstrated by significant others when caring for the patient.
   b. Significant others relate a safe environment in which to care for the patient.
2. Interventions.
   a. Provide education regarding handling the patient.
      (1) Demonstrate how to support extremities when handling the patient.
      (2) Discuss fears related to potential injuries from handling the patient.
   b. Maintain safe environment.
      (1) Assess for proper brace application and fit.
      (2) Discuss potential for injury, for example, fractures due to minor trauma.
      (3) Position pillows to support affected tissues.

V. PRACTICE SETTING CONSIDERATIONS

A. Office/outpatient.

1. Provide parents/guardians with information regarding diagnosis and treatment.
2. Provide parents with information regarding signs and symptoms of pathophysiology, and which symptoms need intervention.

B. Home care.

1. Encourage adequate sunlight exposure.
2. Home environment modified to promote safety.
3. Alternative caregivers instructed by parents in handling of infant or child.

C. Long-term care.

1. Avoid injury, such as fractures related to minor trauma.
2. Support and education regarding appropriate vitamin D supplementation.
3. Long-term dietary alterations

Bibliography

American Society for Bone and Mineral Research. (1996). *Primer on the metabolic bone diseases and disorders of mineral metabolism* (3rd ed.). New York: Lippincott-Raven.

Avioli, L., & Krane, S. (1998). *Metabolic bone disease and clinically related disorders* (3rd ed.). San Diego: Academic Press.

Behrman, R.E., Kliegman, R.M., & Jenson, H.B. (1996). Bone and joint disorders. In *Nelson textbook of pediatrics (16th ed.)* (pp. 2132-2138). Philadelphia: W.B. Saunders Company.

Black, J., Matassarin-Jacobs, E., & Luckman, J. (1997). *Medical-surgical nursing: Clinical management for continuity of care (5th ed.).* Philadelphia: W.B. Saunders Company.

Galsworthy, T.D., & Wilson, P.L. (1996). Osteoporosis: It steals more than bone. *American Journal of Nursing, 96*(6), 27-33.

Guyton, A.C. (1996). Parathyroid hormone, calcitonin, calcium, and phosphate metabolism, vitamin D, bone, and teeth. In A. Guyton & J. Hall. *Textbook of medical physiology* (9th ed. pp. 985-1002). Philadelphia: W.B. Saunders.

Hartman, J. (2000). Vitamin D deficiency rickets in children: Prevalence and need for community education. *Orthopaedic Nursing, 19*(1), 63-69.

Hunt, A.H. (1998). Metabolic conditions. In A.B. Maher, S.W. Salmond, & T.A. Pellino (Eds.), *Orthopaedic nursing* (2nd ed., pp. 431-479). Philadelphia: W.B. Saunders Company.

Kim, T. (1994). Primary hyperparathyroidism. *Orthopaedic Nursing, 13*(3), 17-29.

National Academy of Sciences. (1997). *Dietary reference intakes.* Washington, DC: National Academy Press.

National Institutes of Health. (2000). Optimal calcium intake. *NIH Consensus Statement, 12*(4), 1-31.

Patton, K., & Thibodeau, G. (2000). *Structure and function of the body.* St. Louis: Mosby.

Schoen, D.C. (2000). Musculoskeletal pathology. In D.C. Schoen, *Adult orthopaedic nursing.* (pp. 43-48). Philadelphia: Lippincott.

Siris, E., & Schussheim, D. (1998). Osteoporosis: Assessing your patient's risk. *Women's Health in Primary Care, 1*(1), 99-106.

STUDY QUESTIONS

Anne is a 32-year-old female athlete who runs 5 miles daily and participates in frequent weekend road races and triathalons. She is 5' 7", 100 pounds, and gives a history of amenorrhea, lactose intolerance, moderate alcohol use, and daily vitamin supplementation. Anne is well known to you and presents with a chief complaint of severe allergy symptoms for which she has been treated with steroids in the past. (Questions 1-3)

1. Based on Anne's history, which of the following would **not** be a major concern in gathering more data regarding her current complaint.
   a. Frequency and duration of exercise.
   b. Duration of amenorrhea.
   c. Dietary intake of foods high in calcium
   d. Daily vitamin supplementation.

2. After completing the history and physical examination, it is identified that Anne is a high-risk patient for osteoporosis. Patient education should include an emphasis on:
   a. What can be done now so that osteoporosis does not occur when she is 60 or older.
   b. What can be done to prevent further bone loss and increase her bone mineral density.
   c. Continue high levels of exercise, as weight bearing is essential for reduction of bone loss.
   d. Modifying her home environment to be free of obstacles and other risks of falling.

3. Anne is instructed on the need for adequate calcium intake through dietary ingestion and supplementation. Anne should be encouraged to maintain a calcium intake of:
   a. 500 mg per day.
   b. 1,000 mg per day.
   c. 1,5000 mg per day.
   d. 2,000 mg per day.

Tom is a 42-year-old male who presents to the orthopaedist with a chief complaint of pain that intensifies with walking. He has been referred with a possible diagnosis of Paget's Disease. (Questions 4-6)

4. History and physical examination should include:
   a. History of bacterial infections.
   b. Location and duration of pain.
   c. Change in shoe size.
   d. Leg length discrepancy.

5. Calcitonin is prescribed for Tom. The nurse should teach Tom and his family:
   a. Subcutaneous injection technique and site rotation.
   b. To eat salmon twice weekly.
   c. Need to take calcitonin with meals.
   d. Need to take calcitonin 1/2 hour before breakfast.

6. Which of the following is **not** true about pain associated with Paget's disease?
   a. It may be treated symptomatically with aspirin or NSAIDs.
   b. It worsens with weight bearing.
   c. It may respond to heat therapy or massage.
   d. Severe pain is best treated with rest and narcotics.

Monica, age 52, presents for evaluation of recurrent kidney stones and a history of chronic low back pain. Her serum calcium level was noted to be above 10 mg/dl, which alerted the practitioner to the possibility of hyperparathyroidism. (Questions 7-8)

7. History data taken by the nurse should include:
   a. Family history of parathyroid disease.
   b. Iron intake.
   c. Menstrual history.
   d. Tallest height remembered.

8. A primary goal is to treat symptoms associated with and reduce the serum calcium level. Which of the following is **not** a primary treatment?
   a. Forcing fluids up to 3,000 m/day IV or PO.
   b. Administration of diuretics as ordered.
   c. Administration of plicamycin (Mithracin®) as ordered.
   d. Vitamin D with or without supplemental calcium.

A 9-month-old infant was brought to the doctor because he was becoming increasingly restless and irritable. Upon assessment, it was noted that there was a bowing of his legs with some thickness of his wrists and ankles. His posterior fontanelle remained open. Blood work and x-rays were suggestive of a diagnosis of rickets. (Questions 9-10)

9. According to the pathophysiology of rickets, which of the following statements is correct:
   a. Bone softening is a result of vitamin D deficiency.
   b. Bone matrix is not calcified properly.
   c. Age-related bone loss is caused by increased GI calcium absorption.
   d. Bone developed is affected before birth.

10. Rickets is rare in the United States but occasionally appears. Which of the following situations is **not** related to Rickets?
    a. Breast-fed infants who do not receive vitamin D supplementation.
    b. Overcrowded, urban areas where people receive limited sunlight penetration.
    c. Infants receiving a formula with a non-fortified milk base.
    d. Breast-fed infants who are then switched to a formula at 3 months of age.

Chapter 14 *TRAUMA*

Ann Butler Maher, MS, RN, APNC, ONC

Contents

OBJECTIVES

At the completion of this chapter, the learner will be able to:

- List common traumatic injuries and their incidence across the lifespan.
- Recall the mechanism of injury for common fractures/dislocations.
- Identify the appropriate assessment for common traumatic injuries.
- Discuss therapeutic modalities and interventions for common traumatic injuries.

KEY POINTS

- Trauma is the leading killer of Americans under the age of 45 and the fifth leading cause of death.
- Trauma has a bimodal distribution: high-energy injuries in the young (ages 16-35) and low-energy injuries in elders (age 70-80+).
- Fifty-nine million Americans are injured each year, accounting for 36 million emergency department visits.
- After head injuries, pelvic fractures are the most common cause of traumatic death.
- Pain assessment of the trauma patient is an ongoing process. Neurovascular status, level of consciousness, and progression of symptoms must be evaluated before medicating the patient.
- Pathologic fractures can often precede a patient's fall.
- Many sports injuries can be prevented with attention to key points, warm-up exercises, and not overlooking warning signals:
- Warm-up exercises are essential as they increase muscle temperature and blood supply.
- It is important not to overlook warning signals of persistent pain in muscles, bones, and joints.

CHAPTER 14

TRAUMA

STRAINS

I. OVERVIEW

A. Definition: trauma in which the body of a muscle or the attachment of a tendon has been damaged by overstretching, misuse, or overexertion.

B. Pathology.

1. Chronic: mild to moderately over-stretched muscle or tendon that persists in causing symptomatology for a prolonged period of time. Most often results from improper care of an acute strain, or repeated use of muscle beyond normal capacity. Can result in weakness of the area.
2. Acute: classified according to degree of injury.
    a. First degree: mild stretching of the muscle/tendon.
    b. Second degree: moderate stretching and/or tearing of the muscle/tendon.
    c. Third degree: severe muscle/tendon stretching in which the involved tissue ruptured, tore completely through, or pulled away from the bone.

C. Incidence.

1. May occur in almost any age group or in any musculotendinous unit.
2. Injury to any specific area of the body.
3. Often related to particular types of activity.

D. Considerations across the lifespan.

1. Shoulder tendons in elderly more prone to injury than in younger people.
2. Upper arm strain more common in middle-aged and elderly males than in women or younger men.
3. Injuries to ankle and knee are common at any age, particularly in athletes.

E. Complications: recurrence of injury with greater severity (first degree strain to rupture).

II. ASSESSMENT

A. History. Recent stress of muscles by exercising or working to excess (sudden muscle overload by lifting something heavy).

1. Mechanism of injury.
2. Symptoms.
    a. First degree: gradual onset of symptoms that did not begin to appear until several hours after the overexertion. Feeling of stiffness and soreness of the involved area.
    b. Second degree: overactivity results in sudden, acute, incapacitating pain which subsided, leaving the affected muscle/tendon tender.
    c. Third degree: complaint of feeling a sudden tearing, snapping, or burning sensation in the injured area during the period of overexertion and diminished ability or inability to move a body part.
    d. See Table 14.1.

B. Physical examination. Reproducing the injury by placing the body part/joint through range of motion may produce pain and/or tenderness of the site, limited range of motion.

1. Chronic: pain, limited range of motion, tenderness over site.
2. First degree.
    a. No loss of range of motion.
    b. Tenderness on palpation.
    c. Muscle spasm may be noted.
    d. No edema or ecchymosis.
3. Second degree.
    a. Extreme muscle spasm.
    b. Passive motion results in increased discomfort.
    c. Areas noted to be edematous soon after the injury.
    d. Ecchymosis appears after several hours or days.
4. Third degree.
    a. Muscle spasm.
    b. Point tenderness.
    c. Edema noted.
    d. Inability of the contracting muscle to produce motion.
    e. Ecchymosis will be delayed.
    f. May have muscle bulge above palpable defect.

C. Diagnostic tests. X-rays to rule out an avulsion fracture.

III. COMMON THERAPEUTIC MODALITIES

A. RICE. An acronym for rest, ice, compression, and elevation, RICE has been found to be effective for almost all types of injuries, from a strained muscle to a fracture.

1. Rest.
    a. An area that has been injured and is not placed at rest could extend the recovery period.
    b. Rest includes use of a sling, crutches, immobilizers, and splints.
2. Ice (cryotherapy).
    a. The application of ice decreases bleeding from injured blood vessels by causing them to contract. Ice applied for 20 minutes decreases soft tissue blood flow by 25%.
    b. The more blood that collects in a wound, the longer it takes for the injury to heal. Ice popsicles work well for areas such as the ankle.
        (1) Freeze water in a paper or foam cup.
        (2) Peel away the edges of the cup.
        (3) The remaining part of the cup can be used to hold the popsicle and massage the injured area.

Table 14.1
Common Sports Injuries: Fractures, Sprains, Strains, Dislocations, and Inflammations

Anatomic Area	Mechanism of Injury	Common Athletic Assessment	Activities	Acute Management
UPPER EXTREMITY Clavicle fracture	Fall on shoulder or outstretched arm	• Edema • Crepitus • Unable to raise affected arm above head • Can feel movement of both ends of clavicle	• Contact sports • Cycling • Skiing • Horseback riding	*Adult/Child:* • Sling or shoulder immobilizer • Ice • NSAIDs
Dislocated shoulder joint	• Lifts arm and turns outward to protect body from fall • Falling directly on lateral aspect of shoulder • Posterior: arm caught and turned out and back • Anterior: arm pulled forward and downward	• Pain • Lack of motion • May feel empty socket • Uneven posture in comparison to other shoulder • Affected arm longer • Abduction limited • Diagnose with x-ray	• Rugby • Hockey • Wrestling • Skiing	*Adult/Child:* • Manipulate • Immobilize, sling, swathe • Pendulum exercise in 3 weeks
Shoulder bursitis	• Fall or blow to shoulder, or supraspinatus tendon rupture resulting in inflammation • Repetitive motion causing accumulation of fluid in bursa	• Pain in anterior shoulder • Pain on lifting in abduction and internal rotation	• Baseball • Swimming • Racquet sports	• Rest • Heat • Nonsteroidal medication • Physical therapy
Elbow dislocation	• Falling on a hand with a flexed elbow • Elbow overextended posterior dislocation most common	• Intense pain • Swelling • Limited motion • Deformity • Ecchymosis	• Football • Rugby • Squash • Wrestling • Cycling • Skiing	• Immobilization • Ice • Assess neurovascular status • After 2-5 weeks, start gentle ROM
Radial-ulnar bursitis Epicondylitis	• Continued excessive use of the elbow • Repetitive one-sided movements	• Pain outer aspect of elbow, radiates up and down lateral forearm • Weak wrist • Tenderness over lateral epicondyle • Medial pain triggered by flexion and extension of the forearm	• Tennis • Squash • Badminton • Golf • Baseball pitching	• Cold in acute phase • Heat in chronic phase • Rest • Bracing/wrist splint • Isometric exercise
Wrist sprain/ fracture	• Falling on outstretched arm in an attempt to protect yourself	• Pain, edema • Ecchymosis • Deformity • Limited motion	• Skating • Hockey • Wrestling • Skiing • Soccer • Handball • Horseback riding	• Ice • Elevation • Immobilization • Cast, brace, or external fixation • Gentle ROM after healing, 4-6 weeks

Table 14.1 (continued)
Common Sports Injuries: Fractures, Sprains, Strains, Dislocations, and Inflammations

Anatomic Area	Mechanism of Injury	Common Athletic Assessment	Activities	Acute Management
LOWER EXTREMITY				
Knee sprain	Twisting injury that produced incomplete tear of ligaments and capsule around the joint	• Pain • Limited motion • Edema • Ecchymosis • Tenderness over joint • Joint appears stable	• Basketball • Football • High jump	• Ice • Elevation • Compression (Ace®) • Active ROM • Isometric exercises • May immobilize 2-4 weeks
Knee strain	Result of sudden forced motion causing muscle to be stretched beyond normal capacity	• Pain • Limited motion • Pain aggravated by activity	• Soccer • Swimming • Skiing	• Ice • Elevation • Rest • Gradual return to activities
Meniscal tears of knee	• Sharp, sudden pivot • Direct blow to knee • Forced internal rotation • Wear from repetitive squatting or climbing • Torsional weight-bearing force	• Edema • Medial tear: pain in medial knee occurs in hyperflexion, hyperextension, and turning in of knee with knee flexed • Lateral tear: most common pain in lateral knee on hyperflexion and hyperextension and internal rotation of foot with knee flexed • Displaced fragment: inability to extend knee; locked • Diagnosis with arthroscopy, MRI, physical exam (medial joint line tenderness and + McMurray's sign)	• Hockey • Basketball • Football	Conservative: • RICE • Exercising quadriceps • Hamstring SLR • Resistive exercising • NSAIDs • Physical therapy Surgical: arthroscopy
Tibia/fibula fracture		• Tibia: upper two thirds most frequent • Fibula: usually 2-3 inches above lateral malleolus (Isolated fractures uncommon)	• Running • High jumping • Contact sports	• Ice • Elevation • Cast 4-6 weeks
Ankle sprain	• Foot is twisted, stretching ligaments • ROM has been exceeded	• Pain • Edema • Limited motion • Ecchymosis • On exam, ankle is stable, except third degree sprain	• Tennis • Basketball • Football • Skating	• Ice • Elevation • Support (high-top sneakers, ACE® wraps, air cast, SLC)
Ankle strain	Sudden forced motion stretching muscles beyond normal capacity	• Acute: severe pain • Chronic: achy pain	• Running • All ball sports	• Immobilization in cast, brace • Ice • Elevation • Rest • Gradual return to exercise in 4-6 weeks

Table 14.1 (continued)
Common Sports Injuries: Fractures, Sprains, Strains, Dislocations, and Inflammations

Anatomic Area	Mechanism of Injury	Common Athletic Assessment	Activities	Acute Management
Ankle fracture	• Inward turning on sole of foot and front of foot • Supination with internal rotation or pronation with external rotation	• Pain • Edema • Deformity • X-ray shows fracture	• Contact sports • Tennis • Basketball	• Ice • Elevation • Cast 4-6 weeks • Surgery if fracture is displaced or unstable
Stress fracture	• Occurs with repeated loading of bone, often in an unconditioned extremity • Muscles normally shunt stress forces away from bone • When overuse causes muscle fatigue, bone shielding is lost and a fracture results	• Pain after running long distances without history of impact • Local tenderness and swelling • X-ray may not show fracture until 2 weeks when callus begins to form, but MRI will show stress fracture • Bone scan positive after 3 days	• Running • High jumping • Gymnastics • Ice skating	• Rest • Non-weight bearing • Cast or Una boot
Navicular metatarsal fractures		• Pain with activity • Localized tenderness • Pain • X-ray may show callus in 2 weeks • Bone scan positive	• Running • Over training • Skating	• Rest • Ice • Most are nondisplaced so weight bearing as tolerated • Hard-sole shoe or short leg walking cast for comfort

c. Usually 30 minutes on and 15 minutes off while awake for up to 72 hours after injury.

3. Compression.
   a. The application of some form of compression limits the swelling, which if left uncontrolled could delay healing.
   b. Following trauma, blood, and fluid from the surrounding tissues leak into the damaged area and distend the tissue.
   c. Ace® bandages are the most common type of compression device used and should be applied after icing.
   d. Ace® bandages should be wrapped tightly enough to compress the area and promote venous return but not compromise neurovascular function or arterial blood flow.
   e. If the Ace® bandages are too tight, numbness, cramping, or pain may result. Keep the wrap loosest proximally and tightest distally.
4. Elevation.
   a. Placing the injured part at or above heart level so that gravity drains off excess fluid.
   b. Swelling begins within moments of the injury. Decreased edema facilitates pain relief and allows injured areas to move more freely.
   c. Elevation is contraindicated in the presence of arterial deficiency.

B. First degree muscle strain.

1. Comfort measures, such as local heat applications (after 24 hours), muscle relaxants, mild analgesics, and anti-inflammatory medications.
2. Rest.
3. Immobilization.

C. Second or third degree muscle strains.

1. Elevation of the injured part, if possible, until edema subsides.
2. Ice (to decrease edema and increase comfort) used intermittently for first 24-72 hours. Thereafter, heat may be applied in uncasted patients.
3. 4-6 weeks of limited mobility by:
   a. Internal repair.
   b. External support devices, such as slings, casts, splints, or immobilizers.
4. Muscle relaxants, analgesics, and anti-inflammatory medications.
5. After healing has progressed, active exercises are started and gradually increased until patient has regained normal strength and motion. Physical therapy may be required.

D. See Table 14.1.

IV. NURSING DIAGNOSES, OUTCOMES, AND INTERVENTIONS

A. Pain, acute.
1. Outcome: patient has decreased or relief of pain at the injury site.
2. Interventions.
   a. RICE treatment.
      (1) Rest injured part. Immobilization may be required.
      (2) Ice/cold application for 24-48 hours.
      (3) Compression: Ace® bandages, soft braces.
      (4) Elevation and position for comfort.
   b. After cryotherapy is stopped, heat may be used.
   c. Analgesic, muscle relaxant administration.
   d. Instruct patient on therapeutic value and regimens of cold/heat, rest/immobilization, compression, and elevation.

B. Physical mobility, impaired.
1. Outcomes.
   a. Patient resumes normal activity.
   b. Patient exhibits normal range of motion.
2. Interventions.
   a. Teach proper use of ambulatory devices.
   b. Use methods to conserve energy and maintain immobility of involved area.
   c. Teach patient about healing process, limitation of motion, and prevention of further strains. Rehabilitation is the most important part of preventing future injury.

C. Self-care deficit syndrome: bathing/hygiene, feeding, dressing/grooming, toileting.
1. Outcome: patient resumes normal self-care activities.
2. Interventions.
   a. Assist patient with activities of daily living (ADL).
   b. Educate patient regarding self-care activities while immobilized, using methods to conserve energy and maintain immobility of involved area.
   c. Educate patient regarding selection of clothing that does not require buttoning, zipping, or lacing for the patient with hand involvement. Consider ease of application (zippers, pullovers, buttons, laces).
   d. Teach patient to pass injured extremity through clothing before the uninvolved extremity when dressing.
   e. Promote independence of ADL.

D. Tissue perfusion, altered peripheral.
1. Outcome: resolution of edema at site of injury.
2. Interventions.
   a. Monitor condition of injured part and provide measures to reduce edema.
   b. Monitor patient's neurovascular status. (Do not assess motion of involved joint with a third degree strain.)
   c. Elevate injured areas when possible.
   d. Apply ice or heat, as ordered.

V. HOME CARE CONSIDERATIONS

A. Emphasize to patient need for rest and immobilization to prevent further injury.

B. With athletes, educate concerning varying exercise protocols to allow for muscle rest.
1. First: focus on increasing ROM.
2. Second: strengthen.
3. Third: proprioception.
4. Fourth: return to the sport.

C. Teach patient guidelines for when sports injury should be evaluated by physician.
1. Pain: prolonged, or nonsubsiding; continued pain after 2 weeks.
2. Joints: any injury that occurs in or near a joint.
3. Function: any loss of function.
4. Healing: any injury that is not healed in 3 weeks, or in which the structure is apparently abnormal.
5. Any sign of infection on or under the skin, presence of pus, red streaks, swollen lymph glands, or fever.

SPRAINS

I. OVERVIEW

A. Definition: a type of traumatic joint injury in which the surrounding ligament fibers have been damaged by excessive stretching or exertion.

B. Classification.
1. Mild/grade 1/first-degree sprain is one in which only a few fibers of the ligament have been torn or separated and hematoma formation is minimal and completely localized.
2. Moderate/grade 2/second-degree sprain is more severe than mild sprain with up to half of the ligament fibers torn.
3. Severe/grade 3/third-degree sprain/rupture is a sprain in which the ligament is completely torn through. The torn ends are separated from each other in the belly of the ligament or from the bone at the normal point of attachment which may result in an avulsion fracture.

C. Etiology. Sprains result from trauma, usually described as a sudden, twisting injury or forcible hyperextension of the joint.

D. Incidence.
1. The most common sprains observed in the upper extremities are in the wrist.
2. The most common sprains observed in the lower extremities are of the lateral ligament of the ankle and ligaments of the knee.
3. Extension sprains are common in the cervical spine region.

E. Considerations across the lifespan.
1. Common occurrence in any age group.
2. Frequent occurrence in athletes.

F. Complications.
1. Recurrence.
2. Joint instability.

II. ASSESSMENT

A. History.

1. The patient with an upper extremity sprain will frequently present a history in which the mechanism of injury was:
   a. Participation in a sporting event.
   b. Overstressing joints while working or exercising.
   c. Attempting to break a fall.
   d. Bracing oneself during impact in a vehicular accident.
2. The patient with an ankle sprain frequently presents with a history of stepping on an uneven surface, causing inversion or eversion of the ankle.
3. Knee involvement can be caused by sports injuries, motor vehicle accidents, and missteps.
4. Cervical extension sprains are generally caused by rear end motor vehicle collisions.
5. The degree of disability, decreased joint mobility, and discomfort may be experienced differently by different individuals.
6. See Table 14.1.

B. Physical examination.

1. Dependent on degree of injury.
2. Edema, ecchymosis, and tenderness of the soft tissues around the injured joint.
3. Decreased range of joint motion with second-degree and third-degree sprains.
4. Increased pain upon palpation or application of stress to injured ligament.
5. Joint effusion.
6. Mild/grade 1/first-degree:
   a. Mild pain.
   b. Tenderness and edema.
   c. No joint laxity.
   d. Edema may decrease range of motion.
7. Moderate/grade 2/second-degree:
   a. Greater pain.
   b. More tenderness and edema than first degree.
   c. May have some joint laxity (but with good endpoint).
   d. Edema may impair movement.
8. Severe/grade 3/third-degree:
   a. Severe pain.
   b. Joint laxity with endpoint.
   c. Edema.
   d. Loss of movement/function.

C. Diagnostic tests.

1. Radiographic findings demonstrate the presence of edema without bone injury or displacement.
2. X-ray important to rule out avulsion fracture.

III. COMMON THERAPEUTIC MODALITIES

A. RICE (see Strains).

B. Immediate medical treatment involves elevation and immobilization of the joint followed by applications of ice. Thereafter, treatment depends upon the severity of injury.

C. Grade 1/first-degree sprain.

1. Elastic bandage/cervical collar to provide protection during healing.
2. Crutches may be recommended but weight bearing is allowed in lower extremity sprains.
3. Elevation and intermittent applications of ice may be continued for 24-72 hours.
4. Mild analgesics as needed.
5. Isometric exercises may be prescribed.

D. Grade 2/second-degree sprain.

1. Elastic bandage and splinting of the weakened joint to prevent further tearing and loss of function.
2. Weight bearing may be allowed but crutches are recommended on lower extremity sprains.
3. Intermittent ice applications may be continued for 24-72 hours after injury with heat applications thereafter, according to need.
4. Joint elevation, as needed, to minimize edema.
5. Analgesics, as needed.
6. Isometric exercises may be prescribed.

E. Grade 3/third-degree sprain.

1. Restoration of ligament integrity.
   a. Casting or bracing for approximately 4 weeks to maintain comfort and to aid in approximation of the torn ends as the connective fibrous tissue scar forms.
   b. Surgical approximation of the torn ends as an aid to healing.
2. Ice application intermittently for first 24-72 hours.
3. For the uncasted patient, heat may be applied thereafter as necessary for comfort.
4. Analgesics, as needed.
5. Physical therapy as healing is progressing.

IV. NURSING DIAGNOSES, OUTCOMES, AND INTERVENTIONS (See Strains).

V. HOME CARE CONSIDERATIONS (See Strains).

DISLOCATIONS AND SUBLUXATIONS

I. OVERVIEW

A. Definition/pathology: difference between dislocation and subluxation is one of degree of displacement of articulating surfaces.

1. Dislocation: displacement of a bone from its normal joint position to the extent that articulating surfaces lose contact.
2. Subluxation: displacement of a bone from its normal joint position to the extent that articulating surfaces partially lose contact.

B. Etiology. Force applied to the joint either directly or indirectly.

1. In the upper extremity, dislocations commonly due to a direct blow or to an indirectly applied force resulting from a fall on the outstretched arm or hand.
2. In the knee, dislocations generally caused by a severe twisting or blow to the knee most commonly as a result of a motor vehicle crash.

3. In the hip.
   a. Posterior dislocation is the most common dislocation. A force along shaft of femur when hip is in flexion and adduction (as from a fall or dashboard injury) is the most common cause of posterior dislocation.
   b. Anterior dislocations are rare and occur when the hip is forced into extension, abduction, and external rotation.
   c. Central dislocations occur with severe blows to lateral aspect of the hip, particularly if it is abducted.

C. Incidence. While almost any joint may become dislocated, some joints are more prone to dislocation than others.

1. Most common dislocation is anterior dislocation of the humerus in the shoulder joint; usually occurs in adults.
2. Other joints of the upper extremity do not dislocate as easily as shoulder joints.
   a. The elbow generally does not dislocate without a great deal of force. Soft-tissue damage is marked and includes capsule tearing and possibly neurovascular damage as well as fracture of the radial head.
   b. Subluxation of the radial head (nursemaid's elbow) is the common traumatic elbow injury in children occurring primarily in children ages 2-4.
   c. True dislocations of the wrist joint are rare.
   d. Finger dislocations are common in ball-handling sports.
3. The most common lower extremity dislocation is anterior dislocation of the knee joint. This is an orthopaedic emergency because of associated vascular and neurologic injuries.
4. The adult hip is normally a stable joint..
   a. Severe trauma is required for dislocation and is often associated with multisystem trauma.
   b. Posterior or anterior dislocations may occur with or without associated fractures.
   c. Central dislocations occur only with a fracture of the acetabulum; the femur may or may not be fractured.

D. Considerations across the lifespan.

1. Occur throughout the lifespan.
2. May be present at birth.

E. Complications.

1. Nerve and blood vessel injuries.
2. Ligament laxity which increases the risk of recurrent dislocation
3. Avascular necrosis of the head of the femur which loses circulation when it is dislocated

II. ASSESSMENT

A. History.

1. History of injury.
2. Assess hand dominance with upper extremity injuries; assess prior ambulatory status with lower extremity injuries.
3. Depending on joint involved and direction of dislocation, symptoms may vary widely in intensity from minimal to severe and may be the result of compromised respiration, circulation, or nerve transmission. The dislocation may represent very little danger or could be a life-threatening emergency.
4. The patient with a shoulder dislocation often presents with a complaint of joint pain which increases on attempts at abduction.
5. Following subluxation of the elbow (nursemaid's elbow), the pain quickly subsides and the child may return to play but not use the injured arm.
6. The knee dislocation has a high incidence of spontaneous reduction, so ask about mechanism of injury (hit dashboard with knee, hyperextended knee) in patients who complain of pain with range of motion.
7. The patient with a posterior hip dislocation commonly complains of painful muscle spasm about the hip and pain on extension, abduction, and external rotation, while patients with anterior hip dislocations complain of pain on flexion, adduction, and internal rotation.
8. See Table 14.1.
9. See Table 14.2.

B. Physical examination.

1. Observations made during the physical examination differ depending on the site and direction of dislocation.
2. Neurovascular status.
3. Pain on movement.
4. Tenderness.
5. Obvious deformity.
6. Instability of joint.
7. In shoulder dislocations.
   a. The shoulder may appear elevated.
   b. The normally convex contour may appear flattened or concave
   c. The affected arm may be held in slight abduction and external rotation.
   d. The affected arm may appear longer than the unaffected arm.
8. With subluxation of the radial head (nursemaid's elbow).
   a. The child holds the arm flexed at the elbow with the forearm pronated.
   b. Pain can be elicited in the elbow.
9. Most finger dislocations are dorsal.
10. Knee dislocations can be displaced anteriorly, posteriorly, medially, laterally, or in rotation.
    a. Rotational injuries are recognized by the presence of a skin depression over one of the femoral condyles.
    b. The other types of dislocation involve gross deformities indicative of the type of injury.
11. Posterior hip dislocation is suspected when the leg is held in flexion, adduction, and internal rotation with shortening. Peroneal nerve injury may exist with inability to dorsiflex the ankle and decreased sensation on the dorsum of the foot and base of first and second toes.

Table 14.2
Common Fractures/Dislocations

Fracture/ Dislocation	Mechanism of Injury	Assessment	Treatment	Approximate Healing Time
Skull	• Direct blow, fall, fight, collision.	• Level of consciousness. • Increased intracranial pressure. • Observe for lumps, bumps, indentations, bleeding.	*Adult/Child:* • Conservative: observation and steroids. • Surgical: burr holes. • Surgical: craniotomy to relieve pressure. • Direct pressure to control bleeding.	*Adult/Child:* 4-6 weeks.
Clavicle	• Fall on shoulder or outstretched hand.	• Have patient stand or sit upright without back support for observation. • Majority: middle third of bone. • Palpation: tenderness, swelling, deformity, crepitus. • Inspection: shoulder drops downward, forward, inward. May be tenting around skin.	*Adult:* • Conservative: sling, clavicle strap, soft immobilizer. - In cases where no reduction is required, some patients require soft immobilizer while others need only a sling for support. - Closed reduction followed by immobilization in a soft immobilizer. • Surgical: open reduction is generally avoided unless necessary because surgery increases the incidence of nonunion. Surgery is indicated when the bone is considerably fragmented or when underlying soft tissues must be repaired or explored for damage. *Child:* • Conservative: sling.	*Adult/Child:* Clavicle fractures heal rapidly but it is difficult to maintain immobility during early stages of healing. 3-6 weeks.
Sterno-clavicular joint	• Fall on shoulder or outstretched hand.	• Posterior dislocation move clavicle retrosternally. • Inspection: - Bleeding in area around neck. - Swelling. - Difficulty breathing. - Changes in vital signs.	*Adult:* • Conservative: - Sandbag between scapula will pull medial end out of retrosternal area. - Clavicle strap. • Surgical: internal fixation.	*Adult:* 6-10 weeks. *Child:* 3-4 weeks.
Shoulder dislocation	• Fall on outstretched hand. • Common sport-related injury. • Loose-jointed children can voluntarily dislocate by suppressing the activity of one muscle group.	• Most are anterior. • Inspection: - Position of limb: held in abduction and external rotation. - Swelling: bulge over anterior aspect of shoulder. • Severity of pain and muscle spasm. • Mobility: unable to touch opposite shoulder. Cannot abduct beyond 90 degrees. • Neurovascular assessment.	*Adult/Child* • Conservative: - Reduction with analgesia, conscious sedation, or muscle relaxant if seen shortly after injury. - Reduction under anesthesia if treatment delayed. - Postreduction: sling and swathe, shoulder immolbilizer.	*Adult/Child:* At least 2 weeks.

Table 14.2 (continued)
Common Fractures/Dislocations

Fracture/ Dislocation	Mechanism of Injury	Assessment	Treatment	Approximate Healing Time
Proximal humeral fracture	• Fall on outstretched hand or elbow. • Direct blow.	• Cut away clothing for assessment and treatment: movement may be painful and the motion of bone fragments harmful to soft tissues. • Inspection: local swelling, tenderness, upper third of arm. • Mobility: loss of motion of internal rotation and abduction. • Assess for nerve involvement: axillary, median, radial, ulnar. • Pain. • Crepitus. • Arterial involvement with direct blow. • Neurovascular assessment.	Approximately 85% of proximal humeral fractures are nondisplaced or minimally displaced and are treated conservatively. • Conservative treatment in *adults*: - Few weeks of rest. - Sling and swathe. - Closed reduction may be needed. - Hanging cast. - Program of exercises post-healing. • Surgical treatment: displaced fracture. - Open reduction and internal fixation. • Conservative treatment in *children*: - Sling. - Splint. - Sling and swathe. - Hanging cast should not be used in children under 12 years old.	*Adult:* 4-10 weeks. *Child:* 3-4 weeks.
Supracondylar fracture	• Fall on extended or flexed elbow.	• Injury is obvious, usually displaced. • Vascular and nerve involvement common at injury site. • Neurovascular assessment — displacement may cause compartment syndrome.	*Adult:* • Conservative: closed reduction with casting, posterior splint, and sling. • Surgical: open reduction or percutaneous pinning if fracture unstable. *Child:* • Conservative: closed reduction with casting, posterior splint and sling. • Surgical: percutaneous pinning if displaced.	*Adult/Child:* 4-8 weeks.
Elbow injuries	• Occur more commonly in elderly or children.		Although treatment modalities may vary for differing elbow fractures, the one treatment held in common in all immobilization approaches is prevention of extension contractures by keeping the elbow in at least some degree of flexion during healing. Early motion to prevent contractures.	

Table 14.2 (continued)
Common Fractures/Dislocations

Fracture/ Dislocation	Mechanism of Injury	Assessment	Treatment	Approximate Healing Time
Olecranon fracture	• Direct blow or fall.	• Pain, swelling. • Inability to extend elbow. • Neurovascular assessment.	*Adult:* • Conservative: aspiration of hemarthrosis, sling, traction (skin or skeletal). • Surgical: - Closed reduction with cast from shoulder to wrist, 45-90 degrees flexion. - Open reduction, screw fixation, wiring. *Child:* • Conservative: aspiration of hemarthrosis, sling, traction (skin or skeletal). • Surgical: - Closed reduction with cast. - Closed reduction. Percutaneous wire fixation.	*Adult:* 7-12 weeks. *Child:* 4-6 weeks.
Elbow dislocation	• Fall on outstretched hand with elbow extended • *Children:* Pull on arm can dislocate.	• Apparent early deformity. • Late swelling may mask deformity. • Neurovascular assessment.	*Adult:* • Closed reduction under anesthesia. • Posterior splint and sling or cast. *Child:* • Reduce immediately by supinating and flexing the elbow.	*Adult:* 4-6 weeks. Start gentle ROM after 2 weeks. *Child:* Begin motion in couple of days.
Radius, ulna fractures	• Direct trauma. • Fall on outstretched hand. • Forearm fractures of ulna alone are rare.	• Localized swelling and tenderness. • In adults, often accompanied by significant swelling. • Limitation in ROM: painful pronation-supination. • Neurovascular assessment.	• Nondisplaced: casting, posterior splint for 1-2 weeks followed by a sling and active movement of elbow started. • Displaced: open reduction and internal fixation.	*Adult:* 12 weeks. *Child:* 6-8 weeks.
Colles' fracture	• Fall on outstretched hand.	• Wrist appears puffy and deformed. • Hump deformity seen when wrist is viewed from side. • Neurovascular assessment.	• Nondisplaced: forearm splint or cast, pressure dressing. • Displaced: manual traction, plaster cast, percutaneous pinning, or external fixation.	*Adult:* 4-8 weeks.
Hand fracture	(See Chapter 17, Hand)			
Sternum	• Direct trauma to chest. • Usually motor vehicle accident.	• Swelling over sternum. • Tenderness or pain. • Sternal and rib fractures may cause flail chest: observe for paradoxical breathing. • Evaluate for cardiac and lung contusion.	• Conservative: analgesics.	*Adult:* 6-8 weeks. *Child:* 3-4 weeks.

Table 14.2 (continued)
Common Fractures/Dislocations

Fracture/ Dislocation	Mechanism of Injury	Assessment	Treatment	Approximate Healing Time
Rib	• Direct or indirect trauma to chest usually by blows, crushing injuries, or strains caused by coughing or sneezing. • The fifth to ninth ribs most frequently involved.	• Pain or tenderness to touch. • Respiratory evaluation for shallow respirations and protective guarding. • Subcutaneous emphysema/ crepitations.	• Analgesics. • Pulmonary toileting to prevent respiratory complications. • Severe: regional nerve block for pain relief.	*Adult:* 6-8 weeks. *Child:* 3-4 weeks.
Pelvis	Severe trauma as with motor vehicle crashes, falls from great heights, and crushing injuries.	• Assess for shock: hemorrhagic • Local pain, swelling, tenderness, and crepitus. • Neurovascular assessment. • Assess peripheral pulses: absence of peripheral pulses may indicate a tear in the iliac or femoral artery. • Severe back pain may indicate retroperitoneal bleed. • Ongoing assessment for injuries to bladder, rectum, intestines, and intra-abdominal organs. • Stable fracture: unilateral fracture of superior and inferior pubic rami, single fracture of iliac ring. • Unstable fracture: bilateral or unilateral fracture of the superior and inferior pubic rami and the sacroiliac joint or sacrum, or a fracture or dislocation of sacroiliac joint or sacrum and symphysis pubis-hip deformity present.	• Emergent: external fixation for open book fracture, may be life saving. • Conservative: bed rest until comfortable ambulation with guarded weight bearing • Surgical: open reduction internal fixation; external fixation. • Stable fracture: bed rest several days then progressive ambulation; analgesics. • Unstable fracture: external fixation alone or combined with ORIF (posterior); or ORIF (anterior and/or posterior). • Skeletal traction if patient unable to tolerate surgery.	*Adult:* *6-12 weeks.* *Child:* Assess 6-8 weeks.
Hip fracture	*Adult:* *Femoral Neck:* • Trivial or minor injuries. • Fall: direct blow over greater trochanter. • Lateral rotation injury-head firmly fixed in acetabulum, neck rotates posteriorly, gets caught in acetabulum, and buckles.	• Neurovascular check distal to injury. • Femoral neck: impacted. - Slight pain in groin or along medial side of knee. - Antalgic gait. - Discomfort on ROM. - Muscle spasm: extremes of motion. - May have marked valgus.	• Internal fixation with multiple percutaneous pins: followed by early ambulation with weight bearing as tolerated. • Prosthetic replacement: followed by early ambulation, weight bearing as tolerated. • Open reduction with internal fixation (nails, plates screws), ambulation with weight bearing as tolerated.	*Adult:* 3-6 months.

Table 14.2 (continued)
Common Fractures/Dislocations

Fracture/ Dislocation	Mechanism of Injury	Assessment	Treatment	Approximate Healing Time
Hip fracture (continued)	• Osteoporosis. *Intertrochanteric:* • Fall involving direct and indirect forces to greater trochanter. • Metastatic disease.	Femoral neck: displaced. • Extreme pain in hip region. • Leg externally rotated, abducted, and shortened. • Patient at risk for disruption of blood supply and avascular necrosis. • Marked shortening. • 90 degrees external rotation. • Swelling in hip region, ecchymosis over greater trochanter, risk for great blood loss. • Movement causes groin pain.		
	Child: • Requires great force as with bumper injuries. • Severe trauma: falls from heights, motor vehicle injuries, bicycle accidents.	*Child:* femoral neck. • Pain in hip. • Extremity shortened, externally rotated. *Child:* intratrochanteric. • May only have shortening. • Pain. • External rotation.	• Closed reduction, Knowles pins, screws. • Abduction, hip spica. • Skeletal traction. • Cast.	*Child:* 6-8 weeks.
Hip dislocation	• Considerable force needed. • Anterior: forced abduction and extension. • Posterior: force applied against flexed knee with hip in flexion. • Central: severe blow to lateral hip while in abduction. • Child: under age 5. • Fall: minimal trauma. • Acetabulum largely cartilaginous; soft. • Joint laxity common. • As age increases, so does degree of force required to dislocate.	• Severe pain, especially with movement. • Anterior: thigh extended, abducted externally rotated. • Posterior: thigh flexed, adducted internally rotated, short, possible sciatic nerve injury. • Central: usually with a fracture. • Neurovascular assessment.	*Adult/Child:* • Conservative treatment: - Closed reduction under analgesia, muscle relaxant followed by: a. Anterior: cast/brace to hold leg adducted, internally rotated. b. Posterior: Buck skin traction, hip spica, or brace. *Adult/Child:* • Surgical treatment: - Open reduction under anesthesia when closed does not work followed by hip spica for child. - Central: skeletal traction, or internal fixation.	*Adult:* 2-6 weeks. *Child:* 6 weeks.

Table 14.2 (continued)
Common Fractures/Dislocations

Fracture/ Dislocation	Mechanism of Injury	Assessment	Treatment	Approximate Healing Time
Femur, proximal and distal	• Direct or indirect trauma. • Falls. • Motor vehicle crashes.	• Proximal: external rotation, shortened extremity, acute pain, inability to move leg. • Distal: severe pain, swelling, deformity. • Possible injury to popliteal nerves and vessels; check neurovascular status. • Both have extensive soft tissue damage and considerable blood loss—sometimes severe enough to precipitate shock.	Proximal: • Conservative: skin traction, skeletal traction, cast/cast brace. • Surgical: reduction internal fixation with intramedullary rod. Distal: • Conservative: skeletal traction, cast brace, spica cast. • Surgical: open reduction, internal fixation with intramedullary rod. Note: *children* ages 0-2 years are treated in casts; ages 2-10 years, casting is preferred treatment. Two exceptions: multiple injuries and propensity for extensive shortening.	*Adult:* 8-16 weeks. *Child:* 6-12 weeks.
Patella fracture	• Direct blow or fall, torsional injury. • In older, obese, or poorly conditioned individuals, indirect injury can occur from a bump, descending the stairs, or a forceful squat.	• Pain, swelling, tenderness, effusion. • Frequently are open fractures. • Inability to extend knee. • Audible and painful snap may occur followed by a fall or loss of balance.	*Adult/Child:* • Conservative: ice until swelling subsides. - Without displaced fragments: aspiration of blood, crutches, non-weight bearing, immobilizer to fully extend knee, cast, if unable to prevent flexion. • Surgical: with displacement: open reduction and internal fixation with application on long leg or cylinder cast, or excision.	*Adult/Child:* 4-6 weeks.
Patella dislocation	• Direct blow to medial side. • Severe falls, athletic injuries.	• Knee buckling causing a fall. • Tenderness along medial border. • Severe pain in anterior knee area. • Muscle spasm. • Displaced laterally. • When knee is extended with hips flexed, patella returns to normal position. • May feel "pop" with dislocation and spontaneous reduction. • Patellar instability.	*Adult/Child:* • Conservative: ice, immobilizer, cast (long leg), knee immobilized in extension. • Surgical: if unable to align, repair injured ligaments, knee immobilized in extension.	*Adult/Child:* 6-8 weeks.

Table 14.2 (continued)
Common Fractures/Dislocations

Fracture/ Dislocation	Mechanism of Injury	Assessment	Treatment	Approximate Healing Time
Knee dislocation	• Severe blow with hyper-extension of knee. • Twisting or crushing injury.	• Critical to evaluate and monitor neurovascular status. • Pain on ROM, evaluate for ligament injury. • May be displaced anteriorly, posteriorly, laterally, or medially (anterior most common). • Swelling, effusion, ecchymosis, tenderness. • Puffiness, marked fullness popliteal area could mean popliteal artery injury. • Observe for signs of vascular insufficiency or severe or increasing pain after reduction which may indicate arterial injury.	*Adult/Child:* • Closed reduction with immobilization by cast, knee immobilizer, or posterior splint. • Open reduction to repair soft tissue or vascular damage.	*Adult/Child:* 6-8 weeks.
Tibia, fibula fractures	• Direct trauma to shin area, torsional force, stepping into hole. • Ski boot injury. • Fibula is non-weight bearing bone so fractures of fibula alone are rare. • Fibula fractures often occur in response to ankle fractures. • Open fractures of tibia are more common than any other major bone as much of its surface is just below the skin.	• Usually occurs in both bones. • Angulation/deformity. • Localized pain. • Neurovascular evaluation with attention to signs of compartment syndrome.	*Adult:* • Conservative: - Stable, nondisplaced closed reduction fracture: long leg cast followed by short leg cast. • Surgical: - Comminuted/open: external fixation, open reduction internal fixation, intramedullary (IM) nailing *Child:* • Conservative: long leg cast.	*Adult:* 6-10 weeks.
Ankle fracture	• Inversion/eversion. • Stepping in a hole, walking on uneven surface, platform shoes, skateboards, steps, curbs, inline skating.	• Pain, swelling, ecchymosis, difficulty bearing weight, pain on flexion, extension, rotation. • Ligamentous injury produces same symptoms, fracture is usually accompanied by ligamentous injury. • Neurovascular assessment.	*Adult:* • Conservative: closed reduction, short-leg cast, splint. • Surgical: internal fixation. • Displaced: external fixation. *Child:* • Conservative: long leg cast. • Surgical: open reduction internal fixation may be necessary for Salter: Type III and IV fractures.	*Adult:* 8-12 weeks. *Child:* 4-6 weeks.

Table 14.2 (continued)
Common Fractures/Dislocations

Fracture/ Dislocation	Mechanism of Injury	Assessment	Treatment	Approximate Healing Time
Calcaneus fracture (Don Juan)	• Fall or jump from high place, landing on heels.	• Evaluate for wrist and spine injuries frequently associated with compression fractures, especially T12, L1, L2. • Pain, swelling, ecchymosis. • Heel is broadened. • Hollows beneath malleoli are obliterated. • Movement painful and restricted.	*Adult:* • No reduction - Jones compression dressings. • Reduction: short leg cast. • Non-weight bearing. • If displaced: closed or open reduction with a cast or PRAFO. *Child:* • Bulky dressing.	*Adult:* 6-8 weeks. *Child:* 4 weeks.
Metatarsal fractures	• Direct trauma, crush injury. • Heavy object falls on foot. • Jump or fall on ball of foot.	• Pain, swelling, ecchymosis. • Tenderness on palpation.	• Closed reduction and immobilization in walking short leg cast or hard sole shoe. • Surgical: percutaneous pinning, open reduction with internal fixation.	*Adult:* 4 weeks.
Toe fracture	• Object falling on toe. • Stubbing toe.	• Pain, swelling, ecchymosis. • Tenderness on palpation.	• Tape to adjacent toe to stabilize. • Walking cast or stiff sole shoes may be applied with multiple toe fractures.	*Adult/Child:* 2-4 weeks.
Cervical spine fracture	• Blow to top of head. • Falls landing on head. • Hyperextension - striking head on dashboard. • Hyperflexion - diving in shallow water. • Hyperextension followed by hyperflexion - rear end collision.	• Associate with skull and facial fractures. • Neck pain, tenderness over spinous process. • Neurologic evaluation for paralysis, paresthesia. • Neck pain with motion.	• Immobilize spine, sandbags, or cervical collar. • Spine board. • Tongs and traction, halo body jacket. • Internal fixation/decompression fusion.	*Adult/Child:* 6-8 weeks.
Thoracic lumbar spine fracture	• Acute hyperflexion fall from height, landing on feet or buttocks. • Deceleration forces - seat belt injury.	• Back pain, point tenderness. • Neurologic evaluation to determine deficits: most common in T12, L1, L2. • Observe: ileus; thromboembolic complications.	• Conservative: spine board, firm mattress, logroll, lumbar, thoracic corsets. • Surgical: if unstable fusion, spinal instrumentation. • Decompression	*Adult:* 12-16 weeks. *Child:* 8-16 weeks.

12. Anterior hip dislocations present with the hip held in extension, abduction, and external rotation.

C. Diagnostic tests.

1. X-rays of affected extremity.
2. Often x-ray views of unaffected joint also taken.
3. No arthrogram or ultrasound on infants as bone is not yet visible.
4. Arteriogram or duplex Doppler ultrasound for suspected vascular injuries with knee dislocation.

III. COMMON THERAPEUTIC MODALITIES

A. Shoulder dislocation.

1. Two weeks in a sling if reduction is not necessary.
2. Closed reduction followed by 2-3 weeks of immobilization in Velpeau's bandage, commercial immobilizer, or sling and swathe.
3. Open reduction and internal fixation.

B. Elbow dislocation.

1. Closed reduction under general anesthesia.
2. Sling with gentle range of motion after 2 weeks.

C. Elbow subluxation (nursemaid's elbow).

1. Closed reduction
2. Observe child until arm is used.
3. No immobilization.

D. Wrist dislocation.

1. Closed reduction.
2. Casting varies from 2 weeks to 3 months.
3. Very few wrist dislocations require surgery as long as reduction is completed within 2 weeks of injury.

E. Finger dislocation.

1. Stable dislocations of proximal interphalangeal (PIP) joint and simple dislocation of the metacarpophalangeal (MCP) joint managed with closed reduction and immobilized with dorsal splint in 30 degrees of flexion.
2. Unstable and complex dislocations require surgery followed by splinting in 30 degrees of flexion.

F. Knee dislocation.

1. Closed reduction with gentle, continuous longitudinal traction.
2. Immobilization with a posterior splint in 15 degrees of flexion to avoid tension on the popliteal artery.
3. External fixation if vascular repair is done.

G. Hip dislocation.

1. Posterior dislocation.
   a. Immediate closed reduction to prevent avascular necrosis.
   b. Traction, hip abduction brace, or hip spica with leg in extension, abduction, and external rotation.
   c. Traction with leg in extension for a few days, then ambulatory with crutches and partial weight bearing.
   d. May require open reduction and internal fixation if associated with a fracture or unable to reduce.
2. Anterior dislocation.
   a. Immediate closed reduction to prevent avascular necrosis.
   b. Hip brace or spica cast with leg in flexion, adduction, and internal rotation.
   c. Traction with leg in extension for a few days, then ambulatory with crutches and partial weight bearing.
3. Central fracture dislocation.
   a. Skeletal traction or external fixation for 10-12 weeks.
   b. Open reduction and internal fixation.

IV. NURSING DIAGNOSES, OUTCOMES, AND INTERVENTIONS

A. See Table 14.3.

B. Peripheral neurovascular dysfunction, risk for. Injury, risk for. Tissue perfusion, ineffective; peripheral.

1. Outcomes.
   a. Neurovascular status remains intact.
   b. Joint function restored.
2. Interventions.
   a. Do frequent neurovascular assessment of the soft tissues distal to the injured joint.
   b. The patient should not attempt to move the affected joint.
   c. The extremity must always be supported and the injured area immobilized until diagnosed and treated by a physician.
   d. Teach patient how to protect the affected joint while carrying out ADL.

C. Physical mobility, impaired.

1. Outcome: joint mobility is within normal limits.
2. Interventions.
   a. When ordered, provide passive exercises, as needed, and teach and encourage active exercises when the patient is ready.
   b. Uninjured joints should be actively exercised throughout the healing period, particularly in older patients, so that no loss of function occurs in other joints while the patient awaits healing in the injured area.

V. HOME CARE CONSIDERATIONS

A. Discuss with patient the potential for recurrence of the injury.

B. In young, athletic patients with a high incidence of recurrence of shoulder dislocations, teach which types of movements and activities should be avoided.

FRACTURES

I. OVERVIEW

A. Definition: a break or disruption in the continuity of the bone.

B. Classifications: description is based on physical examination and review of radiographs.

1. Complete: break across the entire section of the bone, dividing it into distinct fragments, frequently displaced (removed from normal position).
2. Incomplete: break occurs only through one cortex.
   a. Greenstick (hickory stick or willow) incomplete fracture with intact side of the cortex flexed. Usually seen in children.

Table 14.3
Common Nursing Diagnoses, Outcomes, Goals, and Interventions for Trauma Patients

Diagnoses	Outcomes	Goals and Interventions
A. Pain, acute	• Patient has decreased pain or pain relief.	• Promote comfort. 1. Assess pain; provide pain relief modalities and evaluate effectiveness. a. Medications: PCA may be desirable for patient with multiple trauma or extensive surgery. b. Positioning: elevation of extremities. c. Relieve areas of undue pressure. 2. Teach relaxation techniques. 3. See Chapter 7, Pain. 4. See Chapter 5, Perioperative Patient Care.
B. Tissue perfusion ineffective: peripheral; fluid volume, deficient	• Patient's circulation is intact; tissue perfusion is adequate	• Promote circulation. 1. Monitor cardiovascular status. 2. Position for optimum peripheral circulation. 3. Elevate extremities. 4. Teach exercises to provide peripheral circulation. 5. Assess for signs of shock: decreased blood pressure, tachycardia, cool clammy skin, decreased urinary output, frank hemorrhage, anxiety, decreased sensorium. Blood loss associated with major fractures is typically 1-3 units for the tibia or fibula, 3-6 units for the femur, and 3-8 units for the pelvis. 6. Monitor intake and output. 7. Relieve pressure caused by tight bandages, casts, or other constricting devices. 8. Monitor for signs of compartment syndrome (see Chapter 8, Complications).
C. Nutrition, imbalanced: less than daily requirement.	• Patient's nutritional needs are met.	• Promote nutrition. 1. Administer intravenous fluids, as ordered. 2. Monitor calcium, vitamin A, D, and C intake. Calcium is needed for bone repair. Vitamin C is vital for bone repair and tissue healing. Vitamin D helps in absorption of needed calcium and plays a part in remodeling of bone. Adequate vitamin A can shorten healing period. 3. Evaluate need for high protein, high carbohydrate diet and supplements: trauma places patient at risk for protein calorie malnutrition.

Table 14.3 (continued)
Common Nursing Diagnoses, Outcomes, Goals, and Interventions for Trauma Patients

Diagnoses	Outcomes	Goals and Interventions
C. Nutrition, altered: less than daily requirement. (continued)	• Patient's nutritional needs are met. (continued)	4. Assess abdomen to determine the presence of bowel sounds, distention, and rule out ileus.
D. Constipation	•Patient has normal or established pattern of bowel elimination.	• Monitor for signs and symptoms of constipation/impaction. 1. Assess for abdominal distention, cramping, flatus. 2. Encourage mobility as per orders to prevent immobility-related constipation. 3. Monitor narcotic administration in relation to side effect of constipation. 4. Assess patient for impaction, as needed. 5. Administer stool softeners, laxatives, enemas, as ordered. 6. Encourage fluids, juices, fruits, and diet with adequate fiber content.
E. Urinary elimination, impaired	• Patient maintains adequate urinary output.	• Monitor urinary output. 1. Maintain urinary output of at least 30 cc per hour. 2. Observe for signs of bladder dysfunction: incontinence, bladder overflow, frequency: risk for urinary dysfunction with pelvic injuries and hip fractures. 3. Assist male patients to stand to void. 4. Position comfortably for use of bed pan. 5. Catheterize under sterile conditions, as needed.
F. Tissue perfusion, ineffective Gas exchange, impaired	Patient exhibits adequate oxygenation; lungs are clear; free from pulmonary and fat emboli.	• Assure adequate oxygenation of tissues. • Maintain adequate pulmonary function. 1. Monitor respiratory status. 2. Position for adequate lung expansion. 3. Adjust bandages/supports that may restrict lung expansion. 4. Teach to turn, cough, and deep breathe frequently. 5 Assess for signs of pulmonary embolism, fat embolism. a. High incidence in long bone fractures, pelvic fractures, and immobilized patients.

Table 14.3 (continued)
Common Nursing Diagnoses, Outcomes, Goals, and Interventions for Trauma Patients

<table>
<tr><th>Diagnoses</th><th>Outcomes</th><th>Goals and Interventions</th></tr>
<tr><td>F. Tissue perfusion, ineffective Gas exchange, impaired (continued)</td><td>• Patient exhibits adequate oxygenation; lungs are clear; free from pulmonary and fat emboli. (continued)</td><td>b. Observe for chest pain, dyspnea, sudden disorientation, tachycardia, and petechiae over chest and axillae, as well as in the conjunctival sac and buccal cavity.
6. Provide respiratory support, as needed, for pulmonary emboli.</td></tr>
<tr><td>G. Skin integrity, impaired peripheral neurovascular dysfunction, risk for</td><td>• Patient is free of skin breakdown; no signs of neurovascular deficit.</td><td>• Prevent loss of skin, tissue, and neurovascular integrity.
1. Skin/tissue.
a. Reposition frequently.
b. Pad pressure areas; keep heels off bed.
c. Keep skin dry and intact.
d. Use lotions/alcohol to keep skin soft and tough.
e. Monitor abrasions/ lacerations for areas of progressive breakdown.
f. Monitor areas of tissue loss for further necrosis and infection. No burning under cast/splint.
g. Help keep fracture fragments immobilized, as needed, for healing.
2. Neurovascular.
a. Assess neurovascular status of extremities.
b. Provide for elevation of extremities to the level of the heart.
c. Monitor progression of deficit and report to physician.</td></tr>
<tr><td>H. Infection, risk for</td><td>• Patient is free of infection.</td><td>• Protect against infection in the absence of an intact first line of defense against infection.
1. Cover open areas with sterile barrier, such as a gauze pad or transparent dressing.
2. Cleanse open areas only with sterile technique.
3. Provide routine sterile pin care, IV site care, surgical wound and decubitus care.
4. Administer antibiotics.</td></tr>
<tr><td>I. Physical mobility, impaired</td><td>• Patient is free of complications of immobility; bone integrity, muscle strength is restored. Maximum mobility is achieved.</td><td>• Promote function/mobility.
1. Monitor activity level; prevent fatigue.
2. Assist with ambulation and the use of required devices.</td></tr>
</table>

Table 14.3 (continued)
Common Nursing Diagnoses, Outcomes, Goals, and Interventions for Trauma Patients

Diagnoses	Outcomes	Goals and Interventions
I. Physical mobility, impaired (continued)	• Patient is free of complications of immobility; bone integrity, muscle strength is restored. Maximum mobility is achieved. (continued)	3. Maintain slings, bandages, splints, or other supports to provide stability/immobilization with ambulation. 4. Assure the patient that function can be returned in the shortest time possible if movement of the fracture site and further injury are prevented until adequate healing has occurred. 5. Teach and encourage exercises, as indicated. Active exercises to uninjured parts. 6. Monitor ability to move injured part(s). 7. Elevate injured area when possible. 8. Apply ice for first 24-28 hours. 9. Administer analgesics to decrease pain of movement. 10. See Chapter 6, Effects of Immobility.
J. Self-care deficit syndrome; home maintenance, impaired	• Patient participates in self-care treatment, and rehabilitation program. Patient returns to full activity and former lifestyle.	• Assist patient to attain optimal level of independence. 1. Assess level of disability and dependence. 2. Collaborate with patient concerning realistic means of contributing to own care. 3. Teach significant others to help the patient regain and maintain optimum independence. 4. Arrange the environment to promote independence in use of materials needed for activities of daily living. 5. Supply special equipment (prism glasses, flexible straws), that enables patient to help him/herself.
K. Self-concept, disturbed	• Patient's positive self-concept and self-esteem are restored.	• Promote positive self-concept. 1. Emphasize remaining skills and strengths: abilities in contrast to disabilities. 2. Provide realistic, yet optimistic feedback concerning functional ability. 3. Allow patient as much control as possible over self-care. 4. Focus on patient as a whole and not just affected part.

Table 14.3 (continued)
Common Nursing Diagnoses, Outcomes, Goals, and Interventions for Trauma Patients

Diagnoses	Outcomes	Goals and Interventions
L. Anxiety; knowledge, deficient	• Patient verbalizes decreased anxiety; Demonstrates knowledge of treatment plan, modified lifestyle; and potential complications.	• Assist in allaying anxiety. 1. Observe for emotional response to injury. 2. Assess degree of anxiety. 3. Provide explanation of treatment. 4. Remain with patient during periods of stress. 5. Serve as a support person for patient; assess patient's support systems. 6. Teach relaxation methods. 7. Evaluate knowledge deficit. a. Determine patient's understanding of fracture and treatment plan. b. Teach patient cast care, use of assistive devices, ambulation techniques, safety hazards in the environment.
M. Diversional activity, deficient	• Patient participates in recreational activities.	• Provide activities to decrease boredom. 1. Assess patient's ability to participate in diversional activities. 2. Select diversional activities according to patient's age, interests, and abilities. 3. See Chapter 10, Therapeutic Modalities. 4. See Chapter 5, Perioperative Patient Care.

b. Partial/fissure fracture occurs in inflexible bone. There is no distinct fragment to be displaced. Usually occurs in adults.

3. Open (compound): bone is broken and external wound leads to fracture site.
   a. Grade I.
      (1) Skin is punctured
      (2) Minimal soft tissue injury and contamination.
      (3) Intact vascular status.
   b. Grade II.
      (1) Accompanied by skin and muscle contusion.
      (2) Moderate wound contamination.
      (3) Comminuted bone fragments.
   c. Grade III.
      (1) Extensive soft tissue damage involving skin, muscles, blood vessels, and nerves.
      (2) Usually associated with massive contamination.
4. Closed (simple): fracture fragments do not extend through mucous membrane or skin.
5. Displaced: fragments malaligned at fracture site.
6. Nondisplaced: fragments aligned at fracture site.
7. Impacted: telescoped, one fragment is driven into the other.
8. Avulsion: separation of a small fragment of bone at the site of attachment of a ligament or tendon.
9. Compression: unusual force applied to bone, causing it to buckle and eventually crack (example: compression fractures of vertebrae).
10. Buckle: impaction injury in childhood. Primarily affecting the developing metaphyseal bone, causing the bone to bulge or bend.
11. Fatigue/stress (March): fracture occurring from repetitive minor stress (metatarsal fractures from marching).
12. Pathologic (spontaneous): fracture occurs with minimal trauma after a pathologic process has weakened the bone.
13. Articular: fracture involves a joint surface.
14. Intracapsular: fracture occurs within joint capsule.
15. Extracapsular: fracture occurs outside joint capsule.

16. Longitudinal: fracture line runs in the direction of the bone's longitudinal axis.
17. Transverse: fracture line runs at approximately a 90-degree angle to the longitudinal axis.
18. Oblique: fracture line is about a 45-degree angle across the longitudinal axis.
19. Spiral: fracture line twists around the bone shaft.
20. Comminuted: more than one fracture line and more than two bone fragments. Fragments may be shattered or crushed.
21. Stellate: fracture lines radiate from one central fracture point.
22. Specific by anatomic location for specific type. Examples:
    a. Colles': fracture within the last inch of the distal radius in which the distal fragment is displaced in a position of dorsal and radial deviation.
    b. Transcondylar: fracture occurs at or close to the condyles of the humerus and partially within the capsule.

C. Etiology.

1. Fractures occur when bone is subjected to more stress than it can absorb.
2. Trauma may be applied by direct force, such as when a moving object directly contacts the area over a bone.
3. Trauma may be applied by an indirect force, such as when a powerful muscle contraction exerts a pulling force on the bone.
4. The amount of trauma required to cause a fracture may vary considerably, depending upon biologic and behavioral factors which may predispose an individual to fracturing.
5. Sternal fractures are usually caused by auto accidents.
6. Rib fractures can occur from direct or indirect trauma.
    a. The fifth to ninth ribs are usually involved.
    b. Rib fractures are very serious in children because it takes tremendous force to fracture their flexible bones.
    c. Underlying organ damage should always be assumed.
7. Most fractures of the upper extremities are caused by either a direct blow or fall onto an outstretched arm or hand.
8. Pelvic fractures are caused by motor vehicle crashes (as a passenger or pedestrian), falls from great heights, and crush injuries.
9. Proximal femur "hip" fractures occur most often in elderly females with osteoporosis and may or may not be associated with a fall.
10. Femoral shaft fractures usually result from tremendous forces (trauma from motor vehicle crashes, gun shot wounds [GSW]).
11. Patellar fractures are frequently associated with compact car motor vehicle crashes, where the knees are subjected to impact on collision; there may be an associated hip fracture and posterior dislocation of the head of the femur.
12. Fractures of the tibia and ankle are most commonly associated with twisting motion, as seen in sports and falls.

D. Predisposing factors.

1. Biologic factors include conditions that alter composition and strength of the bone so that it may be fractured with very little trauma.
    a. Cushing's syndrome.
    b. Neoplasms.
    c. Osteogenesis imperfecta.
    d. Hormonal changes as a result of cortisone therapy or reduction of normal estrogen levels following menopause.
    e. Osteoporosis.
    f. Altered states of health (malnutrition, anorexia).
2. Fractures can occur in healthy bones due to trauma related to behavioral factors, such as curiosity, risk taking.
3. Child or elder abuse also may be a factor in fractures of the very young or the aged.

E. Bone healing.

1. The integrity of the vascular system is interrupted with a fracture.
    a. Small blood vessels normally traversing the bone, periosteum, and adjacent soft tissues are torn and hemorrhage into the fracture site and surrounding tissue, forming a blood clot or hematoma.
    b. Tearing of blood vessels interrupts the blood supply to the Haversian system in cortical bone, creating a zone of necrotic bone distal to the fracture site.
2. Shortly after fracture, reparative cells begin to proliferate and migrate toward the site of injury, laying down a fibrous matrix of collagen (3 days-2 weeks). These cells include:
    a. Fibroblasts in the outer layer of the periosteum and perhaps in nearby connective tissue.
    b. Osteoblasts in the cambium layer of the periosteum.
    c. Similar cells within the bony surface of the marrow cavity.
3. At this time, the needed blood supply is derived mainly from:
    a. Medullary circulation in uncomplicated fractures.
    b. A temporary ingrowth of vascular buds from surrounding soft tissues in complicated fractures.
4. Within several days, as a result of this cellular and vascular proliferation, the fracture site is surrounded by a newly formed, highly vascularized tissue termed a "callus" (2- 6 weeks).
5. The advancing callus pushes the hematoma ahead of it, moving it into the marrow or nearby tissue where it can be broken down and removed by fibrinolysis and phagocytosis.
6. As healing progresses (3 weeks-6 months):
    a. The callus is converted into a loosely woven network of bone, cartilage, and fibrous tissue, which bridges the fracture site.
    b. Debris is removed by phagocytosis, and necrotic bone is resorbed.

c. Callus is gradually replaced by bone.
7. The final steps in healing consist of consolidation and remodeling, which ideally, result in bone healing so completely that it is difficult to identify the original fracture site (6 weeks-1 year).

F. Incidence.

1. Although any bone may be fractured at any age, the incidence varies according to the bone involved.
2. Commonly seen fractures in children.
   a. Clavicle most frequently fractured.
   b. Epicondyle fractures.
   c. Epiphyseal fractures.
   d. Buckle fractures.
   e. Corner and bucket-handle epiphyseal-metaphyseal fractures are seen in victims of physical abuse.
3. Commonly seen fractures in adults.
   a. Femoral shaft fractures occur most often in young or middle-aged adults.
   b. Pelvic fractures occur predominantly in adults.
   c. Fractures of the shaft of the humerus are more common in adults than in children. The older the patient, the more proximal the humeral fracture tends to be.
4. Commonly seen fractures in the elderly.
   a. Proximal femur fractures occur most often in the elderly.
   b. Compression fractures of spine.
   c. Colles' fractures.

G. Considerations across the lifespan.

1. Fractures can occur at any age including in utero although this is rare due to protection by amniotic fluid.
2. Children are skeletally immature.
   a. Most fractures can be treated with closed reduction and casting. The most common exceptions are:
      (1) Fractures of the elbow (supra condylar, epicondylar, and lateral condyle), which frequently require percutaneous pinning.
      (2) Fractures of the proximal femur, requiring open reduction and internal fixation, especially if growth plate is involved.
   b. Injuries to the growth plate in children can result in complications of:
      (1) Limb-length discrepancy.
      (2) Joint incongruity.
      (3) Angular deformities.
      (4) Permanent damage to the growth plate will produce shortening and often progressive angular deformity. Follow-up through skeletal maturity is important for assessment and appropriate intervention.
   c. Fractures through the shaft of a long bone stimulate growth. This is probably due to increased nutrition to the growth cartilage caused by the hyperemia associated with fracture healing. To avoid limb-length discrepancy due to overgrowth, the fracture ends may be set in an overlapping fashion rather than end-to-end in children less than 8 years old.
   d. Immature bone has a thicker periosteum than mature bone, results in less fracture displacement, and tends to increase fracture stability.
   e. Children's bones heal quickly and nonunions rarely occurs; therefore, reduction should be secured early.
   f. Children's bones, which are still growing, have a greater potential to remodel than adults.
   g. Joint stiffness, in most situations, is less of a problem than with immobilized adults and therefore is less of a consideration in the decision to mobilize the extremity.
   h. Children with fractures cannot always be trusted to limit their activities as instructed.
      (1) If there is no pain, the child may return to full activity before the fracture is healed.
      (2) Immobilization should be continued until this risk is past.
   i. Refractures occur in children when the cast is removed too soon and when the fracture has healed with deformity and becomes a stress concentrator.
3. Elderly.
   a. Compression fractures and Colles' fractures are common in patients with osteoporosis.
   b. Osteoporotic bone heals more slowly.
   c. Refractures happen often in this population.
   d. Pathologic fractures may precede an elder's fall.

H. Complications.

1. Impaired mobility.
2. Impaired function.
3. Loss of limb.
4. Neurovascular impairment.
5. Nonunion.
6. Malunion.
7. Limb-length discrepancy; occurs more commonly in children.
8. Post-traumatic arthritis.
9. Infection: osteomyelitis.
10. Skin breakdown under splints/casts.
11. Tetanus/gas gangrene with open fractures.
12. Compartment syndrome.

II. ASSESSMENT

A. History and physical examination.

1. Signs and symptoms can vary considerably, depending upon the site of fracture, the type of fracture, and the amount of trauma that has been sustained by the bone and the surrounding tissue.
2. Mechanism of injury and symptoms experienced.
3. The patient may complain of having experienced acute pain at the time of injury followed by point tenderness.
4. Uncomfortable muscle spasms, increased pain on movement or the application of pressure, or sensations indicative of nerve involvement, such as numbness, tingling, or paralysis.
5. Swelling at the fracture site.
6. Change in the length, shape, alignment, stability, or mobility of the bone.

7. Ecchymosis due to bleeding at the site of injury.
8. Crepitus due to inadvertent movement of bone fragments.
9. Muscle spasm and edema as physiologic response to injury.
10. See Table 14.2.

B. Diagnostic tests.

1. X-rays.
   a. Plain films.
   b. CT scan.
   c. Tomography.
   d. MRI.
   e. Bone scan.
2. Arthroscopy in joint injuries.
3. Laboratory studies.
   a. Urine for occult blood (myoglobinuria).
   b. CBC.
   c. Enzymes.
   d. Pathologic fractures may require additional tests for diagnostic purposes (see Chapter 15, Tumors).

III. COMMON THERAPEUTIC MODALITIES

A. Initial immobilization of injured area.

1. Splints.
2. Bandages.
3. Supportive devices.

B. Closed reduction. Alignment of bone fragments by manual manipulation or traction without surgical intervention. Anesthesia, usually local or conscious sedation, may be used. General anesthesia may be used in some children.

C. Open reduction. Alignment of bone fragments by surgical intervention.

D. Internal fixation. Immobilization of fracture site during surgery with pins, wires, screws, rods, nails, or other types of hardware applied during surgical procedure (usually open reduction). Pins or rods may be inserted percutaneously.

E. Immobilization through use of casts, traction (skin or skeletal), external fixation, splints, supports, or internal fixation. More than one method may be used.

F. Various combinations of the above methods may be used in fracture management.

G. Antibiotics and debridement for open fractures.

H. See Table 14.2.

IV. NURSING DIAGNOSES, OUTCOMES, AND INTERVENTIONS (See Table 14.3)

V. HOME CARE CONSIDERATIONS

A. Maintain joint mobility of all unaffected extremities.

B. Pin site care.

C. Follow prescribed activity program.

D. Avoid safety hazards in the environment.

E. Report unusual symptomatology, such as pain, swelling, changes in neurovascular status, elevation in temperature, drainage, burning (symptom of pressure area under a cast).

SPINAL FRACTURES

I. OVERVIEW

A. Definition/pathophysiology. Best defined by identifying type of injury causing the spinal fracture(s).

1. Flexion.
   a. Posterior ligaments remain intact and cause wedge compression fractures in minor injuries.
   b. Severe injuries are associated with posterior ligament injury and considered unstable.
   c. Spinous processes are separated and kyphotic angulation is noted.
   d. Occurs most often in cervical and lumbar spine.
2. Axial loading.
   a. Also known as burst fractures.
   b. Spinous process is not separated.
   c. Anterior and posterior ligaments are usually intact.
   d. If the fracture fragment causes impingement on the spinal canal, it may cause quadriplegia if the fracture is located in the cervical spine or paraplegia if the fracture is located in the lumbar spine.
   e. If it is not a comminuted fracture, it may be stable.
3. Flexion/rotation.
   a. Fracture dislocation of spine.
   b. Posterior ligament is stretched or torn.
   c. Spinous process separation occurs.
   d. Articular process dislocation and fracture.
   e. Usually associated with paraplegia.
   f. Unstable when located in the thoracic and lumbar spine.
4. Extension
   a. Rare injury.
   b. Most common in cervical spine.
   c. Posterior ligaments intact.
   d. Stable.

B. Etiology.

1. Traumatic origin.
   a. Diving accidents.
   b. Motor vehicle crashes.
   c. Falls or blows to the head.
   d. Falls in a sitting position (race car drivers and pilots who may use ejection seats).
2. Nontraumatic origin.
   a. Osteoporosis.
   b. Multiple myeloma.
   c. Bone cancer: sarcomas, primary and metastatic lesions.

C. Incidence.

1. All ages.
2. Compression fractures most common in midlumbar region.
3. Most frequent compression fracture in thoracic spine is a wedge-type.
4. Most compression fractures are stable.

D. Considerations across the lifespan.

1. Vertebral fractures are more common in adults. In children, the spine is more mobile, and the force is dissipated more easily and over a greater number of segments.
2. Major causes of paraplegia in children and young adults:
   a. Motor vehicle crashes.
   b. Under 2 years of age: child abuse.
   c. Older adolescents: sports such as diving, surfing, and skiing.
3. Osteoporosis is the most common cause of compression fractures in the elderly.

E. Complications.
1. Progressive deformity due to displacement.
2. Pain.
3. Loss of bowel and bladder control.
4. Paraplegia.
5. Quadriplegia.
6. Ileus.
7. Superior mesenteric artery syndrome from TLSO or cast.

II. ASSESSMENT

A. History.
1. Mechanism of injury.
2. Progression of symptoms.
   a. Sensation of extremities.
   b. Motion of extremities.
   c. Level of consciousness.
3. Description of pain.
   a. Severity.
   b. Radiation.
   c. Exacerbated with motion, weight, breathing.
   d. Referred to intercostal space or abdomen.

B. Physical examination.
1. Respiratory function.
2. Position of body: assume cervical injury until x-ray results are available.
3. Neurologic assessment including anal sphincter.
4. Abdominal exam: presence of bowel, bladder function.
   a. Tenderness and/or rigidity.
   b. Distention.
5. Associated injuries, bruising, and lacerations of head are often associated with C-spine fractures.

C. Diagnostic tests.
1. Radiology.
   a. AP and lateral radiographs of entire spine.
   b. CT scan.
   c. MRI.
   d. Tomograms.
   e. Myelogram.
2. Laboratory.
   a. Hemoglobin and hematocrit.
   b. Baseline total protein.
   c. Urea nitrogen.
   d. Blood gases.
   e. Urinalysis.
      (1) Blood; protein.
      (2) Measurement of output.

III. COMMON THERAPEUTIC MODALITIES

A. Nonsurgical treatment: fractures.
1. Cervical: skeletal traction.
   a. Halo apparatus.
   b. Cranial tongs.
   c. Rigid cervical collar/brace.
   d. Cast (Minerva jacket).
2. Thoracic.
   a. Body cast.
   b. Thoracolumbarsacral orthosis (TLSO) until fracture is healed.
   c. Bed rest – logroll.
   d. Progressive mobilization.
   e. Avoidance of sitting.
3. Lumbar.
   a. Bed rest until comfortable.
   b. Lumbar corset/brace.

B. Surgical treatment: unstable fractures. Open reduction internal fixation (ORIF).
1. Decompression fusion.
2. Spinal instrumentation.

IV. NURSING DIAGNOSES, OUTCOMES, AND INTERVENTIONS

A. See Table 14.3.

B. Tissue perfusion, ineffective: spinal.
1. Outcome: proper position maintained.
2. Interventions.
   a. Monitor neurovascular status. Assess neurovascular status of trunk and extremities.
   b. Maintain proper positioning.
      (1) Protect head and spine from excessive flexion and extension.
      (2) Provide immobilization of cervical spine until treatment is initiated.
      (3) Use special turning devices or logroll patients when turning.
      (4) Provide corset/support as needed.
      (5) Infants' and toddlers' heads are of disproportionate size to their bodies. Shoulders/trunk should be elevated with a towel or the neck will be in flexion on a regular back board.

C. Physical mobility, impaired.
Self-care deficit syndrome: bathing/hygiene, feeding/dressing/grooming, toileting.
1. Outcome: patient adjusts to a modified or changed lifestyle.
2. Interventions.
   a. Discuss ways of performing ADL (dressing, hygiene, toileting).
   b. Discuss changes or modifications that may be needed in home environment.
   c. Explore potential need for change in occupation.

D. Role performance, ineffective.
1. Outcome: concerns regarding role disruption/alteration are discussed.
2. Interventions: explore concerns regarding changes

in role.

a. Role performance.
b. Role reversal.
c. Independence vs. dependence.
d. Altered sexuality patterns.

E. Self-concept, disturbed.

1. Outcome:
   a. Verbalizes acceptance of him/herself.
   b. Participates in self-care and rehabilitation activities.
2. Interventions:
   a. Explore concerns regarding changes in self-concept.
   b. Provide realistic and optimistic feedback.
   c. Plan ways for the patient to gain as much control as possible.
   d. Assist patient in understanding that adjustments to changes and rebuilding of self-concept will take time.

V. HOME CARE CONSIDERATIONS

A. Modify home environment to meet patient's needs.
B. Provide adaptive equipment.
C. Explain signs and symptoms of progressive symptomatology that patient must report.
D. Discuss specified activity program.

BULLET INJURIES, BLAST INJURIES, PUNCTURE WOUNDS, CRUSH INJURIES

I. OVERVIEW

A. Definition/etiology/pathophysiology.

1. Bullet injuries.
   a. A low-velocity bullet causes tissue injury by lacerating and crushing the tissue through which it passes.
      (1) The only tissue damaged is that which comes into immediate contact with the bullet.
      (2) There may be an entry wound without an exit wound or both an entry and an exit wound.
   b. A high-velocity bullet often passes completely through the body, leaving both an entry wound and an exit wound.
      (1) This type of missile causes tissue injury by lacerating and crushing the tissue it penetrates, by creating a high-pressure shock wave which penetrates tissues at a distance from the bullet track, and by cavitation.
      (2) In cavitation, the bullet creates a temporary cavity of negative pressure many times the size of the bullet that sucks bacteria and debris into the wound through the bullet entrance and exit openings.
      (3) The temporary cavity collapses, leaving an extensive area of dead tissue around the contaminated bullet track.
      (4) The denser the tissue, the greater the sensitivity to cavitation and the more extensive the wound will be.
      (5) The more elastic the tissue, the greater the resistance to damage will be. Since bone is dense and inelastic, it is susceptible to damage from bullet wounds.
2. Blast injuries.
   a. When explosives are detonated, they are rapidly converted to a large volume of expanding gas, which ruptures the casing and sends fragments outward at high velocity.
      (1) The blast wave moves outward from its source as a rapidly expanding sphere of compressed gas, which quickly loses pressure and velocity as it moves.
      (2) A negative pressure follows along, lasting longer.
      (3) The exploding gases displace an equal volume of air, which blasts along in a mass movement, disrupting human tissue in its path.
      (4) Explosions in confined spaces are far worse than those in the open. Inhalation of toxic gases and smoke add to the trauma.
      (5) Burns may result directly from the fireball created by the burning explosive or secondarily from fires caused by the fireball.
   b. High mortality results from bullet and blast injuries.
3. Puncture wounds.
   a. Puncture wounds may be inflicted with all manner of sharp or dull instruments ranging from fish hooks, knives, and nails to human and animal bites.
   b. The resulting wounds are most prone to infection when contaminated.
   c. Bone may be fractured during the puncture of tissue, or a fragment of the piercing object may become imbedded in the bone.
4. Crush injuries. Crushing of tissues can occur in a number of situations.
   a. In the upper extremity, many crushing injuries are due to catching the hand or arm in machinery.
   b. Often, immense pressures are applied by machines.
   c. The trapped limb is progressively squeezed, causing massive cellular disruption, the bursting or stripping off of skin, comminuted fractures, and traction on tendons and nerves if the rollers reach the shoulder area.
   d. In addition, rollers may be extremely hot, as is the case with mangles in commercial laundries, so that the trapped limb is burned as well as crushed by the machinery.

B. Incidence.

1. Any time; any place.
2. Crush injuries particularly high in industry where heavy machinery is used.

C. Considerations across the lifespan: all age groups.

D. Complications.

1. Compartment syndrome.

2. Loss of extremity.
3. Infection.
4. Loss of limb function due to nerve injury.
5. Loss of life.

II. ASSESSMENT

A. First-aid priorities for bullet and blast injuries, puncture wounds, and crush injuries.

1. Observe for and immediately treat (in order):
   a. Airway obstruction.
   b. Sucking chest wounds.
   c. Hemorrhage.
2. The patient should then be rapidly transferred to a hospital for emergency care.

B. History. Adequate assessment of the damage done to the tissue will depend on specific information. It is of primary importance to know the mechanism of injury.

1. For GSWs, the wound can be better assessed if the type of gun used can be identified.
   a. This can help establish whether a high-velocity or low-velocity bullet produced the wound.
   b. It is also helpful to know the distance between the gun and the victim, the position of the victim in relation to the path of the bullet, whether the bullet passed through anything such as a door or heavy clothing before entering the body, and the direction of the bullet (to help identify the path the bullet took through the tissues and the amount of yaw available to disrupt tissues).
2. In blast injuries, it is helpful to know:
   a. The type of material of which the bomb casing was composed.
   b. Whether the explosion occurred in a closed space or in the open.
   c. The distance between the bomb and the victim.
   d. Whether the victim was in the water or on land (tissue is disrupted at greater distances in water than in the air).
   e. Whether or not the victim was burned by the fireball and its aftermath.
   f. If the victim was very close to the point of detonation, abdominal viscera, the lungs, and the eardrums all may have been damaged as the blast wave traveled through the body (damage to the ear drum being, by far, the most common).
3. In puncture wounds, the mechanism of injury should be identified where not readily apparent.
   a. If a human bite is suspected, efforts should be made to verify this fact. A human bite also may be self-inflicted during eating, gum chewing, or seizures. Human bite injuries have an extremely high incidence of infection.
   b. In cases of dog or cat bite, assessment should include a history of the rabies shot record for the offending animal, if known. Otherwise, the animal should be confined and observed for signs of rabies.
4. Determine the mechanism and setting of trauma in crush injuries.

C. Physical examination.

1. Gunshot wounds.
   a. Typically, the entrance wound is small and deceptive in gunshot wounds. There may be no exit wound, but if present, it may be small or much larger than the entrance wound.
   b. The severity of injury in a projectile wound will depend on the amount of trauma to bone, large blood vessels, and nerves rather than damage done to skin and muscle.
   c. After bleeding has been controlled, potential fractures should be identified.
   d. Often the soft tissue is painless immediately after injury, but a fracture will cause pain.
   e. Additional signs of fracture are abnormal position, length, or shape of the extremity with extreme point tenderness. Abnormal movement, crepitation, and visible bony fragments are also important signs.
   f. If fracture is suspected, the limb is splinted and the assessment continues with the objective of ruling out major injuries to arteries, veins, and nerves.
2. Blast injuries.
   a. Skin, soft tissue, and body injuries are assessed.
   b. In postblast injuries, 12 or more hours after the injury, the patient may suffer from posttraumatic pulmonary insufficiency with mild hemoptysis, cyanosis, behavioral changes, an elevated arterial PCO_2 and decreased PO_2.
3. In puncture wounds where the penetrating object is still in the tissue, it should not be removed, except by a physician.
   a. The wound track may be surgically explored, washed, or probed.
   b. Suspicion of human bite should be high when wounds on the knuckles indicate impact with teeth, as often occurs during a fight.
4. Most industrial crush injuries involve the distal arm and hand.
   a. The hand shows massive subcutaneous and interstitial edema with diffuse oozing of blood.
   b. The entire arm should be immobilized in a splint with the separate fragments aligned to prevent blood vessels from kinking and to protect against further soft tissue damage from fracture fragments.
   c. The arm should be kept constantly elevated.
   d. Tissues should be kept moist with normal saline (see Chapter 17, Hand [Reimplantation] if limb is severed).
   e. Close observation for compartment syndrome.

D. Diagnostic tests.

1. X-rays.
   a. Bullet injuries.
      (1) X-rays: AP and lateral of affected area.
      (2) May require additional views to determine:
         (a) Whether the bullet passed through

one part of the body before lodging in or passed through another part.

(b) If the bullet exited the body or remains in the tissues.

(c) Bone damage and bullet fragments.

b. Blast injuries.
   (1) X-rays: AP and lateral of affected part.
   (2) May require additional views to determine presence of metal fragments from bomb casings, which can act like high-velocity missiles as they pass through tissues.
c. Puncture wounds.
   (1) X-rays: AP and lateral of affected area.
   (2) Visualize imbedded fragments of glass, painted wood, or metal.
   (3) Fractures.
d. Crush injuries.
   (1) X-rays: AP and lateral of affected area.
   (2) Arteriograms/venograms.

2. Laboratory studies in all injuries.
   a. CBC.
   b. ABGs serum.
   c. Urinalysis.
   d. Wound cultures.

III. COMMON THERAPEUTIC MODALITIES

A. Victims injured by projectile of metal casing or high-velocity bullets.

1. Exploratory surgery to remove devitalized tissue.
2. External fixation devices or skeletal traction when high-velocity bullets have fractured bones. Internal fixation is avoided at site of impact.
3. In most cases, the initial surgical wound is left open, covered with dressings, primary suturing delayed for 4-5 days.
4. Broad-spectrum antibiotics started preoperatively and continued into postoperative period after identification of organism.

B. Burns sustained during explosions are treated in the same manner as other burns.

1. Posttraumatic pulmonary insufficiency is treated with endotracheal tube and positive ventilation.
2. In the skin, imbedded foreign objects can result in tattooing. Fine fragments like gunpowder should be removed by vigorous scrubbing. Larger fragments such as bits of metal may be individually extracted with forceps. Removal by scrubbing or extraction should be done at the time of injury before epithelialization occurs.

C. Control of hemorrhage and shock to prevent exsanguination is of prime importance in stab wounds.

1. In most nonemergent cases, foreign bodies are removed under general anesthesia.
   a. Needles may have to be removed under fluoroscopy.
   b. Fish hooks are advanced through the skin until the barbed tip can be cut off. They are then pulled back through the wound and out of the tissues.
   c. Other objects are extracted through the wound with forceps or are not removed at all.
2. After any necessary foreign body removal, the wound is thoroughly cleansed, irrigated copiously, and debrided, as necessary.
   a. Some wounds are sutured and others are not.
   b. Puncture wounds that are deep or grossly contaminated, such as human bites, should never be sutured closed. Instead, after cleansing, they are loosely packed with gauze wicking or a Penrose drain and covered with a sterile gauze dressing.
   c. Treatment for dog bites no longer includes leaving the wound open. These and other superficial wounds are cleansed and sutured.
3. Prophylaxis against tetanus is provided when necessary. This includes a tetanus booster if the last booster was longer than 5 years ago.
   a. Prophylactic antibiotics are used for grossly contaminated wounds.
   b. A series of rabies injections may be necessary for an animal bite when the animal was either found to be rabid or was not captured.

D. Since much soft tissue may remain viable, in crush injuries, only foreign matter and definitely nonviable tissues are debrided initially.

1. Primary closure is usually delayed.
2. Dressing changes and debridement are repeated at 2-3 day intervals until it has been definitely ascertained which tissue is viable. Only then is closure and/or reconstruction attempted.

IV. NURSING DIAGNOSES, OUTCOMES, AND INTERVENTIONS

A. See Table 14.3.

B. Pain, acute.

1. Outcome: patient has decreased or relieved pain.
2. Interventions: after initial efforts to stabilize patient, use measures to control comfort.
   a. Position for comfort.
   b. Apply cold as needed.
   c. Administer analgesics to control pain. If patient is in shock, intramuscular injections of analgesics will not circulate and will provide little benefit. With repeated injections, the drug may be stored in the local tissues only to be released to the general circulation in one massive dose after shock has been resolved. Therefore, analgesics are given intravenously.
   d. Explain to patient or significant others that local anesthetics, while helpful in pain control, may not be appropriate in certain circumstances. Local infiltration, for example, might distort tissues and lead to poor approximation during suturing, which could result in poor cosmetic results.

C. Tissue perfusion, ineffective: peripheral.

1. Outcome: resolution of edema.
2. Interventions.
   a. To control edema and associated discomfort as well as to promote venous circulation, elevation

of the extremity is usually advocated, but here too, individual patient variations must be kept in mind. Elevation of the extremity should not be above heart level.

b. Observe such patients carefully for blanching of the fingers since ischemia may develop rapidly.

D. Nutrition, imbalanced: less than body requirements.

1. Outcome: patient has adequate nutritional intake.
2. Interventions: the patient with multiple traumatic injuries will have nutritional needs far in excess of normal metabolic needs.
   a. Provide supplemental feedings to supply protein and calories.
   b. Provide vitamins and minerals to promote soft tissue healing and bone repair.
   c. Special nutritional planning may be needed because of electrolyte variations. Hyperkalemia, for example, often results from massive crushing injuries, which release intracellular electrolytes into the bloodstream.
   d. Nutritional requirements must be tailored to the individual patient; every effort should be taken to involve the patient in the decision-making process.

E. Infection, risk for.

1. Outcome: no evidence of infection.
2. Interventions.
   a. Adequate debridement is essential. This procedure may be done in the emergency room, operating room, or patient care unit.
   b. Because of interruption of skin integrity as well as possible wound contamination occurring during the traumatic incident, scrupulous care must be taken to prevent infection or additional wound contamination.
   c. Sterile technique for wound care is imperative.
   d. Antibiotics may be applied locally in addition to those administered intravenously or intramuscularly.

F. Physical mobility, impaired.

1. Outcomes.
   a. Patient demonstrates full range of joint motion in all extremities.
   b. Patient maintains an optimal level of independence and control of own activities.
2. Interventions.
   a. Promote mobility within activity limitations and use measures to prevent complications of immobility (see Chapter 6, Effects of Immobility).
   b. Decreased arm/hand/lower extremity immobility and function may present a wide range of problems requiring nursing intervention.
      (1) Emotional reactions to dependency such as feelings of helplessness, anxiety, frustration, or anger may result in the patient's experiencing depression or acting hostile to staff. This may be complicated by post-traumatic stress disorder.
      (2) The patient may become noncompliant or manipulative in efforts to gain some control over the situation.
   c. Help patient to vent unexpressed feelings and work with the patient to help patient gain control over life in more constructive ways.

G. Body image, disturbed.

1. Outcome: patient verbalizes self-acceptance.
2. Interventions.
   a. Assist patient in coping with disturbed body image.
   b. Determine what the disturbance in body image means to the patient and try not to label the individual as "overreacting" or "denying" based on a projection of the nurse's own feelings onto the patient.
   c. Convey to patient that he/she is accepted as is, even though the nurse understands that body changes may not be acceptable to the patient.
   d. Attempts to talk patient out of negative feelings are not therapeutic. Such attempts convey to patient that these very personal feelings are somehow wrong and constitute a form of rejection that reinforces the general feeling of being unacceptable.
   e. In all ways, the patient should understand that, in the eyes of the nurse, he/she is a person of worth.
   f. Use patient support systems and other resources to facilitate coping.

V. HOME CARE CONSIDERATIONS

A. Modifications in home environment and lifestyle to provide for patient accessibility, mobility, and independence.

B. Provide and teach use of adaptive equipment.

C. Discuss specified activity program.

D. Explain progressive symptomatology that patient must report.

E. Instruct patient in use of medications.

Bibliography

Armstrong, J.F. (1999). Bullets: Damage by design. *RN, 62*(1), 38-39.

Berg, E.E. (1998). Open book (AP compression) pelvis fracture. *Orthopaedic Nursing, 17*(2), 59-62.

Blake, R., & Hoffman, J. (1999). Emergency department evaluation and treatment of the shoulder and humerus. *Emergency Medicine Clinics of North America, 17*(4), 859-876.

Brown, F.M. Jr. (1998). Management of Colles' fractures. *Orthopaedic Nursing, 17*(3), 37-40.

Browner, B.D., Alberta, F.G., & Mastella, D.J. (1999). A new era in orthopedic trauma care. *Surgical Clinics of North America, 79*(6), 1431-1448.

Childs, S.G., & Holmes, S.B. (1998). *Guidelines for orthopaedic nursing: Adult trauma.* Pitman, NJ: National Association of Orthopaedic Nurses (NAON).

Green, N.E. (1994). Fractures and dislocations about the elbow. In N.E. Green & M.F. Swiontkowski (Eds.), *Skeletal trauma in children* (pp. 213-256). Philadelphia: W.B. Saunders.

Lappe, J.M. (1998). Prevention of hip fractures: A nursing imperative. *Orthopaedic Nursing, 17*(3), 15-26.

Ludwick, R., Dieckman, B., & Snelson, C.M. (1999). Assessment of the geriatric orthopaedic trauma patient. *Orthopaedic Nursing, 18*(6), 13-20.

Mastey, R.D., Weiss, A-P C., & Akelman, E. (1997). Primary care of hand and wrist athletic injuries. *Clinics in Sports Medicine, 16*(4),

705-724.
Randolph, C.L. (1998). Considerations for the orthopedic nurse in diagnosis and treatment of adolescent sports injuries. *Nursing Clinics of North America, 33*(4), 615-628.
Roberts, D. (1999). Introduction to bone: Structure and function, fractures, and osteoporosis. In *An introduction to orthopaedic nursing* (2nd ed., pp. 3-16). Pitman, N.J.: NAON.
Roberts, D.M., & Stollard, T.C. (2000). Emergency department evaluation and treatment of knee and leg injuries. *Emergency Medicine Clinics of North America, 18*(1), 67-84.
Rudman, N., & McIlmail, D. (2000). Emergency department evaluation and treatment of hip and thigh injuries. *Emergency Medicine Clinics of North America, 18*(1), 29-66.
Snyder, P. (1998). Fractures. In A.B. Maher, S.W. Salmond, & T.A. Pellino (Eds.), *Orthopaedic nursing* (pp. 663-717). Philadelphia: Saunders.
Taggart, H. (1999). Caring for the elderly hip fracture patient. In *An introduction to orthopaedic nursing* (2nd ed., pp. 113-122). Pitman, NJ: NAON.
Whittington, C.F. (1998). Exercise and sport-related injuries. In A.B. Maher, S.W. Salmond, & T.A. Pellino (Eds.), *Orthopaedic nursing* (pp. 746-768). Philadelphia: Saunders.
Williamson, V.C. (Ed.). (1998). *Management of lower extremity fractures.* Pitman N.J.: NAON.

STUDY QUESTIONS

Jimmy Durham, age 12, arrives at the clinic following a fall while inline skating. He complains of knee and shoulder pain, stating that his right lower leg twisted as he fell and he landed on his right shoulder. Preliminary diagnoses based only on physical examination are: (a) second-degree sprain of the right knee, and (b) posterior dislocation of the right shoulder. (Questions 1- 5)

1. Assessment findings consistent with a second-degree sprain would reveal:
   a. Complete range of joint motion.
   b. Lateral displacement of the patella.
   c. Increased compartment pressures.
   d. Joint effusion and ecchymosis.

2. Jimmy's mother asks you to explain why he needs a brace for his knee. Your answer would be based on your knowledge that knee immobilization is used to:
   a. Discourage weight bearing.
   b. Prevents more damage to the soft tissue.
   c. Limit Jimmy's activity.
   d. Maximize healing consistent with Wolff's law.

3. Consistent with a shoulder dislocation, you would anticipate that Jimmy will complain of increased shoulder pain when his right arm is:
   a. Abducted and internally rotated.
   b. Abducted and externally rotated.
   c. Adducted and internally rotated.
   d. Adducted and externally rotated.

4. The diagnostic test used to confirm dislocation is a(n):
   a. MRI.
   b. Radiograph.
   c. Arthrogram.
   d. CT scan.

5. Ice, which is recommended following strains and sprains, is usually applied for
   a. 30-60 minutes every 2 hours.
   b. 15-30 minutes every 2 hours.
   c. 10-20 minutes every 4 hours.
   d. 15-30 minutes every 4 hours.

6. Tennis elbow is characterized by tenderness
   a. Over the medial epicondyle.
   b. On the inferior aspect of the olecranon.
   c. Over the radial head.
   d. Over the lateral epicondyle.

7. A fracture caused by crushing injury that has multiple fracture fragments is classified as
   a. Pathologic.
   b. Comminuted.
   c. Stellate.
   d. Avulsion.

Margaret Jones, aged 66, arrives at your office clutching her arm to her body. She tells you that she tripped while taking her daily walk and fell on her outstretched hand. Her wrist hurts and you suspect a Colles' fracture. (Questions 8-10)

8. A major contributing factor to Colles' fracture in older women is:
   a. Poor physical conditioning.
   b. Changes in articular cartilage.
   c. High rates of carpal tunnel syndrome.
   d. Osteoporosis.

9. The physical finding most indicative of Colles' fracture is:
   a. Loss of motion in the wrist and fingers.
   b. Hump deformity of the wrist.
   c. Absent radial pulse.
   d. Ecchymosis of the hand.

10. Assessment of a patient with a Colles' fracture should include evaluation of the:
    a. Ulnar nerve.
    b. Peroneal nerve.
    c. Radial nerve.
    d. Brachial nerve.

Chapter 15 Tumors of the Musculoskeletal System

Kimberly K. Haynes, MS, RN, CS, ONC

Contents

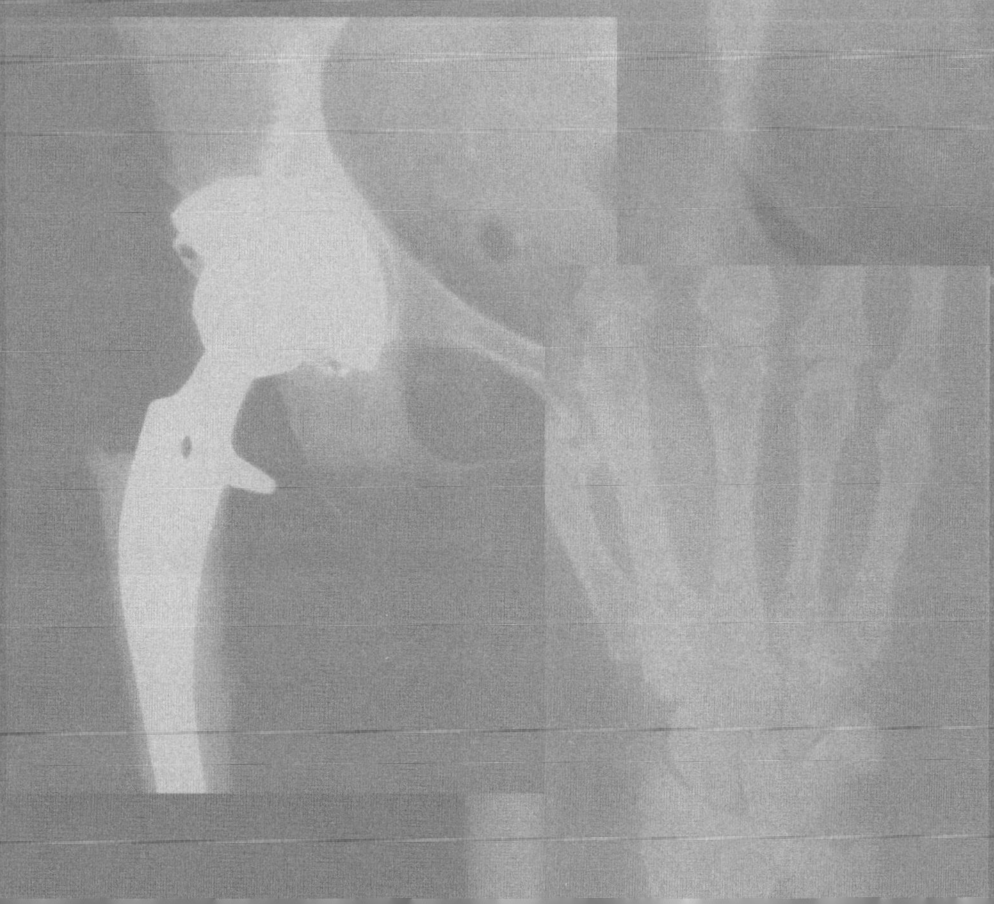

OBJECTIVES

At the completion of this chapter, the learner will be able to:

- Discuss nursing care for patients with sarcomas, metastatic carcinoma, and multiple myeloma.
- Identify surgical options for patients with a malignant bone or soft tissue tumor.
- Describe complications of surgery, chemotherapy, and radiation which may be used individually or in combination as the treatment for sarcomas or metastatic carcinomas.

KEY POINTS

- Patients diagnosed with cancer need an opportunity to verbalize fears and concerns, which may include fears of death, dependency, change in family dynamics, disability, weakness, chemical toxicities, loss of role functions, and financial difficulties.
- Sarcomas affect children and adults. It is estimated that 10,600 new sarcomas will be diagnosed in the year 2000, 2,500 of those being primary bone tumors and 8,100 being primary soft tissue tumors.
- Most drug protocols for bone and soft tissue sarcomas are undergoing changes as more information and results from established protocols are evaluated.
- Surgery is the primary treatment for sarcomas. Chemotherapy and radiation are used neoadjuvantly and adjuvantly depending on the type of sarcoma and the age of the patient.
- Since the 1970s, limb preservation surgery has been the standard of care in the treatment of sarcomas. However, preserving life before limb is most important, therefore amputation may be necessary if good margins cannot be achieved through limb preservation surgery.
- Patients with metastatic carcinoma or multiple myeloma are treated primarily with chemotherapy and radiation. Surgery is used prophylactically to prevent fractures in an area of metastatic deposit to bone, or to stabilize a pathologic fracture through a metastatic deposit to bone.

CHAPTER 15

TUMORS OF THE MUSCULOSKELETAL SYSTEM

PRIMARY TUMORS OF BONE OR SOFT TISSUE

I. OVERVIEW

A. Definition: tumors of the musculoskeletal system are either benign or malignant, and a malignant neoplasm is called a sarcoma.

1. Primary sarcomas are malignant tumors that originate in the bone or soft connective tissue.
2. Benign tumors and tumor-like conditions also originate in bone and soft tissues.
3. Non-neoplastic bone and soft tissue tumors are called tumor-like conditions.

B. Pathophysiology.

1. Sarcomas.
   a. Sarcomas arise from tissues derived from mesoderm or primitive mesenchyme, such as muscle, bone, fat, fascia, and cartilage.
   b. Sarcomas differ from carcinomas by cell origin.
      (1) Common carcinomas are of the breast, lung, prostate, thyroid, and kidney and are derived from ectodermal and endodermal tissues.
      (2) Nerve tumors also arise from ectodermal and endodermal tissues but are characterized as sarcomas because of their behavior.
2. Tumor-like lesion.
   a. Solitary bone cyst (simple or unicameral).
      (1) Cavity filled with clear or sanguinous fluid and lined by a membrane, consisting of connective tissue with scattered giant cells.
      (2) Location: metaphyses, especially proximal humerus and proximal femur.
      (3) Age range: 0-20 years.
   b. Aneurysmal bone cyst (ABC).
      (1) Expanding osteolytic lesion consisting of blood-filled spaces separated by connective tissue.
      (2) Location: long bones of lower extremity.
      (3) Age range: 10-20 years.
   c. Juxta-articular bone cyst (intraosseous ganglion).
      (1) Benign cystic and multiloculated lesion made of fibrous tissue with mucoid change, located in subchondral bone.
      (2) Location: long tubular bones.
      (3) Age range: 20-59 years.
   d. Metaphyseal fibrous cortical defect (nonossifying fibroma).
      (1) Bone lesion with same histologic features of benign fibrous histiocytoma.
      (2) Location: cortically-based in femur and tibia.
      (3) Age range: 0-20 years.
      (4) Theoretically, the most common benign bone tumor, found in approximately 50% of children. However, few are operated on therefore statistics are not accurate.
      (5) Can be self-healing and fill in with mature bone without any intervention.
   e. Eosinophilic granuloma (solitary).
      (1) Lesion with proliferation of reticulohistiocytic elements with leukocytes, lymphocytes, plasma cells, and giant cells.
      (2) Location: diaphyses and flat bones.
      (3) Age range: 1-20 years.
   f. Fibrous dysplasia.
      (1) Lesion, which is developmental in nature, consists of fibrous connective tissue, and it weakens the bone. The tumor has a whorled pattern on x-ray often described as a "ground glass" appearance.
      (2) Location: femur, tibia, and maxillary bones.
      (3) Age range: 0-30 years.
   g. Myositis ossificans.
      (1) Caused by trauma, locally self-limiting ossifying process occurring in the muscle, generally solitary and well circumscribed.
      (2) Location: arm, thigh, and buttocks.
      (3) Age range: 13-30 years, males > females.
3. Primary bone tumor – benign.
   a. Osteoid osteoma.
      (1) Small osteoblastic lesion (less than 1 cm) with demarcated outline and reactive bone formation.
      (2) Location: femur and tibia.
      (3) Age range: 10-25 years.
      (4) Pain at night often relieved by aspirin or NSAIDs.
   b. Osteoblastoma.
      (1) Similar to osteoid osteoma but larger (over 2 cm).
      (2) Location: spine, long bones, and hands.
      (3) Age: 3-78 years, 90% < 30 years old.
   c. Osteoma.
      (1) Benign bony excrescence, well circumscribed, sessile, or pedunculated.
      (2) Location: maxilla and mandible.
      (3) Age: 16-74 years, 3:1 ratio female to male.
   d. Osteochondroma.
      (1) Cartilage-capped bony projection on external surface of bone.
      (2) Most frequent bone tumor.
      (3) Location: metaphyses of long bone, especially proximal tibia and distal femur.
      (4) Age range: 0-30 years.

e. Enchondroma.
 (1) Lesion with formation of mature cartilage but lacking histologic characteristic of chondrosarcoma.
 (2) Most common tumor of the hand.
 (3) Location: hands, feet, humerus, ribs, and femur.
 (4) Age range: 20-40 years.

f. Chondroma.
 (1) Benign cartilage growth, forms between cortex and periosteum.
 (2) Location: small bones of the hand and foot, proximal humeral metaphysis.
 (3) Age: young adults.

g. Chondroblastoma.
 (1) Rare lesion characterized by highly cellular but undifferentiated chondroblast-like cells.
 (2) Location: epiphyses, especially femur, proximal tibia.
 (3) Age range: 5-25 years.

h. Chondromyxoid fibroma.
 (1) Lesion of bone characterized by chondroid and myxoid differentiation of its basic tissue growing in a lobular pattern.
 (2) Location: metaphyses of tubular bones, proximal tibial metaphysis most common.
 (3) Age range: 5-25 years.

i. Desmoplastic fibroma.
 (1) Locally aggressive tumor characterized by abundant collagen fibers.
 (2) Location: mandible most common, metaphysis of long bones.
 (3) Age range: all ages, adolescents and young adults most common.

j. Giant cell tumor or osteoclastoma.
 (1) Benign but aggressive bone tumor with richly vascularized tissue consisting of plump spindle-shaped cells and numerous giant cells.
 (2) Location: distal femur, proximal tibia, distal radius, and proximal humerus.
 (3) Age range: 20-40 years.
 (4) Small potential for malignant transformation but can metastasize without malignant transformation.

4. Primary soft tissue tumors: benign.
 a. Hemangioma.
 (1) Lesion of soft tissue or bone consisting of newly-formed blood vessels, either capillary, cavernous, or venous type.
 (2) Location: head and neck most common, can be intramuscular or intraosseous. Spine is the most common location for bone.
 (3) Age range: all ages.

 b. Benign fibrous histiocytoma.
 (1) Characterized by spindle cell fibrous tissue with a storiform pattern and giant cells, hemosiderin pigment, and lipid-bearing histiocytes.
 (2) Location: skin and most common on extremities.
 (3) Age range: 20-40 years.

 c. Lipoma.
 (1) Tumor of mature adipose tissue with no evidence of cellular atypism.
 (2) Location: upper back, neck, shoulder, and abdomen, then proximal extremities, and buttocks.
 (3) Age range: 40-60 years.

 d. Leiomyoma.
 (1) Tumor arising from smooth muscle.
 (2) Location: genitourinary tract and gastrointestinal tract most common, less common in skin and rare in deep soft tissue.
 (3) Age: all ages.

 e. Rhabdomyoma.
 (1) Tumor arising from striated muscle, less common than its malignant counterpart rhabdomyosarcoma.
 (2) Location: mainly head and neck.
 (3) Age: infants to adults.

 f. Intramuscular myxoma.
 (1) Painless palpable mass, histologically appears very mucoid with loose network of reticular fiber.
 (2) Location: large muscles of thigh, shoulder, buttocks, and upper arm.
 (3) Age: 40-70 years.

 g. Schwannoma (neurilemoma or neurinoma).
 (1) Arises in nerve roots and pain may be progressive.
 (2) Location: spine, retroperitoneum and mediastinum nerve roots.
 (3) Age: 20-50 years but can involve any age group.

 h. Neurofibroma.
 (1) Can be solitary or multiple nodules as in von Recklinghausen's disease.
 (2) Location: extremities or centrally located in body.
 (3) Age: young adults (solitary), children (von Recklinghausen's).

5. Primary bone tumors: malignant.
 a. Osteosarcoma.
 (1) Characterized by formation of bone or osteoid by tumor cells.
 (2) Most common primary malignant bone tumor.
 (3) Location: metaphyses, especially distal femur, proximal tibia, proximal humerus.
 (4) Age range: 10-30 years.
 (5) Involves intramedullary region.

 b. Surface osteosarcoma.
 (1) Tumors arise on surface of bone.
 (2) Three categories: parosteal, periosteal, and high-grade.
 (3) Location: metaphyses, especially distal femur.
 (4) Age range: 20-40 years.

c. Primary chondrosarcoma.
   (1) Characterized by formation of cartilage by tumor cells; has higher cellularity and greater pleomorphism than a chondroma.
   (2) Location: femur, pelvis, ribs, and scapula.
   (3) Age range: 30-60 years.

d. Secondary chondrosarcoma.
   (1) A benign lesion, such as osteochondroma or multiple enchondromatosis, undergoes a malignant transformation.
   (2) Location: pelvis, proximal femur, proximal humerus.
   (3) Age range: 20-40 years.
   (4) Evidence of malignant transformation may include pain, irregular border, or increase in cartilage cap size after patient growth is complete.

e. Mesenchymal chondrosarcoma.
   (1) High-grade malignancy originating in bone 80% and soft tissue 20% biphasic histology, well differentiated round or spindle cell with areas of hyaline cartilage.
   (2) Location: maxilla and mandible, pelvis, femur, shoulder, ribs, and sternum.
   (3) Age: 30-60 years, can be younger or older.

f. Ewing's sarcoma.
   (1) Tumor composed of densely packed small cells with round nuclei.
   (2) Location: diaphyseal regions of long bones and flat bones.
   (3) Age range: 5-15 years.
   (4) Often confused with osteomyelitis as it presents with fever, anemia, leukocytosis, and increased sedimentation rate.

g. Primitive neuroectodermal tumor of bone.
   (1) Tumor resembles peripheral neuroepithelioma of soft tissues.
   (2) Histologically different from Ewing's sarcoma due to neural differentiation.
   (3) Age and location similar to Ewing's sarcoma.

h. Fibrosarcoma of bone.
   (1) Malignant tumor characterized by the formation of spindle-shaped tumor cells of interlacing bundles of collagen fibers and by the absence of other types of histologic differentiation.
   (2) Location: long tubular bones – femur and tibia.
   (3) Age range: 5-80 years.

i. Malignant fibrous histiocytoma of bone.
   (1) Rare tumor with spindle-shaped fibroblast-like cell in storiform or cartwheel pattern.
   (2) Location: long bones – femur and tibia.
   (3) Age range: 12-82 years.

j. Adamantinoma.
   (1) Rare malignant tumor with the presence of circumscribed masses of epithelial cells surrounded by spindle-celled fibrous tissue.
   (2) Location: tibia and fibula.
   (3) Age range: 4-74 years.

k. Malignant lymphoma of bone (non-Hodgkin's lymphoma).
   (1) Tumor cells are rounded, pleomorphic, with many indented nuclei.
   (2) Location: any bone but most common in short bones as ileum, vertebrae, and long tubular bones.
   (3) Solitary osseous lesion without involvement of other osseous or non-osseous sites within 6 months of onset of symptoms. Regional lymph nodes may be present.
   (4) Age range: 10-60 years.

l. Myeloma (see Multiple Myeloma section in this chapter).
   (1) Multiple bone involvement characterized by neoplastic plasma cells with varying degrees on immaturity.
   (2) Associated with abnormal proteins in blood and urine.
   (3) Location: bones with abundant marrow – vertebrae, ribs, skull, pelvis, and sternum.
   (4) Age range: 40-70 years.

6. Primary soft tissue tumors: malignant.
   a. Malignant fibrous histiocytoma.
      (1) Most common soft tissue tumor in late adult life.
      (2) Location: thigh, deep to the fascia.
      (3) Age: mainly in older adults, has been documented in adolescents.
   b. Liposarcoma.
      (1) Second most common soft tissue tumor; characterized by lipoblastic differentiation.
      (2) Location: thigh and retroperitoneum.
      (3) Age range: 40-60 years, males > females.
   c. Synovial sarcoma.
      (1) Occurs around joints of extremities usually in close association with tendon sheath, bursae and joint capsule. Rare inside joint.
      (2) Location: knee region more common then lower thigh.
      (3) Age: 15-40 years, males > females.
      (4) May involve regional lymph nodes.
   d. Epithelioid sarcoma.
      (1) Slow-growing firm tumor arising from fascia or subcutaneous tissue.
      (2) Location: hand and arm.
      (3) Age range: 15-35 years, male to female ratio 2:1.
      (4) May involve regional lymph nodes.
   e. Rhabdomyosarcoma.
      (1) Most common soft tissue sarcoma in childhood, all high grade.
      (2) Location: head, and neck, extremities and trunk.
      (3) Age range: 0-20 years.
      (4) May involve regional lymph nodes.
   f. Fibrosarcoma.
      (1) Formation of tumor cells by interlacing bundles of collagen cells.

(2) Location: thigh and trunk.
(3) Age range: 20-60 years.

g. Dermatofibrosarcoma protuberans.
(1) Nodular cutaneous tumor characterized by a storiform pattern histologically.
(2) Location: most frequently found in trunk and proximal extremities.
(3) Age range: 30-50 years.

h. Leiomyosarcoma.
(1) Tumor of smooth muscle origin.
(2) Location: retroperitoneum and abdominal cavity.
(3) Age: adult life, female > male.

i. Malignant peripheral nerve sheath tumor.
(1) Spindle cell sarcomas arising from nerve or neurofibroma.
(2) Location: along nerves, nerve sheaths.
(3) Age: adult life, 20-50 years.

j. Angiosarcoma.
(1) Malignant tumors characterized by formation of irregular vascular channels lined by one or more layers of atypical endothelial cells and solid masses of poorly differentiated cells.
(2) Location: skin, soft tissues, organs, and bone.
(3) Age range: all ages.

k. Hemangioendothelioma.
(1) Intermediate grade and aggressive tumor characterized by solid cell cords and vascular endothelial structures.
(2) Can metastasize to the lungs, liver regional lymph nodes, and bone.
(3) Location: superficial or deep soft tissue.
(4) Age range: any age but rarely in childhood.

l. Hemangiopericytoma.
(1) Benign, aggressive, and potentially malignant tumor characterized by endothelial-lined vascular channels.
(2) Can metastasize to the lungs and skeleton.
(3) Location: lower extremity, specifically thigh, pelvic fossa, and retroperitoneum.
(4) Age range: primarily in adults, rare in infants and children.

m. Kaposi's sarcoma.
(1) Primitive vasoformative tissue, viral associated or viral induced.
(2) Location: skin and lymph nodes.
(3) Age range: 40-60 years.
(4) Linked with immunosuppression (AIDS, organ transplantation).

n. Lymphangiosarcoma.
(1) See angiosarcoma; cutaneous angiosarcoma associated with lymphedema, most following mastectomies.
(2) Location: extremities, and area near lymph node dissection.
(3) Age: adults.

7. Other: malignant.

a. Chordoma.
(1) Malignant tumor characterized by a lobular arrangement of tissue made up of cords and sheets of highly vacuolated cells and mucoid intracellular material.
(2) Location: proximal and distal ends of vertebral body.
(3) Age range: 30-50 years.

b. Mesenchymoma.
(1) Rare tumor, does not fit into any category, and is characterized by 2 or more unrelated nonepithelial tissue components in same neoplasm.
(2) Location: retroperitoneum and lower extremities.
(3) Age: mostly in > 60 years, but has been reported in children and young adults.

c. Alveolar soft tissue.
(1) Slow growing, painless mass, very rare.
(2) Location: lower extremities, especially thigh in adults, head and neck in infants and children.
(3) Age: 15-35, females > males, can be found in infants and children.

d. Clear cell sarcoma (malignant melanoma of soft parts).
(1) Located deep and near tendons and aponeuroses, lacks epidermal involvement.
(2) Location: extremities, especially foot and ankle.
(3) Age 20-40 years, females > males.

e. Extraskeletal osteosarcoma.
(1) Very rare, progressively enlarging soft tissue mass.
(2) Location: usually thigh and retroperitoneum.
(3) Age: 40 years and older.

f. Extraskeletal chondrosarcoma.
(1) Occurs primarily in deep tissue, slow growing.
(2) Location: extremities.
(3) Age: over 35 but has been reported in children, males 2x > females.

g. Carcinoma (see Bone Metastasis in this chapter).
(1) Primary site: breast, lung, prostate, kidney, and thyroid.
(2) Location: vertebrae, rib, pelvis, and proximal long bones.
(3) Age range: 40 onwards but can occur at any age.

C. Incidence.

1. The incidence of primary sarcomas is low.
2. Approximately 10,600 new sarcomas are diagnosed each year in the United States. Of the 10,600 new tumors, 2,500 are primary bone tumors and 8,100 are primary soft tissue tumors.
3. The occurrence of benign bone and soft tissue tumors is much more common but difficult to actually measure due to the fact many of these tumors are only monitored without surgery.

D. Etiology.

1. Most etiologies unknown.
2. Radiation-induced sarcomas have been identified.
3. Trauma draws attention to lesions already present but is not the cause.
4. Role of virus is being explored (oncogenes in malignancies).
5. Environmental issues such as pollution, exposure to chemicals.
6. Hereditary sarcomas can occur but very infrequently

E. Considerations across the lifespan.

1. Chronicity of disease. Need for periodic follow-up for rest of patient's life.
2. Life-threatening illness treated with chemotherapy, affects developmental goals of each stage of growth and development.
    a. Children:
        (1) Socialization impaired, especially by school absence.
        (2) May experience temporary or permanent developmental delays or regressions.
    b. Adolescents:
        (1) Issues of autonomy vs. dependency; increased reliance on parents; surrender of control; changes in body image; alterations in sexual development.
        (2) Peer relationships suffer.
    c. Young adults:
        (1) Issue of fertility vs. sterility from chemotherapy.
        (2) Marriage and family goals may need to be postponed.
        (3) Ability to find employment and obtain health insurance may be problematic.
    d. Middle age:
        (1) Change in ability to earn a living.
        (2) Career changes may be necessary.
    e. Geriatric:
        (1) Decreased energy.
        (2) Increased dependence on others.
        (3) May be viewed as an early end to productive years.
    f. There is overlap in developmental issues for all age groups. Cancer stigmatizes people, affecting families, friendships, neighborhoods, workplaces, and schools.

F. Complications.

1. Infection in surgical incision.
2. Local recurrence of tumor.
3. Failure of metallic implant or allograft due to fatigue fracture or infection.
4. Permanent toxicities resulting from chemotherapy and/or radiation therapy.
5. Occurrence of metastasis requiring additional treatment.
6. Loss of limb due to infection or uncontrollable recurrence.
7. Death from uncontrolled disease.

II. ASSESSMENT

A. History and physical examination.

1. Duration and onset of symptoms.
2. Pain: usually severe, often occurs at night.
3. Palpable mass: note size, tenderness/swelling.
4. Family history of malignancies.
5. Impaired activity or mobility due to pain or mass.
6. Lymph nodes need to be assessed for enlargement.
7. Liver needs to be assessed for enlargement.

B. Diagnostic tests.

1. Anteroposterior and lateral x-ray of involved area.
2. Computerized tomography (CT) and/or magnetic resonance imaging (MRI) to detect soft tissue involvement and location of tumor and neurovascular structures in transverse or sagittal planes.
3. Bone scintigraphy (bone scan) to rule out multiple osseous lesions or "skip metastasis" (lesion proximal to primary lesion).
4. CT of chest to rule out pulmonary metastases.
5. Ultrasound to rule out cystic tumor.
6. Arteriogram to identify vessel involvement.
7. CBC to rule out infection.
8. Sedimentation rate.
9. Serum electrolytes, including calcium, phosphorus, and alkaline phosphate.
10. Bence-Jones protein in urine to rule out multiple myeloma.
11. Biopsy (see Common Therapeutic Modalities below).

III. COMMON THERAPEUTIC MODALITIES

A. Biopsy.

1. Definition.
    a. Needle biopsy: used in institutions with pathologists well versed in diagnosing sarcomas.
        (1) Done in the operating room or under CT guidance.
        (2) Tissue sample is small therefore open biopsy may be warranted if a diagnostic tissue sample is not received.
    b. Open/incisional biopsy:
        (1) A surgical procedure done in the operating room.
        (2) Procedure in which a small piece of tissue is excised for microscopic examination to determine the type and behavior of the tumor.
    c. Excisional biopsy:
        (1) A surgical procedure in which a small mass, usually benign, is marginally excised.
        (2) Both for definitive treatment and microscopic tissue examination to determine the type of tumor.
2. Indications.
    a. To diagnose a benign versus a malignant mass.
    b. To determine the tissue type to assist with treatment plan.
3. Common anatomic areas.
    a. Any soft tissue mass.
    b. Any bony mass or lesion.
4. Potential problems or complications.
    a. Inadequate tissue for diagnosis (may occur

with needle aspiration or needle biopsy).
b. Delayed wound healing due to infection.
c. Risk of microexpansion of tumor due to tissue contamination.
d. Fracture of biopsied bone due to presence of a stress riser.

B. Limb-salvage or limb-sparing procedures.

1. Definition.
   a. A curative procedure, done as an alternative to amputation, indicated for the surgical ablation of sarcoma.
      (1) The surgical treatment includes removal of the lesion (bone or soft tissue) with a zone of normal surrounding tissue.
      (2) The following are types of limb-salvage currently being performed for bone and soft tissue sarcomas:
         (a) Intracapsular or intralesional excision: a debulking procedure done within the pseudocapsule of the lesion (rarely done and done for palliation only).
         (b) Marginal excision: done en bloc extracapsularly within the reactive zone.
         (c) Wide excision: done en bloc through normal tissue beyond the reactive zone but within the compartment of origin, leaving in situ some portion of the compartment.
         (d) Radical resection: done en bloc of the lesion and entire compartment of origin, leaving no remnant of the compartment of origin.
         (e) Rotationplasty: modified amputation done usually on a skeletally immature child with a malignant tumor near the knee (distal femur or proximal tibia).
            i. It is done due to the tumor's proximity to the growth plate.
            ii. The procedure involves removing the knee joint and tumor, turning the distal portion of the lower leg 180 degrees and attaching the remaining tibia and foot to the distal portion of the remaining femur.
            iii. The ankle joint becomes the new knee joint and the patient will function as a below-the-knee amputee with a special prosthesis.
            iv. Before this technique was developed a child's only option for treatment for a tumor around the knee was an above knee amputation.
   b. Surgical treatment for sarcoma may be combined with:
      (1) Preoperative and/or postoperative chemotherapy.
      (2) And/or radiation therapy.
   c. Bony defects resulting from surgery are replaced with:
      (1) Metal implants.
      (2) Allografts with internal fixation.
      (3) Allografts with metal implant combination alloprosthesis.
      (4) Autografts, such as vascularized or nonvascularized fibular grafts.
   d. Skin or muscle deficits may be covered with:
      (1) Split thickness skin grafts.
      (2) Vascularized or nonvascularized myocutaneous flaps (local or free).
   e. Some benign bone lesions may be:
      (1) Curetted and frozen with liquid nitrogen (known as cryotherapy).
      (2) Painted in the cavity with phenol after the lesion has been removed.
      (3) Both phenol and cryotherapy induce further bone tissue necrosis decreasing the chance of local recurrence.
      (4) Lesions are permanently filled with bone graft (synthetic or autograft).
      (5) Occasionally bone cement (methylmethacrylate) is used to fill the defect, however detection of recurrence is more difficult when bone cement is used.
2. Indications.
   a. Tumors can be totally removed with margins (both grossly and microscopically) tumor-free.
   b. Neurovascular bundle uninvolved.
   c. Skeletal development nearly complete to minimize leg-length discrepancy.
3. Materials for reconstruction.
   a. Allograft:
      (1) Cadaveric human bone transplant to replace resected bone.
         (a) Donor must have no history of infection, cancer, hepatitis, or HIV.
         (b) Allograft is stored in -80 degree Celsius deep-freezer and has negative 10-day cultures. Freezing minimizes immunogenicity so tissue typing or immunosuppressive drugs are not needed.
      (2) Rigid internal fixation is needed and patients are non-weight bearing for 6-12 months.
      (3) Healing by creeping substitution is a slow process whereby cadaver bone is replaced by the patient's own bone, at least at the junction between the patient's bone and the allograft.
      (4) The allograft can be ordered with or without soft tissue attachments (tendons and ligaments). It is called an OA or osteoarticular graft if ordered with the soft tissue attachments.
      (5) Irradiated freeze-dried tissue (allograft) is also available to fill cavities left by small lesions, usually benign.
   b. Autograft:

(1) Replaces resected bone with patients own bone from sites such as iliac crest, fibula, or rib; may be vascularized or nonvascularized fibular graft.
(2) Optimal material, however it is another surgical incision and it is usually very painful.

c. Metallic prosthesis:
(1) May replace joint as well as large part of the shaft of the bone, or the entire bone such as a total femur replacement.
(2) Can be off-the-shelf prosthesis or custom made.

d. Alloprosthesis: combination of metal prosthesis and cadaveric allograft.

5. Resections by site.

a. Upper arm: wide excision or radical resection of tumor within the biceps brachialis, coracobrachialis (anterior), or triceps (posterior).

b. Proximal humerus: wide excision of tumor within humerus with total shoulder replacement or proximal humeral replacement, proximal allograft, or alloprosthesis.

c. Proximal humerus, glenoid (shoulder joint), distal clavicle:
(1) Modified Tikhoff-Lindberg procedure is a wide excision or radical resection of scapula, proximal humerus, distal clavicle, acromion, glenoid cavity, deltoid muscle; attach remaining humerus to clavicle with metal rod and/or Dacron® graft and/or allograft bone.
(2) Flail shoulder results and radial nerve palsy (nerve sacrificed) usually occur.
(3) Hand and elbow are usually functional.

d. Midshaft humerus: wide excision of tumor within humerus with allograft or autograft using vascularized or nonvascularized fibula.

e. Scapula: marginal or wide excision of scapula, or modified Tikhoff-Lindberg procedure or custom total scapular replacement.

f. Ilium, with or without soft tissue component: marginal or wide excision of ilium with or without surrounding soft tissue. In certain cases, femoral head will create a pseudoarthrosis.

g. Acetabulum and medial wall of pelvis, or wide excision of acetabulum, medial wall pelvis, femur; surrounding tissues fuse femur to ilium or ischium using internal fixation. A custom fit pelvic allograft or prosthesis using internal fixation can be inserted (not common due to high risk of failure due to infection).

h. Pubis, ischium, and ischial tuberosity: wide excision of pubis, ischium, and ischial tuberosity.

i. Upper leg/thigh (soft tissue): wide excision or radical resection of quadriceps (with or without femoral nerve) anteriorly, hamstrings (with or without sciatic nerve) posteriorly; adductor compartment medially.

j. Groin (soft tissue): wide excision of femoral triangle with sacrifice of femoral nerve, artery, vein, and inguinal lymph nodes; with possible reconstruction by arterial graft and hamstring transfer.

k. Proximal femur: wide excision or radical resection of proximal femur, reconstruction using proximal femoral replacement prosthesis, total or hemi-joint replacement, or alloprosthesis.

l. Midshaft femur: wide excision with allograft, metal intercalary replacement, or total metal femur replacement.

m. Distal femur:
(1) Wide excision with long stem distal femoral replacement prosthesis with or without proximal tibial prosthetic component, allograft or combination of both, alloprosthesis.
(2) Peroneal nerve may be sacrificed if the popliteal space is involved therefore an ankle foot orthosis will be needed. Some surgeons prefer to perform knee joint arthrodesis using allograft, however patient satisfaction long term is low due to inability to bend knee.

n. Lower leg/calf (soft tissue): wide excision or radical resection of lateral or medial gastrocnemius.

o. Proximal tibia:
(1) Wide excision with proximal tibial/knee replacement, allograft, or combination of both.
(2) Peroneal nerve may be sacrificed if the popliteal space is involved and an ankle/foot orthosis is needed.
(3) Some surgeons prefer to perform knee joint arthrodesis with allograft (see discussion above, m. Distal femur).

p. Midshaft tibia: wide excision with fibular autograft or allograft (vascularized or nonvascularized).

q. Spine: laminectomy with or without internal fixation, rods, and/or bone graft (either allograft or autograft).

C. Amputation.

1. Definition:
a. The removal of part of a limb above, below, or through a joint.
b. Used in the treatment of sarcomas when limb-sparing surgery cannot be performed.

2. Indications.
a. Inability to attain adequate surgical margins for a limb-sparing surgery.
b. Neurovascular bundle involved by tumor.
c. Young child with tumor who would have limb-length discrepancy due to limb salvages.

3. Amputation levels.
a. Symes (just proximal to the ankle).
b. Below the knee (BK).
c. Knee disarticulation (KD).
d. Above knee (AK).
e. Hip disarticulation (HD).

f. Hemipelvectomy (HP).
g. Hemicorpectomy.
h. Below elbow (BE).
i. Above elbow (AE).
j. Shoulder disarticulation (SD).
k. Forequarter amputation.
l. Rotationplasty (see Rotationplasty under Limb Sparing).

4. Potential problems/complications.
a. Flexion contractures.
b. Pressure sore on distal stump from prosthesis.
c. Neuroma at site of amputated nerve.
d. Wound dehiscence or infection.
e. Excessive swelling at stump due to improper stump wrapping or not wearing stump sock.
f. Phantom sensation/pain.
g. Bone overgrowth, especially in children.

D. Radiotherapy.

1. The use of radiation therapy has shown to decrease the chance of local recurrence in some sarcomas that are radioreceptive.
2. Radiation therapy may interfere with tissue healing, cause joint fibrosis, edema, cessation of growth of extremity due to injury to physis, and permanent bone healing problems. However, these risks are reduced with appropriate planning.
3. The use of radiation has not shown significantly to increase overall survival however, retrospective studies show improved overall survival with local control of the sarcoma.
a. Adjuvant bone.
(1) Effective in small, round-cell tumors, such as Ewing's sarcoma, and for lymphoma.
(2) Not effective for spindle cell sarcomas, such as osteosarcoma or chondrosarcoma.
b. Palliative bone.
(1) Objective: pain relief for metastatic bone disease and improved quality of life.
(2) Dose: range from single dose of 8 Gray (Gy) to 40.5 Gy in 15 fractions (treatments).
(3) Pathologic fractures are irradiated after internal fixation to destroy tumor growth and improve pain control, therefore increasing mobility and function for the patient.
c. Adjuvant soft tissue.
(1) Administered preoperatively, postoperatively, or both depending on size of tumor or close margins upon removing tumor (margin is area surrounding tumor).
(2) Intraoperatively to minimize injury to tissues and structures in close proximity, such as bowel or a joint. Must have IORT (intraoperative radiation therapy) suite available in the hospital setting.
d. Brachytherapy.
(1) Interstitial radiation therapy via iridium.
(2) Catheters inserted intraoperatively, if margins are not expected to be tumor-free or to decrease chance of local recurrence.
(3) The patient's catheters are loaded 3-5 days postoperatively.
(4) Treatment continues for 3-5 days while patient is kept in a lead-lined room with minimal exposure to staff and family.
(5) The implants and catheters are removed after the specified dose of radiation has been administered.
e. Neutron beam therapy.
(1) Radiation produced by heavy particle accelerators.
(2) Used in non-resectable tumor (sacrum or vertebrae).

E. Chemotherapy.

1. Rationale for combination chemotherapy: many cytotoxic drugs have synergistic effects when administered together, and a combination of cell-cycle specific and nonspecific drugs has been demonstrated to have the greatest antineoplastic effect.
2. Rationale for preoperative chemotherapy (neo-adjuvant).
a. To shrink the primary tumor, facilitating en bloc resection.
b. To destroy pulmonary micrometastases, or shrink pulmonary macrometastases.
c. To evaluate the efficacy of the cytotoxic drugs given in the preoperative period.
3. Rationale for postoperative chemotherapy in the absence of documented metastatic disease (known as prophylactic or adjuvant chemotherapy).
a. Malignant cells theoretically have entered the bloodstream before surgery and possibly during manipulation of the tumor at the time of surgery.
b. These cells then travel to other parts of the body at a later date, and metastatic disease would appear.
4. Chemotherapy agents for sarcomas.
a. Chemotherapy for sarcomas is continually being evaluated by standardized protocols in the attempt to find the best combination of drugs.
(1) Chemotherapy regimens for bone sarcomas such as osteosarcoma, Ewing's sarcoma and malignant fibrous histiocytoma, have shown to be effective.
(2) For high-grade soft tissue sarcomas in young adults and children (rhabdomyosarcoma, extraosseous Ewing's sarcoma), chemotherapy plays a major role.
(3) However, in the majority of adult soft tissue sarcomas, chemotherapy has shown no increase in the cure rate.
b. Common drugs currently used in standardized protocols are as follows:
(1) Methotrexate.
(2) Cisplatin.
(3) Ifosfamide.
(4) Dactinomycin.

(5) Cytoxin.
(6) Doxorubicin.
(7) Dacarbazine (DTIC).
(8) Mitomycin C.
(9) Etoposide (VP-16).
(10) Vinblastine.
(11) Vincristine.
(12) Leucovorin.
(13) Mesna.

5. Interferon has not been found to be effective at this time.
6. Routes of administration.
   a. Oral, intravenous bolus (push) or drip, or intra-arterial.
   b. Various venous access devices are available to prevent loss of veins from irritating chemotherapy and to permit prolonged administration of vesicant drugs. Either external venous catheter or an implanted subcutaneous port are used.
   c. Multi-day infusions of some drugs can be administered via an external pump as an outpatient.
   d. Arterial infusions of chemotherapy, while not common, are facilitated by placement of arterial ports.
7. Many of the side effects of chemotherapy can be controlled by good assessment skills and preplanning by the nurses.
   a. Common side effects such as nausea and vomiting have decreased, especially with the advent of newer antiemetics such as Zofran® (ondansetron).
   b. Patients may also be premedicated with dexamethasone, diphenhydramine, lorazepam, metoclopramide, and haloperidol but must be monitored closely for sedation, extrapyramidal reactions, anxiety, and diarrhea.
8. Common side effects.
   a. Alopecia and skin changes.
   b. Aches and pains.
   c. Anorexia.
   d. Constipation and/or diarrhea.
   e. Cystitis.
   f. Stomatitis.
   g. Fatigue.
   h. Depression.
   i. Hematopoietic changes (neutropenia, leukopenia, thrombocytopenia).
   j. Toxicities (cardiac, renal, hepatic, oto, neuro, and pulmonary).
   k. Reproductive system dysfunction.
   l. Metabolic alterations.

IV. NURSING DIAGNOSES, OUTCOMES, AND INTERVENTIONS

A. See Table 15.1.

B. Knowledge, deficient.

1. Outcome: verbalizes understanding of disease and treatments.
2. Interventions.
   a. Answer patient questions.
   b. Be aware for opportunities for increasing patient's knowledge by:
      (1) Verbalizes a deficiency in knowledge or skill/request for information.
      (2) Expresses "inaccurate" perception of health status.
      (3) Does not perform correctly a desired or prescribed health behavior.
   c. Explain disease process.
   d. Explain treatment methods.
      (1) Chemotherapy.
      (2) Radiation.
      (3) Surgery.
   e. Explain resection with reconstructions and durability.
      (1) Allograft.
      (2) Implant.
      (3) Arthroplasty.
      (4) Arthrodesis.
   f. Explain amputation and offer option of meeting amputee.

C. Pain, acute.
Pain, chronic.

1. Outcome: verbalizes pain relief.
2. Interventions.
   a. Assess the patient's pain experience; determine the intensity of the pain at its worst and best.
   b. Assess for factors that decrease pain tolerance.
   c. Reduce or eliminate (when possible) factors that increase pain experience.
   d. Assess the effects of chronic pain on the individual's life, using the person and family.
   e. Collaborate with individual to determine what methods could be used to reduce the intensity of the pain.
   f. Provide for optimal pain relief with prescribed medications and other nonpharmacologic pain relievers.
   g. Reduce or eliminate common side-effects of narcotics.
   h. Promote optimal mobility, with assistive devices as needed.
   i. Assist the family to respond optimally to the individual's pain experience.

D. Decreased cardiac output.

1. Outcome: hemaglobin above 8 gms and no signs and symptoms of fainting or fatigue.
2. Interventions.
   a. Monitor CBC and vital signs.
   b. Monitor blood loss intraoperatively and into drain.
   c. Administer iron/blood transfusions, as needed.

E. Tissue integrity, impaired.
Skin integrity, impaired.

1. Outcome: wound intact.
2. Interventions.
   a. Monitor wounds for drainage, erythema, and tenderness.
   b. Monitor temperature.

Table 15.1
Common Nursing Diagnoses, Outcomes, and Interventions for Patients with Tumors of Bone or Soft Tissue

Diagnoses	Outcomes	Interventions
A. Knowledge, deficient 1. Preoperative procedures and evaluation. 2. Diagnosis and definition of tumor type. 3. Tumor stage: localized versus metastatic; aggressive or slow growing. 4. Surgery goals, procedure, pertinent intra-operative aspects. 5. Expected results post-operatively related to function, sensation, tumor control. 6. Potential complications: infection, deep vein thrombosis, delayed wound healing, prosthetic loosening or dislocation, nonunion of bone graft, etc. 7. Further planned treatments: reconstructive surgery, chemotherapy or radiation therapy, physical and occupational therapy. Discharge plans, long-term follow up, and home care.	• Patient has knowledge of diagnosis, procedures, and treatments. • Patient asks questions freely.	• Assess knowledge base and provide patient teaching. 1. Describe diagnostic test/procedure, purpose, adverse effects. 2. Explain difference between benign and malignant tumors. Describe particular tumor type (bone, soft tissue, vascular, synovial, fatty, etc.) 3. Explain if disease is localized or metastatic; if it is a fast or slow growing tumor. 4. Through demonstration, graphic, model, or x-ray, explain the planned surgical procedure, including placement of incision(s), resection of skin, bones, muscles, nerves, and/or vessels. Explain what is to be replaced/reconstructed (muscle transfer, bone graft, total joint, internal fixation). Describe postoperative dressings, wound care, urinary catheter, etc. 5. Describe expected results: decrease in motion (flexion, extension, etc.), decrease in strength, numbness over incision or other areas where sensory nerves are cut, local control of tumor, change in contour of body part if large muscle resection. 6. Explain or reinforce physician's explanation of potential complications, including infection, deep vein thrombosis, delayed wound healing, etc. Observe and monitor patient for adverse signs/symptoms of complications. 7. Educate and review purpose, mechanism of action, expected outcomes, and side effects of chemotherapy or radiation therapy. 8. Coordinate discharge planning. a. List schedule of follow-up appointments with surgeon(s), oncologist, and/or nurse. b. Explain need for close observation for the next 5 years (to check for local recurrence and metastasis). c. Inform patient that periodic x-rays or scans may be done to help with this detection. d. Assure that patient comprehends and is able to demonstrate home-going physical and occupational therapy programs. e. Teach patient signs and symptoms of complications and provide phone number to call if they occur. f. Instruct patient/significant others with any dressing changes or precautions specific to the surgery. g. Arrange for Visiting Nurse Service (VNS) or other home care personnel (American Cancer Society or local agencies), nurses, aides, and special equipment - hospital bed, commode, reclining wheelchair, etc.

Table 15.1 (continued)
Common Nursing Diagnoses, Outcomes, and Interventions for Patients with Tumors of Bone or Soft Tissue

Diagnoses	Outcomes	Interventions
B. Physical mobility, impaired 1. Disease process (mass invading muscle, tendon, bone, fat, skin, joint). 2. Decreased range of motion. 3. Postoperative impairment due to resection, pain.	• Patient ambulates independently with or without ambulatory devices unless bed rest is necessitated by nature of surgical procedure.	• Assist with physical therapy. 1. Instruct and reinforce exercises for range of motion and strengthening of operative extremity and unaffected limbs for general conditioning. Exercises and strengthening of affected extremity may need to be delayed to permit scarring down of reattached muscle groups. 2. Instruct with crutches or walker for ambulation and transfer techniques. 3. Provide and instruct with use of arm sling, splint, or immobilizer for upper extremity surgery; patient may be restricted to avoid abduction for about 6-8 weeks. 4. Support surgical leg during transfers. Patient may need immobilizer or orthosis if a large muscle resection has been done, such as a radical resection of the quadriceps. Prepare patient for vascular engorgement that occurs when limb is placed in a dependent position after prolonged elevation. 5. For total hip/proximal femoral joint replacements, instruct with precautions to prevent dislocation (see Chapter 12, Arthritis and Connective Tissue Disorders: Osteoarthritis).
C. Pain 1. Disease process (tumor invading nerves or vessels, pressure sensation). 2. Postoperative pain. 3. Neurologic trauma. 4. Phantom limb sensation/ pain following amputation.	• Patient verbalizes decreased or relieved pain.	• Promote comfort. 1. Assist with positioning for comfort. 2. Provide analgesics as ordered. 3. Employ therapeutic touch and relaxation techniques to promote comfort. 4. See Chapter 7, Pain.
D. Self-care deficit syndrome 1. Disease process and loss of function resulting from surgical resections. 2. Range of motion restriction. 3. Limp, pain, weakness.	• Patient participates in self-care activities.	• Assist with occupational therapy. 1. Instruct patient with self-care techniques in relationship to ADL. 2. For upper extremity surgery: assist with passive range of motion to arm and axilla; arrange food tray and bed/nightstand on unaffected side. 3. Assist patient having resection of ilium with alteration in clothing, if necessary. 4. Assess layout of home: stairs, support devices (rails) in regard to promoting safety.
E. Coping, ineffective; family coping, compromised 1. Newly diagnosed tumor. 2. Fear of unknown. 3. Expected/real loss of body part. 4. Inadequate support systems. 5. Inadequate or ineffective coping mechanisms. 6. Isolation while afterloaded radiation catheters are in place.	• Patient/significant others use positive coping mechanisms to deal with disease process/ body image.	• Assist with coping. 1. Discuss preoperatively expected loss or alteration of contour of body part; encourage expression of feelings regarding self-concept and body image; discuss ways to enhance appearance; stress the importance of a tumor cure vs. alteration in body part. Discuss radiation safety principles when implant used, time vs. distance; reassure patient that nursing staff is available and good care will be provided. 2. Assess behavioral changes: encourage patient participation in self-care; help patient identify positive changes in progress.

Table 15.1 (continued)
Common Nursing Diagnoses, Outcomes, and Interventions for Patients with Tumors of Bone or Soft Tissue

Diagnoses	Outcomes	Interventions
E. Coping, ineffective; family coping, compromised	• Patient/significant others use positive coping mechanisms to deal with disease process/ body image.	3. Allow time for patient and significant others to vent feelings of despair, shock, and grief over the diagnosis; consult with a social worker to assist with effective coping mechanisms. 4. Acknowledge independency vs. dependency issues as patient is often an adolescent attempt- to assert independence.
F. Sexuality pattern, ineffective 1. Sterility from chemo- therapy. 2. Alteration in self- concept.	• Patient/significant others find means to express sexuality.	• Provide time for patient to discuss issues relating to the impact of the diagnosis and treatment on self- concept and sexuality. 1. Use open-ended statement such as "How has your illness affected your relationship with your spouse, friend, etc.?" to elicit information. 2. Initiate referrals to other health care workers as appropriate.
G. Skin integrity, impaired 1. Large incision. 2. Multiple incisions. 3. Devascularization of skin from muscle resection. 4. Prolonged operating time. 5. Bed rest after plastic reconstructive surgery. 6. Compromised nutri- tional status.	• Patient's skin integrity remains intact: patient tolerates diet and main- tains determined body weight.	• Maintain skin integrity. 1. Assess skin preoperatively for baseline status. 2. Observe wound/incision for erythema, approxi- mation of skin edges, drainage, dehiscence, tenderness, scaling (especially if patient has received chemotherapy or radiation therapy preoperatively). 3. Prevent pressure on bony prominences (sacrum, heels, elbows, ischial tuberosity); apply heel cups, protectors. 4. Apply water, air, or flotation mattress to bed; turn and position. 5. Using sterile technique, cleanse wound and change dressing daily. 6. Observe orders by plastic surgery regarding care of skin grafts or muscle flaps; skin grafts are often covered with vapor permeable barrier, do- nor site often covered with prescribed dressing. 7. Closed wound drainage system remains in place until there is less than 30 cc per day; record drainage accurately. 8. Expose wound to air after drainage is complet- ed and skin grafts and flaps have adhered and healed. 9. Instruct patient that areas having skin grafts should not be exposed to sun. 10. Provide diet high in protein and calories to main- tain patient in anabolic state which promotes healing.
H. Anxiety **Grieving** 1. Anxiety/depression. a. Potential terminal illness. b. Lengthy hospital stay. c. Chronic pain. d. Extended treatments.	• Patient verbalizes feelings freely.	• Support patient during grieving and help alleviate anxiety. 1. Control disruptions in interpersonal relationships with significant others and physicians. 2. Teach the patient about changes in condition to be aware of; signs of progression or wellness. 3. Provide verbal realistic reassurances for the future.

Table 15.1 (continued)
Common Nursing Diagnoses, Outcomes, and Interventions for Patients with Tumors of Bone or Soft Tissue

Diagnoses	Outcomes	Interventions
2. Grieving. a. Loss of limb. b. Alterations in functional ability. c. Changes in body image as a result of surgery and chemotherapy.	• Patient/significant others have adequate support throughout grieving process.	4. Offer choices in regard to decision making (timing of bath, physical therapy, etc.) 5. Begin discharge planning early, involving patient and significant others so that confidence is built upon well thought-out plans. 6. Assist patient/significant others through grieving process.
I. Potential physiologic/ psychologic complications at time of: 1. Chemotherapy. 2. Biopsy. 3. Amputation. 4. Limb salvage.	• Patient has minimal side effects from chemotherapy.	• Provide nursing care for patients receiving chemotherapy. 1. Assure that informed consent is obtained before protocol is implemented. 2. Prevent/assist with treatment of effects (see Common Therapeutic Modalities for specific drugs and their side effects). 3. Administer antiemetics prechemotherapy, intrachemotherapy, and postchemotherapy as ordered. 4. Use relaxation techniques, including hypnosis and guided imagery, to thwart some GI toxicity. 5. Teach patient proper oral hygiene techniques and use of antifungal/antibiotic mouthwashes and topical anesthetics to minimize the complications and discomfort of stomatitis. Avoid commercial mouth preparations that contain alcohol. 6. Teach patient to avoid crowds and children who are ill when WBC count low. 7. Assist with transfusion of blood products as ordered. Monitor for side effects of transfusion; follow protocol for transfusion reactions. 8. Check results of all laboratory work, including WBC, RBC, BUN, and creatinine to detect abnormalities that may necessitate a change in treatment plans. 9. Assist with urine collections for creatinine clearance before administration of nephrotoxic drugs. 10. Assure patient is well hydrated and administer diuretics as ordered to help flush kidneys for nephrotoxic drugs. 11. Teach patient to avoid sun exposure as appropriate. 12. Administer stool softeners prophylactically as ordered to prevent paralytic ileus. 13. Awaken patient during night to void after nephrotoxic drug administration so metabolites do not remain in the bladder for long periods of time. 14. Monitor cardiac status closely with cardiotoxic drug administration. 15. If the patient is scheduled for procedure, notify anesthesiologist if patient has received bleomycin in order to adjust the percentage of oxygen administered. 16. Counsel patient regarding sperm banking as appropriate. 17. Provide birth control information to sexually active patients receiving teratogenic drugs. 18. Assist with auditory testing/assess for hearing loss in patients receiving ototoxic drugs.

Table 15.1 (continued)
Common Nursing Diagnoses, Outcomes, and Interventions for Patients with Tumors of Bone or Soft Tissue

Diagnoses	Outcomes	Interventions
I. Potential physiologic/ psychologic complications at time of: 1. Chemotherapy. 2. Biopsy. 3. Amputation. 4. Limb salvage. (continued)	• Patient will have knowledge of biopsy procedures and results. • Patient demonstrates appropriate protective measures to prevent fractures following biopsy.	• Provide nursing care for patient undergoing biopsy. 1. Preoperative. a. Explain procedure, purpose, site of biopsy; explain time lag (1-3 days) between biopsy and diagnosis. b. Protect fragile lower extremity tumor site by using crutches/walker. 2. Intraoperative. a. Determine if diagnostic procedure only or frozen section diagnosis followed immediately by definitive procedure at same sitting. b. Local vs. general anesthesia. c. Determine if potentially vascular tumor; may use tourniquet for extremity or methyl methacrylate bone cement for bony biopsy. d. Assure proper labeling of pathology specimens. e. Culture tissue to rule out inflammatory process. f. Use separate table of instrumentation if definitive surgery is performed. Possibly the surgical team would rescrub. 3. Postoperative: protect extremities with use of crutches or walker if bone biopsy is done (to prevent fracture).
	• Patient demonstrates normal range of motion/alignment of proximal joint following amputation. 1. Patient's prosthesis is functional. 2. Patient is without skin breakdown following amputation.	• Provide nursing care for patients undergoing amputation. 1. Preoperative. a. Provide comfort measures including analgesics, assistive gait devices, arm slings, splints, and/or reposition extremity. b. Prevent pathologic fracture preoperatively by providing crutches, walker, or cane; instruct with non-weight-bearing status. Cast brace may be prescribed. c. Educate patient about procedure, expectations of phantom limb sensations and/or pain. 2. Intraoperative. a. Verify amputation permit, if needed. b. Elevate limb for exsanguination instead of using Esmarch bandage to decrease manipulation of tumor. c. Assure transport of limb to pathologist or funeral director as indicated preoperatively by the patient. d. May include immediate postoperative fitting of prosthesis/socket in surgery. 3. Postoperative. a. Prevent flexion contracture of proximal joint. (1) Do not place pillow under lower extremity (2) May place bed in Trendelenburg position and raise head of bed to neutral to decrease lower extremity edema. (3) Assist patient to lie prone t.i.d.

Table 15.1 (continued)
Common Nursing Diagnoses, Outcomes, and Interventions for Patients with Tumors of Bone or Soft Tissue

Diagnoses	Outcomes	Interventions
I. Potential physiologic/ psychologic complications at time of: 1. Chemotherapy. 2. Biopsy. 3. Amputation. 4. Limb salvage. (continued)		(4) Instruct patient with limb positioning maintaining leg in neutral rotation while lying, sitting, or ambulating. b. Assist physical therapist (PT) with gait instruction and compliance of exercises for balance, motion, and conditioning of unaffected limbs. c. For patients with hemipelvectomy. (1) Prevent contamination of incision from stool. (2) Provide support (pillow) for sitting to increase balance and comfort until sitting mold is made. d. Instruct patient and significant other with stump wrapping and/or use stump sock (hip spica wrap for hemipelvectomy and hip disarticulation patients). e. Make arrangements and prepare patient for prosthetic fitting (temporary/permanent). (1) When wound healing is demonstrated (5-7 days postoperatively), a plastic socket and pylon may be supplied. In some situations, pylons may be applied immediately postoperatively. (2) The permanent prosthesis fitting may be delayed until postoperative swelling has subsided and postoperative chemotherapy has been completed as stump size may fluctuate during this period. f. Assist with coping measures for patient and significant others concerning loss of limb. Consult with social service as appropriate. 4. Assist patient with coping with phantom limb sensation/pain. a. Differentiate sensation (numbness, tingling) from pain (burning, knife-like, sharp sensations). b. Educate patient as to cause: abnormal firing originating in spinal or other central neurons, after neurons have lost their normal input from the periphery. c. Most intense in distal parts of extremity hand or foot. Limb may assume an uncharacteristic position (leg is bent and pushing through the mattress of the bed). d. Assist patient to differentiate phantom pain from incisional or stump pain. e. See Chapter 7, Pain.
	• Patient has functional ability of limb following salvage procedure.	• Provide nursing care for the patient undergoing limb salvage/limb-sparing procedure. 1. Preoperative. a. Provide comfort measures. b. Educate patient about procedure and expected functional abilities. 2. Intraoperative. a. Assure proper labeling of biopsy sites and specimens. Ascertain if tumor margins are to be checked.

Table 15.1 (continued)
Common Nursing Diagnoses, Outcomes, and Interventions for Patients with Tumors of Bone or Soft Tissue

Diagnoses	Outcomes	Interventions
I. Potential physiologic/ psychologic complications at time of: 1. Chemotherapy. 2. Biopsy. 3. Amputation. 4. Limb salvage. (continued)	• Patient has functional ability of limb following salvage procedure.	b. Provide extra vessel clamps, ties, suture, hemaclips if tumor is vascular. c. Provide sterile tourniquet, special order/custom-made total joint replacements; liquid nitrogen and equipment; allografts with internal fixation as required. d. Verify if plastic surgery will be needed. Provide proper instrumentation and microscope as needed. e. Prevent excessive manipulation of tumor in surgery. Gentle skin prep with scrub; elevate limb for exsanguination instead of using Esmarch bandage. f. If biopsy or bone graft are to be done at same time, use separate table of instruments (so as not to seed tumor into donor bone graft site). g. Assure communication of procedure to other personnel. For example, significant changes in neurovascular status may be a result of surgical procedure. h. Consent should indicate permission for amputation in case en bloc resection is found to be technically unfeasible. i. Maintain use of laminar air flow for bony procedures. 3. Postoperative. a. For resections of acetabulum/medial wall pelvis/proximal femur with fusion to ilium or ischium. (1) Hip spica may be applied to promote fusion. (2) See Chapter 10, Therapeutic Modalities: Casts. b. For resection of pubis, ischium, ischial tuberosity. (1) Promote comfort while sitting by providing support for the affected area. (2) Maintain leg of operative side in abduction to prevent adduction contracture. (3) Prevent contamination of wound from urine or stool.
J. See Chapter 5, Perioperative Patient Care.		

F. **Coping, ineffective.**
1. Outcome: remains functional and verbalizes concerns and fear related to amputation, hair loss, and the cancer diagnosis.
2. Interventions.
   a. Encourage patient to verbalize concerns and fears.
   b. Allow patient to make decisions whenever feasible.
   c. Involve psychologist/chaplain, as needed.

G. **Grieving, anticipatory.**
1. Outcomes: remains functional and verbalizes end of life desires.
2. Interventions.
   a. Discuss patients desires regarding living will and end of life treatments.
   b. Encourage patient to verbalize concerns and fears.
   c. Involve psychologist/chaplain, as needed.
   d. Assist the patient and family in identifying strengths.
   e. Support patient and family with grief reactions.
   f. Promote family cohesiveness.
   g. Promote grief work.
   h. Provide for expression of grief.

H. **Powerlessness.**
1. Outcomes: remains functional and verbalize concerns and fears.
2. Interventions.
   a. Eliminate or reduce contributing factors.
      (1) Increase effective communication between patient and health care providers.
      (2) Explain all procedures and options.
      (3) Allow time to answer questions.
      (4) Keep the patient informed about scheduled events/activities.
      (5) Anticipate questions/interest and offer information.
      (6) Be an active listener by allowing the patient to verbalize concerns and feelings.
   b. Provide opportunities for individual to control decisions.
      (1) Allow person to manipulate surroundings such as deciding what is to be kept where (personal items).
      (2) Keep needed items within reach (call bell, tissue, etc.)
      (3) Keep promises.
      (4) Provide opportunities for person and family to participate in care.
   c. Assist client in deriving power from other sources.
      (1) Self-help groups.
      (2) Support groups.
      (3) Offer referral to religious leader.

I. **Caregiver role strain.**
1. Outcomes:
   a. Caregiver verbalizes fears and concerns and remains able to manage the home situation.
   b. Caregiver will share frustrations regarding caregiving responsibilities.
2. Interventions.
   a. Assess for causative or contributing factors.
      (1) Poor insight.
      (2) Unrealistic expectations.
      (3) Reluctance or inability to access help.
      (4) Insufficient resources (physical and emotional help, financial help).
      (5) Social isolation and/or insufficient leisure.
      (6) Competing roles (spouse, work, caregiver).
   b. Encourage caregiver to verbalize fears and concerns.
   c. Promote realistic appraisal of the situation.
   d. Promote insight into the situation.
   e. Provide empathy and promote a sense of competency.
   f. Assist in identifying where assistance is desired.
   g. Engage the family (separate from caregiver) in appraisal of situation.
   h. Role play how to ask for help with activities identified.
   i. Offer hospice nursing, if appropriate.
   j. Involve social worker as needed for home care needs.
   k. Involve chaplain/psychologist for spiritual and emotional care as needed.

J. **Spiritual distress.**
1. Outcomes: patient able to verbalize less fear and anxiety regarding impending death.
2. Interventions.
   a. Assess for causative and contributory factors.
      (1) Failure of spiritual beliefs to provide explanation/comfort during crisis of illness/suffering/impending death.
      (2) Doubting quality or strength of own faith to deal with current crisis.
      (3) Anger toward God/spiritual beliefs for allowing/causing illness/suffering/death.
   b. Encourage patient to verbalize fears and concerns.
   c. Involve chaplain services as needed.
   d. Discuss patients wishes regarding living will.

BONE METASTASIS

I. OVERVIEW

A. Definition/pathophysiology/incidence/etiology.
1. Bone metastasis represents one of the most frequent and most debilitating sequelae of malignancy and occurs as a result of the spread of malignant cells beyond their primary site of origin.
   a. Sarcomas primarily spread to the lungs and rarely to another bone or soft tissue site.
   b. Carcinomas, however, frequently spread to the bone.
   c. The most common sites and tumors are presented later in this chapter.
2. Bone metastasis occurs by three routes:
   a. Direct extension involves spread from a local

tumor, such as with multiple myeloma, which arises in the marrow cavity and invades the outer bone.
   b. Hematogenous extension is the most common route of spread and results from seeding of micrometastases through the bloodstream.
   c. Lymphatic dissemination (breast carcinoma).
3. Bone metastasis is manifested by two types of lesions characterized by the type of bone cell that is affected.
   a. Lytic lesions occur as a result of increased osteoclastic activity and bone resorption or lysis incited by tumor cells. Bone destruction predominates (as in breast carcinoma).
   b. Blastic lesions are a result of a process similar to callus formation after a fracture in normal bone.
      (1) Tumor activity evokes a protective response by increased blastic activity in which there is "reactive" bone formation.
      (2) Spontaneous or pathologic fracture is less likely to occur than with lytic lesions in which minor stresses can result in fracture (as in prostate carcinoma).
4. Sites of occurrence.
   a. Thorax and vertebrae 50%.
   b. Extremities 34%.
   c. Skull 22%.
5. Most common primary tumors.
   a. Breast.
   b. Prostate.
   c. Lung.
   d. Kidney.
   e. Thyroid.
   f. Bladder.
6. Complications.
   a. Pathologic fracture: fracture resulting from a weakness in the bone due to advanced metastatic disease.
   b. Impending pathologic fracture:
      (1) Condition in which a lesion has destroyed at least 50% of the bone over 2.5 cm in diameter.
      (2) Prophylactic internal fixation is advocated to prevent pathologic fracture and/or relieve pain.

II. ASSESSMENT

A. History and physical examination.

1. Bone pain suggestive if the patient has a history of a bone-seeking tumor, such as breast or prostate.
2. Localized pain hyper-reflexia, gait abnormality, loss of bowel/bladder control.
3. Radicular pain, paresthesias, indicative of vertebral collapse and/or tumor pressure on the spinal cord.
4. Signs of extremity or vertebral fracture. (See Chapter 14, Trauma [Fractures]).

B. Diagnostic tests.

1. Metabolic disturbances, such as hypercalcemia, may be the presenting symptoms.
2. X-ray.
3. Bone scan reveals involved bones.
4. Alkaline phosphatase elevated with increased osteoblastic activity.
5. Biopsy to confirm diagnosis. Monostotic lesion rarely seen.

III. COMMON THERAPEUTIC MODALITIES

A. Overall treatment goals.

1. Halt disease progression.
2. Relieve pain.
3. Prevent pathologic fractures.
4. Prevent metabolic or hematologic complications.

B. Chemotherapy: appropriate cytotoxic agents for the primary tumor type.

C. Radiotherapy promotes rapid destruction of tumor cells followed by bone healing and recalcification in 3-4 months and provides relief of pain.

D. Surgery.

1. Prophylactic fixation to prevent pathologic fracture especially of weight-bearing areas, such as femur. Often with intramedullary rod or internal fixation.
2. Fracture treatment may involve use of intramedullary rods, pins, and plates as well as the use of methylmethacrylate to replace larger segments of diseased bone.
3. Spine.
   a. Determine presence or absence of cord compression and stable or unstable spine.
   b. High dose steroid therapy for acute edema.
   c. Treatment options.
      (1) Asymptomatic: systemic chemotherapy or hormonal therapy.
      (2) Compression fractures or painful lesion: steroid therapy, radiation therapy, and brace if minimal subluxation.
      (3) Traction (halo apparatus) may be needed with marked subluxation.
      (4) Lower thoracic and upper lumbar fracture/dislocation:
         (a) Operative stabilization with metal.
         (b) Methylmethacrylate.
         (c) Autogenous bone.
         (d) Allograft.
      (5) Cord compression:
         (a) Radiotherapy.
         (b) Surgical decompression with stabilization.
         (c) Anterior and/or posterior approach depending upon the site of the tumor fixation with metal,
         (d) Methylmethacrylate.
         (e) Fibular strut autologous bone.
         (f) Allograft.
4. Solitary metastasis treatment options.
   a. Excise lesion.
   b. Internal fixation with intramedullary rods or internal fixation and/or methylmethacrylate.
   c. Endoprosthesis for head, neck, or intertrochanteric fractures of the femoral or humeral head.

d. Total hip, shoulder, or knee replacement.

E. Analgesics: see Chapter 7, Pain.

IV. NURSING DIAGNOSIS, OUTCOMES, AND INTERVENTIONS

A. See Table 15.1.

B. Injury, risk for.

1. Outcome: patient aware of method to prevent pathologic fracture.
2. Interventions.
    a. Note presence and size of lytic lesion on x-ray.
    b. Instruct patient in preventive measures.
        (1) Encourage activity which is not painful.
        (2) No heavy lifting.
        (3) No pushing, pulling, or twisting.
        (4) Keep environment safe.
    c. Evaluate for assistive devices.

C. Physical mobility, impaired.

1. Outcomes.
    a. Regain physical mobility post-pathological fracture.
    b. Neurovascular status remains intact with potential spinal cord compression.
2. Interventions.
    a. Interventions to regain physical mobility following a pathological fracture.
        (1) Monitor pain and response to pain control measures.
        (2) Assess neurovascular status (use dermatome if vertebrae involved).
        (3) Assess positioning and fit of immobilization devices.
        (4) Use logrolling and lift sheet.
        (5) Avoid using trapeze.
        (6) Utilize nursing interventions to decrease affects of immobility.
            (a) Skin assessment, decubitus prevention.
            (b) Pulmonary toilet.
            (c) Anti-constipation medication.
    b. Interventions to maintain neurovascular status with a potential spinal cord compression.
        (1) Monitor for weakness, paresthesia, paralysis, and bowel/bladder dysfunction.
        (2) Notify physician if any symptoms present.
        (3) Administer steroids as ordered.
        (4) Maintain bed rest

D. See Nursing Diagnoses, Outcomes, and Interventions for Primary Tumors of Bone and Soft Tissue, earlier in this chapter.

MULTIPLE MYELOMA

I. OVERVIEW

A. Definition.

1. Multiple myeloma is a malignancy of the plasma cells.
2. B cells proliferate and infiltrate the bone marrow, cause bone destruction and suppress normal hematopoeisis.

B. Pathophysiology.

1. The B cells produce high amounts of monoclonal "M" bands of immunoglobulins.
2. The myeloma cells are not effective in their immune function and also have an osteoclastic effect which may result in pathological fractures and hypercalcemia from increased bone resorption.

C. Incidence.

1. Accounts for approximately 1% of hematologic malignancies in the United States.
2. Multiple myeloma is a disease of middle age and elderly.

D. Etiology.

1. The cause of multiple myeloma is not understood.
2. Many factors such as age, race, environmental factors, occupational exposure and radiation are being investigated.
3. Also family history, alcohol and tobacco use, and immune disorders are being considered as risk factors for the disease.

E. Considerations across the lifespan.

1. A disease of the late middle age and elderly.
2. Can be treated and controlled but not cured.
3. May live several months to several years after diagnosis.

F. Complications.

1. Pain.
2. Pathological fractures.
3. Anemia.
4. Dehydration.
5. Hypercalcemia.
6. Fatigue.
7. Renal insufficiency.
8. Side effects from chemotherapy.

II. ASSESSMENT

A. History and physical examination: see Bone Metastasis in this chapter.

1. Bone pain with or without fracture.
2. Long bone fractures (see Bone Metastasis).

B. Diagnostic tests.

1. Anemia, weakness, infection, weight loss, mental status changes.
2. Bone marrow studies: plasma cell infiltration less than 10%.
3. Serum and urine electrophoresis: monoclonal spikes.
4. Bence-Jones protein in urine is positive.
5. Proteinuria, hypercalcuria with spinal cord compression or renal failure.
6. X-ray: multiple, lytic lesions, plasmacytomas.
7. MRI: used on select patients for more complete skeletal information.
8. Serum B2 macroglobulin is an important prognostic factor.

III. COMMON THERAPEUTIC MODALITIES

A. If the patient is asymptomatic frequent monitoring alone may be the initial treatment.

B. **Monitoring consists of lab work and radiographs. If progression of disease is noted, then there is further treatment with chemotherapy, radiation, and possibly surgery if an impending or pathological fracture is evident.**
   1. Chemotherapy: common drugs used include melphalan, prednisone, VAD (vincristine, doxorubicin, dexamethasone), and interferon-alpha.
   2. Radiotherapy (see Bone Metastasis).
   3. Surgery (see Bone Metastasis).

IV. NURSING DIAGNOSES, OUTCOMES, AND INTERVENTIONS

A. **See Table 15.1.**

B. **Infection, risk for.**
   1. Outcomes: patient will remain free of infection even with myelosuppression and abnormal immunoglobins.
   2. Interventions.
      a. Assess for high temperature, pulmonary congestion, skin breakdown
      b. Teach patient to avoid sources of infection: crowds, etc.
      c. Monitor lab values, especially CBC and differential.
      d. Ensure adequate hydration.
      e. Institute preventive measures for skin problems.
      f. Pulmonary toilet.

C. **Urinary elimination, impaired.**
   1. Outcomes: patient will develop no renal impairment due to increased protein catabolism and hypercalcemia.
   2. Interventions.
      a. Fluid management: force fluids to 2 liters per day to protect kidneys from hypercalcuria, Bence Jones protein, and increased uric acid.
      b. Monitor intake and output if renal insufficiency is present. Note: Patient may not be kept NPO without intravenous support.
      c. Allopurinol may be given to protect kidneys.
      d. Teach patient dietary restrictions, if ordered.
      e. Prompt treatment of hypercalcemia and urinary tract infections.
      f. Avoid nephrotoxic antibiotics and excessive nonsteroidal anti-inflammatory drugs (NSAIDs).
      g. Hypercalcemia management: see content on metabolic bone disorders.

D. **See Nursing Diagnoses for Primary Tumors of Bone and Soft Tissue earlier in this chapter.**

Bibliography

Carpenito, L.J. (1999). *Handbook of nursing diagnosis* (8th ed.). Philadelphia: Lippincott.

Dorfman, H., & Czerniak, B. (1998). *Bone tumors.* St. Louis: Mosby

Enneking, W. (1983). *Musculoskeletal tumor surgery.* New York: Churchill-Livingstone.

Enzinger, F., & Weiss, S. (1995). *Soft tissue tumors* (3rd ed.). St. Louis: Mosby.

Greenlee, R., Murray, T., Bolden, S., & Wingo, P. (2000). Cancer statistics, 2000. *CA - A Cancer Journal for Clinicians, 50*(1), 7-33.

Greenspan, A., & Remagen, W. (1998). *Differential diagnosis of tumors and tumor-like lesions of bones and joints.* Philadelphia: Lippincott-Raven.

Haynes, K. (1998). Neoplasms of the musculoskeletal system. In A. Maher, S. Salmond, & T. Pellino (Eds.), *Orthopaedic nursing.* (2nd ed., pp 769-803). Philadelphia: W.B. Saunders Company.

Huvos, A. (1991). *Bone tumors: Diagnosis, treatment, and prognosis* (2nd ed.). Philadelphia: W.B. Saunders Company.

Itano, J., & Taoka, K. (1998). *Core curriculum for oncology nursing* (3rd ed.). Philadelphia: W.B. Saunders Company.

Malpas, J., Bergsagel, D., Kyle, R., & Anderson, K. (1998). *Myeloma: Biology and management.* Oxford: Oxford University Press.

Mirra, J. (1989). *Bone tumors: Clinical, radiologic, and pathologic correlations.* Philadelphia: Lea & Febiger.

Otto, S. (1997). *Oncology nursing* (3rd ed.). St. Louis: Mosby.

Perez, C.A., & Brady, L.W. (1998). *Principles and practice of radiation oncology* (3rd ed.). Philadelphia: Lippincott-Raven.

Piasecki, P. (1996). Nursing care of the patient with metastatic bone disease. *Orthopaedic Nursing, 15*(4), 25-33.

Rubins, R.D., & Fogelmann, I. (1991). *Bone metastases: Diagnosis and treatment.* London: Springer-Verlag.

Schoen, D.C. (2000). Musculoskeletal pathology. In D.C. Schoen, *Adult orthopaedic nursing* (pp. 43-84). Philadelphia: Lippincott.

Simon, M., & Springfield, D. (1998). *Surgery for bone and soft-tissue tumors.* Philadelphia: Lippincott-Raven.

Theriault, R. (1993). Hypercalcemia of malignancy, pathophysiology, and implications for treatment. *Oncology, 7*(1), 47-55.

Yang, J.C. , Chang, A.E., Baker, A.R., Sindelar, W.F., Danforth, D.N., Topalian, S.L., DeLaney, T., Glatstein, E., Steinberg, S., Merino, M., & Rosenberg, S. (1998). Randomized prospective study of the benefit of adjuvent radiation therapy in the treatment of soft tissue sarcomas of the extremity. *Journal of Clinical Oncology, 16*(1), 197-202.

STUDY QUESTIONS

Becky, a 10-year-old, is found to have a painful mass in her right proximal tibia. Her orthopaedic surgeon tells her and her parents that he needs to do an open biopsy to rule out Ewing's sarcoma. (Questions 1-5)

1. Which of the following symptoms can be seen with Ewing's sarcoma?
   a. Elevated temperature.
   b. Normal sedimentation rate.
   c. Elevated red blood count.
   d. Normal white blood count.

2. Histologically Ewing's sarcoma cells are described as:
   a. Fibrous, spindle shaped.
   b. Small, round cells.
   c. Filled with collagen.
   d. Mixed intracellular material.

Once Becky's diagnosis was confirmed, chemotherapy and local treatment options were discussed.

3. Which of the following is **not** a primary use for chemotherapy?
   a. Shrink the primary tumor size.
   b. Diminish pulmonary metastasis.
   c. Facilitate potential for limb salvage surgery.
   d. Kill tumor cells and destroy the tumor.

4. The side effects of radiation include:
   a. Growth acceleration in involved limb.
   b. Pathologic fracture in first 8 weeks.
   c. The development of joint fibrosis and edema.
   d. Nausea and vomiting for 3 hours after treatment.

5. Surgical options are difficult due to Becky's age and include rotationplasty and above-knee amputation. Which of the following is the least important in considering the surgical options?
   a. Body image disturbance.
   b. Quality of life following surgery.
   c. Amount of skeletal growth left.
   d. Her gender and goals in life.

Edith, a 39-year-old nursing administrator, presented to her orthopaedist's office with complaints of pelvis and hip pain. She was limping. Her radiographs revealed lytic lesions of the hip and pelvis. Her surgeon ordered a bone scan to rule out carcinoma as she was a smoker. The scan showed abnormality in many bones. (Questions 6-7).

6. Which of the following is an **uncommon** site to observe carcinomas of the bone?
   a. Rib.
   b. Vertebra.
   c. Pelvis.
   d. Sternum.

After a biopsy revealed metastatic adenocarcinoma from her lung, the orthopaedist talked toEdith about her risk for fracture.

7. Which of the following is not a priority in determining an impending pathologic fracture?
   a. A lesion has destroyed 50% of the bone.
   b. Severe pain in the affected extremity.
   c. Inability to bear weight on involved extremity.
   d. X-rays that show bone metastasis in the area.

Larry, age 16, complained to his mother for 3 weeks about his knee pain. She took him to his primary care physician. An x-ray revealed a bone-forming lesion in his femur. (Questions 8-10).

8. Examination of a patient with tumor should include:
   a. Pain assessment.
   b. Liver scan.
   c. Gait analysis (computerized).
   d. Lymph node biopsy.

Larry's doctor mentioned both benign and malignant tumors. A biopsy would be necessary to differentiate between osteosarcoma and osteoid osteoma.

9. An osteoid osteoma is a benign tumor that:
   a. Requires surgical excision in 90% of the patients.
   b. Causes night pain, but can be relieved by aspirin.
   c. Usually develops into a large osteoblastic lesion.
   d. Occurs most often in the spine and femur.

10. Which of the following is the most common primary malignant bone tumor?
   a. Osteoblastoma.
   b. Chondrosarcoma.
   c. Osteosarcoma.
   d. Osteochondroma.

Chapter 16 THE SHOULDER

Cindy Bagwell-Crum, MEd, BSN, RN, CNOR, CST

Contents

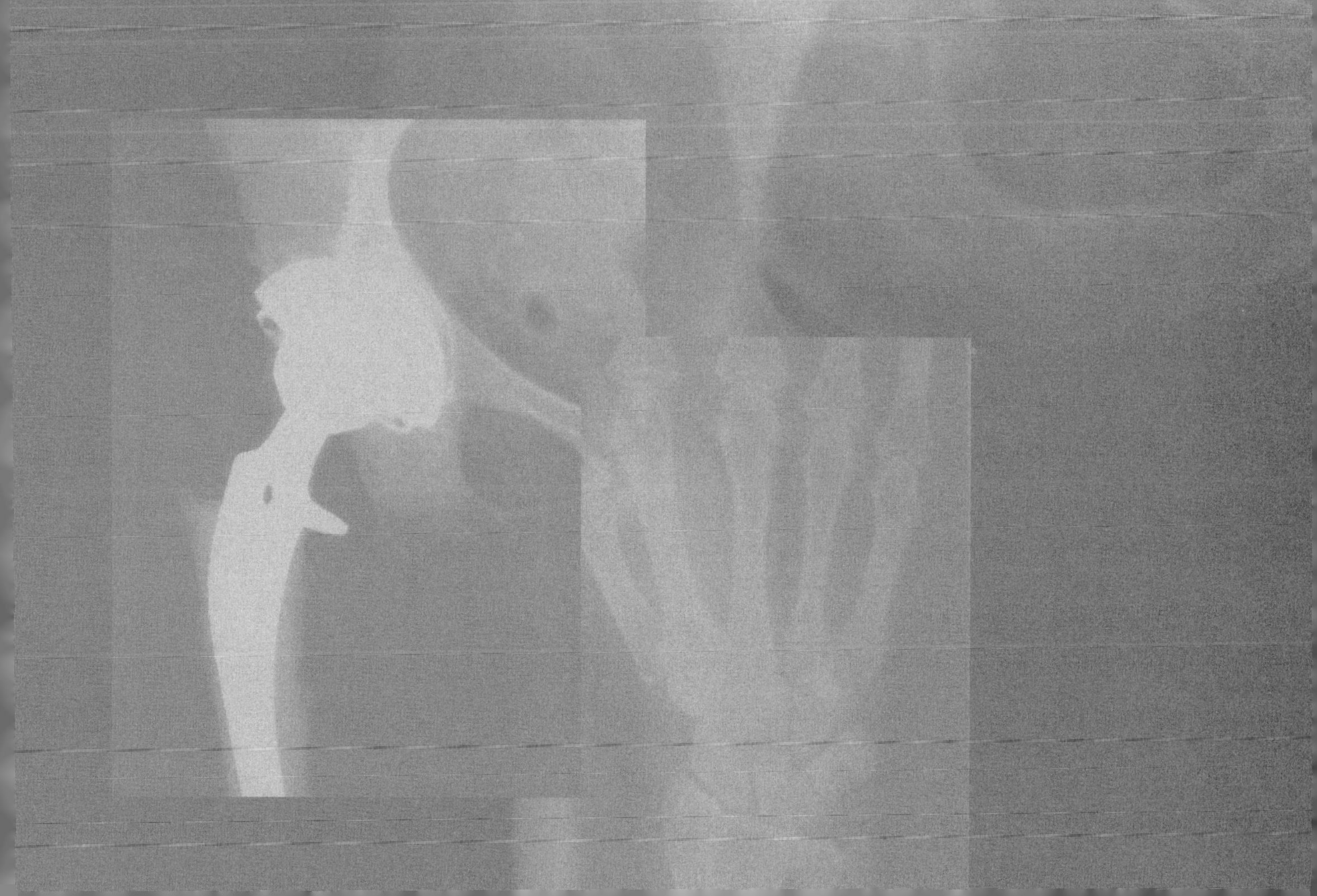

OBJECTIVES

At the completion of this chapter, the learner will be able to:

- Explain the mechanism of injury for common shoulder dislocations/instability.
- Discuss the key aspects of assessment for a patient with shoulder pathology.
- Explain home care considerations for the patient with a shoulder condition.
- Identify nursing interventions for managing patients with shoulder pathologies.
- Discuss nonsurgical and surgical management for the patient with a shoulder problem.

KEY POINTS

- The shoulder is the most frequently dislocated joint in the human body. The sternoclavicular joint is the most frequently used joint in the body because all movement of the upper extremities requires its movement.
- Dislocation is commonly due to a direct blow or is indirectly due to force from a fall on the outstretched arm or hand.
- Diagnosis of glenohumeral instability occurs more frequently since the development of arthroscopy.
- Pain in the shoulder is exceeded in frequency only by low back and neck pain.
- Shoulder girdle complex describes the shoulder joint more accurately.
- The shoulder is difficult to assess due to the vast number of structures located in such a confined space.
- The shoulder has a greater range of motion but is less stable than the hip joint.

CHAPTER 16

THE SHOULDER

ROTATOR CUFF TEARS

I. OVERVIEW

A. Definition: a rotator cuff tear is a tear in the muscles that make up the rotator cuff.
1. The rotator cuff is a musculotendinous cuff that stabilizes the humeral head as it moves against the glenoid labrum and acts as a fulcrum.
2. The rotator cuff allows the deltoid muscle to elevate (abduct) the arm without impingement between the superior humeral head and the acromion process of the scapula.
3. The rotator cuff is composed of the four muscles that originate from the scapula.
4. The four muscles and their tendons that make up the rotator cuff can be remembered by the acronym "SITS." The arm hanging at the side:
   a. **S**upraspinatus lies directly under the acromion and provides abduction and in forward elevation of the arm.
   b. **I**nfraspinatus is posterior to the supraspinatus and assists the teres minor in rotating the humerus (and thus the arm) externally.
   c. **T**eres minor is immediately posterior to the supraspinatus and infraspinatus muscles and assists the infraspinatus in rotating the humerus (and thus the arm) externally.
   d. **S**ubscapularis is located anteriorly (and is not palpable) and provides for internal rotation of the humerus.
5. Of the muscles of the rotator cuff, the supraspinatus is the most commonly ruptured, especially near its insertion.

B. Etiology.
1. Rotator cuff normally undergoes some degenerative changes with advanced age, leaving asymptomatic "worn out" spots in the cuff.
2. Tears occur as the result of a sudden adduction force being applied to the cuff while the arm is being held in abduction.
3. Traumatic tears of the cuff can occur as a result of minor trauma such as:
   a. A fall on the shoulder.
   b. Throwing an object.
   c. Lifting a heavy object.
4. Tears in younger people are usually the result of substantial trauma.
5. Repeated impingement resulting from encroachment of the acromion coracoacromial ligament or acromioclavicular joint on the rotator cuff tendons and subdeltoid bursa or on the coracoid process (see Table 16.1).

C. Pathophysiology.

Table 16.1
Factors in Development of Impingement Syndrome

1. Form of Acromion
   a. Type 1 Flat
   b. Type 2 Concave
   c. Type 3 Hooked
2. Vascularization of rotator cuff
3. Function of rotator cuff and biceps muscles
4. Glenohumeral joint stability
5. Condition of acromioclavicular joint
6. Occupation and hobbies of patient

1. Degenerative changes due to aging.
2. A weakened rotator cuff may eventually lead to a partial or complete tear.
3. There is almost always a rupture of tendon of long head of biceps.

D. Incidence.
1. The supraspinatus is the most commonly affected, then the external rotators (infraspinatus and teres minor which work as a team), and lastly the subscapularis.
2. Usually seen in patients over 40 years of age.
3. Women have a greater incidence.

E. Consideration across the lifespan.
1. In younger patients (less than 50), trauma tends to stretch rather than tear the cuff tendons.
2. In older patients, tears are more common.
3. Stages of tears:
   a. Stage 1: patients younger than 25 years old.
   b. Stage 2: patients between the ages of 25-40.
   c. Stage 3: patients over 40 years of age.

F. Complications.
1. Contractures, of the shoulder and elbow if the patient does not follow the exercise and rehabilitation regime.
2. 4% of all full rotator cuff tears develop glenohumeral arthritis.
3. Post-surgical complications:
   a. Damage to or detachment of deltoid.
   b. "Pulling out" of repair is major concern.

II. ASSESSMENT

A. History.
1. Presenting symptoms.

a. Pain and tenderness of shoulder.
   (1) Primarily anterolateral and superior aspect of shoulder, increasing at night.
   (2) Pain may refer to/radiate to the insertion of the deltoid muscle in the upper humerus.
b. May report physical activities/limitations.

2. Mechanism of injury:
   a. Sports: overhead, repetitive motions: swimming, racquet sports (tennis, racquetball), baseball (especially pitching).
   b. Trauma: fall on outstretched hand, blow to upper arm.
   c. Work: repetitive overhead motion, heavy lifting.

B. Physical examination.

1. Local pain at anterior aspect of shoulder, especially where the tear comes in contact with the coracoacromial ligament when the arm is in abduction or externally rotated.
   a. Patient complains of pain at night, inability to lay flat, and finds sleeping in a recliner or in a semi-sitting position best.
   b. Tenderness may be noted over the cuff.
   c. Swelling with atrophy of the supraspinatus and infraspinatus muscles.
2. Positive (but not always) drop test.
   a. Patient is instructed to fully abduct his/her arm.
   b. Ask him/her to slowly lower it to the side.
   c. The arm will drop to the side from a position of about 90 degrees abduction.
   d. Patient is unable to lower arm smoothly and slowly no matter how many attempts.
   e. If the patient is able to hold his/her arm in abduction, a gentle tap on the forearm will cause the arm to fall to the side.
3. When the arm is passively abducted at the shoulder, the patient still may be unable to sustain the position and the arm will drop to the side.
   a. Patient is unable to initiate or maintain active abduction of the arm at the shoulder joint.
   b. Efforts to abduct the arm produces characteristic shoulder shrugging.
   c. Active abduction at the glenohumeral joint is severely impaired with a complete tear of the supraspinatus tendon.
4. Active range of motion with resistance:
   a. There may be weakness of shoulder, but good motion and function even in the most severe tears.
   b. Pain elicited in patients with weakness suggests a tear.
5. Complete neurovascular assessment.
6. Compare affected extremity with unaffected side.
7. Full mobility of the shoulder joint is not lost because the scapula is not affected.
   a. Active or passive arm elevation only 90 degrees.
   b. Passive external rotation 60 degrees.
   c. Glenohumeral abduction 40 degrees.
   d. Internal rotation 20 degrees.
   e. Resisted abduction and very weak external rotation.
8. Subacromial crepitus, palpable or audible when the shoulder is rotated in the abducted position.
9. Impingement test:
   a. Local anesthetic is injected into the subacromial space.
   b. After a short waiting period patient is reevaluated.
   c. If pain persists, either the injection is in the wrong place or there is another source of the pain.
   d. If pain is relieved, motion is usually improved, and it is considered a positive impingement test.
   e. Stages of impingement according to Neer:
      (1) Stage 1: reversible small bleeding and edema in the rotator cuff.
      (2) Stage 2: fibrosis and tendinitis of rotator cuff.
      (3) Stage 3: osteophytes of the acromion and acromioclavicular joint and partial tear of rotator cuff.

C. Diagnostic tests.

1. Plain radiographs:
   a. Often normal.
   b. Views would show:
      (1) Collapse of proximal humeral head.
      (2) Erosion of glenoid cavity.
      (3) Spur formation along the anterior edge of the acromion.
      (4) Displaced fracture of the tuberosity.
      (5) Greater tubercle and both acromioclavicular joint surfaces: an acromiohumeral interval on the anteroposterior film of less than 7 mm is helpful in diagnosis of chronic complete rotator cuff tears.
2. Arthrogram: demonstrates leakage of the contrast material from the shoulder joint capsule into the subacromial bursa (see Chapter 4, Diagnostic Studies).
3. MRI: study of choice due to being more definitive and shown to have a 93%-100% accuracy.
4. CT (see Chapter 4, Diagnostic Studies).

III. COMMON THERAPEUTIC MODALITIES

A. Objective of treatment: reduction of pain and increased joint function.

B. Nonsurgical treatment.

1. Home program.
   a. Rest the shoulder with specified exercise program.
   b. Modification of home activities.
   c. Nonsteroidal anti-inflammatory oral medication
   d. Analgesics and mild narcotic if necessary.
   e. Heat application
2. Office setting: subacromial injection.
   a. Injection of local anesthetic is helpful in localizing pain to a specific anatomical region.

b. Process.
   (1) 8-10 cc of local anesthetic is injected into the subacromial space.
   (2) After 5-10 minutes the pain should have decreased by 50%.
   (3) If not, 2-3 cc local anesthetic may then be injected into the acromioclavicular joint to provide accurate diagnosis.

C. Surgical treatment.

1. Primary indication is significant pain resulting in disability and functional limitations that are intolerable to the patient.
2. Surgery is usually considered after an adequate trial of conservative management, usually 6-8 months.
   a. Arthroscopic debridement of nonviable rotator cuff tissue without attempting a direct repair.
   b. Anteroinferior acromioplasty: involves the resection one-half of the thickness of the anterior acromion and tapering the resection posteriorly; the rotator cuff is then mobilized and repaired.
   c. Arthroscopically assisted subacromial decompression (acromioplasty) and cuff repair: provides satisfactory clinical results in a patient with small tears involving only one tendon.
   d. Procedures that utilize:
      (1) Autogenous or allograft tendon grafts.
      (2) Active tendon transfers.
   e. Distal clavicle resection (open or arthroscopically).

IV. NURSING DIAGNOSES, OUTCOMES, AND INTERVENTIONS

A. See Table 16.2.

B. Physical mobility, impaired.

1. Outcome.
   a. Patient plans activities appropriate for restrictions.
   b. Patient resumes normal activities.
   c. Patient exhibits normal range of motion.
2. Interventions.
   a. Discuss activity limitations.
   b. Teach (and demonstrate as appropriate) patient, family, and significant others the purpose and objective of the shoulder immobilizer.
   c. Instruct on and plan activity program to aid in strengthening muscles and maintaining function.
   d. Discuss (and demonstrate as appropriate) exercises:
      (1) Muscle setting exercises
      (2) Finger exercises.
      (3) Pendulum exercises twice a day.
      (4) Exercises for the elbow twice a day.
      (5) Resistive exercises after 8 weeks.
   e. Stress the patient's responsibility in doing the exercises and rehabilitation.
   f. Explain the potential effect on balance and walking of immobilized arm.
   g. When assisting the patient, make sure not to support the patient under the affected elbow or put pressure on his/her affected shoulder.

C. Self-care deficit syndrome.

1. Outcome: patient resumes normal self-care activities.
2. Interventions.
   a. Educate patient about self-care activities while shoulder immobilizer is in place.
   b. Teach patient to pass injured arm through clothing before uninvolved extremity when dressing.
   c. Teach patient to get out of bed on the unaffected side.

V. PRACTICE SETTING CONSIDERATIONS

A. Office/outpatient.

1. Cryotherapy.
2. Gentle active assisted range of motion.
3. Physical therapy (heat, cold, exercises).

B. Home care considerations.

1. Emphasize importance of modification of activities to prevent exacerbation.
2. Activities should be simple and easily performed.
2. Passive motion early after repair and then progression.
3. Plan of care is surgeon preference.
4. Review guidelines for seeking physician evaluation.

C. Rehabilitation.

1. Complete rehabilitation takes a minimum of 6 months-1 year.
2. Patient's dedication to the exercise regime will greatly determine outcome.

TENDINITIS OF THE SHOULDER

I. OVERVIEW

A. Definition: inflammation of the tendons in the shoulder girdle complex. The most common cause of shoulder pain is rotator cuff tendinitis (also known as impingement syndrome). Other tendons in the shoulder girdle complex are also affected.

B. Etiology.

1. Calcium salt deposits.
2. Repeated impingement such as in throwing or swimming causing edema and hemorrhage followed by inflammation and fibrosis.

C. Pathophysiology.

1. Rotator cuff impinges against the under surface of the acromion and the coracoacromial ligament as the arm is raised, and often involves the supraspinatus tendon.
2. Bicipital tendinitis is the inflammation of the long head of the biceps tendon and its sheath in the coracoacromial arch.
3. Calcific tendinitis is a degenerative process involving the supraspinatus tendon.

D. Incidence.

1. Rotator cuff tendinitis.
   a. Age range from teens to 40 years of age.
   b. Often athletically active.
2. Calcific tendinitis: seen in women over 30 years of age

Table 16.2
Common Nursing Diagnoses, Outcomes, and Interventions for Shoulder Patients

Diagnoses	Outcomes	Interventions
A. Physical mobility, impaired	• Patient has increased mobility and muscle strength. • Patient has no joint deformities.	• Promote mobility and muscle strength within restrictions. 1. Discuss, provide equipment to assist with mobility. 2. Conduct exercise/activity program to strengthen muscles and maintain function. a. Physical Therapy consult as indicated. b. ROM exercises maintain function. c. Exercise program increases muscle strength. 3. Promote use of unaffected extremities.
B. Role performance, altered	• Patient demonstrates activities associated with family role. • Patient manages home/work roles. • Verbalizes needed adaptations when symptoms interfere with role performance.	• Explore patient's feelings and concerns related to changing role responsibilities and impact on self-concept. • Promote family cohesion. 1. Identify typical family coping mechanisms. 2. Promote care of patient by family members. • Assist the patient/family to readjust role expectations as necessary. • Assess for functional deficits, which may require lifestyle changes and occupational therapy. • Assess for economic impact of treatments and functional impairments. 1. Adequacy of insurance coverage. 2. Loss of income due to impairments.
C. Self-care deficit syndrome; home maintenance, impaired	• Patient performs ADL with maximum independence. • Necessary home maintenance activities are accomplished. • Environment facilitates optimal independence.	• Promote independence in self-care and assist as needed. • Set realistic goals with patient for maximum independence. 1. Assess functional abilities. 2. Assess activity tolerance. 3. Assist patient in accepting and realizing when activities extend beyond self-care capacity • Structure environment to maximize patient independence. • Allow sufficient time to complete self-care activities. • Provide a consistent program for improvement of ADL skills to be followed at home.

Table 16.2 (continued)
Common Nursing Diagnoses, Outcomes, and Interventions for Shoulder Patients

Diagnoses	Outcomes	Interventions
C. Self-care deficit syndrome; home maintenance, impaired (continued)	• Patient performs ADL with maximum independence. • Necessary home maintenance activities are accomplished. • Environment facilitates optimal independence. (continued)	• Augment self-care devices with assistive devices, if needed. 1. Instruct patient in the use of adaptive devices and ADL skill programs. 2. Provide clothing that uses Velcro® fasteners instead of buttons, snaps, or zippers.
D. Noncompliance	• Patient participates in the treatment plan.	• Promote adherence to the treatment plan. 1. Identify the level of compliance with the prescribed regimen. 2. Assess the level of understanding regarding the condition and treatment. 3. Identify the difficulties the patient experiences in carrying out the home regimen. • Collaborate with the patient to develop the treatment plan. • Assist the patient in identifying sources of supports and available resources.
E. Coping, ineffective; family coping, compromised; family process, altered	• Patient demonstrates adequate coping mechanisms to deal with stressors imposed by illness/therapeutic regime. • Patient identifies specific sources of stress.	• Promote adaptation/coping. 1. Assist patient in verbalizing concerns, feelings, and fears. 2. Provide current information on condition and changes in condition. 3. Prepare patient for prolonged course of therapy and permanent disability, as necessary. 4. Help patient establish realistic goals. 5. Involve patient in treatment decisions. 6. Reinforce adaptive mechanisms successfully used. 7. Acknowledge patient strengths and effective coping strategies. 8. Assist patient to identify support systems and community resources. • Enhance management of disease process. 1. Teach patient about diagnosis/management. 2. Assess level of understanding and compliance with treatment plan. 3. Teach patient in home care needs/techniques.

Table 16.2 (continued)
Common Nursing Diagnoses, Outcomes, and Interventions for Shoulder Patients

Diagnoses	Outcomes	Interventions
F. Pain, acute; Pain, chronic	• Patient demonstrates maximal degree of comfort.	• Assess patient's pain level related to joint degeneration/trauma, operative/incisional pain. • Observe for nonverbal communication. • Promote patient comfort. 1. Relieve pain with appropriate techniques: moist heat, muscle relaxants, antispasmodics, analgesics, relaxation, etc. 2. Encourage diversional activities 3. Control environmental factors that precipitate or increase the pain experience. 4. Discuss coping methods with the patient. • Assess for limited joint motion and proper functional alignment. • Use physical modalities for pain relief and joint protection before and after activity.
G. Anxiety	• Patient will express fears and concerns related to diagnosis and treatment. • Patient will understand the following: 1. Underlying pathology. 2. Treatment plan. 3. Availability of community resources.	• Develop a plan of care to minimize patient anxiety. 1. Allow patient to express fears and concerns related to diagnosis and treatment plan. 2. Include patient/family in decision-making process. 3. Provide education regarding: a. Underlying pathology. b. Treatment. c. Community resources.

E. **Consideration across the lifespan: from teenagers through geriatrics.**

F. **Complications.**
1. With infiltration injections, caution should be taken as the following complications could occur:
   a. Promotion of degeneration and rupture in already compromised structures.
   b. Production of tendon atrophy.
   c. Decreased ability of damaged tendon to heal.
2. Tendinitis in younger patients (less than 50) can result in shoulder dislocation.

II. ASSESSMENT

A. **History.**
1. Presenting symptoms in rotator cuff tendinitis.
   a. Acute pain in the shoulder.
   b. Recurrent or chronic pain of the shoulder.
2. Presenting symptoms in calcific tendinitis.
   a. Acute, disabling attack of shoulder pain.
   b. Chronic, less severe pain may also occur.
3. Presenting symptoms in bicipital tendinitis: an anterior shoulder pain that resembles rotator cuff tendinitis and may co-exist with bicipital tendinitis.

B. **Physical examination.**
1. Rotator cuff tendinitis.
   a. Pain is aggravated by activity.
   b. Sharp catches of pain when arm is elevated overhead.
   c. Impingement sign:
      (1) The patient forcibly elevates the arm while the examiner pushes the shoulder against the greater tuberosity and the anterior acromion.
      (2) Facial grimacing and pain indicate entrapment of the supraspinatus tendon/muscle or bicipital tendinitis.
2. Calcific tendinitis.
   a. Interferes with activities of daily living (ADL).

b. Arm is held close to the side.
c. Any type of motion is severely limited by pain.
d. Tenderness is maximum at the tip of the acromion.
e. Inflammation may extend to the subacromial bursa.

3. Bicipital tendinitis: tenderness is maximal in the bicipital groove over the intertubercular sulcus.
   a. With arm at the side and elbow flexed 90 degrees.
   b. Ask the patient to supinate the forearm against resistance.
   c. Increased pain in the bicipital groove indicates bicipital tendinitis.

C. Diagnostic tests.
1. Radiographs.
2. Arthrography.
3. MRI.
4. Ultrasonography must be an adjunct with the physical examination.

III. COMMON THERAPEUTIC MODALITIES

A. Objective of treatment: reduce pain.

B. Nonsurgical treatment.
1. Narcotic analgesics.
2. NSAIDs.
3. Exercise.
4. Friction massage for 6-8 sessions.
5. Infiltrations:
   a. One corticosteroid injection is usually all that is needed to be effective.
   b. Place the arm in a sling for 3-4 days and limit activities after the injection.
   c. After 10 days increase activity and recheck in 2 weeks.
      (1) For bicipital tendinitis, the infiltration is placed within the tendon sheath.
      (2) For calcific tendinitis, the infiltration is placed in the subacromial space.
6. Ice or infrared heat.
7. Needle or puncture aspiration for calcific tendinitis.

C. Surgical treatment.
1. Inspection and synovectomy.
2. Repair of partial tears.

IV. NURSING DIAGNOSES, OUTCOMES, AND INTERVENTIONS

A. See Table 16.2.

B. Pain.
1. Outcome: patient demonstrates increased comfort levels.
2. Interventions.
   a. Assess patient's pain level.
   b. Observe for nonverbal signs of discomfort.
   c. Promote patient comfort
      (1) Instruct how to control environmental factors that increase pain
      (2) Discuss coping methods with the patient.
   d. See Chapter 7, Pain.

ARTHRITIS OF THE SHOULDER

I. OVERVIEW

A. Definition: arthritis is defined as inflammation of the joint. There are two common types of arthritis that are generally considered when discussing the shoulder joint: rheumatoid and osteoarthritis.
1. Osteoarthritis is a localized, progressive, noninflammatory disease, also known as degenerative joint disease (DJD).
2. Rheumatoid arthritis is a chronic systemic inflammatory disease that primarily has a symmetrical distribution of the peripheral joint.
3. Bursitis, inflammation of a bursa is the primary condition of pain in shoulder for most patients with rheumatoid arthritis.

B. Etiology.
1. Rheumatoid arthritis:
   a. Unknown.
   b. The most common theories of cause are autoimmune response and infection.
   c. Genetic disposition and trauma are also thought to be causes.
   d. See Chapter 12, Arthritis and Connective Tissue Disorders.
2. Osteoarthritis:
   a. Primary cause unknown.
   b. Secondary cause is predisposing events such as:
      (1) Trauma.
      (2) Lifestyle-specific factors (pitcher's shoulder).
      (3) Aging (wear and tear).
   c. Presently there is some thought that it could be due to immune response.
   d. See Chapter 12, Arthritis and Connective Tissue Disorders.

C. Pathophysiology.
1. Rheumatoid arthritis:
   a. In the shoulder, rheumatoid arthritis almost always starts at the glenohumeral joint.
      (1) Articular manifestations of joint destruction.
      (2) Joint inflammation and effusion.
      (3) Redness, swelling, and painful motion of the joint.
   b. Nonarticular manifestations include:
      (1) Fatigue.
      (2) Malaise.
      (3) Shoulder weakness.
   c. Damage to ligaments, tendons, cartilage, joint capsule and bone.
2. Osteoarthritis:
   a. In the shoulder, osteoarthritis appears primarily in the acromioclavicular joint and less often in the glenohumeral joint.
   b. As a noninflammatory and nonsystemic disease affecting articular cartilage, the articular cartilage is worn away and the bone ends rub together.

c. With cartilage degeneration there is bone degeneration and the development of spurs.
d. Pain, due to osteoarthritis is usually relieved by rest.

D. Incidence.

1. Rheumatoid arthritis:
   a. Greater incidence in females with a 3:1 ratio.
   b. Gender difference disappears with age.
   c. Affects all races.
2. Osteoarthritis:
   a. Over age 55, it affects twice as many women as men.
   b. Most common form of disabling disease in the United States.
   c. Begins as early as 2nd decade and peaks between 5th and 6th decades.
   d. Lifestyle/occupational patterns may lead to involvement of joints not usually affected such as factory workers and baseball pitchers with repetitive motion.
   e. Developed after trauma or other disorder.
   f. More prevalent in Caucasians than African-Americans.
   g. Acromioclavicular joint is one of the joints that demonstrates early degenerative changes.

E. Considerations across the lifespan.

1. Rheumatoid arthritis: age of onset usually between 20-50 years of age with the average being 40 years of age.
2. Osteoarthritis:
   a. Generally occurs in the elderly.
   b. Patterns vary as to the extent of immobility presented.
   c. Increased incidence in obese individuals.

F. Complications.

1. Rheumatoid arthritis.
   a. Joint instability and subluxation resulting from:
      (1) Joint destruction.
      (2) Loss of supporting structures.
      (3) Muscle atrophy.
   b. Acute depression and anxiety.
2. Osteoarthritis.
   a. Decreased joint range of motion.
   b. Loss of joint function.
   c. Loss of independence in ADL.
   d. Pain: characterized as aching pain that can become debilitating.

II. ASSESSMENT

A. History.

1. Rheumatoid arthritis.
   a. History of fatigue, malaise, weakness.
   b. Reports vague arthralgias and myalgias.
   c. Reports joint pain and stiffness lasting an hour or more.
   d. Pain at rest, especially night.
2. Osteoarthritis.
   a. Stiffness in the shoulder joint. Become stiffened for 20-30 minutes at a time and increases in severity with changes in the weather.
   b. Paresthesias.
   c. Joint crepitation with motion. (Patient may complain of hearing a "popping, cracking, or grinding" sound.)

B. Physical examination.

1. Rheumatoid arthritis.
   a. Swelling, redness, warmth.
   b. Pain, tenderness, nodules.
   c. Fever.
   d. Anemia.
   e. Note comparison of two extremities for size, shape, color, and symmetry.
   f. Note joint mobility, crepitus, function, sensation.
   g. Assess muscular strength and for presence of muscular spasms.
2. Osteoarthritis.
   a. Localized pain and when direct pressure is applied to joint.
   b. Pain with activity that improves with rest and is then followed by stiffness.
   d. Usually not much swelling.
   e. No systemic symptoms.
   f. Deformity of joint due to:
      (1) Loss of articular cartilage.
      (2) Collapse of subchondral bone.
      (3) Overgrowth of bone.
      (4) Atrophy of adjacent muscles.

C. Diagnostic tests.

1. Rheumatoid arthritis.
   a. Joint aspiration with synovial fluid analysis.
      (1) Milky, cloudy, or dark yellow.
      (2) Increased WBC.
      (3) Significant increase in ESR (erythrocyte sedimentation rate).
   b. Bone scan can detect early joint changes and more readily confirm diagnosis.
   c. X-rays help to confirm disease activity and monitor treatment results.
2. Osteoarthritis.
   a. CT, arthrography, and MRI used to evaluate integrity of rotator cuff and the degree of glenoid bone loss and glenoid version.
   b. Synovial fluid analysis, the best method for differentiating between osteoarthritis and rheumatoid arthritis (clear and yellow).
   c. Plain films are used for checking for sign of joint space narrowing.
   d. Bone scan, radionuclide imaging, used to determine skeletal distribution of osteoarthritis.

III. COMMON THERAPEUTIC MODALITIES

A. Main objective of treatment: pain relief and maintaining joint function.

B. Nonsurgical treatment.

1. Rheumatoid arthritis.
   a. Medications.
      (1) Anti-inflammatory.
         (a) Salicylates are drug of first choice.
         (b) NSAIDs (nonsteroidal anti-inflammatory drugs).

(2) Analgesics.
(3) Intra-articular steroid injections.
(a) Temporary suppression of inflammation.
(b) Limited use of four (4) times per year per joint.
(4) Investigative agents (alkylating or antineoplastic drugs).
(5) See Chapter 12, Arthritis and Connective Tissue Disorders.

b. Exercise: preservation of joint motion and maintenance of muscle strength requires a balance of rest and activity.
(1) Range of motion (ROM).
(a) Passive ROM for stretching tightened muscles and preventing flexion contractures during acute inflammation.
(b) Active ROM for stretching when pain and inflammation are not present.
(c) Isometric techniques to sustain muscle strength and mass with mild resistance exercises.

c. Total lymph node irradiation (TLI).

d. Physical therapy.
(1) Heat lamps.
(2) Heat/cold compresses to decrease inflammation.

2. Osteoarthritis: majority of patients can be successfully managed conservatively.
a. Self-care modifications.
b. Medications.
(1) NSAIDs: combine anti-inflammatory properties with analgesic and antipyretic properties.
(2) Corticosteroid injections.
(3) See Chapter 12, Arthritis and Connective Tissue Disorders.
c. Exercise:
(1) ROM exercises 3-4 times per day.
(2) Strengthening exercises once a day.
(3) Gradually increase number of repetitions.
(a) Gradual progression is important.
(b) After careful evaluation of progression, an endurance exercise program can be included.

C. Surgical treatment

1. Goal of this treatment is:
a. Pain relief.
b. Joint stabilization.
c. Correction of deformity.
d. Improvement of function.

2. Rheumatoid arthritis.
a. Synovectomy: removal of synovial membrane in accessible joints and tendon sheaths.
b. Tenosynovectomy: surgical repair or removal of damaged tendons.
c. Arthrodesis: surgical fusion of the joint.
d. Hemiarthroplasty is the replacement of the humeral head with a prosthesis, used in the treatment of:
(1) Certain acute fractures of the proximal humerus (see Fractures of the Shoulder, this chapter).
(2) Painful, chronic glenohumeral incongruities.
e. Total arthroplasty, a replacement of the humeral head and the glenoid surface with prostheses, is indicated when:
(1) There is severe destruction of the joint from a disease process such as rheumatoid arthritis or arthritis after instability surgery.
(2) Other reasons for performing arthroplasty are:
(a) Fractures that may culminate in avascular necrosis.
(b) Chronic glenohumeral incongruence due to:
i. Sickle cell infarction.
ii. Irradiation necrosis.
f. Resection arthroplasty: a salvage procedure in which there is severe bone loss.
(1) Secondary to tumor.
(2) Chronic osteomyelitis or septic osteomyelitis.
(3) Failed prior arthroplasty.

3. Osteoarthritis:
a. Surgery is considered when there is:
(1) Pain, especially nocturnal pain.
(2) Diminishing capacity to carry out ADL independently.
(3) Progressive and irreversible loss of joint function.
(4) There needs to be an innervated and intact deltoid.
(5) In addition, there needs to be satisfactory periscapular muscular control.
b. Four basic surgical procedures.
(1) Osteotomy: cutting through the bone to realign the bones of the shoulder joint.
(2) Debridement of the shoulder joint done arthroscopically.
(3) Arthroplasty: replacement of the humeral head and the glenoid surface with prostheses (see Rheumatoid Arthritis above).
(4) Arthrodesis: surgical fusion of the shoulder joint.

4. Contraindication for surgical treatment is a recent history of bacterial infection within the joint or osteomyelitis.

5. Complications of surgery.
a. Postoperative infection.
b. Loosening of prosthesis in shoulder arthroplasty.
c. Loss of motion or strength due to improper component size, overcorrection of muscular reconstruction, or instability of the shoulder joint.
d. Reduced function in the elbow joint.
e. Impingement syndrome.
f. Nerve injuries.

IV. NURSING DIAGNOSES, OUTCOMES, AND INTERVENTIONS

A. See Table 16.2.

B. Pain.

1. Outcome: patient will remain comfortable with pain relief measures.
2. Interventions:
   a. Regional block for pain relief for the first 12 hours postoperatively.
   b. Pain medications:
      (1) Patient controlled analgesic (PCA) pump administration of narcotics.
      (2) Intramuscular administrations (morphine, meperidine, or ketorolac).
      (3) After 24 hours, oral analgesics (Vicodin® or Tylenol with Codeine #3®).
   c. Correct position to reduce stress on the shoulder.
      (1) Elevate the head of the bed.
      (2) Support the arm with a pillow.
      (3) Keep the shoulder correctly aligned while the patient is in bed.
   d. Apply ice near the incision to reduce swelling and discomfort.

C. Physical mobility, impaired.

1. Outcomes:
   a. Patient will have increased mobility and muscle strength in upper extremity.
   b. Patient will be able to abduct operative shoulder to 90 degrees in 7-10 postoperative days.
2. Interventions.
   a. Make sure the sling, sling and swathe, or shoulder immobilizer is properly in place. (Note, if reconstruction of rotator cuff was also done, an adduction humeral splint or cast shell may be used).
   b. Patient may use the trapeze to readjust self in bed, but only with the unaffected arm.
   c. Ambulate the patient on first postoperative day with orthosis on operative arm.
      (1) Assist the patient out of bed.
      (2) Because patient cannot use immobilized arm and due to lack of swing, the patient will need to adjust to a change in balance.
   d. Teach the patient how to do required exercises.
      (1) Start with finger and thumb exercises.
      (2) Gentle passive exercises (and then active) exercises of wrist/hand.
      (3) Patient will begin internal rotation of operative arm after third postoperative week, with permission.
      (4) Finally operative shoulder exercises as prescribed.
      (5) Begin internal rotation of operative arm after third postoperative week, with permission.
      (6) Some patients will utilize a continuous passive motion (CPM) machine.
   e. Conduct an exercise program to strengthen muscles and maintain function.

D. Role performance, ineffective.

1. Outcomes: patient manages home/work roles.
2. Interventions.
   a. Assist patient/family in readjusting role expectations as necessary.
   b. Assess for functional deficits which may require lifestyle and/or work changes.
   c. Occupational therapy as needed.

E. Self-care deficit syndrome.

1. Outcomes: patient performs ADL with maximum independence.
2. Interventions.
   a. Promote independence in self-care and assist as needed.
   b. Assist patient to accept and realize when activities extend beyond self-care capacity.
   c. Home care assistance for activities beyond patient capabilities.

F. Noncompliance.

1. Outcomes: patient will participate in the treatment plan.
2. Interventions.
   a. Promote adherence to the treatment plan.
   b. Collaborate with the patient to develop treatment plan.
   c. Assist the patient in identifying sources of supports and available resources.
   d. Encourage the patient to stay with the plan. (To a great degree, functional recovery depends on implementing a comprehensive postoperative rehabilitation regime and patient adherence to the plan).

V. PRACTICE SETTING CONSIDERATIONS

A. Office/outpatient.

1. For long-term rehabilitation exercise regimen, patient must be dedicated and compliant.
2. Instruct the patient about the long-term rehabilitation regimen.
3. Assist patient/family in identifying sources of supports and available resources.

B. Hospital.

1. Shoulder position should remain in the required abducted position with the shoulder immobilizer for 1 week, then at night for 4 weeks.
2. Radiographs are taken in the recovery room.
3. Deep vein thrombosis (DVT) prophylaxis.
4. Neurovascular checks postoperatively every 2 hours for 24 hours.
5. Continuous passive motion (CPM) and active exercises are begun.
6. Limitations include no internal rotation for 3 or more weeks postoperatively to avoid the possibility of joint disruption.

C. Home care considerations.

1. Refer to home care nurses for wound care and assistance with ADL as needed.
2. Instructions as to follow-up physical therapy and physician appointment.

INSTABILTY OF THE SHOULDER

I. OVERVIEW

A. Definition: shoulder instability encompasses both subluxation and dislocation.

1. Dislocation completely separates the articular surfaces of the joint.
2. Subluxation is an incomplete or partial dislocation of one bone from the joint surface.

B. Etiology.

1. Instability may occur following an acute injury.
2. Repetitive stretching of the shoulder with overhead activities can also cause instability.
3. Dislocations can be caused by either direct or indirect forces.
   a. Anterior/posterior.
   b. Medial/lateral.
4. Subluxations may be caused by loose surrounding support structures due to:
   a. Congenital problems.
   b. Trauma to tendons and ligaments.
   c. Joint effusions due to infection.
   d. Disuse atrophy due to prolonged joint immobilization.

C. Pathophysiology.

1. Subluxation in late cocking phase, the anterior and anterior/inferior aspects of the shoulder endure tremendous tension. Structures in the posterior aspect of the joint are compressed.
2. Dislocations in traumatic cases are caused by force applied against the abducted and externally rotated shoulder. The result of the blow is that the head of the humerus is malpositioned anterior to the shoulder joint.
3. Recurrent dislocations can be due to congenital weaknesses of the shoulder structures. In traumatic instances, once the capsule is torn recurrent dislocations can easily happen.

D. Incidence.

1. Anterior dislocation.
   a. Is usually an athletic injury from a fall on the extended arm.
   b. Glenohumeral joint: area of most common upper-extremity injuries and is the most common dislocation of a major joint. Four types of anterior glenohumeral dislocations:
      (1) Subcoracoid: accounts for 90% of all anterior dislocations.
      (2) Subglenoid: accounts for 7%. This position differs from inferior dislocations because there is contact of the humeral head with the scapula at the posterioinferior rim of the glenoid rim.
      (3) Subclavian: rare; usually seen in multiple traumas. The subclavian is present when the humeral head is medial to the coracoid and inferior to the clavicle.
      (4) Intrathoracic: rare; usually seen in multiple traumas. The humeral head extends through the ribs onto the thoracic cavity in this type of dislocation.
   c. Of all shoulder dislocations, 95% are anterior.
   d. Of the anterior dislocations, 50%-70% are suffered by patients under 30 years of age.
   e. Recurrent anterior dislocations:
      (1) Appear in 90%-95% of patients under 20 years of age, but with immediate care, the risk of recurrence is decreased 25%-35%.
      (2) Rate for those over 40 years of age is 10%-15%.
   f. Sternoclavicular dislocations occur in isolation approximately 40% of the time. For patients with sternoclavicular dislocation, 55% will present with some form of clavicle fracture.
   g. Sternoclavicular dislocations are graded as to the degree of damage:
      (1) Grade I – incomplete (this is a stable injury).
      (2) Grade II – unstable.
      (3) Grade III – rupture of both the sternoclavicular and costoclavicular ligaments and is considered a complete dislocation.
2. Posterior dislocation.
   a. Rarely occurs.
   b. When it does occur, usually in a patient with seizures in which the extended arm is abducted and internally rotated.
   c. Rarely seen by itself; it is seen more commonly in combination with anterior and inferior instability (complex instability).
   d. Literature reveals that nearly 50% of the time, this type of dislocation is missed on initial evaluation.
   e. Three varieties:
      (1) Subacromial.
      (2) Subglenoid.
      (3) Subspinous.
3. Inferior instability.
   a. Usually significant soft-tissue injuries such as avulsion of the supraspinatus, pectoralis major, and teres minor muscles.
   b. In inferior dislocation there is no contact between the humeral head and glenoid rim.
4. Superior dislocations are extremely rare.
5. Complex (multi-directional) instability: occurs often, is in two or more directions, and may be a combination of anterior, posterior, or inferior instabilities.

E. Considerations across the lifespan.

1. Anterior dislocation is a common (90%-95%) recurrent injury especially for patients under 20 years of age.
2. In patients between 20-40 years of age, there is only 10%-15% recurrence of anterior dislocations.

F. Complications.

1. With anterior dislocations:
   a. Damage to the major nerves of the arm or to the axillary nerve occurs 5%-14% of the time.
   b. With axillary nerve injury, the disability varies

from slight weakness of the deltoid muscle and hyperesthesia over the upper outer aspect of the arm to complete paralysis, and usually clears up within a few weeks to several months.

2. Bony lesions occur 38% of the time.
3. Tears of the rotator cuff.
4. Avulsion fractures of the greater tuberosity.
5. Recurrent shoulder dislocations.
6. Post-surgical complication can be punctate calcification of the acromioclavicular and coracoclavicular ligament resulting in an impingement syndrome.
7. Associated injuries that may occur with a posterior dislocation include fractures of the posterior rim of the glenoid fossa and the greater and lesser tuberosities as well as labral and capsular tears. Humeral head fracture can occur during relocation.

II. ASSESSMENT

A. History.

1. Pain in shoulder.
   a. In anterior dislocations, pain especially is felt during late cocking phase.
   b. Pain during accelerating phase is evidence of impingement syndrome.
   c. Pain can radiate to fingertips and usually disappears quickly.
2. For posterior instability there is a perception of dislocation when performing activities with the arm flexed, adducted, and internally rotated.

B. Physical examination.

1. Assess for loss or change of normal contour of the joint by comparing extremities and palpation. Deformity is evident in the anterior dislocation but difficult to visualize in the posterior dislocation.
   a. The humeral head is palpable along the lateral aspect of the chest in an inferior instability. It is palpable anteriorly in the subcoracoid region.
   b. In anterior dislocation there is a flattening of the normally rounded shoulder contour.
   c. The acromion is prominent with fullness anteriorly.
   d. In inferior dislocations, the humeral head is easily palpated on the lateral thorax.
   e. In superior dislocations, the humeral head is typically superior to the fossa with the arm adducted and shortened.
2. Assess for change in the length of the extremity.
3. Check mobility of the affected extremity. Patient with anterior dislocation usually resists any attempt at passive movement or active abduction of the arm.
4. Neurovascular checks. If the axillary nerve is involved, there will be paralysis of the deltoid muscle and an area of anesthesia on the lateral aspect of the arm.

C. Diagnostic tests.

1. Stability tests (throwing tests).
2. Apprehension Test: affected shoulder is positioned in 90 degrees of abduction and external rotation with the elbow in 90 degrees flexion. The shoulder is pushed gently into external rotation. Patients with instability become apprehensive and feel a sensation of impending dislocation.
3. See Table 16.3 for subclassifications of shoulder instability.
4. X-rays are essential to establishing whether the humerus has been displaced anteriorly or posteriorly in relation to the glenoid fossa. Most often an AP, lateral "Y," and axillary views are taken.
   a. Reveals a Hill-Sachs lesion which is a defect on the humeral neck caused when the humeral neck strikes glenoid rim during dislocation.
   b. Bankart lesion is a defect on the glenoid rim.
   c. For posterior dislocations, the "Y" or axillary view radiograph is the best diagnostic test.

Table 16.3
Subclassifications of Shoulder Instabilities

1. **Type**
   a. Dislocation
   b. Subluxation
   c. Dislocation/subluxation
2. **Direction**
   a. Anterior
   b. Posterior
   c. Inferior
   d. Superior
   e. Multidirectional
3. **Etiology**
   a. Traumatic
   b. Atraumatic
      (1) Spontaneous primary and recurrent dislocation
      (2) Recurrent voluntary dislocation/subluxation

III. COMMON THERAPEUTIC MODALITIES

A. Objective of treatment: decreased pain and increased joint stability and mobilization while decreasing anxiety.

B. Nonsurgical treatment.

1. Reduction of dislocation as soon as possible with or without anesthesia.
   a. Without anesthesia requires muscle relaxation.
      (1) Use of weights plus the muscle relaxer can reduce.
      (2) If not, countertraction can be accomplished by the physician placing a hand in the axilla and lifting the humerus laterally with gentle internal and external rotation. Grade III injuries may require surgical treatment should closed techniques not work.
   b. With anesthesia may be the technique of choice or as an alternative if the first method failed.
2. Immobilization of joint.
   a. Soon enough to prevent permanent limitation of motion.

Table 16.4
Classification of Acromioclavicular Joint Injury

Type I	Painful but stable joint. The ligament is stretched but with an incomplete disruption.
Type II	Some degree (less than half the diameter of the clavicle) of subluxation and joint separation. The ligament is intact.
Type III	Displacement greater than 5 mm. Coracoclavicular disruption is usually ligamentous, but may present with a coracoid avulsion fracture.
Type IV	Injuries with an extreme posterior displacement of the distal clavicle.
Type V	These are rare and similar to Type III injuries.
Type VI	Very rare. It involves a complete disruption of the acromioclavicular and coracoclavicular ligaments.

b. Long enough for the damaged tissues to heal.
c. Type of immobilizer depends on the age of the patient.
   (1) Young patients may use a collar and cuff or Velpeau bandage, and maintained for 3-6 weeks to allow soft tissues and muscles to heal.
   (2) Over 50 years of age, recurrent dislocation is less but permanent shoulder stiffness is higher.
      (a) Shoulder is either not immobilized or immobilized for a short period of time.
         i. Grade I injuries may need a sling.
         ii. Grade II injuries placed in a sling with a figure-of-eight bandage or swathe for 1-2 weeks.
      (b) Gentle active and assisted movements as soon as tolerated is the course of action.

3. Cryotherapy is used during first 24-48 hours post-trauma or surgery when it is most effective in reducing inflammation. (Do not place ice bags on the incision site.)
4. RECIPE (rest, elevation, compression, ice, proper exercise).
5. Analgesics as needed.

B. Surgical treatment.

1. Surgical repair is necessary for permanent correction of recurrent dislocations.
2. The procedure depends on the patient's age and activity level and the degree of damage to the glenoid.
3. In the instance of Type IV, V, and VI acromioclavicular joint dislocations, surgery is recommended immediately (see Table 16.4).
4. Surgical procedures.
   a. Bankart procedure: securing the anterior rim of the glenoid fossa.
   b. Capsulorrhaphy: the anterior capsule is overlapped to strengthen the capsule and stabilize the humeral head.
   c. Putti-Platt: procedure to reattach the lateral portion of the muscle to the anterior rim of the glenoid fossa to limit external rotation.
   d. Bristow-Helfet: procedure to secure the coracoid process with attached tendon of biceps and coracobrachialis muscle to the glenoid rim.
   e. Manson and Stack: procedure in which the anterior capsulomuscular wall is tightened.
   f. Eden-Hybbinette: procedure placing a bone graft against the anterior aspect of the neck of the scapula and the rim of the glenoid cavity.
5. Potential complications.
   a. Infection.
   b. Circulatory impairment.
   c. Shoulder joint stiffness.

IV. NURSING DIAGNOSES, OUTCOMES, AND INTERVENTIONS

A. See Table 16.2.

B. Physical mobility, impaired.

1. Outcomes: patient has increased mobility and no joint deformities.
2. Interventions.
   a. Promote mobility and muscle strength within restrictions.
   b. Discuss exercise program to promote mobility.
   c. Promote use of unaffected extremities during mobility restrictions.
   d. Promote exercise program. (Note: the type of exercises and when they begin depends on the type of surgery.)
      (1) Gentle range of motion exercises.
      (2) Pendulum exercises where the patient:
         (a) Leans forward.
         (b) Allows the arm to hang down and away from the body.
         (c) Slowly swings the arm from side to side.
      (3) No internal or external rotation movements until allowed by physician.

V. HOME CARE CONSIDERATIONS: The type of immobilizer and length of immobilization will depend on the surgery that was performed.

A. Instruct to avoid long, uninterrupted car rides.

B. Inspect and instruct on sitting in appropriate chairs in order to rise from them.

C. Pendulum or gentle range-of-motion exercises without weights or external rotation. Exercises to increase over time as tolerated.

ADHESIVE CAPSULITIS

I. OVERVIEW

A. Definition: fibrosis of the glenohumeral joint capsule (also known as frozen shoulder.)

B. Etiology: slow, gradual onset characterized with pain and stiffness and progressive limitation of motion. Specific causes unknown but prolonged bed rest or immobilization of shoulder joint may be predisposing factors. Secondary causes are fracture dislocation and arthritis.

C. Pathophysiology: condition related to fibroblastic proliferation of collagen and nodular bands that causes shrinking of the capsule and thickening of the glenohumeral ligaments.

D. Incidence.

1. Occurs in patients age 50-70 years of age.
2. 25% of these patients have diabetes mellitus.

E. Complications.

1. Rotator cuff can become weakened if intra-articular injections are not kept to a minimum dosage.
2. Atrophy of muscles of glenohumeral girdle may occur.

II. ASSESSMENT

A. History.

1. Patient complains of diffuse, dull, aching pain in the shoulder.
2. Progressive restriction of motion.
3. Over 2 months, pain eventually radiates to forearm with complaints of pain at night.

B. Physical examination.

1. No localized tenderness upon palpation.
2. Either presents with arthritis bilaterally or appears first on one side and later on the other side.
3. Diffuse, dull aching pain in shoulder:
    a. Pain may become constant and disabling.
    b. Pain may radiate down the arm and the back to the scapula.
4. Loss of movement, particularly abduction and rotation.
5. Atrophy of the muscles of the shoulder girdle may be apparent.

C. Diagnostic tests.

1. Routine x-rays.
2. Arthrographs are diagnostic and reveal a very small joint space.

III. COMMON THERAPEUTIC MODALITIES

A. Objective of treatment: relieve pain and joint inflammation while increasing mobility.

B. Nonsurgical treatment.

1. Intra-articular injections with weak corticosteroid solution.
2. Distention therapy is a local intra-articular injection with amount of solution being greater than joint cavity can hold.
    a. Goal is to break adhesions between capsule and humeral head.
    b. Immediately increases motion and decreases pain.
    c. Gentle ROM during every waking hour.
    d. Heat and assistive exercises.
    e. Analgesics.

C. Surgical treatment.

1. Manipulation under general anesthesia gives more favorable results.
2. In severe cases, surgical release of adhesions.

IV. NURSING DIAGNOSES, OUTCOMES, AND INTERVENTIONS

A. See Table 16.2.

B. Physical mobility, impaired.

1. Outcomes: patient has increased mobility.
2. Interventions.
    a. Promote physical mobility of the arm and shoulder within restrictions.
    b. Heat and assistive exercises in the beginning.
    c. Pain medications may need to be given before exercising.
    d. Later an exercise program to regain range of motion and strength within the shoulder and arm.
    e. Instruct and support patient regarding the prognosis of the condition: self-limiting with symptoms decreasing within 6 months-2 years.

C. Pain.

1. Outcomes: patient demonstrates maximal degree of comfort.
2. Interventions.
    a. Assess patient's pain level.
    b. Promote patient comfort with correct positioning.
    c. Utilize distraction activities to help with pain relief.
    d. Anti-inflammatory drugs.
    e. Oral pain medications.

FRACTURES OF THE SHOULDER

I. OVERVIEW

A. Definition: a fracture is a break in one or more cortices of a bone, frequently with associated soft-tissue injuries.

B. Etiology.

1. Fall on affected shoulder
2. Moderate to severe blow to site
3. Weakened area in bone from tumor or lack of proper vitamins or minerals, especially calcium.

C. Pathophysiology.

1. Osteoporosis is a large reason for the great number of humeral fractures. In displaced fracture of humeral neck, the pectoral muscles pull distal fragments inward and forward and the deltoid muscle pulls it upward.
2. Fall is usually on outstretched hands from standing height.
3. Clavicular fractures are usually direct trauma to shoulder laterally.

4. Scapula fractures are direct trauma usually from motor vehicle accidents, high-impact sports or hard impact of strenuous occupational duties.

D. Incidence.

1. Most common fracture of the shoulder is the proximal humerus.
2. Scapula fractures account for 1% of fractures.

E. Considerations across the lifespan.

1. Proximal humeral fractures are more common in elderly.
2. Clavicular fractures are more common in children.
3. Scapula fractures are typically seen in patients 40-60 years of age.

F. Complications: humeral neck fracture may cause axillary nerve damage.

II. ASSESSMENT

A. History: activity when incident occurred.

B. Physical examination.

1. Pain in shoulder: specific area; clavicle, scapula, proximal humerus.
2. Assess mobility.
   a. Clavicle: inability to raise arm.
   b. Proximal humerus: inability to move arm.
   c. Scapula: pain with shoulder movement.
3. Note swelling, discoloration, temperature, crepitation.
4. Compare affected extremity with unaffected side to note deformities.
   a. Clavicle: protrusion of inner half of clavicle.
   b. Scapula: bone displacement on palpation.
5. Neurovascular examination: in scapula fractures, the radial nerve may be damaged as demonstrated by decreased sensation in the web space and inability to extend thumb, fingers, and wrist.

C. Diagnostic tests: x-rays.

III. COMMON THERAPEUTIC MODALITIES

A. Objectives of treatment: maximal degree of comfort and stability.

B. Nonsurgical treatment.

1. Cold packs: for first 24 hours to aid in decreasing inflammation.
2. Analgesic medication to alleviate pain.
3. Type of immobilization and length of immobilization of the extremity depends on extremity involved.
   a. A clavicular fracture is usually self-healing, so they do not require elaborate splinting, usually only a sling, a figure-of-eight bandage, or both.
   b. Scapular and humeral fractures requires a sling and swathe.
   c. Humeral fractures:
      (1) Sling and swathe.
      (2) Sometimes a Velpeau bandage for 3 weeks.
      (3) A hanging arm cast or lateral traction apparatus that maintains forward flexion and traction may be used until a soft callus forms.
      (4) A closed reduction may be used, but for more severe cases or fractures of the surgical humeral neck, open reduction and internal fixation is usually indicated.

B. Surgical treatment: the goal of surgery in more complex displaced fractures is to achieve a painless and stable shoulder.

1. Choice of technique and devices to treat the fractures depends on several factors:
   a. Type of fracture.
   b. Quality of bone and soft tissue.
   c. Age of patient.
   d. Reliability of patient.
2. Open reduction internal fixation (ORIF) is indicated if displacement of the fragments is too severe to return extremity to function. Several devices may be used to achieve an ORIF.
   a. Intramedullary (IM) nails.
   b. Plates and screws.
   c. Staples.
   d. Wires.
   e. Suture material.
3. Arthroplasty.
   a. See Arthritis of the Shoulder, this chapter..
   b. Other reasons for performing arthroplasty.
      (1) Fracture that may culminate in avascular necrosis.
      (2) Chronic glenohumeral incongruency due to:
         (a) Sickle cell infarction.
         (b) Irradiation necrosis.
4. Hemiarthroplasty: the replacement of the humeral head with a prosthesis.
   a. Performed in the case of a humeral neck fracture in which the glenoid is not involved and is functionally sound.
   b. Used in the treatment of certain acute fractures of the proximal humerus (see Chapter 14, Trauma [Fractures]).
      (1) Replacement of the proximal humerus is done for fracture-dislocations and for the treatment of fractures in which reduction is almost impossible and the articular fragment is likely to undergo avascular necrosis.
      (2) Need surgery as soon as possible, as a delay of 10-14 days or longer results in:
         (a) Increased scarring.
         (b) Contractures of the muscles and other soft-tissue structures.
         (c) Increased osteoporosis of the bone fragments.

IV. NURSING DIAGNOSES, OUTCOMES, AND INTERVENTIONS

A. See Table 16.2.

B. Fear.

1. Outcomes.
   a. Patient will express fears and concerns related to condition.
   b. Patient will understand the treatment plan and availability of community resources.
2. Interventions.

Table 16.5
Categories of Sternoclavicular Joint Dislocations

Grade I	A stable injury in which the ligamentous complex is stretched but not disrupted.
Grade II	An unstable injury in which there is a rupture of the sternoclavicular ligament and some subluxation of the medial clavicular head.
Grade III	A rupture of both the sternoclavicular and costoclavicular ligaments with a complete dislocation. This results in a gross displacement of the medial clavicular head.

a. Provide education regarding treatment, community resources, and pathology.
b. Allow patient to express fears and concerns related to treatment plan.
c. Express need for compliance with treatment and rehabilitation regimen.
d. Encourage and reinforce stringent adherence to exercise regimen.

V. PRACTICE SETTING CONSIDERATIONS

A. Hospital.
1. PCA pump for pain.
2. Instruct as to the change in balance when ambulating due to arm being close to the chest. Reassure and explain the need to prevent falls or injuries to affected shoulder.
3. Proper positioning to decrease pain and promote healing such as elevation and exercises.
4. Immobilization at all times except when exercising. Passive exercises on day of surgery.
5. Finger and thumb exercises as soon as possible, all other joints on day of surgery.
6. Gentle passive exercises including forward flexion and external rotation of shoulder.
7. Head of bed (HOB) elevated 30 degrees for comfort.
8. CPM (continuous passive motion) machine.

B. Home care considerations.
1. Pendulum exercises 10 days postoperatively.
2. Should not actively elevate arm for 6-8 weeks postoperatively or until deltoid muscles are declared healed.
3. Alternatives and resources for aid in ADL.

C. Complications.
1. Postoperative infection.
2. Instability of glenohumeral joint after total shoulder arthroplasty (TSA).

SPRAINS, STRAINS, AND CONTUSIONS

I. OVERVIEW

A. Definition:
1. Sprain is a wrenching or twisting of a joint with partial rupture of its ligaments.
2. A sprain is more serious than a strain, which is the overstretching of a muscle without swelling.
3. Contusion is the injury to tissues without breakage of skin or a bruise.

B. Etiology: these injuries occur by the same mechanisms as dislocations. They are less severe and self-limiting than dislocations.

C. Pathophysiology.
1. In an acromioclavicular joint injury, subclassification of the injury depends on amount of injury sustained to the acromioclavicular joint and the coracoclavicular ligaments (see Table 16.4).
2. In a sternoclavicular joint injury, the degree of damage sustained by the supporting ligaments and the final position of the clavicular head determines the category (see Table 16.5).

II. ASSESSMENT

A. History.
1. Shoulder pain.
2. Mechanism of injury.

B. Physical examination.
1. Assess for:
   a. Swelling.
   b. Discoloration.
2. Assess mobility.
   a. Difficulty in doing ADLs.
   b. Disability of function may or may not be evident.

C. Diagnostic tests: x-rays may or may not show abnormalities.

III. COMMON THERAPEUTIC MODALITIES

A. Objective of treatment: maximal comfort.

B. Nonsurgical treatment.
1. Cold packs for 24 hours.
2. Analgesic medications for pain.
3. Immobilization with a sling if desired to protect the extremity.

IV. NURSING DIAGNOSES, OUTCOMES, AND INTERVENTIONS

A. See Table 16.2.

B. Pain.
1. Outcomes: patient will demonstrate maximal degree of comfort.
2. Interventions.
   a. Assess patient's level of pain.
   b. Relieve pain with positioning.
   c. Utilize a sling to immobilize and relieve pressure from the weight of the arm.
   d. Utilize heat and cold therapy, as appropriate.
   e. Pain medications when needed.
   f. Muscle setting exercises.

V. HOME CARE CONSIDERATIONS: Encourage as much activity as possible within activity restrictions.

SPRENGEL'S DEFORMITY

I. OVERVIEW

A. Definition: a congenital anomaly characterized by a high, small mal-rotated scapula. It is usually associated with other anomalies such as scoliosis, spina bifida, clavicular malformation, etc.

B. Etiology: it may be a compression of the brachial plexus and the vessels between the scapula and the first rib, creating a thoracic outlet syndrome.

II. ASSESSMENT: Physical examination

A. Scapulothoracic motion is limited.

B. Glenohumeral motion is usually normal.

III. COMMON THERAPEUTIC MODALITIES

A. Objectives of treatment: increase mobility.

B. Nonsurgical treatment. Depends on the degree of disability and loss of motion as well as the age of the child and associated abnormalities.

C. Surgical treatment.

1. Usually is not indicated before 3-4 years of age.
2. The procedures entail relocating the scapula at a lower position.

IV. NURSING DIAGNOSES, OUTCOMES, AND INTERVENTIONS

A. See Table 16.2.

B. Coping, ineffective.
Family coping, compromised.

1. Outcomes: patient demonstrates adequate coping mechanisms to deal with illness.
2. Interventions.
   a. Promote adaptation/coping.
   b. Reinforce adaptive mechanisms that are being used successfully.
   c. Assist patient/family in verbalizing concerns, feelings, and fears.

CONGENITAL DYSPLASIA OR HYPOPLASIA OF THE GLENOID

I. OVERVIEW

A. Definition: an uncommon condition in which there is a failure during embryonic stages of the formation of either the upper or lower glenoid epiphysis. Usually it is the lower glenoid epiphysis that is not formed.

B. Etiology: this condition may be associated with various other congenital anomalies, but usually it is an isolated one that occurs bilaterally.

II. ASSESSMENT

A. History.

1. Asymptomatic in early childhood.
2. Symptomatic when child reaches mid-teens.

B. Diagnostic tests: usually discovered on routine x-ray.

III. COMMON THERAPEUTIC MODALITIES

A. Objectives of treatment: coping with illness/deformity.

B. Nonsurgical treatment: exercises.

C. Surgical treatment: osteotomy of the neck of the scapula with interpositional bone graft to improve the glenoid contour and reduce symptoms.

IV. NURSING DIAGNOSES, OUTCOMES, AND INTERVENTIONS

A. See Table 16.2.

B. Coping, ineffective.
Family coping, compromised.

1. Outcomes: patient demonstrates adequate coping mechanisms to deal with illness.
2. Interventions.
   a. Promote adaptation/coping.
   b. Reinforce adaptive mechanisms successfully used.
   c. Assist patient/family in verbalizing concerns, feelings, and fears.

REFERRED VISCERAL-SOMATIC PAIN

I. OVERVIEW. Definition: other medical conditions can present with the initial complaint of shoulder pain. These conditions have nothing to do with the shoulder girdle complex other than lying within the dermatome, myotome, or sclerotome that innervates both areas.

II. ASSESSMENT: Referred Pain Diagnosis

A. Cardiac.

1. Anginal.
2. Hand-shoulder syndrome.

B. Gallbladder/hepatic injury/hepatitis.

C. Lung tumor.

D. Cervical (spondylosis).

E. Splenic injury.

F. Pleuritis/pneumonia/pulmonary embolus.

G. Diaphragmatic irritation.

H. Ruptured viscus.

Bibliography

Altizer, L.L. (1998). Degenerative disorders. In A.B. Maher, S.W. Salmond, & T.A. Pellino (Eds.), *Orthopaedic nursing* (2nd ed., pp. 480-544). Philadelphia: W.B. Saunders Company.

Bates, B. (1995). *A guide to physical examination and history taking* (6th ed.). Philadelphia: J.B. Lippincott Company.

Berg, E.E. (1995). Posterior shoulder (glenohumeral) dislocation. *Orthopaedic Nursing, 14*(1), 47-49.

Berg, E.E. (1997). Calcific tendonitis of the shoulder. *Orthopaedic Nursing, 16*(6), 68-69.

Calliet, D.C. (1991). *Shoulder pain* (3rd ed.). Philadelphia: F.A. Davis Company.

Deuschle, J. A. & Romeo, A.A. (1998). Understanding shoulder arthroplasty. *Orthopaedic Nursing, 17*(5), 7-15.

Gregory, B. (1994). *Orthopaedic surgery.* St. Louis: Mosby Year Book.

Heveron, B., & Kaempffe, F.A. (1995). Tears of the rotator cuff. *Orthopaedic Nursing, 14*(6), 38-41.

Iannotti, J.P., & Williams, G.R. (1999). *Disorder of the shoulder: Diagnosis and management.* Philadelphia: Lippincott Williams & Wilkins.

Kelley, M.J., & Clark, W.A. (1995). *Orthopaedic therapy of the shoulder.* Philadelphia: J.B. Lippincott Company.

Long, J.S. (1996). Shoulder arthroscopy. *Orthopaedic Nursing, 15*(2), 21-31.

Maher, A.B. (1996). Trauma. In S.W. Salmond, N.E. Mooney, & L.A.Verdisco (Eds.) *NAON: Core curriculum for orthopaedic nursing* (3rd ed., pp. 415-449). Pitman, NJ: National Association of Orthopaedic Nurses.

Maher, J., & Childs, S.G. (1999). The shoulder. In S.G. Childs (Ed.), *The upper extremity: Traumatic injuries and conditions* (pp. 53-72). Pitman, NJ: National Association of Orthopaedic Nurses.

McFarland, E.G., Leigh, A.C., Urguhart, M.W., & Kellam, K. (1997a). Shoulder immobilization devices. Part 1: The Sling. *Orthopaedic Nursing, 16*(4), 17-20.

McFarland, E.G., Leigh, A.C., Urguhart, M.W., & Kellam, K. (1997b). Shoulder immobilization devices. Part 2: Shoulder immobilizers. *Orthopaedic Nursing, 16*(5), 66- 71.

McFarland, E.G., Leigh, A.C., Urguhart, M.W., & Kellam, K. (1997c). Shoulder immobilization devices. Part 3: Abduction pillows and braces. *Orthopaedic Nursing, 16*(6), 47-54.

Mourad, L. (1995). Orthopaedic nursing. In K.V. Gettrust (Series Ed.), *Plans of care for specialty practice.* New York, NY: Delmar Publishers, Inc.

Murphy, M., & Hahn, G.V. (2000). Orthopedic surgery. In M.L. Phippen & M.P. Wells (Eds.), *Patient care during operative and invasive procedures* (pp. 502-567). Philadelphia: W.B. Saunders Company.

Petrone, R.A. (1995). *Athletic injuries of the shoulder.* New York: McGraw-Hill, Inc.

Post, M., Flatow, E.L., Bigliani, L.U., & Pollock, R.G. (1998). *The shoulder: Operative technique.* Baltimore, MD: Lippincott Williams & Wilkins.

Schoen, D.C. (2000). Care of the patient with shoulder and elbow injuries. In D.C. Schoen (Ed.), *Adult orthopaedic nursing* (pp. 403-442). Philadelphia: Lippincott.

Sheehy, S.B., & Lombardi, J.E. (1995). Extremity trauma. In S.D. Sheehy & J.E. Lombardi (Eds.), *Manual of emergency care* (pp. 552-576). St. Louis: C.V. Mosby.

Warren, R.F., Craig, E.V., & Altcheck. D.W. (1999). *The unstable shoulder.* Philadelphia: Lippincott-Raven Publishers.

Winkel, D. (1997). *Diagnosis and treatment of the upper extremities.* Gaithersburg, MD: Aspen Publishers, Inc.

Zimmer, Inc. (1991). *Fracture and fracture management.* Warsaw, IN: Zimmer, Inc.

STUDY QUESTIONS

1. George Carpenter, age 52, arrives at the clinic complaining of left shoulder pain. While obtaining a medical history, he states his shoulder began hurting approximately 2 months ago and has rapidly gotten worse during arm movement. The pain now radiates to his forearm and hurts at night. He has had no previous immobilization or trauma. Preliminary diagnosis is a frozen shoulder. The treatment that gives a more favorable result would be:
   a. Intra-articular injections.
   b. Distention therapy.
   c. Immobilization.
   d. Manipulation under general anesthesia.

Susie Hamilton, age 18, is a member of the high school swim team. She has presented to the sports medicine clinic with complaints of right shoulder pain. The pain came on suddenly after the state swim match in which Susie set the state record in the butterfly event. Physical examination revealed pain with the arm elevated overhead and the appearance of edema to the right shoulder. (Questions 2-3)

2. From the presenting information, what would be the most likely diagnosis?
   a. Bicipital tendinitis.
   b. Rotator cuff tendinitis.
   c. Calcific tendinitis.
   d. Bursitis.

3. Another name for this condition would be:
   a. Impingement syndrome.
   b. Acromioclavicular arthritis.
   c. Frozen shoulder.
   d. Adhesive capsulitis.

John Simpson, age 37, was admitted to the emergency room after a fall at work. He was complaining of severe pain to the left shoulder. Upon exploring the mechanism of the injury, it was noted that a piece of heavy machinery malfunctioned and to avoid being hit, Mr. Simpson had to dive to the ground upon which he fell on his left shoulder which was tucked to his side. The physical examination revealed swelling, hematoma, and gross deformity to the left shoulder. He was unable to raise his arm or stretch it across his chest. Initial diagnosis after radiographs showed displacement of the acromioclavicular joint. (Questions 4-6)

4. From the presenting information, what would be the most likely diagnosis?
   a. Dislocation.
   b. Subluxation.
   c. Glenoid fracture.
   d. Arthritis.

5. Mr. Simpson's radiographs showed an extreme posterior displacement of the distal clavicle. How was this injury classified?
   a. Type I.
   b. Type II.
   c. Type III.
   d. Type IV.

6. What would be the initial treatment for this type of injury?
   a. Anti-inflammatory medications.
   b. Immediate surgical interventions.
   c. Cold pack.
   d. Physical therapy.

Jason Phillips, age 14, arrived in the emergency room with complaints of pain to his right shoulder area and his arm held closely to his body. He states he was playing soccer when a team member ran into him and caused him to land on his right arm. Upon physical examination, he is unable to raise his arm and there is evidence of swelling and hematoma with some deformity and crepitus over the clavicular area. (Questions 7-8)

7. How would this injury be classified?
   a. Clavicular fracture.
   b. Glenoid fracture.
   c. Humeral head fracture.
   d. Scapula fracture.

8. What should be the initial treatment for this injury?
   a. Open reduction internal fixation.
   b. Sling to support the arm.
   c. Arthroplasty.
   d. Exercise.

9. Other medical conditions can manifest complaints of shoulder pain. These conditions have nothing to do with the shoulder girdle complex except that it is innervated by the same nerves that innervate the true area of pain. This phenomenon falls under the heading of:
   a. Referred visceral-somatic pain.
   b. Hyperchondriac.
   c. Congenital anomalies.
   d. Impingement syndrome.

10. Mrs. Walker, age 70, tripped and fell on her outstretched right arm. She presented to the emergency room with gross swelling and discoloration of her right shoulder. Upon viewing the radiographs, the physician's diagnosis was a humeral neck fracture and rheumatoid arthritis. What should be the initial treatment for this injury?
    a. Sling and swathe.
    b. Cold pack.
    c. Arthroplasty.
    d. Open reduction internal fixation.

Chapter 17 Nursing Care for Hand and Wrist Problems

Sharon G. Childs, MS, CRNP-CS, ONC

Contents

OBJECTIVES

At the completion of this chapter, the learner will be able to:

- Recognize three interventions to provide safety and prevent injury to the hand/wrist.
- Describe the pathophysiology of common hand conditions or traumatic injuries.
- Identify assessment criteria for each hand/wrist condition or injury including history and physical examination techniques.
- Select common provocative diagnostic tests performed to establish definitive diagnoses.
- State common therapeutic modalities and complications that occur in hand/wrist conditions or injuries.
- Recall nursing standards and nursing diagnoses for hand/wrist conditions or injuries.
- State specific nursing interventions to meet the needs of the patient with a hand/wrist condition or injury.
- Discuss outcome criteria based on the patient's physical condition and home care considerations.

KEY POINTS

- Prevent hand injuries through use of ergonomic principles in product design; organization of work, home, and recreational environment; and development of safety instructions and programs.
- Always compare the neurovascular (NV) status of the affected hand/wrist to the unaffected side.
- Monitor contracted digits for moisture from perspiration. This can cause skin maceration.
- To recover amputated parts:
    1. Place part in a slightly dampened normal saline or dry sterile gauze, if available.
    2. Place part in a watertight sealed bag/container.
    3. Do not place amputated tissue in water, saline, iodine, or any solution.
    4. Place watertight sealed bag/container in ice. Never use dry ice.
    5. Note time ice applied and when cooling of tissue began.
- With children, attempts are made to replace parts even with severe injury because of the child's developmental needs.
- The hand/wrist is splinted and placed in the functional position.

CHAPTER 17

Nursing Care for Hand and Wrist Problems

DUPUYTREN'S CONTRACTURE

I. OVERVIEW

A. Definition: a progressive thickening of the palmer fascia that results in fibrosis and eventual contracture of the ring and small fingers at the level of the metacarpal phalangeal (MCP).

B. Etiology.

1. Seen mostly in Caucasians with Northern European extraction.
2. Associated with heredity, in gout, rheumatoid arthritis (RA), diabetes mellitus (DM), Human Immunodeficiency Virus (HIV), epilepsy, and cigarette smoking.
3. Autosomal dominant.
4. Associated with alcoholism and its metabolic effects on fat and prostaglandin.

C. Pathophysiology.

1. At the cellular level, platelet derived and fibroblast growth factors promote dense myofibroblast and collagen synthesis that causes fibrosis and thickening of palmer aponeurosis (fascia). Inflammatory process is associated with chronic overuse and local free-radical generated microvascular ischemia.
2. Flexion contracture develops slowly and progressively from spontaneous proliferation of connective tissue and formation of large amounts of collagen resulting in cord-like structures in palmer fascia.
3. Nodules form in fatty subcutaneous layers between the MCP and proximal interphalangeal (PIP) flexor creases.
4. Cords attach to flexor tendon sheathes, joint capsules, interosseous fascia, periosteum, and skin.
5. Neurovascular (NV) bundles become entwined pulling diseased tissue toward center of the digit.
6. In later state, collagen adheres to tendons and as it ages, shrinks causing contracture further limiting function in involved digits.

D. Incidence.

1. Affects about 2% of the population.
2. More prevalent in white males of northeastern European ancestry (Irish, Scandinavian).
3. Occurs bilaterally in majority of cases but when unilateral, the right hand is affected twice as frequently as the left.
4. When more than one finger is contracted, the ring and little fingers are more often involved.
5. 5% of clients may have a similar condition in the plantar fascia of the foot.

E. Considerations across the lifespan: occurs most frequently in late 40s or early 50s; however, has been reported in younger and older patients.

F. Complications.

1. Skin breakdown related to moisture beneath flexed digit.
2. Infection/incisional separation.
3. Postsurgical bleeding/hematoma.
4. Incomplete release of contracture.
5. Scarring if motion not instituted early.
6. Reoccurrence of contracture.
7. Neurovascular injury.

II. ASSESSMENT

A. History.

1. No history of trauma.
2. May or may not have a dull ache in the palm. No complaints of severe pain.
3. Numbness, tingling, cramping, and stiffness of affected fingers in the morning.
4. Family history.
5. Alcohol intake.
6. Hand dominance.

B. Physical examination.

1. Palpate palmer crease opposite ring or affected finger where thickened and contracted band may be palpated in palmer fascia.
   a. Loss of fat tissue occurs with formation of hard nodules and induration or dimpling of the skin.
   b. "Knuckle pads" are common on the dorsum of (PIP) joint.
2. Perform range of motion (ROM).
   a. In the early stage, there is a decrease in ROM.
   b. In the later stage, well-developed flexion contracture interferes with activities of daily living (ADL).
3. Observe for moisture from perspiration beneath contracted digit that will cause skin maceration.
4. Assess and document NV status.

C. Diagnostic tests: x-ray to rule out bone mass/lesion.

III. COMMON THERAPEUTIC MODALITIES

A. Finger strengthening and stretching exercises.

B. Continuous extension/elongation surgical preparatory techniques.

C. Surgical excision is treatment of choice.

1. Resection of thickened palmer fascia is performed during the early stage and is often done as an outpatient ambulatory care surgical procedure.
2. Postoperative bulky dressing with or without splint for 5-7 days.
3. Finger and hand exercises begin in 24-48 hours and continue for several months.

Table 17.1
Common Nursing Diagnoses, Outcomes, and Interventions

Diagnoses	Outcomes	Interventions
A. Injury, risk for	• Patient will use safety precautions and avoid repetitive motion strain (RMS), traumatic, and chronic injuries to the hand.	• Provide individual patient and community education to promote safety and avoid occupation-related hand injuries. 1. Avoid repetitive motions or sustained positions, such as wrist flexion or hyperextension (seamstress, carpenter, machine operator, typist, computer operator, guitarist, painter, etc.) 2. Reduce speed, force, and number of repetitive motions. 3. Avoid lifting heavy objects with hands only. 4. Alternate work and rest periods. 5. Alternate which hand is being used. 6. Rotate work activities. 7. Alternate hard and easy tasks. 8. Use the whole hand and fingers to grasp objects to avoid strain on digits or wrists. 9. Organize recreational activities, home, and work areas so height and distance of objects prevent stretching or overreaching. 10. Perform exercises that strengthen the hand and arm. 11. Encourage patient to read new product information for safety precautions. 12. Prevent falls. 13. Review power equipment and vehicular safety precautions. • Work with companies to develop specific occupational safety criteria for personnel and safety instructions for clients. • Work with manufacturers to design ergonomic products (hand tools, lawn mower guards, saw blade guards, power tools, etc.)
B. Tissue perfusion, ineffective; peripheral neurovascular dysfunction, risk for	• Neurovascular status will remain intact.	• Compare injured hand with unaffected hand. • Compare preoperative baseline with postoperative status. • Elevate and support the extremity as ordered. • Apply ice/cold packs as ordered. • Assess each digit separately when multiple digits are involved.

Table 17.1 (continued)
Common Nursing Diagnoses, Outcomes, and Interventions

Diagnoses	Outcomes	Interventions
B. Tissue perfusion, ineffective; peripheral neurovascular dysfunction, risk for (continued)	• Neurovascular status will remain intact. (continued)	• Differentiate arterial and venous vascular assessment. • Observe dressing/wound for bleeding and monitor hemoglobin and hematocrit. • Prevent constriction from dressings, casts, or splints.
C. Skin integrity, impaired	• Patient heals without evidence of infection and skin breakdown.	• Assess and monitor skin integrity. • Assess preoperatively with range of motion (ROM) to ensure adequate surgical skin coverage and healing. • Keep skin clean and dry to prevent breakdown beneath contracted/deformed parts of the hand.
D. Physical mobility, impaired; self-care deficit syndrome: **• Bathing/hygiene** **• Feeding/toileting** **• Dressing/grooming**	• Patient will demonstrate the use of adaptive devices and modified techniques to maintain independence in self-care and activities of daily living (ADL). • Patient achieves maximal potential of function.	• Assess and monitor hand function, self-care limitations, and ADL. • Note ROM, strength, atrophy, and fine motor coordination. • Test motor function ONLY IF ORDERED by the physician immediately postoperative in tendon repairs, vascular and nerve grafts, and skin grafts. • Observe ability to perform movements necessary for self-care and ADL related to feeding, hygiene, dressing, toileting, occupation, and recreation. • Teach the use of assistive devices.
E. Post-trauma response; anxiety	• States reduced anxiety related to conservative/surgical treatment.	• Alleviate anxiety. • Assess degree of anxiety and patient perception of the injury (functional loss, hand dominance, cosmesis, occupational and social concerns). • Provide explanation of diagnostic procedures. • Provide preoperative teaching and explanations of postoperative regimes. • Offer reassurance and support. • Allow time to answer patient's questions.
F. Pain, acute; pain, chronic	• Decreased pain and adequate pain relief.	• Assess pain status. • Believe the patient's pain; hand/finger injuries are very painful. • Instruct patient in noninvasive pain relief techniques. • Keep extremity elevated. • See Chapter 7, Pain.

Table 17.1 (continued)
Common Nursing Diagnoses, Outcomes, and Interventions

Diagnoses	Outcomes	Interventions
G. Infection, risk for	• No complications will develop related to the injury or treatment provided.	• Prevent and monitor for infection. • Perform preoperative skin preparation as ordered. • Administer preoperative antibiotic as ordered. • Monitor temperature elevation. • Monitor white blood cell count, C-reactive protein, and sedimentation rate. • Perform sterile dressing changes. • Note any purulent drainage, foul odor, hematoma, erythema, warmth, and wound dehiscence. • Obtain wound culture as ordered.

IV. NURSING DIAGNOSES, OUTCOMES, AND INTERVENTIONS (See Table 17.1)

V. HOME CARE CONSIDERATIONS (See Table 17.2)

MALLET FINGER (JERSEY FINGER)

I. OVERVIEW

A. **Definition: mallet finger is most often a closed tendon injury of the distal extensor apparatus of the distal interphalangeal (DIP) joint.**

B. **Etiology.**
   1. Seen in the patient who has fallen on a digit.
   2. Injury may also occur during environmental and/or occupational activities.
   3. Commonly related to sport injury (being struck by a ball, pulling at a jersey of another player).

C. **Pathophysiology.**
   1. Sudden forceful flexion/extension of a digit.
   2. Disruption of the insertion of the flexor/extensor apparatus onto the dorsal/volar base of the DIP.
   3. Forceful disruption of tendon structure may avulse a fragment of bone that is then referred to as an avulsion fracture.

D. **Incidence.**
   1. Mallet finger is seen in the patient who falls, jamming the digit.
   2. More common in dominant hand.
   3. Mallet finger/jersey finger affects the DIP joint only and accounts for 18% of finger sprains.
   4. Common in middle/ring/small fingers.

E. **Considerations across the lifespan.**
   1. Teenagers and young adults are the most common population.
   2. Elderly individuals often do not seek treatment which may lead to a dysfunctional finger which disrupts ADL.

Table 17.2
Home Care Considerations for People with Hand Injuries/Conditions

1. Instruct patients about signs and symptoms of complications to report to their health care provider (edema, erythema, increased or severe pain, numbness or paresthesias, coolness of the hand/wrist, bloody/purulent drainage, and fever).
2. Instruct patients about wound/dressing care (prospective time for suture removal, how to shower and manage personal hygiene, etc.).
3. Instruct patients about the use of cast/splints/slings for elevation and alignment (rationale for use, how to apply, and how to care for the orthopaedic devices).
4. Reinforce the use of assistive devices and instruct in modified methods of performing self-care in ADL (eating utensils, zippers vs. buttons, loafers vs. ties, reachers, sponges, rest vs. activity, etc.).
5. Reinforce instructions given by the health care provider for activity restrictions and rehabilitative exercises.
6. Encourage patient compliance with regimen, and follow-up with health care provider, occupational/ physical therapist, and community resources.

F. **Complications.**
   1. Avulsion fracture and/or delayed treatment may result in loss of normal functioning of the digit.
   2. Cosmetic deformity of the digit.
   3. Protracted pain and disability secondary to delayed/non-union of fracture or complete rupture of the tendon.
   4. Joint instability.

II. ASSESSMENT

A. History.

1. May or may not complain of pain and/or deformity to DIP joint.
2. Patient describes the mechanism of injury to the joint.
3. Unable to grasp or make a fist.

B. Physical examination.

1. Ecchymosis present.
2. Swelling present to DIP joint.
3. Pain with active and passive ROM (unable to flex/extend DIP joint).
4. Digit is NV intact.
5. Note open skin lesions about injury that indicates an open fracture.

C. Diagnostic tests: A/P, lateral, oblique x-rays to rule out avulsion fracture.

III. COMMON THERAPEUTIC MODALITIES

A. Relocation of DIP if dislocated.

B. If open injury, give tetanus prophylaxis.

C. Irrigate wound.

D. Apply dry sterile dressing.

E. Soft tissue sprains treated by PRICEMM (protection, rest, ice, compression, medications, and modalities).

1. **P** = protection by altering ROM, modifying sport/work/activities by way of splint/support.
2. **R** = rest of injured DIP to decrease stress loading on joint and allow tissue repair.
3. **I** = ice/cold compresses to decrease swelling and relieve pain.
4. **C** = compression of DIP with tape/splint to control edema, provide support/comfort/stability.
5. **E** = elevate hand to decrease swelling by mobilization of post-inflammatory fluid.
6. **M** = medications such as nonsteroidal anti-inflammatory drugs (NSAIDs) to decrease the effects of the local inflammatory mediators, decrease swelling/pain; narcotics for pain relief.
7. **M** = modalities such as PT/OT after sufficient time in splint to gently mobilize DIP joint, regain mobility/flexibility/strength.

IV. NURSING DIAGNOSES, OUTCOMES, AND INTERVENTIONS (See Table 17.1)

V. HOME CARE CONSIDERATIONS

A. See Table 17.2.

B. Instruct patient/parent on correct use of splint.

C. Explain rationale/side effects of NSAIDs and narcotics.

D. Monitor injury for increased pain or deformity.

TRIGGER THUMB/FINGERS

I. OVERVIEW

A. Definition: locking or snapping of thumb or finger in a flexed position due to stenosis and thickening of tendon sheath.

B. Etiology.

1. Possible congenital origin: familial tendency such as trisomy 13.
2. Trauma.
3. Repetitive/forceful hand/finger movements.

C. Pathophysiology.

1. Repeated injury and inflammation cause the tendon sheath to become stenosed, tendon enlarges, forming a nodule or diffuse mass.
2. As tendon passes through stenosed tendon sheath, in extension the nodule will catch and make a "snap" or a "pop." This "trigger" mechanism is usually located at the level of the A-1 pulley about the metacarpal head, and may be palpated on the volar aspect of the hand.
3. Frequently mechanical tenosynovitis develops.

D. Incidence.

1. 30% have spontaneous resolution.
2. Hand dominance.
3. Bilateral occurrence common.
4. May have more than one digit involved.
5. More common in women.
6. Possible reoccurrence if treated conservatively.
7. Seen in DM, RA, gout, and metabolic disorders.

E. Considerations across the lifespan: occurs in all ages.

1. Newborns and infants: thumb most commonly involved.
2. Predominantly between ages of 40-70: thumb most commonly involved followed in frequency by middle finger and ring finger.

F. Complications.

1. Digital nerve injury: in child, make a shallow incision as digital nerves are very close to midline incision area.
2. Infection.
3. Transection of A2 pulley.
4. Incomplete release of A1 pulley.
5. Hematoma.
6. Bow stringing posture of flexor pollicis longus if distal pulley not preserved.

II. ASSESSMENT

A. History.

1. Trauma to finger or thumb.
2. Digit locking in flexed position.
3. Pain when gripping items.
4. Familial history.
5. Occupation with repetitive digital movements.
6. Hand dominance.
7. Medical morbidity (DM, RA, gout, metabolic disorders).

B. Physical examination.

1. Palpable nodule over extensor tendon.
2. Evidence of thumb/finger locking in flexed position.
3. A popping sound when extending thumb/finger.
4. Tenderness over tendon sheath.
5. Assess NV status.
6. Assess digital skin integrity.
7. Pain while attempting to extend digit.

C. **Diagnostic tests: x-ray to rule out bony pathology and differentiate diagnosis from that of hypoplastic and arthrogrypotic thumb.**

III. COMMON THERAPEUTIC MODALITIES

A. **Infant/child.**
   1. At birth may be passively extended, splint for 6 weeks. Use sequential casts/splints to achieve full extension.
   2. Under 1 year, if trigger mechanism continues or reoccurs with conservative splinting, consider surgery.
   3. Over 1 year, consider surgical transection of pulley.

B. **Adult.**
   1. Injection of local anesthetic and corticosteroid.
   2. Gentle active ROM exercises.
   3. Surgical transection of A1 pulley.
   4. Application of cool alternating with warm compresses.

IV. NURSING DIAGNOSES, OUTCOMES, AND INTERVENTIONS (See Table 17.1)

V. HOME CARE CONSIDERATIONS

A. **See Table 17.2.**
B. **Instruct patient/parent in use of sequential cast/splint in infant.**
C. **Explain action and side-effects of corticosteroid injection and assist with procedure.**
D. **Observe and report signs of infection or increased pain.**

DeQUERVAIN'S TENOSYNOVITIS

I. OVERVIEW

A. **Definition: DeQuervain's is a tenosynovitis of the extensor pollicus brevis and abductor pollicus longus tendons located in the first dorsal compartment in the wrist.**

B. **Etiology.**
   1. This condition is seen in people between 30-50 years of age.
   2. Caused by repetitive and forceful exertions of the wrist/hand.
   3. Occurs in individuals who hold manual labor-type jobs, typists, machinists, brick masons.

C. **Pathophysiology.**
   1. Awkward, forceful, and repetitive use of tendinoligamentous structures precipitate fatigue and accumulation of metabolic waste products.
   2. Acute and chronic re-injury causes recurrent inflammation, pain, and fibroblastic changes in the tendon and tendon sheath.
   3. Fibroblastic changes may lead to permanent scarring.

D. **Incidence.**
   1. Seen more commonly in women.
   2. Dominant hand/wrist most often affected.
   3. May occur in the weekend athlete or the homeowner who overdoes weekend chores.
   4. DeQuervain's as a work-related musculoskeletal disorder (WRMD) accounts in part for 56% of all occupational injuries.

E. **Considerations across the lifespan.**
   1. May see increased incidence in aging population.
   2. Frequently seen postpartum (repetitive lifting of an infant).

F. **Complications of nontreatment.**
   1. If untreated, may lead to progressive loss of hand function.
   2. May lead to chronic wrist/hand pain.

II. ASSESSMENT

A. **History.**
   1. Determine prior history of trauma and repetitive strain injury.
   2. Exclude non-occupational reasons for this condition.
   3. Patient complains of increased pain with repetitive wrist/hand movements.
   4. Elicit location, duration, and intensity of pain.

B. **Physical examination.**
   1. Positive Finkelstein's test (ulnar deviation of hand with thumb flexed against palm).
   2. Pain with palpation about the radial styloid and/or at the base of the thumb.
   3. Mild swelling and warmth palpated.
   4. Positive pain with active and resistive ROM of the wrist/hand.

C. **Diagnostic tests.**
   1. Finkelstein's test.
   2. Radiographs are not generally warranted unless significant blunt trauma or twisting/ torque has occurred to the wrist.

III. COMMON THERAPEUTIC MODALITIES

A. **Ergonomic adjustment of wrist/hand postures.**
B. **Wrist/hand splinting in early inflammatory phase.**
C. **Administration of NSAIDs.**
D. **PRICEMM (see Mallet/Jersey Finger in this chapter).**
E. **Cortisone injection.**

IV. NURSING DIAGNOSES, OUTCOMES, AND INTERVENTIONS (See Table 17.1)

V. HOME CARE CONSIDERATIONS (See Table 17.2)

GANGLION

I. OVERVIEW

A. **Definition: a cystic structure adjacent to a joint or tendon sheath.**

B. **Etiology.**
   1. Pathogenesis is related to chronic repetitive stress, and synovial herniation.
   2. Trauma or degenerative changes in fibrous joint

capsule are thought to be contributing factors.

3. May be associated with rotatory subluxation of the scaphoid (RSS).
4. Depending on the location, may compress the median nerve causing carpal tunnel syndrome (CTS).

C. Pathophysiology.
1. Cystic structure is found on:
   a. Dorsoradial wrist.
   b. Volar radial wrist.
   c. Seed ganglia may erupt on dorsal DIP joint, or palmer surface of the digits.
2. Consists of clear mucinous gel-like material encased in fibrous capsule.
3. Swelling is non-inflammatory in nature.
4. Benign.

D. Incidence.
1. Most common soft tissue tumor in hand.
2. Females have a higher predisposition (3:1) than males.
3. Reoccurrences are common.

E. Considerations across the lifespan.
1. Most frequently seen in people 15-50 years of age.
2. Rarely seen in elderly.

F. Complications (post-surgical).
1. Compression of median nerve secondary to post-surgical edema.
2. Infection.
3. Hematoma.

II. ASSESSMENT

A. History.
1. Gradual or abrupt onset.
2. May be post-traumatic.
3. Reported loss of function is rare.
4. Pain: present/absent.
5. Soft tissue mass.
6. Numbness and tingling in thumb, index, and middle fingers if associated with CTS.
7. Hand dominance.

B. Physical examination.
1. Local pain and feeling of weakness exacerbated by dorsiflexion of wrist.
2. Mass is more prominent on wrist when it is flexed.
3. Usually freely movable.
4. Size of ganglion may vary.
5. Altered ROM.

C. Diagnostic studies: A/P and oblique x-ray views of wrist and hand to rule out additional pathology.

III. COMMON THERAPEUTIC MODALITIES

A. Aspiration of ganglion followed by injection of corticosteroid.

B. Application of pressure dressing and splinting.

C. NSAIDs.

D. Surgical excision with postoperative dressing and splint immobilization for 3 weeks followed by active exercises.

IV. NURSING DIAGNOSES, OUTCOMES, AND INTERVENTIONS (See Table 17.1)

V. HOME CARE CONSIDERATIONS (See Table 17.2)

CARPAL TUNNEL SYNDROME (CTS)

I. OVERVIEW

A. Definition: CTS is a median nerve entrapment neuropathy. The median nerve is compressed beneath the transverse carpal ligament in the wrist.

B. Etiology.
1. Most common entrapment neuropathy in the upper extremity (UE).
2. May be seen in those with arthritis, lipomas, ganglion, after a fracture or trauma.
3. Often seen during premenstrual period, pregnancy, menopause, in DM, when there is thyroid dysfunction (which suggests hormonal changes may play a part), and in systemic conditions that lead to fluid retention.

C. Pathophysiology.
1. Carpal tunnel is composed of carpal bones and transverse carpal ligament.
2. Median nerve travels over carpal bones and under transverse carpal ligament.
3. CTS may occur in any disease or thickening of the tendon sheaths, which causes pressure on the median nerve.

D. Incidence.
1. Occurs in women five times more frequently than in men. Rationale is related to hormonal variances related to menses, pregnancy, and menopause.
2. Dominant extremity is most often affected, but may be bilateral.

E. Considerations across the lifespan: usually occurs between 30-50 years of age.

F. Complications.
1. Infection.
2. Hematoma.
3. Neurovascular injury (rare).
4. Incomplete division of the transverse carpal ligament.
5. Symptom resolution:
   a. Post surgery.
   b. May be less in women under 40 years old.
   c. May be related to women returning to workforce and the same job after surgery.
   d. Hormonal variances as stated under D. Incidence (above).
6. Untreated CTS may lead to progressive loss of motor function and finite finger sensibility.

II. ASSESSMENT

A. History.
1. Display sensory/motor median nerve symptoms of:
   a. Burning pain.
   b. Paresthesias.
   c. Numbness in the thumb, index, middle fingers, and half of the ring finger.

d. May radiate to the forearm/shoulder.
2. Causes nocturnal discomfort.
3. Pain is initially relieved by repositioning and/or movement of the hand/wrist.
4. Increased pain and paresthesia:
   a. With rapid, repetitive and forceful hand flexion.
   b. Or, hyperextension, vibration, forceful gripping.
   c. Positions are often work-related (dentist, seamstress, machine operator, writer, knitter, bowler, typist, computer operator, guitarist, carpenters, painter etc.).
5. Complains of:
   a. Progressive weakness.
   b. Inability to perform fine motor activities.
   c. Drops small objects or cannot grasp large objects.
   d. Has decreased tactile discrimination.
6. Generally in dominant hand.

B. Physical examination.
1. Positive Tinel's sign: percussion over the volar wrist crease elicits symptoms such as numbness, tingling, and paresthesias.
2. Positive Phalen's test: symptoms are elicited when patient holds his/her wrists in flexion for 60 seconds.
3. In advanced cases, weakness and atrophy of small muscles innervated by median nerve (thenar muscle of the thumb, etc.) may be seen.

C. Diagnostic tests.
1. X-rays (A/P, lateral) needed to rule out bony abnormality (about the hand and wrist).
2. Nerve conduction studies determine latency in nerve conduction and rule out lesions more proximal to spinal cord (both invasive and non-invasive types available).
3. Electromyelogram (EMG) detects decreases in muscle conduction velocities.
4. Carpal compression tests reveal amount of pressure necessary to elicit symptoms of CTS.
5. C-Spine x-ray may be needed to rule out cervical pathology causing referred pain to the hand/wrist.

III. COMMON THERAPEUTIC MODALITIES

A. Treatment of the underlying pathology or functional cause.

B. Splinting and immobilization to rest affected limb (occupational and night splinting).

C. Injection of corticosteroids to decrease edema.

D. Administration of NSAIDs.

E. Osteopathic manipulative treatment with "opponens roll" maneuver and self-stretching.

F. Self-laser/acupuncture treatments at home.

G. Modifying work environment to ergonomically correct tools and work station

H. Surgical decompression of median nerve through release of the transverse carpal ligament performed as an open or endoscopic procedure.
1. Postoperative interventions.
   a. Use postoperative dressing for 1 week, volar splint for 14-21 days with open procedure.
   b. Use smaller postoperative dressing; a splint may or may not be used with an endoscopic procedure.
2. Rehabilitative exercises:
   a. Use hand actively.
   b. Exercise each digit (gentle flexion/extension) as soon as possible, and as prescribed by the surgeon.

IV. NURSING DIAGNOSES, OUTCOMES, AND INTERVENTIONS

A. See Table 17.1.

B. Sleep pattern disturbance.
1. Outcome: sleep will be uninterrupted during night.
2. Interventions.
   a. Evaluate quality sleep patterns.
   b. Pain is often the cause of sleep disorder; re-evaluate pain management and modify as necessary.
   c. Splint extremity at night.
   d. Provide sedation/hypnotics at night.

C. Noncompliance, potential.
1. Outcome: complies with splinting and therapeutic activity restrictions.
2. Interventions.
   a. Explain rationale for treatment and consequences of noncompliance.
   b. Associate therapeutic regimes with positive beliefs and values of patient.

V. HOME CARE CONSIDERATIONS (See Table 17.2)

REPLANTATION

I. OVERVIEW

A. Definitions.
1. Total replantation: microvascular surgical procedure to restore hand/digit to its original site.
2. Revascularization:
   a. Reconstruction of microcirculation that has been damaged in order to prevent ischemic tissue from becoming necrotic.
   b. Term also describes restoration of incomplete amputation, a technically more difficult procedure than total replant.
3. Complete amputation: a hand/digit that has been totally severed from body.
4. Incomplete/partial amputation: a hand/digit that has become partially severed from body, with part of vital neurovascular structures remaining intact.
5. Warm ischemia time: amount of time since amputated part was severed (without adequate cooling).
6. Cool ischemia time: amount of time severed part is maintained on ice.
7. Total ischemia time: sum of warm and cold ischemia times or the time elapsed from the loss of blood flow to the amputated tissue to the beginning of surgical

intervention.

B. Etiology: multiple traumatic injuries.

1. Trauma: vehicular (car/motorcycle), occupational (farm industry/mechanics), and home (lawn mowers/power tools).
2. Self-imposed suicide attempts.

C. Pathophysiology.

1. Consists of reattachment of partially or completely severed tissue or parts.
2. In larger proximal injuries, reconstructive flaps of free tissue transfers (autografts) may be needed to provide essential NV structures, muscle, and skin to cover large tissue defects and salvage wrist/hand.
3. Procedure must be performed as rapidly as possible after amputation to inhibit bacterial growth and avoid muscle ischemia, which is irreversible after 6 hours warm ischemia time.
   a. Digital/distal parts may be replaced beyond this time from 24-36 hours based on total ischemia time and viability of the tissue.
   b. Proximal digit replant may be contraindicated except in multiple digit amputation; proximal amputations at the palm and wrist levels generally result in good hand function.

D. Incidence.

1. Upper extremity.
   a. Upper extremity is most often traumatically amputated and replaced.
   b. Function is not dependent on length of replanted extremity.
2. Proximal/digital location of injury.
   a. Digital (80%-90%) viability and distal replants have higher success rate.
      (1) Digital functional return is approximately 85%.
      (2) Digits contain less muscle and have lower metabolic needs.
   b. Proximal replants with large muscle mass have higher failure and function rate because of:
      (1) Increased ischemia.
      (2) High metabolic needs.
      (3) Poor reinnervation.
      (4) Lack of sensibility and proprioception.
3. Type of injury.
   a. Clean cut (guillotine) has the best prognosis.
   b. Severely crushed/avulsed – not replanted because of:
      (1) Nerve stretching.
      (2) Massive soft tissue and vascular bed damage.
      (3) Massive contamination.
      (4) Associated comminuted/segmental fracture patterns and open fracture.
      (5) Multilevel amputation.
      (6) Missing pieces of amputated parts.

E. Considerations across the lifespan: all age groups.

1. May be less successful in children.
   a. When successful, function better than adults because of capacity for reinnervation and adaptation.
   b. Digits usually grow to 80% of their adult length.
   c. Support and assurance are needed for child, parents, and sibling(s).
   d. Attempts are made to replace parts even with severe injury because of child's developmental needs.
2. Cosmesis is an issue for all age groups; hand/digit function is important for certain populations such as artists, musicians.
3. In elderly.
   a. Careful attention is given to underlying systemic disease.
   b. Ability to withstand prolonged surgical time under anesthesia.
   c. Metabolic demands of limb.

F. Complications.

1. Arterial occlusion (thrombosis).
   a. Aggressive pharmacotherapy with heparin, fibrinolytic agents (streptokinase, urokinase) and vasodilators (papaverine).
   b. Surgical re-exploration/revision.
2. Venous congestion, the most common.
   a. Manual massage of digit.
   b. Medicinal leech therapy.
      (1) Each leech removes approximately 5 ml of blood from area.
      (2) It also secretes hirudin, an enzyme with anticoagulant properties that assists in vascular patency causing the wound to ooze 50 ml of blood for 24-48 hours after detachment.
   c. Surgical re-exploration/revision.
3. Regional/systemic sepsis.
4. Acute renal failure:
   a. Associated with proximal injury.
   b. Systemic inflammatory response.
   c. Shock.
5. Decreased cold tolerance.
6. Serial surgeries to gain maximal function.
7. Functional disabilities/contractures and loss of finite sensibility and proprioception.
8. Retardation of bone growth, which can be treated by bone stimulators and distraction procedures.
9. Donor site morbidity:
   a. Infection.
   b. Tissue necrosis.
   c. Poor/inefficient wound healing.
   d. Extensive scarring.
10. Replant failure/amputation.
11. Post-traumatic stress disorder/psychoemotional dysfunction.
12. Complex regional pain syndrome (previously referred to as reflex sympathetic dystrophy [RSD]).

II. ASSESSMENT

A. See Table 17.3.

B. Emergency assessment at the scene (first aid/EMT/paramedics).

1. Evaluate ABCs.

Table 17.3
Replantation: Assessment and Interventions

Assessment:
1. Emergency care at the scene
   a. ABCs.
   b. Evaluate for injury to other organ systems.
   c. Estimate blood loss and control bleeding.
   d. Assess for signs and symptoms of shock.
   e. Assess residual limb and amputated part(s) based on criteria.

2. ER/preoperative care
   a. Repeat steps A-E above.
   b. Diagnostic tests-lab, EKG, X-ray, possible arteriogram.

3. Postoperative care
   a. Assess NV status.
   b. Assess pain level.
   c. Assess for signs or symptoms of infection.
   d. Assess patient's psychoemotional status.
   e. Assess patient's needs for home care and social support.

Nursing Interventions:
1. Emergency care
   a. Resuscitate.
   b. Apply direct pressure and elevate extremity to control bleeding.
   c. Keep patient warm; elevate lower extremities.
   d. Insert IV for fluid resuscitation.
   e. Recover and package tissue parts. Dress/splint as indicated.
   f. Rapid transport to Trauma/ER/Replant Center.

2. Trauma/ER/preoperative care
   a. Repeat steps A-D above.
   b. Prepare patient for OR.
   c. Cleanse/irrigate topical contamination.
   d. Administer antibiotic, tetanus prophylaxis.
   e. Administer analgesics.
   f. Perform diagnostic tests.
   g. Maintain calm atmosphere.
   h. Begin preoperative teaching with patient/family/significant other.

3. Postoperative care
   a. Monitor circulation clinically/electronically and/or prevent vasoconstriction to prevent arterial occlusion/venous congestion/vasospasm. Administer medications on schedule without interruption. Notify physician of changes immediately. EMERGENCY!!!
   b. Provide pain relief promptly.
   c. Maintain sterile technique.
   d. Direct nursing actions to the phase which patient is undergoing to provide emotional support and assist in the reintegration process. Provide psychological counseling.
   e. Provide patient teaching and discharge planning. Encourage compliance with wound care, therapy, and exercises, protection of the limb and follow-up with the surgeon/health care provider.
   f. Assist patient with self-care and vocational counseling, etc. to maintain independence.

2. Assess for injury to vital organs.
3. Estimate blood loss.
   a. Completely severed vessel ends constrict.
   b. Partially severed vessel ends remain open resulting in hemorrhage.
4. Assess for shock.
5. Preliminary assessment of residual limb and amputated part(s).

C. Emergency department/preoperative assessment.
1. Repeat steps 1-4 above.
2. Reassess residual limb and amputated part.
3. Criteria for replantation: realistic goals should be based on expected outcomes for injured part and person as a whole.
   a. Function and form improved: major criterion.
   b. Warm/cool/total ischemic time/viability of amputated tissue/part.
   c. Level of amputation: distal/proximal.
   d. Number of digits amputated.
      (1) One digit may not be replaced.
      (2) Multiple digits: replace as many as possible.
      (3) Thumb replaced: responsible for 50% of hand function.
   e. Bilateral amputation/associated with contralateral disability or paralysis.
   f. Hand dominance.
   g. Type injury: clean (guillotine)/crushed, avulsed.
   h. Age.
   i. Hemodynamic, stability related to other acute injuries; ability to withstand anesthesia time.
   j. Pre-existing systemic disease (DM, hypertension, atherosclerosis, peripheral vascular disease, collagen-vascular disease, bleeding disorders, chronic pulmonary disease, renal disease, and immunocompromising diseases etc.).
   k. Smoking history, alcohol, and drug abuse.
   l. History of active psychoaffective illness or motivational problems.

D. Diagnostic tests.
1. Laboratory:
   a. CBC, SMA18, PT, PTT.
   b. Type and cross-match, as ordered.
2. Electrocardiogram (EKG).
3. X-rays:
   a. Amputated tissue and proximal stump.
   b. Chest x-ray
   c. Arteriogram to determine vascular status.

III. COMMON THERAPEUTIC MODALITIES

A. Surgical replantation by a team that includes microvascular, orthopaedic, and/or plastic surgeons.
1. A two-team approach may be used.
   a. One cares for patient and residual limb.
   b. Other prepares the amputated part(s).
2. Surgical repair.
   a. Microsurgical identification and tagging of tendioligamentous and NV structures in residual limb and amputated part.

b. Soft tissue debridement.
c. Bone: preparation by shortening, fixation, and periosteal repair.
d. Tendon: repair of extensor and flexor tendon.
e. Vascular reanastomosis (arteries/ veins).
   (1) Arteries are anastomosed first.
   (2) More veins are anastomosed than arteries: use flap donor site or free transfer if needed.
f. Nerves: repair and/or transfer.
g. Muscle: repair and possible fasciotomies.
h. Skin (grafting may be needed).
i. Digital transposition and/or toe to thumb transfer.
j. Pollicization.
k. Temporary ectopic revascularization of site to preserve the part until secondary transfer recipient site is ready (deep inferior epigastric vessels).

IV. NURSING DIAGNOSES, OUTCOMES, AND INTERVENTIONS

A. See Table 17.1.

B. Grieving, anticipatory.
Grieving, dysfunctional.

1. Outcome: patient will function adequately with ADL.
2. Interventions.
   a. Acknowledge patient's grief
   b. Allow time for patient to express feelings and concerns; encourage verbalization.
   c. Offer therapeutic support – teach/reinforce effective coping techniques.

C. Nutrition, imbalanced: less than body requirements.

1. Outcome: patient shows signs of improved nutritional status by evidence of progressive wound healing and stable serum/metabolic parameters.
2. Interventions.
   a. Monitor wound healing.
   b. Monitor serum electrolytes, glucose, albumin, transferrin, WBC.
   c. Discuss with patient his/her ability to prepare meals at home.

D. Post-traumatic response.

1. Outcome: patient will resolve stress response by using therapeutic coping techniques.
2. Interventions.
   a. Encourage discussion of traumatic situation so patient is able to connect feelings with the event.
   b. Utilize antidepressant and antianxiety medications.
   c. Obtain psychiatric consult for patient and family.

E. Injury, risk for (postoperative).

1. Outcome:
   a. No disruption of replant/graft site.
   b. Vascular/nerve and tissue anastamoses will be maintained at surgical site.
2. Interventions.
   a. Reinforce preoperative instructions to prevent pulmonary complications.
      (1) Deep breathing exercises every 2 hours.
      (2) Incentive spirometry and respiratory treatment as ordered.
   b. Monitor hemoglobin and hematocrit (H/H). Low H/H may precipitate vasoconstriction and ischemic pain.
   c. Monitor donor and recipient site for infection.
   d. Provide adequate nutrition to meet metabolic needs for healing. Give high-calorie, high-protein diet.
   e. Promote comfort. Administer analgesics promptly. Pain triggers vasospasm.
   f. Monitor NV status through clinical evaluation and technical equipment so circulation will be maintained and to prevent vasoconstriction and possible ischemia.
      (1) Patients are not asked to demonstrate motor/sensory function. A deficit is expected immediately postoperatively.
      (2) Monitor for signs of arterial occlusion.
         (a) Replanted part is pale/pallor.
         (b) Slow capillary refill: more than 2 seconds or not observable.
         (c) Tissue turgor is abnormal.
         (d) Replanted part is cool.
         (e) Serum rather than blood obtained when dermal bleeding tested.
      (3) Monitor for signs of venous occlusion.
         (a) Replanted part is cyanotic.
         (b) Increased capillary refill (instantaneous).
         (c) Tense, distended turgor.
         (d) Replanted part is cool.
         (e) Bleeds briskly for extended time when dermal bleeding is tested. Color: dusky (dark blue to purple).
      (4) Elevate extremity above heart level since there are more problems with venous outflow. However, lower arm if arterial occlusion or compartment syndrome is suspected.
      (5) Use Doppler to discern pulse.
      (6) Use pulse oximetry to measure arterial blood oxygen saturation to detect tissue hypoxemia before visible signs and symptoms develop.
      (7) If using a temperature probe, monitor temperature readings along with NV status. Compare temperature of uninjured parts with injured part. If temperature of injured digit is less than 30° C, there is poor perfusion of replanted digit. Also report more than 5° C difference between normal and replanted extremity and a drop of 2° C in an hour. Check lead/probe placement.
      (8) If using muscle contraction monitoring (evoked M wave) in free flaps, monitor reading when performing NV assessments.
      (9) Fluorometry readings may be performed by injecting 0.5 ml of fluorescein, an IV

dye rapidly absorbed that penetrates all perfused tissue. (Venous congestion gives a high reading; arterial occlusion gives an abnormally low reading on monitor). Perform with NV assessments. *Notify physician of changes in the above immediately. Emergency!!!*

(10) Assure administration of thrombolytic agents to decrease accumulation of platelets at site of small vessels. ASA® (acetylsalicylic acid), Persantine®, and low molecular dextran are commonly used. Dextran enhances microvascular flow by expanding plasma volume and reducing blood viscosity. Use for approximately 5 days. Do not interrupt for other medications. Anticoagulant therapy (heparin or low molecular weight products) is sometimes given. Caution should be used as heparin may potentiate active bleeding. Check clotting test results. Hyperbaric oxygen therapy, Vasodilan®, and Thorazine® are used by some institutions to promote vasodilation.

(11) Maintain room temperature 78-80° F. Prevent drafts. Some institutions use heat cradles or light heating pads if ordered. Caution must be used to prevent injury related to sensory deficit.

(12) No smoking and smoke-free environment are needed (patient, roommate, family/visitors, or staff). Nicotine causes vasospasm and local microvascular collapse.

(13) No caffeine (coffee, tea, colas, chocolate).

(14) Monitor intake and output and keep well hydrated – 3,000 cc per day unless contraindicated. Dehydration increases blood viscosity and impedes flow.

(15) Encourage limited activities and rest first week postop.

(16) Avoid alcohol.

F. Individual coping, ineffective potential (postoperative).

1. Outcome: patient will adjust to potential changes in body and lifestyle.
2. Interventions.
   a. Provide psychoemotional support based on the phase patient is undergoing.
   b. Undergoes shifts in phases similar to those in grief process.
      (1) Pre-accidental: often has stressful life event or unresolved conflict that causes or relates to postoperative emotional state (guilt, blame, and developmental crisis).
      (2) Initial shock (early hospitalization).
         (a) Seems calm because of numbness, shock, dreamlike state.
         (b) Walls off fear of dying.
         (c) Often does not grasp what is said, leading to communication difficulties.
         (d) Sees amputated part as irretrievable.
      (3) State of uncertainty.
         (a) Has anxiety about disruption of body integrity.
         (b) May not look at limb.
         (c) If looks at original swollen/discolored limb, may doubt ownership, completeness of self. Feels conspicuous/visible, vulnerable.
         (d) Refers to self as the broken part, "the hand," since replanted limb receives the attention.
         (e) Fears for survival of part and its function. Perceives situation as "touch and go." Magnifies minor changes. Feels limb is dead due to sensory/motor loss.
         (f) Wonders how replanted limb will affect occupation, income, role and acceptance by family/friends, appearance, and sexual attractiveness. Susceptible to outside suggestions and influence.
      (4) Recognition of loss.
         (a) Occurs when some degree of disability, appearance, and loss of function become apparent.
         (b) Displays sadness, depression, anger, frustration, hopelessness, and helplessness and mourns based on emotional significance and meaning of restored part to the individual.
      (5) Acceptance and reintegration.
         (a) Begins to give up uninjured form and reintegrate new altered part into the body schema. Accepts more readily if emotionally well adjusted prior to injury and receives family support.
         (b) Feels everything was tried even if failure occurs. Reluctant to have amputation if limb viable but nonfunctional.
   c. Counseling by team nurse/physician psychotherapist.

V. SPECIFIC SITE INTERVENTIONS

A. Emergency care at the scene (first aid/EMT/paramedic).

1. Resuscitate (ABCs).
2. Assess vital signs for signs of shock and evaluate for evidence of injury to other vital structures.
   a. Elevate lower extremities if not contraindicated by patient's condition.
   b. Keep warm.
   c. Start IV fluid resuscitation.
   d. Give 100% oxygen by non-rebreather mask or nasal cannula.
3. Control bleeding.
   a. Gently remove topical debris.
      (1) Do not remove impaled objects.
      (2) Secure impaled objects with tape, wraps, dressing to prevent object from moving about in the tissue.
   b. Apply direct pressure with sterile dry dressing.

c. Do not use tourniquet unless patient is hemorrhaging. If absolutely necessary, then place as proximal to injury as possible.
d. Elevate injured part.
4. Recover all amputated tissue and part(s).
a. Cover with slightly moistened normal saline or dry gauze, if available.
b. Place tissue/part(s) in watertight sealed bag/container.
c. Do not immerse tissue/part(s) in any solution. Do not apply any antiseptic ointment/cream.
d. Place watertight sealed bag/container on ice. Note time ice applied.
e. For incomplete/partial amputation repeat steps 1-3 and apply ice to distal extremity. Splint to prevent further disruption of osseous and vascular tissue, immobilize fracture, and prevent kinking/overstretching of nerves and vessels.
f. Transport immediately to trauma/emergency department/replant center.

B. Emergency department/preoperative care.
1. Continue resuscitation and care to stabilize life-threatening situations (ABCs).
2. Treat injuries to other organ systems.
3. Control bleeding by direct pressure, elevation of affected extremity; apply and monitor pneumatic compression (B/P) cuff as prescribed by physician.
4. Monitor for hypovolemic shock: administer IV fluid replacement (crystalloids/ blood/dextran, etc.).
5. Continue assessment of residual limb and part(s) based on criteria in Section IV., E. Injury, risk for (postoperative).
a. Cleanse/irrigate with physiologic solution to remove gross contamination.
b. Debridement, at any stage of care, is generally performed by advanced practitioners and physicians on replantation team.
c. Maintain hypothermia of amputated tissue.
6. Administer medications.
a. Emergency drugs, as needed.
b. Tetanus toxoid.
c. Cephalosporins and/or broad-spectrum antibiotics as indicated.
d. Analgesics for pain.
7. Prepare for diagnostic tests.
8. Provide preoperative instructions and preparations.
a. NPO for surgery.
b. Possibility of prolonged surgery.
c. Cough and deep breathing exercises.
d. Pain management.
9. Provide emotional support and alleviate anxiety.
a. Allow patient/family to discuss feelings concerning situation or event and decision to undergo replantation (shock, numbness, blame, guilt, anger, etc.).
b. Maintain calm atmosphere.

C. Postoperative nursing care (see Table 17.1).
1. Success of replantation is unpredictable. It is measured by survival and in the maximal return of sensory/motor function and form the patient achieves. Some patients have significant disability. Global hand function can be evaluated by scoring systems (Tamai, Mellesi, others).
2. Short-term goals have been successful if:
a. No evidence of hypovolemia.
b. Tissue pink, warm, good turgor, and capillary refill.
c. Therapeutic clotting times.
d. No signs of infection.
3. Long-term functional outcomes depend on:
a. Patient's motivation and need to use.
b. Emotional stability.
c. Adaptability of lifestyle.
d. Job requirements.
e. Acceptance by family and friends.
f. Participation during lengthy rehabilitation period.
4. Verbalizes ways to protect limb from potential injury.
5. Begins to reintegrate altered body part into self-concept and describes methods of changing lifestyle as needed.
6. Economic outcomes influence patients and institutions.

VI. HOME CARE CONSIDERATIONS

A. See Table 17.2.
B. Avoid direct/indirect trauma to limb (collision/contact sports, sharp objects, extremes of ambient temperature, restrictive clothing with elastic bands, etc.).
C. Reinforce need to prevent vasoconstriction.
D. Arrange for vocational counseling as needed.
E. Explain community services available.
F. Reinforce compliance with exercise.

ARTHROPLASTY

I. OVERVIEW

A. Definition: arthroplasty is partial or total replacement of the joint surface, with metal and polyethylene plastic or silastic (silicone); the purpose is for pain relief and to improve functional flexibility/mobility in the hand/fingers or wrist. Restoration of motion and function is less predictable than pain relief.

B. Etiology.
1. Surgical procedure performed in patients with osteoarthritis (OA) and rheumatoid arthritis (RA).
2. May also be performed after failed arthrodesis, nonunion post-trauma, avascular necrosis, and malignant bone tumors.
3. 500,000 total joint arthroplasties (of all joints) performed each year.

C. Pathophysiology.
1. Patients with rheumatic arthropathies such as RA, ankylosing spondylitis, psoriatic arthritis, enteropathic arthropathy, and systemic lupus erythematosus develop varying articular and soft tissue structural involvement that leads to joint destruction, joint instability, and loss of functional capacity of the involved joint.

2. Some of the mediators of inflammation which affect articular cartilage, joint capsule, and tendinoligamentous structures in the inflammatory arthropathies are: bioactive lipids (prostaglandins, leukotrienes, lipoxegenase products, platelet activating factors, thromboxane); complement components; cytokines (interleukins, tumor necrosis factor, colony stimulating factors, growth promoting factors); coagulation factors; proteinases; activated platelets; and oxygen-derived free radicals (superoxide anion, hydrogen peroxide, and hydroxyl radical).
3. Wear and tear of a joint surface related to non-inflammatory OA creates articular changes, pain, and loss of joint functioning. Trauma, falls, automobile crashes, and other unforeseen injuries precipitate joint and surrounding tissue damage leading to osteoarthritic joint modifications (joint space narrowing, osteophytes, sclerosis).

D. Incidence.
1. Arthroplasty performed more often in female population.
2. Most common surgical procedure for joint restructuring after failed arthrodesis.
3. Performed in any gender post-trauma.

E. Considerations across the lifespan.
1. Arthroplasty is generally done in the older adult population.
2. Arthroplasty in children and adolescents has a higher incidence of failure and necessity of repeat joint replacement.

F. Complications (post-surgical).
1. Infection.
2. Implant fracture.
3. Neurovascular damage.
4. Recurrent deformity.
5. Complex regional pain syndrome (RSD).
6. Poor wound healing (persons with inflammatory arthridities may be prescribed corticosteroids or immunosuppressive agents that alter tissue healing).
7. Bone absorption about implant resulting in implant loosening.
8. Dislocation of prosthesis.
9. Spread of silicone to other tissues (silicosis).
10. Synovitis of joint due to fragmentation of implant.
11. Failure requiring repeat arthroplasty.

II. ASSESSMENT

A. History.
1. Obtain prior history of hand/wrist surgery.
2. Obtain family history to distinguish inflammatory versus non-inflammatory arthritis, (RA versus OA), early familial degenerative osteoarthritis.
3. Ask focused questions regarding nature of patient's symptoms: pain, joint stiffness, when does it occur, what irritates it, what joints are involved, how long through out the day does it last?
4. Ask the patient to describe constitutional symptoms (malaise, weakness, fever, fatigue) which may indicate an inflammatory arthritis.

B. Physical examination.
1. Observe and evaluate deformation about affected joints.
2. Pain may or may not be present with active or passive ROM.
3. Symmetric joint involvement seen in rheumatic-type arthridities.
4. The DIP and PIP joints are involved in OA (Heberden's and Bouchard's nodes) and some inflammatory arthridities.
5. Skin is usually intact, however various lesions of the integument may be present.
6. Digits are neurovascularly intact.
7. Joints may be unstable with active stressing.
8. MCP joints are involved in RA.

C. Diagnostic tests.
1. Plain radiographs demonstrate in OA: subchondral cysts, sclerosis, osteophytosis, joint space narrowing.
2. Plain radiographs show in rheumatic-type arthridities: erosions, osteoporosis, varying joint space collapse.

III. COMMON THERAPEUTIC MODALITIES

A. Therapeutic medication regimens for rheumatic-type arthritis and OA.
B. Intraarticular injections of corticosteroids, hyaluronic acid products (Synvisc® or Hyalgan®).
C. Administration of analgesics for pain.
D. Arthrodesis may be attempted prior to arthroplasty.
E. Physical and occupational therapy.
F. Dynamic and static finger splints post-surgery.
G. A trial of Neutriceuticals (glucosamine) may be warranted.
H. Arthroplastic surgery.

IV. NURSING DIAGNOSES, OUTCOMES, AND INTERVENTIONS (See Table 17.1 and Replantation section)

V. HOME CARE CONSIDERATIONS (See Table 17.2)

FINGER FRACTURES – BENNETT'S AND ROLANDO

I. OVERVIEW

A. Definition: Bennett's fracture is an oblique intra-articular fracture of the first metacarpal (MCP) of the thumb. Rolando's fracture is also an oblique/intra-articular fracture of the first metacarpal in the thumb that contains more comminuted fracture fragments.

B. Etiology.
1. Thumb fracture occurs from direct axial loading onto the digit.
2. It may also occur when falling forward onto an outstretched hand and while the thumb is stuck in abduction during axial compression.

3. Bennett's/Rolando's fracture may occur during an industrial injury, motor vehicle crash, sports, and other traumatic events.

C. Pathophysiology.

1. During axial loading and/or forced abduction, dislocation of the articular surface causes the bone to split at the main portion of the metacarpal from the volar beak.
2. Concomitant opposing pulling forces by the volar ligament and abductor pollicus longus tendon predisposes this fracture to comminution.
3. These fractures result in obvious deformity secondary to tearing of the volar plate, and oppositional traction forces of the abductor and adductor ligaments about the metacarpal head.
4. Comminuted fragments, malunion, and recalcitrant subluxation predispose the first (MCP) joint to secondary arthritis, significant pain, weakness, and hand dysfunction (grip strength, pincer movements, and ADL).
5. Frayed and torn tendioligamentous structures avulsed during the traumatic event may become entrapped within the aponeurosis (fascia); this is referred to as a Stener's lesion.

D. Incidence.

1. More common in the dominant hand.
2. May occur during contact sports (football, basketball, hockey, wrestling, soccer).

E. Considerations across the lifespan. This fracture can occur at all ages, from the young athlete to the elderly individual.

F. Complications.

1. Delayed treatment will result in loss of normal hand function (grip/pinch).
2. Cosmetic deformity of the thumb.
3. Persistent pain, hand dysfunction.
4. May develop post-traumatic OA.
5. First MCP joint instability.

II. ASSESSMENT

A. History.

1. Describe the mechanism of injury precipitating the event.
2. Ascertain hand dominance.
3. Past medical history related to hand injury (sports, occupational, domestic).

B. Physical examination.

1. Pain about base of the thumb during active and passive ROM.
2. Unable to abduct or adduct the thumb.
3. Swelling, ecchymosis present to thumb and about the hypothenar eminence.
4. Digit is neurovascularly intact.
5. Note punctured/abraded skin lesions about fracture that may indicate open fracture.
6. Obvious deformity about first MCP.
7. Crepitus may be palpated about fracture.
8. Inability to use affected hand.

C. Diagnostic tests.

1. A/P, lateral, and oblique radiographs.
2. Comparison view in pediatric/adolescent patients.
3. CT scan may be necessary.

III. COMMON THERAPEUTIC MODALITIES

A. Splinting of the affected hand above and below the level of injury.

B. Initial attempt by emergency department medical staff and/or orthopaedist or hand specialist to relocate thumb if grossly malaligned.

C. If wound open, tetanus toxoid, wound irrigation, apply dry sterile dressing.

D. May require oral/parenteral antibiotic therapy.

E. Analgesics for pain.

F. PRICEMM (see Mallet/Jersey Finger in this chapter).

G. Application of thumb spica cast.

H. Percutaneous pinning (K/C wire).

I. Surgery for open reduction internal fixation.

1. Early hand rehabilitation.
2. Post-op cast, wound, and dressing instructions.

IV. NURSING DIAGNOSES, OUTCOMES, INTERVENTIONS

A. Physical mobility, impaired.

1. Outcome: patient will maintain finger flexibility/strength.
2. Interventions.
   a. Have patient demonstrate post-op hand exercises.
   b. Instruct patient and family in dressing changes and maintenance of cast/splint.

B. See Table 17.1.

IV. HOME CARE CONSIDERATIONS (See Table 17.2)

BOXER'S FRACTURE

I. OVERVIEW

A. Definition: Boxer's fracture is a fracture of the forth or fifth metacarpal neck sometimes involving the head of the MCP.

B. Etiology.

1. This fracture occurs when the individual strikes an object such as a wall or another person with a closed fist.
2. Not common in sports injury, but may occur during a fall (football, rugby).
3. May be seen in industrial/occupational injuries.

C. Pathophysiology.

1. Fracture results from longitudinal focused forces along the long axis of the MCP.
2. During the mechanism of injury, part of the radial base of the MCP remains articulated with the hamate; the remaining section of the MCP is subluxed proximally and dorsally.
3. Striking forces generated in this fracture cause transcortical and/or spiral fracture of the MCP.
4. Fracture may be rotated, shortened, or angulated due to traction exerted by the intrinsic musculature and flexor tendons.

D. **Incidence.**
   1. Second most common fracture in the hand.
   2. Commonly seen following an altercation.
   3. Most common in dominant hand.

E. **Considerations across the lifespan: generally occurs in the younger population.**

F. **Complications.**
   1. Cosmetic deformity to dorsum of hand about fracture site.
   2. Mal-union, non-union of fracture.
   3. Decreased hand grip/fist closure secondary to angulated healing.
   4. If surgery required, possible post-op infection (wound/pin site).
   5. Possible local or systemic sepsis. Laceration/bite to skin over MCP resulting in suppurative tenosynovitis, a deep space wound infection that requires a surgical incision and drainage, tetanus prophylaxis, and oral/parenteral antibiotic therapy. Treated as an orthopaedic emergency!!

II. ASSESSMENT

A. **History.**
   1. Obtain thorough mechanism of injury; patient may be embarrassed about how the fracture occurred and not relay accurate information.
   2. Ascertain prior hand injury or surgery.
   3. Obtain hand dominance.

B. **Physical examination.**
   1. Complains of pain about MCP.
   2. Obvious to subtle MCP deformity.
   3. Unable to make a fist.
   4. Decreased active and passive ROM.
   5. Affected digits are neurovascularly intact.
   6. Integument may be lacerated, abraded, or open fracture may be present.
   7. Swelling, ecchymosis to involved MCP.
   8. Kanavel's signs are present if there is deep-space wound infection. These signs are:
      a. Pain with passive extension of digits/hand.
      b. Hand/digits are in rested/flexed posture.
      c. Fusiform swelling present about dorsum and volar aspect of the hand.
      d. Pain about involved tendon sheath.

C. **Diagnostic tests.**
   1. A/P, lateral, oblique radiographs.
   2. CT scan.

III. COMMON THERAPEUTIC MODALITIES

A. **Closed reduction to anatomic alignment (up to 30 degrees of angulation post-reduction may be acceptable).**

B. **Ulnar gutter splint with or without buddy taping of the other digits.**

C. **Sufficient padding between digits to prevent sweat excoriation.**

D. **Analgesics for pain; NSAID therapy.**

E. **If open fracture, patient requires oral/parenteral antibiotic therapy, tetanus toxoid, and thorough wound cleansing and dressing management.**

F. **Surgery (ORIF), percutaneous pinning; arthrodesis may be performed.**

G. **PRICEMM (see Mallet/Jersey Finger in this chapter).**

H. **Physical/occupational therapy to prevent finger/hand stiffness.**

IV. NURSING DIAGNOSES, OUTCOMES, INTERVENTIONS

A. **See Table 17.1.**

B. **Infection, risk for (open fracture).**
   1. Outcome: absence of infection as evidenced by normal WBC, body temperature, and negative wound cultures.
   2. Interventions.
      a. Monitor temperature and vital signs
      b. Wound surveillance for evidence of infection (erythema, warmth, purulent exudates).
      c. Monitor laboratory values (WBC, differential).

V. HOME CARE CONSIDERATIONS (See Table 17.2)

SCAPHOID FRACTURE

I. OVERVIEW

A. **Definition: a scaphoid fracture involves the scaphoid (navicular) bone that is located in the wrist.**

B. **Etiology.**
   1. Most common wrist fracture.
   2. This fracture is known for increased incidence of non-union.
   3. Most often occurs after a fall on an outstretched hand.

C. **Pathophysiology.**
   1. Fracture occurs from forceful hyperextension of the wrist.
   2. Scaphoid is classified as a proximal carpal bone yet it extends into the distal carpal row.
   3. Specific type of fracture (wrist, proximal, distal, tubercle) depends on the position of the forearm at the time of injury.
   4. Scaphoid (wrist) fracture occurs when the wrist is in hyperextension, radial deviation, and the fall has caused axial loading onto the wrist.
   5. Since the scaphoid crosses two carpal rows, persistent dorsiflexion stressors and normal tension loading of the carpal structures predisposes the scaphoid to fracture during axial loading on an outstretched dorsiflexed hand/wrist.

D. **Incidence.**
   1. Most common carpal bone fracture.
   2. Often seen following falls (sports, motorcycle).
   3. Seen more often in females 20-40 years old.

E. **Considerations across the lifespan: rarely seen in children; the epiphysis of the distal radius is weak and will fracture before the scaphoid fails. Resulting fracture is generally classified as a Salter I/II of the distal radius.**

F. Complications.

1. Due to intrinsically poor blood supply, scaphoid fracture is subject to delayed union, and avascular necrosis.
2. Missed injury/diagnosis predisposes the patient to persistent chronic wrist pain.
3. Loss of wrist ROM.
4. Decreased grip strength.
5. Cosmetic deformity about wrist.
6. Post-surgery, possible wound infection.

II. ASSESSMENT

A. History.

1. Ascertain correct mechanism of injury and when injury occurred.
2. Obtain hand dominance.

B. Physical examination.

1. Patient may or may not complain of moderately severe pain about the anatomic snuffbox in the (radial) wrist.
2. Gripping may be painful.
3. Swelling may or may not be present.
4. Hand is neurovascularly intact.
5. Axial compression of the thumb and radial deviation of the wrist precipitate pain.

C. Diagnostic tests.

1. A/P, lateral, scaphoid views of the wrist. Comparison views may be warranted. Initial radiographs may not rule out fracture.
2. Repeat radiographs in 2-3 weeks if patient still complains of pain.
3. Bone scintigraphy (bone scan) in cases of continued pain or repeat negative radiographs.

III. COMMON THERAPEUTIC MODALITIES

A. PRICEMM (see Mallet/Jersey Finger in this chapter).

B. Analgesics for pain.

C. Long arm thumb spica cast.

D. ORIF (screws, bone graft).

E. Arthrodesis of wrist.

F. Carpectomy.

IV. NURSING DIAGNOSES, OUTCOMES, INTERVENTIONS (see Table 17.1)

V. HOME CARE CONSIDERATIONS (see Table 17.2)

Bibliography

American Society for Surgery of the Hand. (1990). *The hand* (3rd ed). New York: Churchill Livingstone.

Ballas, M., Tycko, J., & Mannarino, F. (1998). Common missed orthopaedic problems. *American Family Physician, 57*(2), 267-274.

Bas, H., & Deinert, J. (1999). Anatomic variations in sensory innervations of the hand and digits. *Journal of Hand Surgery, 24*(6), 1171-1184.

Benson, L., Williams, C., & Kahle, M. (1998). Dupuytren's Contracture. *Journal of the American Academy of Orthopaedic Surgeons, 6*(1), 24-35.

Boulas, J. (1998). Amputations of the fingers and hand: indications for replant. *Journal of the American Academy of Orthopaedic Surgeons, 6*(2), 100-105.

Brown, P. (1999). Pointers for managing common hand injuries. *Journal of Musculoskeletal Medicine, 16*(12), 675-680.

Chen, H., Buchman, M., & Wei, I. (1999). Free flaps for soft tissue coverage of the hand and fingers. *Hand Clinics, 15*(4), 541-554.

Childs, S.G. (1999). *The upper extremity: Traumatic injuries and conditions.* Pitman, NJ: Anthony J. Jannetti, Inc.

Childs, S.G. (1999). *Finger injury.* Lippincott's Primary Care Practice, 3(4), 397-403.

Childs, S.G., & Holmes, S. (1998). *Guidelines for orthopaedic nursing: Adult trauma.* Pitman, NJ: Anthony J. Jannetti, Inc.

Dellon, L., & Keller, K. (1997). Computer-assisted quantitative sensorimotor testing in patients with carpal tunnel syndromes. *Annals of Plastic Surgery, 38*(5), 493-502.

Dellon, E., Keller, K., Moratz, V., & Dellon, L. (1997). Validation of cutaneous pressure threshold measurements for the evaluation of hand function. *Annals of Plastic Surgery, 38*(5), 485-492.

Dionysian, E., & Eaton, R.G. (2000). The long-term outcome of volar plate arthroplasty of the proximal interphalangeal joint. *Journal of Hand Surgery, 25*(3), 429-437.

Herbert, R., Gerr, F., & Dropkin, J. (2000). Clinical evaluation and management of work-related carpal tunnel syndrome. *American Journal of Industrial Medicine, 37*(1), 62-74.

Katzman, B., Klein, D., & Mesa, J. (1999). Immobilization of the mallet finger: Effects on the extensor tendon. *Journal of Hand Surgery, 24*(1), 80-84.

Leddy, J. (1998). Soft tissue injuries of the hand in the athlete. *Instructional Course Lectures, 47*, 181-186.

Maher, A., Salmond, S., & Pellino, T. (1998). *Orthopaedic nursing* (2nd ed). Philadelphia: W.B. Saunders.

Merle, M., & Doutel, G. (1997). Advances in digital replantation. *Clinics Plastic Surgery, 24*(1), 87-105.

Massy-Westropp, N. (2000). A systematic review of the clinical diagnostic tests for carpal tunnel syndrome. *Journal of Hand Surgery, 25*(1), 125-127.

Palmer, L.M. (2000). Management of the patient with a total joint replacement: The primary care practitioner's role. *Lippincott's Primary Care Practice, 3*(4), 419-427.

Provinciali, L., Giattini, A., Splendiani, G., & Logullo, F. (2000). Usefulness of hand rehabilitation after carpal tunnel surgery. *Muscle Nerve, 23*(2), 211-216.

Pyne, J., & Adams, B. (1992). Hand tendon injuries in athletics. *Clinics in Sports Medicine, 11*(4), 833-849.

Putnam, M. (1996). Post-traumatic stiffness in the hand. *Clinical Orthopaedics and Related Research, 327*, 182-190.

Rayan, G. (1999). Clinical presentation and types of Dupuytren's disease. *Hand Clinics, 15*(1), 87-96.

Resende, L., Adamo, A., & Bonani, A. (2000). Test of a new technique for the diagnosis of carpal tunnel syndrome. *Journal of Electromyography Kinesiology, 10*(2), 127-133.

Roth, M. (1994). Metacarpophalangeal joint implant arthroplasty. *American Operating Room Nurses Journal, 60*(6), 929-946.

Snider, R. (1997). *Essentials of musculoskeletal care.* Rosemont, IL: American Academy of Orthopaedic Surgeons.

Schmitt, M. (1999). Part 2: Common wrist and hand problems. *Patient Care for the Nurse Practitioner, 10*, 38-42, 47-48.

Schoen, D. (2000). Care of a patient with hand and wrist surgery. In D.C. Schoen, *Adult orthopaedic nursing* (pp. 381-402). Philadelphia: Lippincott.

Slade, J.F., Mahoney, J., Dailinger, J., & Baxamusa, R. (1999). Wrist and hand injuries. In musicians: *Management and prevention. Journal of Musculoskeletal Medicine, 16*(9), 542-550.

Sternberg, Z., & Klienman, W. (1999). Occult scapholunate ganglion: A cause of dorsal radial wrist pain. *Journal of Hand Surgery, 24*(2), 225-231.

Takami, H., Takahashi, S., & Ando, M. (2000). Operative treatment of mallet finger due to intraarticular fracture of the distal phalanx. *Archives of Orthopaedic Trauma and Surgery, 120*(1-2), 9-13,

Thornburg, L. (1999). Ganglions of the hand and wrist. *Journal of the American Academy of Orthopaedic Surgeons, 7*(4), 231-238.

Wilgis, E.F. (1997). Distal interphalangeal joint silicone interpositional arthroplasty of the hand. *Clinical Orthopaedics and Related Research, 342*, 38-41.

Zucker, R. (2000). Clinical diagnosis of carpal tunnel syndrome. *Journal of the American Medical Association, 283*, 4.

STUDY QUESTIONS

Mr. Carter is a 40-year-old right-hand dominant factory worker. He goes to his health care provider with pain in his hand. He complains of intermittent numbness and paresthesias over his thumb, index and middle fingers, and half of the ring finger. The pain frequently wakes him up at night. He has no history of systemic disease, however, his work requires frequent forceful repetitive movements and hyperextension of his wrists. He states that his hand "goes to sleep," often feels weak, and he occasionally drops objects. Physical examination reveals a flattening of the thenar muscle at the base of the thumb. (Questions 1-3)

1. The most common entrapment neuropathy that best fits the above clinical manifestations is:
   a. Ulnar tunnel syndrome affecting the ulna nerve.
   b. Carpal tunnel syndrome affecting the median nerve.
   c. Anterior interosseous syndrome affecting the radial nerve.
   d. Quervain's syndrome affecting the tibial nerve.

2. Physical diagnostic evaluation tests to determine Mr. Carter's diagnosis would include positive:
   a. Anterior Drawer and Allis sign.
   b. Galleazi's sign and Barlow's maneuver.
   c. Tinel's and Phalen's sign.
   d. Finkelstein and Bronson's sign.

3. Which of the following would **not** be a treatment for carpal tunnel syndrome?
   a. Vigorous daily repetitive wrist exercises.
   b. Immobilization and night splinting.
   c. Local injections of corticosteroids.
   d. Surgical decompression of median nerve.

Mr. Garrick is a 55-year-old male who immigrated to the United States from Ireland. His medical history reveals type 2 diabetes. He has noticed a nodule gradually forming in the distal palmer crease at the base of his ring finger on his dominant right hand. A fibrous cord extends from the finger to the palm and keeps the finger "locked" in a flexed position. Mr. Frank finds many of his activities of daily living difficult to perform, including using tools for his wood-working hobby. (Questions 4-5)

4. The clinical manifestations above best describe which diagnosis?
   a. Mallet finger.
   b. Dupuytren's contracture.
   c. DIP joint ganglion.
   d. Radial tunnel syndrome.

5. The goal of treatment for Mr. Garrick's condition is to restore normal hand function. This is best done by:
   a. Conservative finger splinting only.
   b. Tendon and nerve transfers.
   c. Series of steroidal injections.
   d. Surgical partial palmer fasciectomy.

6. Mrs. Greenberg is a 32-year-old who has been told that she has a ganglion on the dorsum of her left wrist. Which of the following pieces of information would it be necessary to provide for Mrs. Greenberg' patient education?
   a. Surgery is the only treatment method that can cure this condition.
   b. Ganglia are cancerous cysts that occur during early childhood.
   c. Ganglia erode through tissue causing infection and destruction of vital structures
   d. Ganglia are more common in females and reoccurrences are common.

7. Mr. Dason has a condition known as flexor stenosing tenosynovitis or "trigger finger" in the ring finger of his nondominant hand. Which clinical manifestation would you anticipate that he would have?
   a. Finger stiff and locked in extension upon awakening.
   b. A nodule in the tendon pulley that becomes locked when extension is attempted.
   c. Pain when bending or flexing his affected digit.
   d. No family or trauma history, and work that does not involve repetitive motion activity.

8. The hand serves many functions including finite movement and prehension. The hand allows the person to perform an intricate ballet of movement for daily needs; it "reads" for the blind and "speaks" for the deaf. Prevention of hand injuries is a very important role for the nurse. What information should not be included in safety programs to prevent hand injuries or exacerbation of chronic disorders:
   a. Avoid forceful repetitive motions or sustained positions for lengthy periods.
   b. Organize work and home sites that utilize products based on ergonomic principles.
   c. Reorganize type of work activities to prevent hand rotation and provide rest periods.
   d. Ergonomics is not a concern for home/recreation activities due to shortness of time.

As you pull in your driveway from your work as a nurse, you see Mr. Hammil, your 32-year-old right-hand dominant neighbor who is a construction worker, cutting up a fallen tree with a chain saw. Suddenly he cries out loudly for help. You go over to see him and find that he has amputated the thumb, index, and middle fingers on his left hand. The laceration is jagged yet clean and blood is spurting from the hand. You make Mr. Hammil lie down. Another neighbor accesses the 911 system, while you assess his airway, breathing, and circulation. (Questions 9-15)

9. Based on these findings, you would assess that Mr. Hammil has:
   a. An occult hand fracture.
   b. A ligamentous injury with a hematoma.
   c. Partial hand and finger amputations with a lacerated artery.
   d. An erythematous eruption of the skin and soft tissues.

10. Which of the following initial nursing interventions would you perform to control the bleeding?
    a. Elevate the victim's arm above his heart level only and keep him lying down.
    b. Apply direct pressure to the wound with a clean material while elevating the extremity.
    c. Apply a tourniquet as far from the wound as possible to occlude arterial flow.
    d. Apply ice directly to the soft tissue to cause vasoconstriction and halt blood flow.

11. Once the bleeding was controlled and the paramedics stabilized Mr. Hammil's general condition, the amputated fingers and thumb were located. Transport these digits with Mr. Hammil to the hospital by placing them in:
    a. A container with skin directly on ice cubes, and note the time the parts were amputated.
    b. A container with a liquid antiseptic solution to bathe the parts.
    c. A container with a salt-water solution to bathe the parts.
    d. A water-tight sealed plastic bag placed into a container with ice and note the time.

Postoperatively Mr. Hammil returns to the unit in a splint with tips of digits and thumb exposed with a bulky mitt hand dressing. Orders are to monitor the neurovascular status that ordinarily includes color, temperature, capillary refill, sensation, and movement.

12. Which of these neurovascular check measures would you **not** perform in the replantation patient immediately postoperatively?
    a. Sensibility and motor function tests.
    b. Temperature probe readings.
    c. Doppler and/or pulse oximetry monitoring.
    d. Fluorometry readings.

13. Which of the following medications is **not** commonly administered after surgery to promote adequate circulation?
    a. Low molecular dextran/heparin.
    b. Vasodilan®/Thorazine®.
    c. Aspirin/Persantine®.
    d. Nicotine/Vascar®.

14. The nurse observes that the index finger is becoming cool, skin is tense and distended, and nailbeds have a bluish color. These are signs of:
    a. Arterial occlusion.
    b. Venous congestion.
    c. Vascular claudication.
    d. Vasospasms.

15. Mr. Hammil's physician has ordered medicinal leeches be placed on the index finger. Leech therapy acts by:
    a. Removal of approximately 25 cc of blood by each leech.
    b. Secretion of hirudin, an enzyme that serves as an anticoagulant and causes bleeding.
    c. Strong sucking action serves as a method of manual stimulation to increase blood flow.
    d. Providing an antibacterial effect to decrease potential for infection.

Chapter 18 THE SPINE

Margaret Hickey, MS, RN, ONC
Mary Faut Rodts, MS, MSA, RN, ONC

Contents

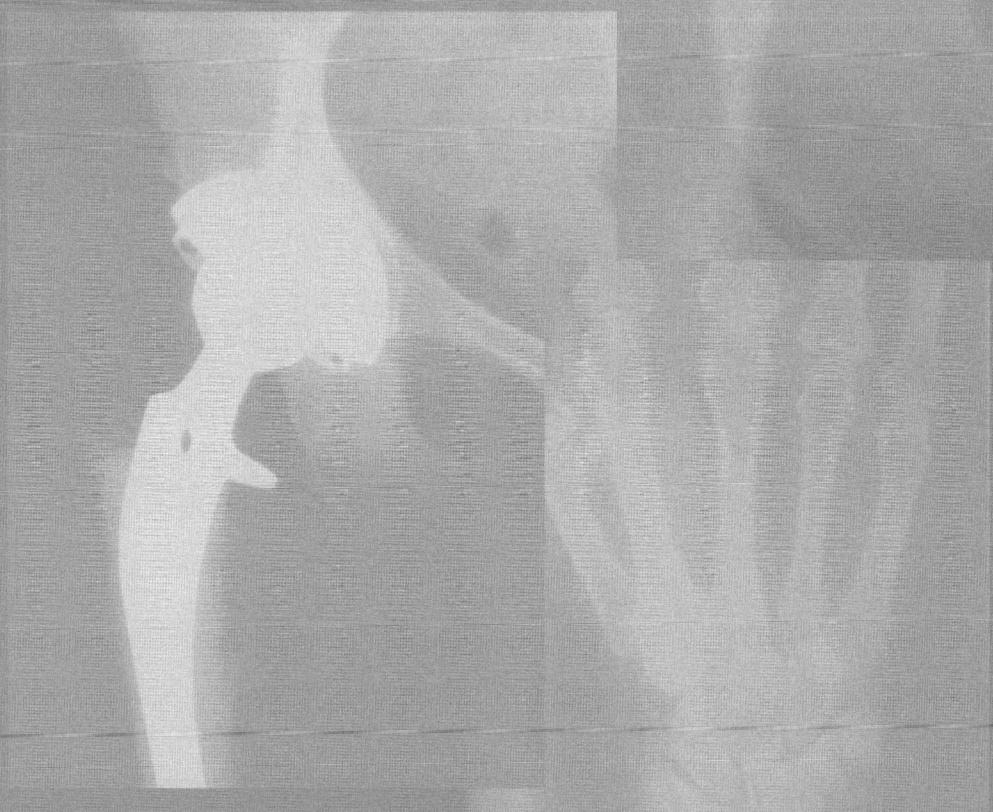

OBJECTIVES

At the completion of this chapter, the learner will be able to:

- Define common terms relating to spine pathology including: scoliosis, kyphosis, herniated nucleus pulposus, spinal stenosis, degenerative disc disease, spondylolysis/spondylolisthesis, and failed back syndrome.
- Discuss the essential aspects of assessment of the patient with spine pathology.
- Discuss common conservative and surgical treatment options for the patient with spine pathology.
- Discuss pre-operative, intra-operative, and postoperative nursing management of the patient with spine pathology.
- Identify home care considerations following spine surgery.

KEY POINTS

- All patients with spinal disorders need a thorough musculoskeletal/neurologic assessment.
- Assessment includes reflexes and motor and sensory function of both the upper and lower extremities. Baseline data are established and then monitored and recorded throughout treatment.
- When assessing patients for a suspected spinal disorder, evaluation for other non-orthopaedic causes of symptoms needs to be included.
- Spine surgery should be considered only after conservative management has failed. The exceptions to this include cauda equina syndrome or progressive neurologic compromise, which require urgent evaluation and surgical intervention.
- Pain management should include teaching about modalities and medications to manage pain.

CHAPTER 18

THE SPINE

SPINE ASSESSMENT: AN OVERVIEW

I. ASSESSMENT

A. History.

1. Chief complaint.
2. Date of onset.
3. Detailed history of incident.
4. Outline of treatment attempted and outcomes of treatment.
5. Pain.
   a. Location.
   b. Quality or type.
   c. Back/leg versus neck/arm pain.
   d. Duration/frequency/intensity.
   e. Aggravating/alleviating factors.
   f. Utilization of a pain drawing.
6. Medications.
   a. Current prescription and over-the-counter/herbal medications.
   b. Medications previously tried and response.
7. Past medical/surgical history.
8. Allergies.
9. Occupational history.
10. Lifestyle history including activities of daily living and recreational activities.
11. Alcohol/drug history.
12. Smoking history.
13. Pregnancy/last menstrual history.
14. "Red Flags."
    a. Bowel/bladder loss of control.
    b. Saddle anesthesia.
    c. Weight loss.
    d. Fevers/night sweats.
    e. Night pain.
    f. Arm/leg weakness.
    g. Headaches/dizziness.
    h. Abdominal tenderness.

B. Physical examination.

1. Height/weight.
2. Vital signs.
3. Gait.
4. Able to walk on toes and heels.
5. Range of motion.
6. Straight leg raise.
7. Strength/reflexes/sensation.
   a. Grade.
   b. Symmetry.
   c. Dermatomal distribution.
8. Non-organic physical signs.

II. RADIOGRAPHIC EVALUATION

A. X-ray.

1. AP and lateral views.
2. Oblique views.
3. Flexion/extension views if question of instability.

B. Computerized tomography (CT scan).

1. Computerized x-ray image to produce an image of a cross-sectional plane of an area of the body.
2. Demonstrates bony anatomy.
3. Good for evaluation of spinal stenosis.
4. Has been replaced by MRI as the gold standard for evaluation.

C. Magnetic resonance imaging (MRI).

1. A magnetic field and radiofrequency impulses produce a signal which is processed through a computer producing sagittal and axial images of the spine.
2. Visualization of soft tissues, bones, discs, nerves.
3. Can demonstrate tumor/infection.
4. Gadolinium (contrast) enhancement is used:
   a. To differentiate scar tissue from a new problem, if prior spine surgery has been performed.
   b. Used to diagnose some tumors.

D. Myelogram.

1. An invasive study in which dye is injected into the subarachnoid space and allowed to fill out along the spinal column and nerves.
2. Demonstrates spinal cord compression and nerve impingement.
3. Can miss a far lateral disc herniation.

E. Discogram.

1. Dye is injected into the center of the disc under fluoroscopic guidance.
2. Allows for visualization of disc morphology.
3. Reproduction of pain can aid in determining symptomatic disc level(s).

F. Bone scan/gallium scan.

1. Nuclear medicine scan.
2. Evaluates inflammatory process in bone such as tumor, infection, or acute fracture.

III. CONSERVATIVE TREATMENT

A. Attempted prior to considering surgical management. The exceptions to this which require immediate surgical management include:

1. Cauda equina syndrome-compression of the cauda equina resulting in saddle anesthesia, acute paraplegia, and/or bowel or bladder incontinence.
2. Neurologic dysfunction such as worsening motor or sensory function.
3. Infection.
4. Tumor.

B. Types of conservative management.

1. Oral medications.
   a. Nonsteroidal anti-inflammatory medications.
   b. Steroids: dose pack or taper.
   c. Neuroleptics.
   d. COX-2 inhibitors.

e. Muscle relaxants.
f. Analgesics: narcotic or non-narcotic.
g. Antidepressants.
2. Physical therapy.
a. Goal is to decrease pain and increase function/strength/flexibility.
b. Should be active, however, modalities often used as a comfort measure.
3. Injections.
a. Intramuscular injections.
(1) Narcotic analgesic for acute pain.
(2) Steroids.
b. Epidural injection.
c. Selective nerve root block.
d. Facet injection.
e. Sacroiliac injection.
f. Trigger point injections.
4. Acupuncture.
5. Chiropractic care.
6. Massage therapy.
7. Herbalist.
8. Other: anything that is not harmful which helps the pain.

IV. SURGICAL INTERVENTION

A. Performed urgently if:
1. The diagnosis is cauda equina syndrome.
2. There is progressive neurologic deficit.

B. Rapid evaluation and treatment must be performed for:
1. Fracture.
2. Tumor.
3. Infection.

C. Elective surgery is performed:
1. ONLY in the presence of a surgically treatable problem.
2. WITH correlating diagnostic testing and corresponding physical findings.
3. AND when conservative management fails to alleviate the pain.

D. Patient needs to have a clear understanding of the:
1. Surgical plan.
2. Goal of surgery.

E. Expectations of surgery need to be realistic.

F. Risks and potential complications need to be clearly outlined.

G. Discussion of work/occupational issues.
1. Realistic expectations of time frame for return to work.
2. Realistic expections regarding lifting/work restrictions.

H. Involve family/significant others as appropriate.

I. Discuss postoperative home management prior to surgery.

SCOLIOSIS

I. OVERVIEW

A. Definition: scoliosis is a lateral curvature of the spine with vertebral rotation.

B. Etiology.
1. Idiopathic.
a. There is no known cause.
b. There is an apparent familial pattern in most cases.
c. Many theories have been researched, such as:
(1) Vestibular dysfunction.
(2) Alteration in collagen metabolism.
(3) Muscular weakness.
(4) No consensus reached.
2. Congenital.
a. Early in embryonic life (6-8 weeks).
b. A malformation occurs in the development of the vertebral structures.
c. Creating structural problems in the bony architecture, such as:
(1) Hemivertebra.
(2) Congenital bar.
(3) Block vertebra.
3. Paralytic.
a. Polio.
b. Muscular dystrophy.
c. Cerebral palsy.
d. Spina bifida.
e. Various myopathies may cause a curvature of the spine secondary to muscular imbalance.
d. The curve is different in presentation in that it is generally a long sweeping curve.
4. Neurofibromatosis.
a. A sharp angulated curvature is frequently seen in conjunction with neurofibromatosis.
b. Unusually thin ribs, scalloping of vertebra, and café au lait spots also are seen in most cases.
5. Traumatic/radiation:
a. Traumatic injury to bony column.
b. Iatrogenic injury to the growth centers of the vertebra secondary to asymmetric radiation can result in curvature of the spine.
6. Sciatic: curvature with a significant trunk shift secondary to nerve root irritation (herniated nucleus pulposus, tumor).
7. Hysterical: although very rare, a nonstructural scoliosis has been reported as the result of emotional disturbance.

C. Pathophysiology.
1. A curve may present in any area of the spine: cervical, thoracic, thoracolumbar, lumbar.
2. The most common curve pattern is a right thoracic.
a. Produces a rib prominence.
b. As the spine begins to curve:
(1) The vertebral column rotates around its long axis.
(2) This causes ribs in the thoracic region to become prominent on the convex side.
c. Thoracic hypokyphosis may be present, and if severe, decreases the space between the vertebral bodies and the sternum, affecting pulmonary and cardiac function.
d. A lumbar curve is usually a left curve.
(1) Produces an asymmetric waistline.

(2) Is a primary curve or compensatory curve of a right thoracic curve.

D. Incidence (idiopathic).

1. 3%-5% of children screened for scoliosis will have positive examinations.
2. 0.6% require treatment (females – 1.0%, males – 0.1%).

E. Considerations across the lifespan.

1. Infantile idiopathic scoliosis.
   a. 1 to 3 years old.
   b. Males are affected more often.
   c. More commonly seen in Great Britain.
   d. Curve often corrects itself with no treatment.
2. Juvenile.
   a. 3-9 years old.
   b. Occurs equally in males and females.
   c. High risk of progression of curve due to significant growth potential.
3. Adolescent.
   a. 10 years through maturity.
   b. Occurs equally in males and females.
   c. In females, curves are more progressive, thus requiring treatment more often.
4. Young adult.
   a. 20-40 years old.
   b. Curves under 40 degrees generally remain stable.
      (1) No symptoms.
      (2) No treatment indicated.
   c. Curves greater than 40 degrees may demonstrate progression.
      (1) May still be asymptomatic.
      (2) Surgery required if progression is documented.
5. Adult.
   a. 40 years or older.
   b. Curves under 40 degrees continue to remain stable.
      (1) No symptoms.
      (2) No treatment.
   c. A progressive curve in the thoracic spine (greater than 65 degrees) may be responsible for:
      (1) Shortness of breath and fatigue.
      (2) Cor pulmonale is only seen in severe thoracic scoliosis.
      (3) Surgery is indicated.
   d. A progressive curve in the lumbar spine may be responsible for:
      (1) Low back fatigue and pain.
      (2) Early degenerative changes.
      (3) Spinal stenosis.
         (a) With nerve root entrapment.
         (b) Surgery is indicated.

F. Complications.

1. Progressive scoliosis that is untreated can result in significant deformity.
2. Cardiopulmonary compromise if in the thoracic area with a curve greater than 65 degrees.
3. Debilitating back pain if in the lumbar area.

II. ASSESSMENT

A. History and physical examination.

1. Usually asymptomatic in children. However, in severe thoracic scoliosis, shortness of breath may be noticed.
2. Adults may experience fatigue, back pain, and shortness of breath depending on location of curve.
3. Not noticed until identified during a school screening examination, regularly scheduled physical, or while trying on clothing.
4. Difficulty fitting clothing (hemline uneven, different lengths of pant legs).
5. May or may not be a family history of scoliosis.
6. Progression of deformity noted.
7. Pain, numbness, tingling, weakness may be present. Requires further work-up.
8. Menstrual history.
9. Clothing must be removed to adequately assess spine.
   a. A gown that opens posteriorly.
      (1) A bathing suit of neutral colors (girls).
      (2) Gym trunks (boys).
   b. Provides the necessary visualization of the spine while still providing privacy for patient.
10. Prominent scapula.
11. Asymmetric waistline or prominent hip.
12. Asymmetry in the level of the shoulders.
13. Prominent breast or anterior rib cage.
14. Plumb line hung from C7 does not pass through gluteal crease.
15. On forward bend test, if rib (thoracic area) or paravertebral muscle (lumbar area) prominence is noted, scoliosis is suspected.
16. Leg-length discrepancy can cause functional scoliosis.
17. Neurologic examination to rule out any underlying neurologic problem causing the scoliosis.

B. Diagnostic tests.

1. Observation/school screening protocol.
   a. Inspect spine in upright and forward flexed position from:
      (1) Behind the patient.
      (2) In front of the patient.
      (3) To the side of the patient.
   b. Use a scoliometer at apex of curvature to quantify a prominence. (Scoliometer reading of greater than 10 degrees requires physician referral.)
2. Radiographs of spine.
   a. Initial radiographs should be obtained:
      (1) In patients with a positive assessment.
      (2) Follow-up radiographs should be taken only after examination and progression is suspected.
   b. Radiographs should be taken posterior to anterior to decrease x-ray exposure to thyroid, breasts, reproductive organs.
   c. Appropriate shields should be used to protect breasts and reproductive organs.
   d. Standing posterior anterior (PA) view of spine to decrease radiation exposure to the breasts.

e. Standing lateral view of spine.
f. Side bending radiographs, in most cases, are only required for preoperative planning.
3. Somatosensory evoked potentials (SSEPs) and Motor Evoked Potentials (MEP).
   a. Obtained prior to surgery to be used as a baseline.
   b. Used intraoperatively to monitor spinal cord function.
4. Pulmonary function testing (PFT).
   a. For curves in the thoracic area greater than 65 degrees.
   b. For neuromuscular scoliosis.

III. COMMON THERAPEUTIC MODALITIES

A. Observation.

1. Curves less than 15-20 degrees are observed for progression because many of these curves will never progress past that point.
2. Clinical examination to rule out progression of curvature.
3. Postural exercises may be prescribed; however, there are no data to support the theory that exercises can correct or prevent a structural scoliosis.

B. Brace.

1. Curves between 20 and 40 degrees in a growing child will require:
   a. Use of a brace to prevent further progression of the curvature.
   b. The brace may temporarily correct the scoliosis while the child is under brace treatment.
   c. However, maintenance of curvature at pre-brace degree is considered successful treatment.
2. Exercises are prescribed in conjunction with bracing to maintain trunk muscle strength and hamstring stretching.
3. Bracing is ineffective in the mature patient.
4. Contraindications.
   a. Cervicothoracic or high thoracic curves do not respond well to bracing.
   b. Thoracic hypokyphosis.
   c. Curves over 40 degrees.
   d. Emotional intolerance.

C. Surgery (see Table 18.1).

1. Recommended for curves above 40 degrees.
   a. Posterior spinal fusion with instrumentation
      (1) Most common approach for treatment of adolescent idiopathic scoliosis.
      (2) Performed for moderate adult scoliosis.
   b. Anterior spinal fusion may consist of a disc excision with no instrumentation to mobilize the spine prior to posterior correction with instrumentation or anterior spinal fusion with instrumentation.
      (1) Generally used as first stage of a two-stage procedure for severe scoliosis or paralytic scoliosis.
      (2) Anterior spine fusion with instrumentation may be recommended as the only procedure for adolescent scoliosis.
   c. Thoracoscopic approach for thoracic curves.
      (1) Used for disc excisions and fusions in conjunction with the posterior approach.
      (2) Early investigation of thoracoscopic approaches with instrumentation for thoracic scoliosis being done in some centers.
      (3) Thoracotomy is still the treatment of choice.
   d. Combined anterior and posterior surgery may be recommended for adults or children with severe curvatures.
      (1) Variations of surgical plans may be recommended for complex scoliosis patients.
      (2) Traction devices are used infrequently due to better surgical technique and instrumentation. Halo gravity traction is the treatment of choice for severe, rigid scoliosis that requires slow manipulation of spine.
2. Need for postoperative casting has decreased due to better spine fixation. Immobilization, when indicated, is achieved by a removable thoracolumbar sacral orthosis (TLSO).

IV. NURSING DIAGNOSES, OUTCOMES, AND INTERVENTIONS

A. See Table 18.2.

B. Injury, risk for.

1. Outcome: patient will not experience a neurologic deficit following spinal surgery.
2. Interventions: monitor for signs and symptoms of a neurologic deficit following spinal surgery.
   a. Muscle strength of upper and lower extremities.
   b. Sensation of upper extremities, torso, and lower extremities.
   c. Complaints of numbness, tingling, and increased radiating pain in the extremities or torso; heaviness in the extremities.
   d. Urinary incontinence, inability to void or loss of rectal tone.
   e. Explain to the patient the necessary neurologic checks that will be required as the preoperative assessment is being done (sensation, strength, reflexes, motion to upper and lower extremities, Stagnara wake-up test, and somatosensory monitoring [SSEP]) and motor evoked potentials (MEP).

V. HOME CARE CONSIDERATIONS (See Table 18.3, page 476)

KYPHOSIS

I. OVERVIEW

A. Definition: kyphosis is normal in the thoracic spine. It becomes abnormal when curvature is above 45 degrees.

B. Etiology.

1. Postural kyphosis.

Table 18.1
Common Surgical Procedures

Surgical Procedure	Indications	Procedure	Risks
Percutaneous discectomy	Bulging or herniated lumbar disc	A probe is placed into the center of the disc under fluoroscopic guidance through a small incision. The herniated disc is removed using a cutting cannula at the end of the probe and removing a portion of the center of the disc so that the bulging or herniated disc retracts back taking pressure off of the nerve.	Nerve root injury, infection, hematoma, no improvement of symptoms
Microdisectomy/limited approach discectomy/ laminotomy and discectomy	Herniated lumbar disc	A small incision is made, a hole is made in the lamina (laminotomy), and, with the assistance of magnifying glasses or microscope, the herniated portion of the disc is removed.	Nerve root injury, infection, dural tear, hematoma, no improvement of symptoms
Intradiscal electrothermal therapy (IDET)	Degenerated or bulging disc causing discogenic low back pain	The symptomatic disc level is confirmed by discography prior to proceeding. A needle is placed into the disc under fluoroscopic guidance and a catheter is then threaded through and coiled around the center of the disc. The catheter heats the center of the disc in an effort to thicken and contract the disc wall to oliminate it from being a pain generator.	Nerve root injury, infection, no improvement of symptoms
Laminectomy	Central herniated disc or spinal stenosis	The lamina is removed to either access the area of a centrally herniated disc so that the disc herniation can be removed OR the lamina is removed to relieve pressure caused by spinal stenosis.	Nerve root injury, infection, hematoma, dural tear, no improvement of symptoms
Posterior spinal fusion	Instability which can be attributed to a variety of causes such as degenerated or multiple herniated discs, spinal stenosis which requires extensive decompression, spondylolisthesis	Bone graft material is placed laterally between the transverse processes and over a period of time, heals or "fuses" to create a fusion mass which provides stability to the area.	Nerve root injury, infection, hematoma, dural tear, no improvement of symptoms, failure of the fusion to heal, or transitional instability at adjacent segments

Table 18.1 (continued)
Common Surgical Procedures

Posterior spinal fusion with instrumentation	As above	As above with the addition of spinal instrumentation being placed in an effort to immobilize the fused level to aid in the healing of the fusion mass. (Pedicle screw fixation is not FDA approved for all surgical indications.)	As above with the addition of nerve root injury at the time of placement of the instrumentation, breakage of the instrumentation system, or need for removal of the system in the future.
Anterior spinal fusion	Instability attributable to a variety of reasons creates anterior instability	An abdominal approach is used to expose the spine and a fusion is created using bone graft material or a cage filled with bone material.	Nerve root injury, retroperitoneal hemorrhage, failure of the bowels to regain normal function, sterility in men, failure of the fusion to heal. If cages are used, dislodgement of the cage resulting in injury to the nerves or the aorta, as well as the need for additional surgery.
Anterior cervical discectomy and fusion (ACDF)	Cervical herniated disc, stenosis, or instability	An incision is made in the front of the neck and the cervical disc is removed. Bone is then placed to create a fusion. This may be done with or without instrumentation.	Nerve root injury, respiratory distress or failure, hematoma, failure of the fusion to heal, no improvement of symptoms

a. Overcorrects on hyperextension of spine.
b. Patient is able to straighten spine by good posture.

2. Scheuermann's disease.
   a. Unable to correct spine on hyperextension.
   b. Wedging of at least three of the apical vertebra of the kyphosis of more than 5 degrees.
   c. Irregular vertebral endplates.
   d. Narrowing of intervertebral disc space.
3. Congenital.
   a. Early in embryonic life (6-8 weeks).
   b. A malformation occurs in the development of the vertebral structures.
   c. Creating structural problems in bony architecture of spine.
4. Paralytic kyphosis.
   a. Secondary to polio.
   b. Muscular dystrophy.
   c. Cerebral palsy.
   d. Spina bifida.
   e. Some of the myopathies may cause a kyphosis secondary to muscle weakness.
5. Traumatic/radiation.
   a. Traumatic injury to the bony column.
   b. Iatrogenic injury to the growth centers of vertebra secondary to asymmetric radiation can result in curvature.
6. Postlaminectomy: following laminectomy for spinal cord tumors, cysts, or syringomyelia, kyphosis often develops.

C. Pathophysiology. Kyphosis may be present in any area of the spine but most commonly describes the thoracic spine.

D. Incidence.

1. 1% of the population will have a kyphosis during adolescence.
2. Incidence increases for females after menopause.

E. Considerations across the lifespan.

1. Congenital, paralytic, or traumatic kyphosis is seen in juvenile patients.
2. Postural kyphosis and kyphosis secondary to Scheuermann's disease is seen most commonly in adolescence.
3. Adult progressive kyphosis occurs in the female after menopause secondary to softening of the bone and compression fractures.
4. Post-laminectomy kyphosis can be seen at any age.

F. Complications.

1. Postural kyphosis left untreated can result in a fixed kyphosis and deformity.
2. Kyphosis secondary to Scheuermann's disease without treatment may result in a significant deformity.
3. Severe thoracic kyphosis may cause cardiopulmonary problems and pain.

Table 18.2
Common Nursing Diagnoses, Outcomes, and Interventions for Spinal Disorders

Diagnoses	Outcomes	Interventions
A. Observation 1. Coping, ineffective.	• Patient/family verbalizes the rationale for observation and warning signs of progressive scoliosis requiring earlier evaluation.	• Provide support for coping due to uncertainty of future treatment requirements. • Answer questions about future treatment honestly. • Do not promise that surgical treatment will not be required.
B. Bracing as initial therapy or bracing/casting as post-operative therapy 1. Comfort, altered: pain. a. Cast/brace contact. b. Restrictions. c. Postoperative pain. 2. Skin integrity, impaired. a. Incision. b. Pressure area from brace/cast. 3. Gas exchange, impaired. a. Inability to deep breath b. A tight brace/cast. 4. Coping, ineffective. a. Knowledge, deficient. 5. Activity intolerance. 6. Body image, disturbed. 7. Nutrition, imbalanced: less than body requirement. a. Loss of appetite. b. Esophageal reflux. 8. Elimination patterns, impaired.	• Patient verbalizes comfort in brace/cast. • Patient is able to perform self-care activities (skin care, application/removal of brace). • Patient's respiratory status remains unchanged. • Patient demonstrates ability to cope with brace/cast wearing. • Patient demonstrates increasing activity within established limitations. • Patient verbalizes acceptance of altered body image. - Patient describes the importance of wearing the brace/cast as prescribed. • Patient demonstrates good nutrition as evidenced by no weight loss and good intake. • Patient verbalizes ability to care for personal needs (elimination).	• Promote comfort. 1. Have brace/cast modified, if indicated. 2. Gradually increase time in brace as comfort allows. 3. Develop goals for the patient to help identify the optimal bracing time. 4. Medicate postoperative patients as necessary to help achieve brace/cast wear. • Maintain skin integrity. 1. Assess skin breakdown or irritation. 2. Assess brace/cast for proper fit. 3. Have brace/cast modified if necessary. 4. Increase time in brace gradually. 5. Instruct patient to avoid lotion that softens the skin and use alcohol rubs to toughen the skin in reddened areas. 6. Tape cast edges and protect skin from rough cast edges. 7. Instruct patient to keep cast dry and avoid cracks.
C. Post Surgery 1. Pain, acute 2. Nutrition, imbalanced: less than body requirement. a. Nothing by mouth/clear liquids postoperative status. b. Potential for ileus. 3. Infection, risk for. a. Alteration in physical regulation b. Magnitude and length of procedure. 4. Constipation. a. Limited intake. b. Use of narcotic analgesics. c. Decreased mobility.	• Patient's pain is controlled as evidenced by ability to rest and participate in prescribed activities. • Patient maintains adequate intake and weight. • Patient has no signs or symptoms of infection. • Patient is able to have bowel movements without difficulty. • Patient's urine output is at least 30 cc per hour. 1. Patient is able to void without difficulty. 2. Patient does not have incontinence.	• Preoperatively, discuss the surgical procedure, preoperative testing and postoperative management with patient/significant others. 1. Explain all preoperative tests. 2. SSEP and MEP monitoring. 3. Explain the Stagnara wake-up test. (After the spine has been straightened and instrumentation completed, the anesthesia is diminished and the patient is asked to move his/her extremities. Following confirmation of good motor function, anesthesia is reinstituted and the wound closed. Decreased or absent motor function would require

Table 18.2 (continued)
Common Nursing Diagnoses, Outcomes, and Interventions for Spinal Disorders

Diagnosis	Outcomes	Interventions
C. Post Surgery (continued) 5. Urinary elimination, altered pattern. a. Decreased urine output following hypotensive anesthesia. b. Sodium retention with decreased glomerular filtration rate and effective renal blood flow. c. Potential for neurologic injury. 6. Fluid volume deficit. a. Magnitude and length of surgical procedure. b. Blood loss. 7. Gas exchange, impaired. a. Atelectasis. b. Anesthesia. c. Pain. d. Narcotics. e. Surgical manipulation of chest geometry. 8. Injury, risk for: neurologic. 9. Coping, ineffective. 10. Activity, intolerance for. 11. Physical mobility, impaired. 12. Self care, deficient. 13. Growth and development, altered: spinal fusion. 14. Body image, disturbed.	• Patient's vital signs remain stable. 1. Hemoglobin and hematocrit within normal range following a major surgical procedure. 2. No signs or symptoms of hypovolemia are present. 3. Normal amount of drainage seen on dressing and from drainage tubes. • Patient maintains adequate ventilation. 1. Breath sounds clear. 2. Temperature within normal range following a major surgical procedure. • Patient's neurologic status remains intact. 1. No signs or symptoms of sensory or motor loss. 2. No changes in bowel or bladder pattern. • Patient verbalizes decreased anxiety about surgical procedure, postoperative routines, and follow-up care. • Patient increases activities of self-care as tolerated and limitations placed secondary to surgical procedure. • Patient/family verbalizes understanding of the effects of a spinal fusion on growth. • Patient discusses feelings about new body image.	instrumentation removal after reinstitution of anesthesia.). Also explain SSEP and MEP testing. 4. Discuss the need of the intensive care unit and what can be expected; explain visiting restrictions and rationale. 5. Discuss postoperative equipment that can be anticipated (IVs, arterial line, urinary drainage system, cardiac monitor, and turning frame). Anterior fusion patients may require nasogastric tube and chest tube. If a ventilator is under consideration, this *must* be discussed with the patient. 6. Explain to the patient the necessary neurologic checks that will be required as the preoperative assessment is being done (sensation, strength, reflexes, motion to upper and lower extremities). 7. Teach logrolling, coughing, and deep breathing. If a turning frame is to be used, show the patient how it works and assist with a trial ride on the frame to reduce fear. 8. Provide reassurance regarding progress. 9. Attend to needs of the patient and be available. 10. Provide diversional activities. 11. Develop a trusting relationship with the patient. • Promote comfort: assess patient's pain status and provide comfort measures (analgesics, muscle relaxants, position change). • Provide nutrition. 1. Administer IV fluids as ordered. 2. Assess abdomen to determine the presence of bowel sounds, distention, and rule out ileus. 3. Observe for signs and symptoms of superior mesenteric artery syndrome (cast syndrome). 4. Progress diet slowly and continue to monitor for signs and symptoms of ileus. 5. Prior to discharge, discuss nutritional requirements to promote fusion healing.

Diagnoses	Outcomes	Interventions
		• Monitor for signs and symptoms of infection. 1. Assess temperature. 2. Assess wound for redness, hematoma, drainage, dehiscence, and inordinate amount of pain. 3. Administer antibiotics as ordered. 4. Assess for change in neurologic status secondary to increasing hematoma. • Observe for signs and symptoms of constipation or impaction. 1. Obtain a baseline assessment of bowel function. 2. Assess patient for abdominal distention, cramping, and passage of flatus. 3. Administer stool softeners as ordered. 4. Encourage oral intake of fruits and juices. 5. Decrease narcotics when patient demonstrates reduced complaints of pain. 6. Assess patient for impaction in the absence of bowel movement. 7. Administer enemas as indicated to relieve constipation. • Monitor urinary output/integrity. 1. Obtain a baseline assessment of bladder function. 2. Provide fluids. 3. Maintain urine output of at least 30 cc per hour. 4. Expect diminished urine output for the first 24-48 hours in those patients who have had hypotensive anesthesia. 5. Observe for any signs of incontinence or bladder distention. • Watch for signs and symptoms of hypovolemia. 1. Assess vital signs as indicated. 2. Assess status of hemoglobin/hematocrit. 3. Assess and record drainage from surgical drains, chest tubes, and dressing. 4. Administer blood replacement and IV fluids as ordered. • Assess respiratory status. 1. Provide pulmonary hygiene (deep breathing, coughing, tri-flow, IPPB).

Table 18.2 (continued)
Common Nursing Diagnoses, Outcomes, and Interventions for Spinal Disorders

Diagnoses	Outcomes	Interventions
		2. Provide comfort measures to help encourage pulmonary hygiene (administer analgesics prior to exercise, instruct patient on splinting wound). 3. After thoracoabdominal surgery chest tubes are used. (1) Monitor patency of tubes. (2) Output. 4. Encourage ambulation when tolerated. • Monitor for signs and symptoms of neurologic/neurovascular impairment. 1. Assess color, temperature, movement, and sensation of extremities. 2. Assess for bowel and bladder changes. • Develop schedule of activities to restore routine. 1. Logroll the patient from side to side as ordered every 2-4 hours or as needed to provide comfort. 2. Encourage elevation of head of bed as soon as tolerated. 3. Provide quiet periods throughout the day to encourage rest. 4. Encourage diversional activities. 5. Progress patient's return to normal activities and self-care when tolerated. • Explain decreased growth of the spine over those segments of the spine that are fused prior to completion of spinal growth. • Encourage patient to discuss concerns regarding surgical outcome.

II. ASSESSMENT

A. History and physical examination.

1. Postural kyphosis will usually be asymptomatic in children.
   a. However, in severe thoracic kyphosis, shortness of breath may be noticed.
   b. Patients with Scheuermann's disease will describe thoracic back pain and fatigue.
2. Adults may experience fatigue, back pain, and shortness of breath depending on severity of the curve.
3. Not noticed until identified during a school screening examination, regularly scheduled physical, or while trying on clothing.
4. Family thought posture was normal for age group.
5. May or may not be a family history of kyphosis.
6. Clothing must be removed to adequately assess spine.
   a. A gown that opens posteriorly.
   b. A bathing suit of neutral colors (girls).
   c. Gym trunks (boys).
   d. Provides necessary visualization of spine while maintaining privacy for patient.
7. Increased thoracic rounding.
8. May have shoulder asymmetry if scoliosis is also present.
9. May have abdominal creases with significant kyphosis.
10. On forward bend test, increase thoracic rounding when viewed from side.
11. Tight hamstrings with inability to touch toes.
12. Neurologic examination to rule out any underlying neurologic problem causing the kyphosis.

B. Diagnostic tests.

1. Observation/school screening protocol.
   a. Inspect spine in upright and forward flexed positions.
   b. From behind, in front of, and to the side of the patient.
2. Radiographs of the spine.
   a. Initial radiographs should be obtained on patients with a positive assessment. Follow-up radiographs should be taken only after examination and if progression is suspected.
   b. Radiographs should be taken posterior to anterior to decrease x-ray exposure to thyroid, breasts, reproductive organs.
   c. Appropriate shields should be used to protect breasts and reproductive organs.
   d. Standing lateral view of spine.
   e. Standing PA view of spine to fully assess spinal condition at first evaluation.

III. COMMON THERAPEUTIC MODALITIES

A. Observation.

1. Curves less than 45 degrees are observed for progression.
2. Clinical examination to rule out progression of the curvature.
3. Postural exercises may be prescribed to correct the kyphosis.

B. Brace.

1. Curves above 45 degrees in a growing child will:
   a. Require use of a brace to prevent further progression of curvature.
   b. Different from brace treatment for scoliosis.
   c. Correction achieved through bracing is often maintained if brace is worn until end of growth.
2. Exercises are prescribed in conjunction with bracing to maintain trunk muscle strength and hamstring stretching.
3. Bracing is ineffective in the mature patient.

C. Surgery. Anterior and posterior spine fusion is necessary for kyphosis (see Table 18.1).

1. Recommended for curves above 65 degrees.
   a. Posterior spinal fusion with instrumentation. Luque rods with sublaminar wires are generally reserved for paralytic curvatures.
   b. Anterior disc excision and spinal fusion or anterior spinal fusion with a strut graft. Graft may be taken from the fibula or rib; or cadaver bone may be used.
   c. Combination anterior and posterior fusion with instrumentation is necessary to achieve correction.
2. Variations of surgical plans may be recommended for complex patients.
3. Traction devices are used infrequently due to better surgical technique and instrumentation. Halo gravity traction is the treatment of choice for severe, rigid kyphosis that requires slow manipulation of spine.
4. The need for postoperative casting has decreased due to better spine fixation. Immobilization is achieved by use of a Milwaukee brace or TLSO with neck ring attachment.

IV. NURSING DIAGNOSES, OUTCOMES, AND INTERVENTIONS

A. See Scoliosis, this chapter.

B. See Table 18.2.

V. HOME CARE CONSIDERATIONS (See Table 18.3)

HERNIATED NUCLEUS PULPOSUS

I. OVERVIEW

A. Definition: protrusion of the center portion of the disc (nucleus pulposus through a crack in the outer cartilagenous ring (annulus fibrosis).

B. Etiology.

1. Trauma.
2. Repetitive stress.
   a. The annulus develops cracks or fissures due to repetitive stress to the area.
   b. Allows for protrusion of disc material.
3. Degeneration of the disc.

Table 18.3
Common Home Care Considerations for Spinal Disorders

A. Observation.
1. Discuss the signs and symptoms of neurologic compromise and progressive symptomatology.
2. Explain wound care procedures and signs of possible wound complications. Wound complications should be caught early and treated aggressively.
3. Caution patients to avoid bending, twisting, or lifting until permitted by the physician.
4. Encourage increase in walking activity as tolerated.
5. Patients who have undergone lumbar surgery are typically more comfortable lying on their backs with a pillow under the knees or lying on their side with a pillow between the legs. Patients who have undergone cervical surgery are typically more comfortable with the head and the neck in a neutral position.

B. Brace/casting.
1. Brace philosophy and use is physician specific.
2. Assist patient in becoming comfortable getting the brace on and off.
3. Discuss clothing and how to wear brace to increase compliance and comfort.
4. Encourage walking activity as tolerated in the brace.
5. After cervical surgery, the neck and shoulders should be supported when changing position.

C. General home care considerations.
1. Provide written and verbal discharge instructions.
2. Involve significant others early in the treatment and teaching.
3. Encourage patient to write down questions as they arise.
4. Discuss the importance of a healthy diet on healing.
5. Instruct patients on the use of pain medicines as prescribed.
6. Caution patients to avoid driving and alcohol consumption while on pain medicines.
7. Fusion patients should be advised to stop smoking and avoid anti-inflammatory medicines while the fusion heals since both have been shown to compromise fusion consolidation.
8. Caution patients that they may fatigue quickly for the first few weeks until they build up their stamina.
9. Discuss sexual activity and limitations (dependent upon the surgery location and procedure).
10. Encourage patients to contact the physician's office to discuss any questions or concerns after discharge from the hospital.

a. As a person ages, the annulus degenerates causing cracks or fissures.
b. The nucleus pulposus can herniate through the fissure.

C. Pathophysiology.
1. The intervertebral disc consists of two parts.
   a. The inner portion of the disc is the nucleus pulposus, which is a gelatinous material with a high water content.
   b. This is surrounded by cartilaginous/fibrous layers of tissue called the annulus fibrosis.
   c. The disc functions as:
      (1) A cushion or "shock absorber" between the vertebrae.
      (2) Aides in giving flexibility to the spine.
2. When a disc herniates:
   a. The nucleus pulposus herniates out through a crack in the annulus fibrosis.
   b. The disc herniating into the spinal canal can create pressure on the passing nerve roots as well as an inflammatory response.

D. Classification of herniated discs.
1. Bulging: an out-pouching of the disc.
   a. Terminology can be confusing.
   b. This is not considered a disc herniation by most practitioners
   c. Bulging is considered a normal part of the aging process.
2. Protrusion is the herniation of the disc that does not protrude past the posterior longitudinal ligament.
3. Extrusion is the herniation of the disc through the posterior longitudinal ligament.
4. Sequestered: free fragment is where the herniated portion of the disc is no longer attached to the annulus.

E. Incidence.
1. Men are more commonly affected possibly related to occupational influences.
2. Most commonly affected disc levels:
   a. L4-5 and L5-S1.
   b. C6-7 and C5-6.

F. Complications.
1. The most acute and life-altering potential complication is cauda equina syndrome.
2. A disc herniation can be a life-altering disorder; it is not a life-threatening condition.
3. Patients may experience financial strain due to lost time from work and a change in occupation may be necessary if the patient's job requires heavy physical labor.

II. ASSESSMENT

A. History and physical examination.
1. History.
   a. Symptoms.
      (1) History of onset: can be acute or gradual.
      (2) Characteristics/location of pain in leg(s) or shoulder/arms.
      (3) Previous history.

(4) Aggravating/alleviating factors.
(5) If onset is related to accident/injury: how did it happen; when; where?
(6) If related to an auto accident: when; seat belted; driver or passenger; how much damage to car?

b. Occupational history.
c. Lifestyle: quality of life/activities of daily living (ADL).
d. Social history.
(1) Alcohol/drug use.
(2) Cigarette use.
e. Family history.
f. Past medical history.

2. Subjective complaints.
a. Influenced by mechanism of injury and area of the herniation.
b. May complain of a sudden onset of pain after a specific traumatic event or may present with a long history of progressively worsening pain.
c. Many patients will have attempted to treat symptoms with home remedies or alternative therapies prior to presenting for evaluation and treatment.
d. Sciatic pain will follow the distribution of the nerve into the affected extremity on the side of the herniation.
e. Central disc herniations may produce more neck/back pain or pain into both or alternating extremities of the affected region.
f. Lumbar pain is usually aggravated by:
(1) Standing.
(2) Walking.
(3) Bending.
(4) Coughing/sneezing.
(5) Other activities, which may increase pressure in the affected area.
(6) It is usually relieved by rest.
g. Cervical pain is usually aggravated by:
(1) Neck flexion.
(2) Extension.
(3) Rotation.
(4) Lateral bending.
(5) Axial loading.
(6) It is usually relieved by rest.

B. Physical examination.

1. Lumbar herniations.
a. Limited forward flexion.
b. List away from the affected side noted during standing or ambulation.
c. Positive straight leg raising test on the affected side. There maybe a positive contralateral straight leg raising test as well.
d. Sensory, motor, or reflex changes in the affected dermatome.
(1) L3-4 herniations.
(a) Sensory deficit in the anterior thigh and at medial aspect of ankle and foot.
(b) Diminished or absent patellar reflex.
(2) L4-5 herniations.
(a) Difficulty heel walking.
(b) Decreased strength of the extensor hallucis longus.
(c) Sensory deficit in the lateral aspect of the thigh and anterior aspect of the lower leg and space between the great and second toe.
(3) L5-S1 herniations.
(a) Difficulty toe walking.
(b) Sensory deficit lateral and posterior aspect of the lower leg, foot, and last three toes.
(c) Diminished or absent achilles reflex.

2. Cervical herniations.
a. C5-6 herniations.
(1) Sensory deficit of lateral forearm, thumb, index finger, and half of middle finger.
(2) Weakness of wrist extensors.
(3) Decreased brachioradialis reflex. Biceps reflex may be slightly weak.
b. C6-7 herniations.
(1) Sensory deficit of ring and little finger and medial forearm.
(2) Weakness of wrist/tricep flexors and finger extensors.
(3) Decreased triceps reflex.

C. Diagnostic tests.

1. Spine x-rays are used to rule out any other concomitant cause of pain.
2. Magnetic Resonance Imaging (MRI) is used to demonstrate nerve root compromise due to the herniated disc.
3. Myelogram is used to show nerve root cut off or compromised at the level affected by the herniation. Used less frequently since MRI is available.
4. Computerized Tomography is used to demonstrate nerve root compromise. Has been replaced by MRI as the diagnostic tool of choice.
5. Discogram is used in an attempt to reproduce the patient's pain.
6. Electromyography (EMG) is used to demonstrate sensory deficit at the affected nerve root level.

III. COMMON THERAPEUTIC MODALITIES

A. Conservative treatment. Used as initial treatment in the absence of cauda equina symptoms.

1. Conservative treatment is usually attempted for at least 6 weeks unless neurologic deficit is present and progressing.
2. Up to 80% of patients with symptomatic disc herniations will improve in the first 6 weeks with conservative care.
a. Activity modification within comfort levels. Avoid absolute bed rest.
b. Exercises to strengthen and condition muscles.
c. Traction.
(1) Cervical: for cervical herniations.
(2) Pelvic: for lumbar herniations (is seldom used)
(3) Heat or ice to area for comfort: based on

patient comfort and physician preference.

d. Comfort modalities such as diathermy, ultrasound, massage, and transcutaneous electrical nerve stimulation (TENS) are often used in combination with physical therapy.

e. Pharmacologic treatment.
   (1) Analgesics are used in the short-term management of the acute episode.
   (2) Nonsteroidal anti-inflammatory medications (NSAIDs) or COX-2 inhibitors are used to decrease the inflammation of the affected nerve(s).
   (3) Muscle relaxants are sometimes used to decrease muscle spasms in the acute pain phase.
   (4) Steroids such as prednisone or a medrol dose pack are sometimes used short-term to decrease the inflammation that is creating acute pain.

f. Brace or corset may be used for comfort on a short-term basis. Long-term use of a corset or brace will weaken the muscles of the affected area.

g. Epidural steroid injections administer a combination of a steroid and local anesthetic to the epidural space to locally decrease inflammation and resulting pain.

h. Selective nerve root block may be administered to deliver a steroid and local anesthetic directly to the affected nerve root.

i. Facet blocks.

B. Surgical intervention (see Table 18.1).

1. Cervical laminectomy/discectomy.
   a. Herniated nucleus pulposus is removed, usually through an anterior approach.
   b. An associated fusion is often performed to stabilize the affected disc level. This is based on physician practice and surgical philosophy
2. Lumbar surgery.
   a. Percutaneous discectomy.
   b. Microdiscectomy/limited approach discectomy.
   c. Lumbar laminectomy.
   d. Laminectomy and spinal fusion.
      (1) Recurrent disc herniation.
      (2) Concomitant instability.

IV. NURSING DIAGNOSES, OUTCOMES, AND INTERVENTIONS

A. See Table 18.2.

B. Pain.

1. Outcomes.
   a. Patient's pain controlled or alleviated.
   b. Patient experiences as little discomfort as possible during the pre and postoperative period.
2. Interventions.
   a. Provide comfort measures.
      (1) Discuss an individualized plan of care with the patient to alleviate pain using modalities, medications, relaxation, and activity modification.
      (2) Lumbar herniations.
         (a) Patients are usually more comfortable lying with knees flexed. Walking and standing should be performed as tolerated. Sitting for long periods will usually increase discomfort.
         (b) Teach patients to keep their weight down and maintain their muscle tone as much as possible to prevent deconditioning.
      (3) Cervical herniations.
         (a) Support the cervical area when changing positions.
         (b) Use cervical support/collar for short-term management to promote comfort.
      (4) See Chapter 7, Pain.
   b. Provide postoperative general care and care specific to the surgical procedure being performed.
      (1) See Chapter 5, Perioperative Patient Care.
      (2) Provide care for patient undergoing cervical discectomy/laminectomy.
         (a) Assess respiratory status for any wheezing, distress, or stridor as a potential sign of edema or hematoma.
         (b) Provide humidity to help thin secretions.
         (c) Have a tracheotomy tray available in the event of respiratory distress.
         (d) Maintain cervical support as ordered.
         (e) Assess neurovascular status of the upper and lower extremities.
      (3) Provide care for patient undergoing lumbar laminotomy/laminectomy and discectomy or percutaneous discectomy.
         (a) Logroll.
         (b) Increase activity as directed by physician and as tolerated.
         (c) Limit duration of sitting.
         (d) Assess wound for any signs of infection, dehiscence, or hematoma.
         (e) Assess neurovascular status.
         (f) Assess bowel and bladder function for any loss of sensation or control.
      (4) Provide care for patient undergoing a laminectomy and fusion.
         (a) Bed rest may be indicated in the immediate postoperative period. Increase activity as directed by physician and as tolerated by patient.
         (b) Teach appropriate body mechanics and logrolling.
         (c) Lumbar support as indicated by physician preference.
         (d) Assess neurovascular status.

IV. HOME CARE CONSIDERATIONS

A. See Table 18.3.

B. Avoid sitting in low chairs and avoid sitting for long periods.

C. Increase activity as tolerated using proper body mechanics and avoiding any bending, twisting, or lifting until advised by the physician that these activities are permitted.

D. Assess wound for any signs of infection.

SPINAL STENOSIS

I. OVERVIEW

A. Definition: any type of narrowing of the spinal canal or intervertebral foramina.

B. Etiology.

1. Congenital/developmental-hereditary.
2. Acquired.
   a. Degenerative.
   b. Spondylolisthetic.
   c. Iatrogenic: after surgery.
   d. Post-traumatic.
   e. Metabolic.
3. Combination of congenital and acquired.

C. Pathophysiology.

1. Congenital stenosis usually includes the entire canal; acquired stenosis is usually limited to one or several segments.
2. Stenosis can be the result of bony changes causing:
   a. Narrowing.
   b. Spondylolisthesis, resulting in narrowing of the canal.
   c. Post-surgical changes in the canal.
   d. Trauma.
   e. Metabolic changes such as Paget's disease.
3. Can occur at any level in the spine. Most commonly seen in the lower cervical or lumbar segments.

D. Complications.

1. Cauda equina syndrome is a medical emergency and needs to be ruled out as a sequelae of spinal stenosis.
2. Sometimes confused with vascular insufficiency.
3. May require activity modification.

II. ASSESSMENT

A. History and physical examination.

1. Often a gradual onset: usually over a period of years.
2. Low back pain and/or leg pain that increases with walking/standing and decreases with sitting.
3. Forward flexed postures (such as shopping while leaning on a grocery cart or sitting) are usually comfortable since the posture opens up the canal slightly and alleviates pressure on the nerves.
4. Pain may radiate into lower extremities (neuroclaudication) or follow a specific nerve root distribution of an affected nerve.
5. Bowel or bladder may be affected. Weakness may be present. These problems require more immediate evaluation/treatment.
6. Sometimes confused with vascular claudication or diabetic neuropathy. A lower extremity vascular evaluation is necessary on all patients.
7. Lumbar extension usually exacerbates typical pain complaints.
8. Check for lower extremity edema and pedal pulses.

B. Diagnostic tests.

1. Radiographs.
   a. AP, lateral, and oblique x-rays.
   b. Flexion/extension x-rays will demonstrate any concomitant instability.
2. Myelogram/CT will show the area and severity of stenosis (though MRI is usually adequate for this purpose).
3. MRI will evaluate the neural structures.
4. Electrophysiologic tests. An EMG will help to differentiate the cause of arm or leg complaints: neuropathy, peripheral/vascular disease, diabetic neuropathy, or radicular complaints.

III. COMMON THERAPEUTIC MODALITIES

A. Decreasing pain and maximizing function is a major goal of treatment.

B. Maintaining independence is a primary goal since it is most commonly seen in older patients.

C. Activity should be within comfort levels.

1. Advise patients to sit and rest when necessary.
2. Typically, sitting and resting for a few minutes will enable the patient to continue with his/her activity.

D. Anti-inflammatory medications are used for short-term management of the acute phases of pain or for more long-term management in an attempt to avoid surgery.

E. Avoiding extension activities.

F. Injections (epidural steroid) are indicated for management of acute pain episodes.

G. A corset or brace may be used for acute pain episodes.

1. Long-term corset will weaken back and abdominal musculature.
2. This may or may not be a concern depending upon the patient, his/her age, activity level, and treatment goals.

H. Physical therapy and/or aquatic therapy may be prescribed to aid in maximizing functioning and decreasing pain.

I. Surgical intervention (see Table 18.1).

1. In the absence of neurologic compromise or cauda equina symptoms, surgery is a last resort.
2. Surgery should be undertaken when the patient is unhappy with the quality of life due to pain, all conservative options have failed, and the patient understands the risk involved in proceeding with surgery.
3. Since this is usually an older population, the assurance that the patient is medically stable to undergo the surgery is imperative.
4. Decompressive laminectomy is performed to relieve the narrowing and resulting pressure.

5. A concomitant fusion is performed when there is an associated instability present or the decompression will create instability.

IV. NURSING DIAGNOSES, OUTCOMES, AND INTERVENTIONS (See Table 18.2)

V. HOME CARE CONSIDERATIONS (See Table 18.3)

DEGENERATIVE DISC DISEASE

I. OVERVIEW

A. Definition. Wear and tear/degeneration of the disc over time.

B. Etiology.

1. A process of aging.
2. Thought to be a normal variant unless accompanied by back pain.

C. Pathophysiology.

1. Normal disc has good height and serves as a cushion between the vertebrae.
2. A degenerated disc can cause pain, instability, or narrowing of the neural canal (stenosis).

D. Incidence.

1. Incidence increases with age.
2. Up to 95% of people have degenerative disc changes by age 50.
3. Degeneration begins in the 20s and progresses at varied rates from person to person.
4. Sometimes not diagnosed until there is a trauma or event resulting in back pain.

E. Considerations across the lifespan.

1. May be present but not symptomatic until there is a trauma.
2. Controversy exists because this diagnosis is often made after a motor vehicle accident or work-related accident. In cases such as these, it is often determined that the symptoms and pain are an aggravation of a pre-existing condition.

F. Complications.

1. Not a life-threatening condition.
2. Pain often subsides with activity modification.
3. Neurologic examination is warranted to rule out concomitant radicular symptoms.

II. ASSESSMENT

A. History and physical examination.

1. Back pain with or without radiculopathy.
2. Usually a gradual onset with increasing severity which eventually warrants evaluation.
3. Physical examination may be normal.
4. May have flattening of the lumbar contour in the acute phase related to spasms.
5. Range of motion of the spine is often painful.

B. Diagnostic tests.

1. AP, lateral films will demonstrate disc space narrowing.
2. Flexion/extension films will reveal any concomitant instability.
3. MRI or myelo/CT will show any effect upon the neural structures.
4. Discogram/CT will reproduce the patient's typical pain at the symptomatic disc level. Especially useful in cases in which there are multiple levels of involvement.

III. COMMON THERAPEUTIC MODALITIES: Conservative treatment

A. Activity modification within comfort levels until the acute symptoms resolve.

B. Exercises to strengthen the back and abdominal musculature.

C. Anti-inflammatory medications during the acute pain.

D. Heat or ice as comfortable.

E. Epidural injection or selective nerve root block if there is associated radiculopathy.

F. Surgical intervention

1. See Table 18.1
2. Intradiscal electrothermal therapy (IDET).
3. Fusion with or without instrumentation.
   a. Can be performed anteriorly or posteriorly.
   b. Goal is to stabilize the segment to eliminate it from being a pain generator.
   c. Laminectomy is done along with the fusion if there is an associated stenosis.

SPONDYLOLYSIS/SPONDYLOLISTHESIS

I. OVERVIEW

A. Definition.

1. Spondylolysis is a unilateral or bilateral defect in the pars interarticularis.
2. Spondylolisthesis is the anterior translation of one vertebra on top of another.

B. Etiology.

1. Spondylolysis.
   a. Has a definite hereditary predisposition.
   b. May be traumatic in origin, as a result of repetitive stress. Children involved in certain sports activities, such as gymnastics or wrestling, have a higher incidence related to repeated hyperextension stress.
2. Spondylolisthesis.
   a. Cause is dependent upon type of spondylolisthesis.
   b. Types.
      (1) Dysplastic: an elongation and attenuation of the pars with or without lysis (congenital)
      (2) Isthmic: lysis of a previously normal pars. Often seen in young athletes who participate in sports which require repetitive hyperextension movements such as gymnastics, wrestling, or football.

(3) Degenerative: degenerative changes in the vertebrae and disc cause the vertebrae to slip forward.
(4) Traumatic: related to injury to the area.
(5) Pathologic: resulting from a pathologic process such as tumor or infection.

c. Classification.
(1) Grade 1: up to 25% vertebral translation.
(2) Grade 2: 26%-50% vertebral translation.
(3) Grade 3: 51%-75% vertebral translation.
(4) Grade 4: 76%-100% vertebral translation.
(5) Grade 5: spondyloptosis – complete translation.

C. Pathophysiology.

1. Spondylolysis most often occurs at the L4-L5 or L5-S1 vertebra. It may or may not be associated with spondylolisthesis.
2. Spondylolisthesis may occur at any level of the spine; however, it commonly occurs at L4-L5 or L5-S1.

D. Incidence.

1. Spondylolysis.
   a. Equal occurrence among males and females.
   b. 5% of the population have a spondylolysis, most often asymptomatic.
   c. Among pediatric patients, it is diagnosed most frequently in early teen years.
2. Spondylolisthesis.
   a. Males 5%-6%, females 2%-3%.
   b. Occurs more frequently in gymnasts, weight lifters, and football linemen.
   c. Does not become symptomatic until late childhood or early adolescence.

E. Considerations across the lifespan.

1. Spondylolysis.
   a. Defects in the pars interarticularis appear most frequently between ages 6-10.
   b. Often is present but not symptomatic until there is a traumatic event and resulting back pain. The defect is then noted on oblique x-ray films.
2. Spondylolisthesis.
   a. Commonly diagnosed between ages 7-10.
   b. Often, increased athletic activities of adolescence in combination with growth at that age will cause a complaint of back pain and the resulting diagnosis.
   c. Spondylolisthesis may go undetected until adulthood and can be an incidental finding on a pre-employment physical examination or noted on x-ray after a bout of back pain.
   d. Asymptomatic spondylolisthesis does not warrant intervention.

F. Complications.

1. Spondylolysis.
   a. Not a life-threatening illness.
   b. May require alterations in lifestyle or occupation.
2. Spondylolisthesis.
   a. Severe pain with radicular symptoms may occur in an acute spondylolisthesis.
   b. Pathologic causes of spondylolisthesis need to be ruled out.
   c. Bowel and bladder dysfunction can occur secondary to severe spondylolisthesis and resulting nerve impingement.
   d. Weakness in lower extremities may be seen.

II. ASSESSMENT

A. History and physical examination.

1. Low back pain may be acute or may be a chronic condition, which has gradually worsened.
2. Pain is usually low back pain, which may or may not radiate into one or both legs.
3. Neurologic examination may or may not be normal.
4. Bowel and bladder changes require emergent evaluation and treatment.
5. Gait may be slow or waddling.
6. Increased lumbar lordosis and protuberance of abdomen may be present in more severe slips. Hamstring tightness may produce a false positive straight leg raise test.
7. Buttocks may appear more prominent in severe slips and is described as heart-shaped buttocks.
8. A palpable step off in spinous processes of lumbar spine may be palpated in patients with a severe slip.
9. Torso may appear shortened with a severe slip.
10. Forward flexion may be limited.
11. Muscle spasm in lower back.

B. Diagnostic tests.

1. Radiographs.
   a. AP, lateral, and obliques of the lumbosacral spine.
   (1) Lateral views will enable you to determine the degree of slip.
   (2) Oblique views will enable you to view the pars defect as represented by the "scotty dog" appearance.
   b. Flexion/extension films to determine stability/movement.
2. Lumbar MRI or myelogram/CT scan may be ordered to evaluate the neural structures if neurologic changes are present on examination or prior to surgical intervention.
3. Electromyogram will help determine associated nerve root irritation.

III. COMMON THERAPEUTIC MODALITIES

A. Activity should be modified until the acute pain resolves. Absolute bed rest is typically not indicated.

B. Restriction of activities may include avoiding repetitive bending, twisting, and heavy lifting.

C. Immobilization with a lumbosacral corset or lumbosacral orthosis may be ordered for a limited period to help alleviate the acute pain.

D. Analgesics may be ordered during the acute episodes of pain. Anti-inflammatory medications may be used for long-term pain management.

E. Epidural steroid injections may be ordered in an

attempt to decrease nerve root irritation related to the instability.

F. **Physical therapy may be prescribed in an effort to help develop and maintain strong abdominal and back musculature.**

G. **Surgery may be indicated if pain continues/progresses despite conservative treatment.**

H. **Surgical intervention/options (see Table 18.1).**
   1. Posterior spinal fusion with or without instrumentation.
   2. Anterior spinal fusion with bone graft or anterior cage device.
   3. Combination anterior/posterior fusion.
   4. Surgical approach is dependent upon type and degree of slip and surgeon philosophy, skill, and preference.

IV. NURSING DIAGNOSES, OUTCOMES, AND INTERVENTIONS (See Table 18.2)

V. HOME CARE CONSIDERATIONS (See Table 18.3)

FAILED BACK SYNDROME

I. OVERVIEW

A. **Definition: low back and/or associated leg pain of a chronic, nonmalignant nature. Usually associated with low back pain, which has failed to respond to surgical treatment.**

B. **Etiology.**
   1. Incorrect diagnosis of spinal disorder.
   2. Incorrect surgical treatment.
   3. Failure to respond to surgical treatment.
      a. Re-herniation of intervertebral disc.
      b. Failure of spinal instrumentation.
      c. Failure of spinal fusion.
   4. Unknown cause.

C. **Pathophysiology.**
   1. Refer to preexisting condition.
   2. Formation of excessive scar tissue from previous spinal surgery may compress nerves and cause pain.
   3. Ongoing pain and inability to receive adequate measures to relieve pain may contribute to psychological overlay.

D. **Incidence: affects a relatively small number of patients considering the high incidence of low back pain.**

E. **Considerations across the lifespan: primarily occurs in the adult population.**

F. **Complications.**
   1. Chronic pain.
   2. Narcotic dependence/substance abuse.
   3. Depression.
   4. Difficulty with interpersonal relationships/social isolation.

II. ASSESSMENT

A. **History and physical examination.**
   1. History.
      a. Symptoms.
         (1) Characteristics.
         (2) Onset.
         (3) Relieving/aggravating factors.
      b. Surgical history.
      c. Occupational history.
      d. Lifestyle: quality of life/ADL.
      e. Social history.
         (1) Alcohol use.
         (2) Cigarette use.
         (3) Social supports/significant others.
      f. Familial history.
      g. Past medical history.
      h. History of prescription medication use.
   2. Physical examination.
      a. Subjective assessment.
         (1) Pain in lower back and/or legs.
         (2) Numbness and/or paresthesias in the legs and/or feet.
         (3) Pain in sitting versus standing positions.
         (4) Pain with walking.
      b. Objective assessment.
         (1) Symptoms may vary with each patient.
         (2) Local tenderness in lower back region upon palpation.
         (3) Tenderness at sciatic notch upon deep palpation.
         (4) Deep tendon reflexes may not be intact.
         (5) Guarding.
         (6) Positive straight leg raise test (bowstring test may be negative).
         (7) Pain upon forward bending.
         (8) Muscle spasm.
         (9) Muscle weakness.

B. **Diagnostic tests.**
   1. X-rays.
   2. CT scan.
   3. MRI.
   4. Myelogram.
   5. EMG.
   6. SSEP.
   7. White blood cell count.
   8. ESR.
   9. C-reactive protein.
   10. Discogram.
   11. Bone scan.
   12. Psychological evaluation.

III. COMMON THERAPEUTIC MODALITIES

A. **Conservative treatment.**
   1. Short period of activity modification within comfort levels.
   2. Corset/brace.
   3. Local heat or cold application depending upon patient and physician preference.
   4. TENS.
   5. Physical therapy.

6. Acupuncture
7. Back school: a formalized program to teach proper body mechanics.
8. Medications.
   a. NSAIDs.
   b. Muscle relaxants or narcotic analgesics for short-term management of acute episodes.
   c. Antidepressant medications.
9. Pain clinic for comprehensive, multidisciplinary pain management.

B. Surgical treatment.

1. Dependent upon the diagnosis.
2. Dependent upon the presence of a surgically treatable problem.
3. Risk versus benefit of surgical intervention needs to be discussed as well as patient's expectations and realistic goals of surgery since surgical outcome has failed to be optimal in the past.

IV. NURSING DIAGNOSES, OUTCOMES, AND INTERVENTIONS

A. See Table 18.2.

B. Pain, chronic.
Activity intolerance.

1. Outcome: patient learns to cope with effects of chronic pain on activities.
2. Interventions.
   a. Provide alternative means of pain relief.
   b. Encourage participation in activities which promote mobilization and self-care.
      (1) Participate in supervised exercise to maintain mobility.
      (2) Use of corset or brace, as indicated by physician and based on individual relief of symptoms.
      (3) Pace activities to provide rest intervals.
   c. Provide occupational counseling.

V. HOME CARE CONSIDERATIONS (See Table 18.3)

SPINE FRACTURES

(See Chapter 14, Trauma)

SPINAL TUMORS

(See Chapter 15, Tumors)

Bibliography

Andersson, G., & McNeill, T. (1989). *Lumbar spine syndromes: Evaluation and treatment.* New York: Springer-Verlag.

Andersson, G., & McNeill, T. (1992). *Lumbar spinal stenosis.* St. Louis: Mosby Yearbook.

Baldus, C., & Blanke, K. (1997). Pre-operative nursing care. In K.H. Bridwell & R.L. DeWald (Eds.), *The textbook of spinal surgery* (2nd ed., p. 3-10). Philadelphia: Lippincott-Raven.

Borenstein, D.G., Weisel, S.W., & Boden, S.D. (1995). *Low back pain: Medical diagnosis and comprehensive management* (2nd ed.). Philadelphia: Saunders.

Bridwell, K.H., & DeWald, R.L. (1997). *The textbook of spinal surgery.* Philadelphia: Lippincott.

Brown, K.L. (1998). Cauda equina syndrome: implications for the orthopaedic nurse in a clinical setting. *Orthopaedic Nursing, 14*(5), 35-36.

Crowther, C.L. (1999). *Primary orthopaedic care.* St. Louis: Mosby.

Garfin, S.R., & Vaccaro, A.R. (Eds.). (1997). *Orthopaedic knowledge update – spine.* Rosemont, IL: North American Spine Society/American Academy of Orthopaedic Surgeons.

Freymoyer, J.W. (Ed.). (1997). *The adult spine: principles & practice, 2nd edition.* Philadelphia: Lippincott-Raven.

Nance, D., & Hickey, M. (1999). Spondylolisthesis in children. *Orthopaedic Nursing, 15*(1), 41-46.

Rodts, M.F. (1998). Disorders of the spine. In A.B. Maher, S.W. Salmond, & T.A. Pellino (Eds.), *Orthopaedic Nursing.* Philadelphia: Saunders.

Rodts, M.F. (1997). Perioperative and postoperative nursing care for the spinal surgery patient. In K.H. Bridwell & R.L. DeWald (Eds.), *The textbook of spinal surgery* (2nd ed., p. 11-30). Philadelphia: Lippincott-Raven.

Rothman, R.H., & Simeano, F.A. (Eds.). (1999). *The spine* (4th ed.). Philadelphia: W.B. Saunders.

STUDY QUESTIONS

George V., a 21-year-old college student, presented to the school health center with severe, incapacitating low back pain. Upon questioning, he states he has a 3-year history of low back pain. George is on the school weight-lifting team and competes throughout the country. He notes pain after he completes his daily workout or any excessive physical activity. He denies any leg pain or loss of bowel or bladder control. Upon examination, it is noted that George has a palpable step-off in the area of the lumbar spine. He has a waddling gait pattern and his left buttock is more prominent than his right buttock. He has a positive straight leg raising on the right side. All muscle groups are equally intact. Deep tendon reflexes are intact bilaterally. George is diagnosed as having spondylolisthesis. (Questions 1-3)

1. Spondylolisthesis is:
   a. Protrusion of disc material onto the spinal nerve root that cause a waddling gait.
   b. Narrowing of the spinal canal from severe osteoarthritis causing leg pain.
   c. A defect in the pars interarticularis with a forward slip of one vertebra on another.
   d. A curvature of the thoracic spine that leads to difficulty in doing straight leg raises.

2. Which of the following, from George's health history, might be a cause of his spondylolisthesis?:
   a. Smokes one pack of cigarettes per week.
   b. Weighs 20% more than standard for his height.
   c. Regularly lifting weights since he was 15 years old.
   d. Fell off a ladder during his senior year in high school.

3. Which of the following is **not** a common treatment for spondylolisthesis?
   a. Use of nonsteroidal anti-inflammatory drugs for acute episodes of pain.
   b. Immobilization with a lumbosacral corset or lumbosacral orthosis.
   c. Restricted activities such as bending, stooping, or lifting.
   d. Bed rest for 2-4 weeks with pelvic skin traction.

Harry Z. is a 37-year-old white male who works in construction. He is 6' 0", weights 250 pounds, smokes 1fi packs of cigarettes daily, and drinks 2-3 beers per month. He has a past history of occasional back pain following heavy exertion activities. He has no other significant medical history. Two weeks ago he lifted a ladder at work and experienced severe incapacitating low back pain with pain radiating down the right leg from the buttocks along the lateral thigh and calf. He has numbness and tingling in the right great toe. He denies loss of bowel or bladder function. Upon examination, it is noted that Harry has muscle spasm in the paraspinal region, a positive straight leg raise sign on the right side, and difficulty bending forward. Harry is unable to walk on his heels but he is able to walk on his toes. The deep tendon reflexes are intact bilaterally. Muscle strength is intact to all muscle groups. (Questions 4-6)

4. Which risk factor is most likely to contribute to Harry's development of a herniated nucleus pulposus?
   a. Harry is overweight.
   b. Harry smokes 2 packs of cigarettes daily.
   c. Harry is in a high-risk occupation.
   d. Harry drinks 2-3 beers per week.

5. What should Harry do to relieve discomfort?
   a. Begin a rigorous exercise routine immediately.
   b. Maintain complete bed rest for 3-4 weeks.
   c. Use NSAIDs as prescribed by his physician.
   d. Wear a cervical collar while at work.

6. Which disc appears to be causing Harry's symptoms?
   a. L3-L4
   b. L4-L5
   c. L5-S1
   d. C6-C7

Jennifer is a 12-year-old premenarchal female who was noted by her ballet teacher to be unable to stand straight. On examination by the pediatrician, a 30 degree scoliosis was diagnosed. The maternal grandmother had a severe scoliosis. The neurologic examination was normal. (Questions 7-9)

7. Idiopathic scoliosis:
   a. Is lateral curvature of the spine with vertebral rotation.
   b. Is thoracic rounding of the spine.
   c. Is the result of malformation of the vertebra.
   d. Begins in the juvenile age group.

8. The appropriate initial diagnostic study for Jennifer would be:
   a. MRI of the entire spine.
   b. Upright PA and lateral x-rays of the entire spine.
   c. Upright side bending x-rays of the entire spine.
   d. CT of the complete spinal column.

9. The correct treatment for Jennifer is:
   a. Posterior spinal fusion instrumentation.
   b. Traction followed by spinal fusion.
   c. Bracing.
   d. Observation.

Jeff is a 14-year-old with complaints of thoracic back pain. While the pain is more significant following sports activities, he has some pain almost all the time. His mother reminds him to stand up straight and becomes concerned after seeing her son in a photograph with friends. His shoulders appeared to be rounding forward. On examination by his doctor, he was found to have rounding of his back. (Questions 10-11)

10. The appropriate diagnostic tests would be:
    a. Upright PA x-ray of the spine followed by MRI.
    b. Upright PA x-rays and standing lateral of the spine
    c. Standing lateral of the spine and myelogram of the spine
    d. Physical examination and MRI of the complete spine.

11. Bracing for kyphosis:
    a. Corrects the deformity.
    b. Often prevents the deformity from worsening.
    c. Is used in children under age 10.
    d. Is never prescribed.

Chapter 19 *THE HIP, FEMUR, AND PELVIS*

Luann M. Theis, BSN, RN, ONC

Contents

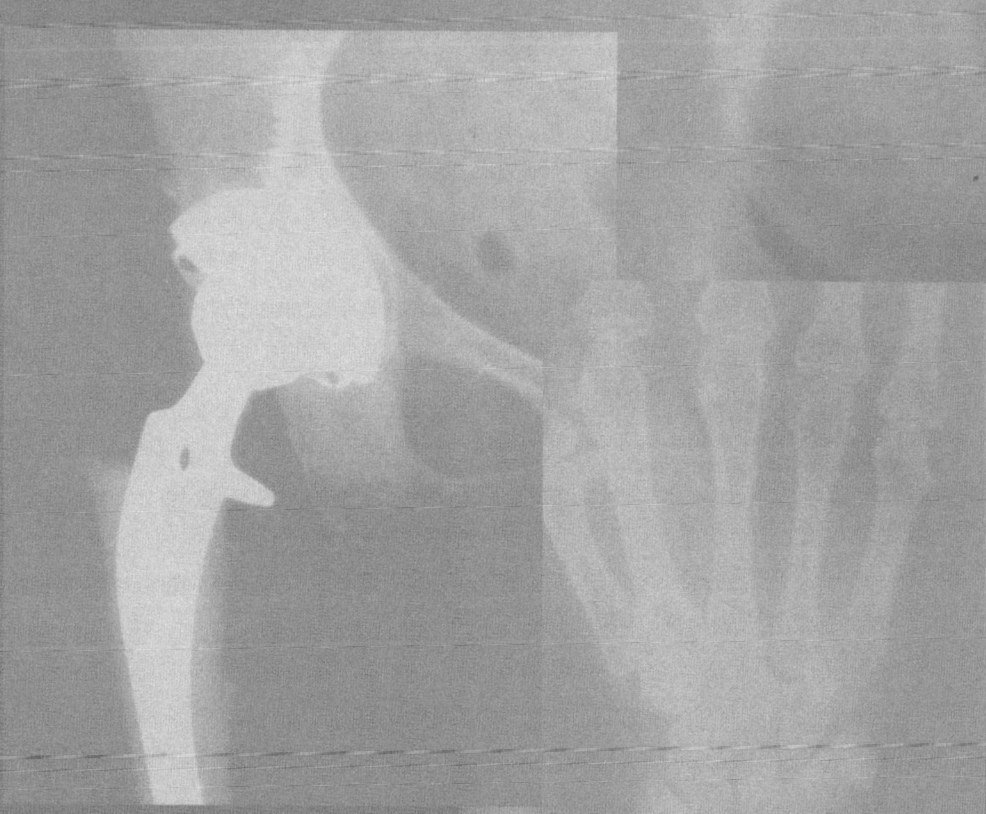

OBJECTIVES

At the completion of this chapter, the learner will be able to:

- Define hip fracture, arthroplasty, dislocation, Girdlestone, osteotomy, and arthrodesis.
- Describe key aspects of assessment and evaluation for the patient with hip diagnoses.
- Discuss surgical management options for the above diagnoses.
- Identify nursing interventions for the management of hip patients.
- Review considerations across the lifespan for patients with hip diagnoses.
- Discuss surgical management options and nursing interventions for femur fractures.
- Discuss key aspects of assessment for the patient with a pelvic fracture and potential treatment options.

KEY POINTS

- More than 300,000 elderly adults will experience a hip fracture each year. This acute event can have major lifestyle changes on the person with only one-half returning to their pre-fracture level of function.
- Surgical repair of hip fractures should occur within 24 hours and the patient should be mobilized as quickly as possible.
- Total hip arthroplasty is one of the most common orthopaedic surgeries. The goal of the procedure is to provide a pain-free functional joint, allowing patients a more normal lifestyle. A wide variety of implants provide a more individual fit with better patient outcomes.
- Following a hip arthroplasty one of the key success factors is using hip precautions which include avoiding: hip flexion beyond 90 degrees, hip adduction, and internal rotation.
- Dislocations are uncommon: the adult hip is a stable joint and a large amount of force is needed for it to dislocate. Following a hip arthroplasty, periarticular muscle tone is weaker due to surgical damage making the patient more prone to dislocation until healing occurs. This fact has significant nursing implications.
- A hip arthrodesis or hip Girdlestone are surgical treatment options that can be used when other methods have failed and provide the patient a partially functional hip with improved lifestyle.
- Femur fractures usually result from major trauma and can have severe complications such as large volume blood loss or fat emboli. Femur fractures can require prolonged rehabilitation and an altered lifestyle for the younger adult who may have a higher incidence related to higher risk activities.

CHAPTER 19

THE HIP, FEMUR, AND PELVIS

HIP FRACTURES

I. OVERVIEW

A. Definition.

1. A break or disruption in the continuity of the proximal portion of the femur.
2. The proximal portion is the portion of the femur that includes the head, femoral neck, greater and lesser trochanters.
3. The proximal femur, together with the acetabulum of the pelvis forms a ball-and-socket joint.

B. Etiology.

1. Most prevalent in the elderly related to a combination of risk factors.
   a. Diminished equilibrium.
   b. Slowed reflexes.
   c. Muscular atrophy.
   d. Diminishing bone tensile strength.
   e. Decreased cognitive functioning and decreased sensorium.
2. Falls are the major cause.
3. Vehicular accidents.
4. Lateral rotation injury can occur when the head of the femur is fixed in the acetabulum, the neck rotates and buckles causing a fracture.
5. Pathologic causes:
   a. Osteoporosis.
   b. Metastatic disease.
   c. Paget's disease.

C. Pathophysiology.

1. The head of the femur is covered by a layer of cartilage and fits into the cup or acetabulum of the pelvis.
2. Vascular supply to femoral head.
   a. Comes from a series of arteries that enter at the junction of the head and neck.
   b. Fractures may tear the blood vessels.
   c. Damage to blood vessels may cause moderate to severe blood loss or avascular necrosis.
3. Hip muscles.
   a. Major hip muscles provide for abduction, adduction, flexion, extension, and rotation.
   b. See Table 19.1.
   c. Tend to displace fracture fragments.
   d. Are responsible for some clinical signs of hip fracture.
4. Weakened bone from pathology related to osteoporosis or metastatic disease may increase risk of fracture.
5. More bone is being resorbed daily than rebuilt in the elderly population (> 55).

D. Incidence.

1. As of 2000, it was expected that hip fractures would rise to 300,000 per year.
2. Average age is close to 80 years.
3. By age 90, one-third of women and one-sixth of men will suffer a hip fracture.
4. Elderly women have higher incidence than men, often due to osteoporosis.
5. About one of every 15 falls in the elderly results in a hip fracture.

E. Considerations across the lifespan.

1. Hip fracture is an acute event that produces a crisis for the elder and family.
2. Only one-half or less of fracture victims return to their pre-fracture level of function.
3. Life style changes post-fracture are a major factor and can affect multiple family members.
4. Need to identify special risk factors of elderly and develop prevention measures.

F. Complications.

1. Delayed union/nonunion.
2. Avascular necrosis.
3. Pulmonary embolism/thrombophlebitis.
4. Post-op infection.
5. Altered lifestyle.

II. ASSESSMENT

A. History.

1. Presenting symptoms.
   a. Leg length shortening.
   b. Pain in affected extremity.
   c. Inability to walk, bend, or move the injured leg when lying supine.
   d. Extremity in position of comfort rather than anatomic alignment.
   e. Leg rotated externally or internally depending on fracture.
2. Circumstances of the fall.
3. Time between injury and arrival at the emergency department.
4. Pre-injury mental status.
5. Pre-injury functional status.
6. Home environment.
7. Support system.
8. Chronic health problems.

B. Physical examination.

1. Examination should be done with minimal joint movement since there is usually severe pain in the hip and leg.
2. Physical findings.
   a. Shortening of the affected leg, usually visibly detectable, compared to uninjured leg.
   b. External rotation of injured leg most common.
   c. Swelling around site of injury.
   d. Discoloration of surrounding tissues, which may extend into groin or down affected thigh.
   e. Complaint of pressure over greater trochanter.

Table 19.1
Major Hip Muscles

Muscle	Insertion	Action
Gluteus minimus	Greater trochanter	Hip abduction and extension
Gluteus medius	Greater trochanter	Hip abduction and rotation
Gluteus maximus	Gluteal tuberosity of the femur	Hip extension and rotation
Iliopsoas	Lesser trochanter	Hip flexion
Adductor magnus, longus and brevis	Linea aspera of femur	Hip adduction
Gracilis	Medial surface of tibia	Hip adduction
Pectineus	Line between lesser trochanter and linea aspera of femur	Hip adduction and flexion

Reprinted with permission from the National Association of Orthopaedic Nurses (NAON). (1999). *An introduction to orthopaedic nursing* (2nd ed., p. 115). Pitman, NJ: NAON.

3. Neurovascular assessment of the affected leg compared to the unaffected leg for a baseline (see Chapter 3, Musculoskeletal Assessment).
4. Assess bony prominences on hip and leg for skin breakdown or bruising.

C. Diagnostic tests.

1. Laboratory tests.
   a. CBC.
   b. Metabolic panel.
   c. Protime/INR.
   d. Type and crossmatch.
2. Radiographs.
   a. Hip: AP and lateral.
   b. Chest: for surgery if indicated.
   c. Bone scan may be ordered if pathologic fracture is being ruled out.
   d. MRI: if avascular necrosis or metabolic disease is suspected.
3. ECG.

D. Types of hip fractures.

1. Intracapsular fractures are located within the joint capsule.
   a. Femoral neck fractures classified here also.
   b. Displaced.
   c. Nondisplaced.
2. Extracapsular fractures located outside the joint capsule.
   a. Intertrochanteric – between trochanters.
   b. Subtrochanteric – below lesser trochanter.
   c. Also classified as stable or unstable.
3. Neck fractures more common in women and frail elderly.
4. Extracapsular more common in males and more active elderly, usually related to greater trauma/force and increased physical activity.
5. Acetabular fracture which is part of true pelvis.

III. COMMON THERAPEUTIC MODALITIES

A. Conservative.

1. Nondisplaced, stable, or impacted fracture may not need surgical repair.
2. May be chosen if patient has dementia, resides in extended care and wasn't ambulatory pre-fracture.
3. May be chosen if patient has poor prognosis to return to functional level of mobility.

B. Preoperative.

1. Buck's traction to decrease muscle spasm and immobilize the leg.
2. IV fluids as ordered.
3. NPO per anesthesia protocol.
4. Pain management with a goal of optimum pain relief without oversedation.
5. Skin care.
6. Repositioning.
   a. Between back and side lying on unaffected extremity.
   b. Physician order to turn on affected hip.
   c. Keep legs abducted with pillow.
7. Relieve patient anxiety, answer questions.
8. Complete surgical permit and preparation.

C. Surgery.

1. Scheduled within 24 hours of the time the patient arrives in emergency.
2. Goal is to repair fracture and return patient to pre-fracture functional level.
3. Operative choice based on type of fracture.
   a. Intracapsular/femoral neck.
      (1) Threaded pins.
      (2) Compression hip screw.
      (3) Femoral head replacement with prosthesis or hemiarthroplasty.
      (4) Primary total hip replacement.
   b. Intertrochanteric repaired with open reduction and internal fixation.
      (1) Nail.

(2) Pin.
(3) Compression hip screw.

c. Subtrochanteric.
(1) Open reduction and internal fixation with intramedullary nail, sliding nail plate or fixed plate.
(2) Closed reduction with nail insertion.

4. Type of fracture, bone integrity, and stability of repair will dictate weight-bearing status postoperatively.
   a. Internal fixation may limit weight bearing up to 6 months.
   b. Hemiarthroplasty or primary total hip will allow more rapid progress with weight bearing.

IV. NURSING DIAGNOSES, OUTCOMES, AND INTERVENTIONS

A. See Table 19.2.

B. See Chapter 5, Perioperative Patient Care.

C. Health maintenance, altered.

1. Outcomes.
   a. Return to pre-fracture living arrangements with support from family and friends.
   b. Patient involved in planning for and accepting of discharge disposition.
2. Interventions.
   a. Assess home arrangements and support systems.
   b. Coordinate discharge planning consult pre-op or immediately post-op.
   c. Assist patient/family in reviewing options of home care, residential facility, community-based rehabilitation facility (CBRF), and/or subacute facility.
   d. Communicate plans with physician.
   e. Support patient/family in decision-making and coping with potential lifestyle changes.

V. PRACTICE SETTING CONSIDERATIONS

A. Office/outpatient.

1. Coordinate hospital admission and preoperative diagnostics if patient is seen preoperatively in this setting.
2. Coordinate follow-up post-surgical care.
3. Explain surgery and recovery to patient.

B. Hospital.

1. Provide emergency, preoperative and postoperative care.
2. Assist in coordinating discharge plans.
3. Teach patient and significant other per Table 19.2.

C. Home care considerations.

1. Assess home situation for safety and functional ability of patient.
2. Reinforce mobility and exercise plans.
3. Monitor lab values or medications as indicated.
4. Teach patient/significant others home activities of daily living (ADL) management.
5. Monitor/assist with and teach incision care

HIP ARTHROPLASTY

I. OVERVIEW

A. Definition.

1. As a broad term, "arthroplasty" refers to resection, reconstruction, or replacement of a joint.
2. Hip arthroplasty refers to surgical reconstruction of an arthritic or damaged hip with artificial (metal, ceramic, polyethylene) femoral and acetabular components.
   a. Total hip arthroplasty replaces the femoral and acetabular structures.
   b. Hemiarthroplasty replaces the femoral structure.
   c. Revision arthroplasty refers to replacing a joint that was previously replaced and went on to failure.

B. Etiology.

1. Most common reason for hip arthroplasty is osteoarthritis (see Chapter 12, Arthritis and Connective Tissue Disorders).
2. Performed after more conservative measures have failed to improve joint motion and/or decrease pain. These can include pharmacologic treatment, therapeutic modalities, an exercise program, dietary weight management, and nontraditional techniques/alternative therapies.
3. General indications for arthroplasty.
   a. Debilitating joint pain.
   b. Loss of hip motion.
   c. Degenerative joint disease (primary/secondary osteoarthritis).
   d. Inflammatory arthritis.
   e. Avascular necrosis.
   f. Neoplastic disease or pathologic fractures of the femoral neck.
   g. Sepsis.
   h. Trauma.
   i. Failure of previous internal fixations or arthroplasties.
   j. Pseudarthrosis.
   k. Joint instability/immobility.
   l. Congenital deformities/dislocations.
4. Contraindications.
   a. Acute/chronic infection (exception is resectional or revision arthroplasty due to sepsis).
   b. Patient history of noncompliance such as severe mental disorders/senility or learning limitations where maintenance of activity restrictions would be difficult.
   c. Age (less then 50 if deemed appropriate).
   d. Pain not incapacitating.
   e. Gainfully employed in manual/heavy labor.
   f. Neuropathic joint.
   g. Participation in active sports.
   h. Poor vascularity in affected extremity; clotting disorders.
   i. Severe uncontrolled systemic disease.
   j. Bone marrow disease such as multiple myeloma or Gaucher's disease.

Table 19.2
Common Nursing Diagnoses, Outcomes and Interventions for Hip Disorders

Diagnoses	Outcomes	Interventions
A. Pain, acute	• Patient's pain is controlled as evidenced by ability to rest and participate in activities. • Patient progresses from IV/IM/ epidural medication to use of oral medication at time of discharge.	• Position hip/leg in proper alignment and according to surgical procedure. • Apply ice to incision. • Encourage the use of relaxation techniques. • Administer epidural/IV/PCA/ IM medications as ordered and needed. • Assess level of pain control and document same. • Transition to use of oral medication as patient tolerates. • Communicate level of comfort to physician and care providers. • Administer pain medication prior to activity.
B Physical mobility, impaired	• Patient will be able to perform bed-to-chair transfer with minimal assistance. • Patient will be able to ambulate a functional distance with assistive device based on needs of discharge setting (home, rehab, subacute). • Patient will be able to perform exercises with assistance at time of discharge; patient/significant other will verbalize exercise program.	• Assess preoperative level of mobility. • Encourage bed mobility; provide overhead frame/trapeze to facilitate. • Instruct in correct positioning of affected extremity; most hip patients should keep leg abducted. • Reinforce exercise program as instructed by physical therapy. • Instruct in use of assistive device such as walker/crutches/cane. • Assist in obtaining walker/crutches for discharge. • Progress mobility from bed-chair transfers to ambulating increased distances.
C. Peripheral neurovascular dysfunction, risk for	• Patient will exhibit normal neurovascular function of affected extremity. • Patient will verbalize signs of compromised neurovascular function and correct reporting.	• Assess affected extremity for circulation, motion, sensation, and temperature per postoperative protocol. • Report alterations in neurovascular status to physician. • Teach patient signs of altered neurovascular status and how to report.
D. Skin integrity, impaired	• Skin remains intact without pressure areas or open breakdown. • Incision healing with edges well approximated.	• Assess skin per protocol. • Reposition every 2-4 hours, alternate (between back and side-lying on unaffected) hip; physician order usually needed to lay on affected hip. • Use pressure relief measures for bony prominences. • Monitor incision for tape blisters or signs of skin infection.

Table 19.2 (continued)
Common Nursing Diagnoses, Outcomes and Interventions for Hip Disorders

Diagnoses	Outcomes	Interventions
E. Tissue perfusion, ineffective	• Patient will maintain adequate tissue perfusion to lower extremities. • Patient will be free from deep vein thrombosis.	• Teach patient exercises including ankle pumps (flexion and extension), foot circles, and quadriceps sets. • Encourage bed mobility. • Assist with ROM exercises to lower extremities. • Maintain correct use of physical devices such as elastic compression stockings and sequential compression devices. • Administer anticoagulants as ordered such as warfarin, heparin, low-molecular weight heparin. • Monitor lab values obtained for anticoagulation such as INR or protime.
F. Fluid volume, deficient; fluid volume, excess	• Patient's intake and output adequate and balanced. • Patient's vital signs remain stable. • Patient's hemoglobin/ hematocrit within range of normal for surgical procedure. • Patient exhibits no signs/symptoms of hypovolemia. • Patient exhibits no signs of excess bleeding from incision or drainage tubes.	• Assess for localized pain, tenderness, redness, and/or swelling in the lower extremity, assess for Homan's sign if above noted. • Assess vital signs per postoperative protocol. • Monitor intake/output each shift and evaluate 24-hour totals. • Monitor hemoglobin/hematocrit for signs of hypovolemia. • Monitor incision dressing and drainage devices for excess bleeding/drainage and report to physician. • Maintain IV fluids as ordered. • Monitor/administer blood products from autotransfusion devices. • Administer blood products as ordered – autologous or banked.
G. Self-care deficit syndrome	• Patient increases ADL/self care as tolerated. • Patient manages ADL/self care within limitations of surgical procedure.	• Assist with ADL as needed; progress with types/amount as tolerated. • Obtain occupational therapy referral as appropriate. • Teach/reinforce restrictions of activity/ADL related to surgical procedure. • Assist in obtaining home care items such as shower bench, elevated toilet seat/ commode, long-handled accessories such as shoe spoon and shower sponge, long-handled reacher. • Review home setting for safety.

Table 19.2 (continued)
Common Nursing Diagnoses, Outcomes and Interventions for Hip Disorders

Diagnoses	Outcomes	Interventions
H. Knowledge, deficient	• Patient verbalizes/demonstrates postoperative care and follow-up; significant other can do same if necessary.	• Teach patient/significant other: 1. Home medications. 2. Incision/dressing care. 3. Activity instructions/limitations. 4. Use of anticoagulants and lab studies. 5. Signs/symptoms of infection. 6. Follow-up care/appointments. • Return demonstration by patient/ significant other as needed.
I. Constipation	• Patient will maintain normal bowel elimination pattern.	• Assess elimination pattern prior to hospitalization. • Maintain intake. • Encourage a diet high in fluids, bulk. • Administer laxatives as ordered/ needed. • Assess GI status per protocol to monitor for postoperative ileus.
J. Urinary elimination, impaired	• Patient will maintain normal urinary elimination pattern.	• Assess for elimination pattern prior to hospitalization. • Provide fluids. • Maintain output of at least 30 cc per hour. • Observe for signs of incontinence or bladder distention. • Obtain order for/perform catheterization as necessary.
K. Respiratory function, risk for ineffective	• Patient maintains adequate ventilation with clear breath sounds.	• Assess respiratory status per protocol. • Instruct/assist with coughing and deep breathing. • Instruct/assist with use of incentive spirometer as ordered. • Encourage mobility and ambulation as tolerated and ordered. • Monitor narcotic use for alteration of respiration. • Request respiratory therapy referral as needed.

C. Pathophysiology.

1. Most common cause of joint damage is primary or secondary osteoarthritis (see Chapter 12, Arthritis and Connective Tissue Disorders).
2. Damage to the articulating surfaces of the hip causes decreasing range of motion and increasing pain.
3. Arthroplasty provides reconstructed articulating surfaces which decrease/eliminate pain and improve joint range of motion.

D. Incidence.

1. Prevalence of total joint arthroplasty has increased annually since the 1980s.
2. One of the most common orthopaedic surgeries.
3. Generally seen in the 60-plus age group; majority of patients in the 70-80 year age range.

E. Considerations across the lifespan.

1. Generally seen in the elderly population.
2. If arthroplasty is done in a younger adult (< 55) the need for a revision related to use and long-term wear is likely.
3. If arthroplasty is done in a younger adult, consideration must be given to alter sports activities and employment/occupation if heavy labor is involved.
4. Type of implant used (cemented or noncemented) is a greater consideration in a younger patient.

5. Patients with a history of Developmental Dysplasia of the Hip (DDH), Legg-Calvé-Perthes Disease or Slipped Capital Femoral Epiphysis may require a total hip arthroplasty at a younger age (see Chapter 11, Pediatric/Congenital Disorders). Often a non-cemented prosthesis is used.

F. Complications.

1. Dislocation.
2. Wound infection.
3. Hematoma.
4. Neurovascular compromise of the extremity.
5. Thromboembolism.
6. Loosening of components.
7. Periprosthetic fracture.
8. Instability and subluxation of components.
9. Prosthetic joint wear (adhesive/abrasive/corrosive wear of the surfaces).
10. Calcar resorption.
11. Ectopic ossification.
12. Peroneal nerve palsy/footdrop.

II. ASSESSMENT

A. History.

1. Presenting symptoms.
   a. Groin or anterior thigh pain radiating toward knee.
   b. Pain is generally insidious, increasing over a period of months and associated with a variety of activities.
   c. Decreased range of motion of the joint.
   d. Gait change to accommodate loss of joint motion and pain.
2. Review pain related to location, intensity, and precipitating activities.
   a. Pain may present along major nerve paths of the hip area.
   b. Pain may be severe enough to awaken the patient from sleep.
3. Assess the affect of the hip arthritis on ADL.
4. Obtain information on predisposing factors such as steroid use, significant trauma, or congenital/developmental factors.
5. Obtain general health history.

B. Physical examination.

1. See hip assessment in Chapter 3, Musculoskeletal Assessment.
2. Progressive degeneration of the hip commonly results in a Trendelenburg gait.
3. Gradual loss of motion of the hip occurs with the position of comfort being flexed at 20-30 degrees. Over time a flexion contracture can occur.
4. Passive range of motion of the joint can exacerbate the symptoms.
5. Shortening of the affected extremity can occur due to erosion of the joint and muscle contractures.
6. Muscle atrophy due to disuse and decreased range of motion.

C. Diagnostic tests.

1. Laboratory tests.
   a. CBC.
   b. Metabolic panel.
   c. Protime/INR.
   d. Type and crossmatch.
   e. Urinalysis and culture and sensitivity, if indicated.
2. Radiographs.
   a. Hip: AP and lateral to evaluate joint space, articular surfaces, osteophyte and cyst formation, and subchondral collapse.
   b. Chest if indicated per anesthesia protocol.
   c. MRI to stage avascular necrosis.
3. ECG.

III. COMMON THERAPEUTIC MODALITIES

A. Preoperative.

1. Review discharge/rehabilitation options post-surgery.
2. Preoperative physical.
3. Appointment with pre-admission center or attendance at total joint class.
4. Physical therapy evaluation and teaching.
5. Occupational therapy evaluation and teaching.
6. Autologous blood draws.
7. Epoetin injections if chosen.

B. Types of implants.

1. Femoral component and acetabular component comprise a total hip implant.
2. Metal with polyethylene liner refers to a metal femoral component articulating with a polyethylene acetabular component; most common type.
3. Ceramic refers to a ceramic femoral head on a titanium stem articulating with a ceramic acetabular component.
4. Metal-on-metal refers to both articulating surfaces being metal; new type of component.
5. Porous coated refers to the surface of the components which allows for bony ingrowth of the prosthesis where it articulates against the bone.
6. Cemented versus noncemented refers to the use of polymethylmethacralate bone cement usually in the femoral shaft with the femoral component.
7. Hybrid refers to a cemented femoral component and porous coated acetabular component for bony ingrowth.
8. Modular components refers to each part of the prosthesis being separate (stem, head, cup, liner) so best fit can be achieved.
9. Custom fit prosthesis.
   a. Created in the OR during surgery which eliminates the need to fit a pre-made femoral component to the femoral cavity.
   b. Mold of the femoral cavity is measured with laser, with the data being fed into a computer to design the implant.
   c. Prosthesis is milled in about 40 minutes and can be cemented or uncemented.
10. Long-stem prosthesis refers to a longer femoral stem used to surpass a periprosthetic fracture, perform a revision arthroplasty, or support a stress riser for fracture.
11. Constrained acetabular component refers to incor-

porating a ring to capture the femoral head eliminating the possibility of dislocation.

C. Surgery.

1. Goal is to provide a functional, pain-free joint.
2. Surgical approach.
   a. Anterolateral results in more muscle damage but is less prone to dislocation. Postoperatively, this patient must avoid:
      (1) External rotation.
      (2) Adduction.
      (3) Hip hyperextension.
   b. Posterolateral approach results in less muscle damage but may be more prone to dislocation. Post-op, this patient must avoid:
      (1) Internal rotation.
      (2) Adduction.
      (3) Hip hyperflexion.
   c. Two other less common approaches are the direct lateral and the transtrochanteric.
3. Bone grafting.
   a. Bone grafting may be necessary when there is inadequate bone stock to support implanted components.
      (1) Allograft.
      (2) Autograft.
      (3) Banked bone may also be used.
   b. Most often this is necessary for patients with:
      (1) Rheumatoid arthritis.
      (2) Congenital dislocated/subluxed hip.
      (3) Nonunion of acetabular fracture.
      (4) Previous unsuccessful surgery requiring a revision arthroplasty.
      (5) Previous infection.
4. Some surgeons prefer to perform an intertrochanteric osteotomy prior to total hip or hemiarthroplasty.
   a. Major advantage is to provide better visualization.
   b. By reattaching the trochanter distally and slightly outward, normal abductor muscle tension is restored, and loads acting on the hip joint are reduced.
   c. Indications include:
      (1) Congenital dislocated hip.
      (2) Previous hip fusion or ankylosing joint.
      (3) Severe joint disintegration.
      (4) Revision arthroplasty.
   d. Potential problems/complications include:
      (1) Increased OR time.
      (2) Increased blood loss.
      (3) Requires fixation for the trochanter, usually wire.
      (4) If trochanter nonunion occurs, patient will be unable to fully bear weight and will have a limp.
      (5) Patient more likely to dislocate prosthesis if trochanter doesn't heal.
      (6) Bursitis may develop over wires.
      (7) Wire breakage, requiring removal.
      (8) Delayed weight bearing and joint range of motion.
      (9) Trochanteric failure.
5. Non-cemented prosthesis.
   a. Avoids problems with loosening due to cement fractures or poor cement bone interface.
   b. Requires more protected weight bearing initially than with a cemented prosthesis.
6. Cell savers are often used in these cases during OR.
7. The extremity is evaluated for length, motion, and stability, and is put through a full range of joint motion.
8. Radiographs are done to verify prosthesis placement and alignment.
9. Surgical technique may be different and surgical time is longer with a revision arthroplasty.
   a. Blood loss is greater.
   b. The method depends on whether it was mechanical failure, amount/type of bone stock, type of original prosthesis, signs of infection and patient age.
   c. Outcomes may not be as good as with primary arthroplasty.
10. Heterotrophic ossification may occur after surgery in a patient with a prior history of the same or a history of ankylosing spondylitis (see Chapter 12, Arthritis and Connective Tissue Disorders).
    a. May require treatment with radiation or indomethacin.
    b. May cause decreased hip range of motion and stiffness postoperatively.

IV. NURSING DIAGNOSES, OUTCOMES, AND INTERVENTIONS

A. See Table 19.2.

B. See Chapter 5, Perioperative Patient Care.

C. Physical mobility, impaired.

1. Outcomes.
   a. Patient able to ambulate a functional distance with use of assistive device (walker, crutches, cane) independently.
   b. Patient's joint function is maintained using postoperative precautions.
2. Interventions.
   a. See Table 19.3.
   b. Instruct patient on correct weight-bearing status.
      (l) Cemented or hybrid components allowed full weight bearing with assistive device unless bone grafting was used that requires protected weight bearing.
      (2) Cementless components allowed partial weight bearing per surgeon instruction with assistive device.
   c. Teach/reinforce isometric exercises.
      (1) Quadriceps setting.
      (2) Gluteal setting.
      (3) Dorsiflexion/plantarflexion (ankle pumps).
      (4) Ankle circumduction exercises.
      (5) Therapy will instruct in additional exercises.
   d. Reinforce hip precautions.

D Infection, risk for.

1. Outcome.

Table 19.3
Postarthroplasty Positioning and Mobility Consideration

Diagnoses	Outcomes	Interventions
A. Total hip replacement (THR)	• Replacement of both the femoral head and resurfacing of the acetabulum. 1. Can be cemented or cementless. 2. Patient prone to dislocation may be placed in a spica cast or abductor brace.	• Prevent dislocation through proper positioning. 1. Abduct operative hip at all times using abductive devices. a. Abduction pillows. b. Regular pillows. c. Skin traction. d. Abduction slings.
B. Hip hemiarthroplasty	• Replacement of femoral component.	e. Splints. 2. Maintain hip in abduction, neutral rotation, or slight external rotation. 3. Avoid hip flexion over 60-90 degrees per surgeon. 4. Avoid adduction. 5. Avoid internal rotation. 6. General policy is to turn to operative side only. a. Maintain abduction with pillows. b. Physician may order turning to nonoperative side. 7. Move extremity gently when transferring or turning in bed. • Assess for symptoms of dislocation. 1. Acute groin pain in operative hip. 2. Shortened extremity in external rotation. 3. Patient may hear or feel a "popping" sensation. • Positioning considerations. 1. Maintain good body alignment in abduction devices. 2. Turn with pillows or supports to maintain abduction. 3. Have patient lie flat several times per day to prevent hip flexion contractures. 4. Head of bed generally not raised more than 45-60 degrees based on surgeon preference. • Activity/exercise regimen. 1. Out of bed to chair. a. Orthopaedic chair (high chair) and elevated toilet seat to prevent excessive flexion. b. Do not elevate the affected extremity when sitting in chair; may flex the knee.

Table 19.3
Postarthroplasty Positioning and Mobility Consideration

Diagnoses	Outcomes	Interventions
B. Hip hemiarthroplasty (continued)	• Replacement of femoral component. (continued)	c. Out of bed to chair beginning any time from night of surgery to first postoperative day. 2. Ambulate partial weight bearing with gait device to full weight bearing per surgeon's protocol. 3. Reinforce exercise regimens. 4. Instruct/reinforce "total hip don'ts." a. Don't flex hip more than 60-90 degrees as per surgeon. b. Don't cross legs. c. Don't sit in a low chair.

Adapted from: Flynn, R., & Carolini, P. (1996). Arthritis disorders. In S.W. Salmond, N.W. Mooney, & L.A. Verdisco (Eds.), *NAON Core Curriculum for Orthopaedic Nursing* (3rd ed., p. 254). Pitman, NJ: NAON.

a. Patient remains free of incisional or joint infection.
b. Patient verbalizes lifelong joint care for infection control.

2. Interventions.
    a. Maintain strict sterile technique in OR.
    b. Reduce circulating particles in the air during OR using a low traffic policy and/or laminar flow.
    c. Administer IV antibiotics as ordered pre and postoperatively.
    d. Assess for signs and symptoms of infection.
    e. Remove indwelling catheters as soon as possible.
    f. Perform sterile dressing changes.
    g. Instruct patient in appropriate wound care.
    h. Instruct patient in lifelong care.
        (1) Inform physicians and dentists of arthroplasty.
        (2) Notify physician if infection is suspected.
        (3) Obtain antibiotics for dental work or minor surgical procedures as directed by surgeon.

V. PRACTICE SETTING CONSIDERATIONS

A. Office/outpatient.

1. Assist patient/significant other to evaluate discharge needs and home arrangements; offer options, and make referrals as needed.
2. Review/discuss advance directives.
3. Assist in obtaining necessary equipment.
4. Coordinate preoperative appointments for history and physical examination, lab work, x-rays, blood donations, and therapy evaluations.
5. Provide preoperative teaching materials; coordinate appointment with preadmission center or joint class.
6. Identify/treat existing infections prior to surgery.
7. Assist with postoperative follow-up care; monitor lab tests as ordered, especially with anticoagulants.

B. Hospital.

1. Provide postoperative care per protocol.
2. Teach hip precautions per Tables 19.2 and 19.3.
3. Assist in coordinating discharge plans.

C. Home care considerations.

1. Assess home situation for safety and functional ability of patient.
2. Reinforce mobility and exercise plans; progress same.
3. Monitor lab values or medications as indicated.
4. Teach patient/significant other home ADL management.
5. Monitor/assist with and teach incision care.

HIP DISLOCATIONS

I. OVERVIEW

A. Definition.

1. Displacement of the femur from the acetabulum so articulating surfaces lose contact.
2. Hip subluxation is a lesser form where articulating surfaces lose partial contact.

B. Etiology.

1. Traumatic injury.
    a. Posterior dislocation most common. Force along the shaft of the femur when the hip is flexed and adducted such as a fall or dashboard injury in a motor vehicle accident (MVA).

b. Anterior dislocations are rare and occur when the hip is extended, abducted, and externally rotated.
c. Central dislocations can occur with a severe blow to the lateral aspect of the hip, especially if the hip is abducted.
2. Post arthroplasty.
a. Occurs when hip is placed in position of extreme flexion, adduction or internal rotation.
b. Patient may complain of feeling a "pop," or hearing a cracking sound.
c. Patient is unable to bear weight on the leg, and it is shortened and externally rotated.
d. Need to notify the surgeon immediately.

C. Pathophysiology.
1. The adult hip is normally a stable joint.
2. In trauma cases:
a. Posterior or anterior dislocations may occur with/without fractures.
b. Central dislocations are associated with an acetabular fracture, but the femur may/may not be fractured.
3. Following hip arthroplasty positions of extreme flexion, adduction, or internal rotation are the least stable related to surgical muscle damage and need to rebuild periarticular muscle tone.

D. Incidence.
1. Not a common occurrence from trauma since severe trauma/force is generally required.
2. Post-arthroplasty dislocations occur in approximately 2% of patients and are more likely in the first 8 weeks postoperatively.

E. Considerations across the lifespan.
1. Can occur throughout the lifespan.
2. Post-arthroplasty would likely be in an elderly person who may have the repeated effects of hospitalization and surgery and potential complications.

F. Complications.
1. Nerve injuries.
2. Loss of hip motion.

II. ASSESSMENT

A. History.
1. Presenting symptoms.
a. Pain, usually severe and increases with movement.
b. Restricted movement.
2. Onset of symptoms; traumatic versus post-arthroplasty.
3. If post-arthroplasty, obtain surgical history.

B. Physical examination.
1. Inspect the extremity for shortening or leg rotation.
2. Assess joint range of motion.
3. Assess neurovascular status of extremity.

C. Diagnostic tests.
1. Hip AP and lateral to determine joint condition and any fractures.
2. Pelvis x-ray or CT may be needed to clearly view some central dislocations associated with an acetabular fracture.
3. Laboratory tests as required if a surgical candidate.

III. COMMON THERAPEUTIC MODALITIES

A. Reduction should be done as rapidly as possible to minimize potential nerve damage and alleviate pain.

B. Treatment goals.
1. Reduce the hip to normal anatomical alignment.
2. Full hip function without neurovascular compromise.

C. Conservative treatment.
1. Closed reduction with analgesia and muscle relaxant.
2. Reduction is followed by:
a. Brace to hold hip in desired alignment based on type of dislocation.
b. Hip spica cast.
c. Buck skin traction.

D. Surgical treatment.
1. Open reduction under anesthesia if closed reduction fails.
2. Open reduction with revision of hip arthroplasty.
3. Open reduction is followed by:
a. Brace to hold hip in desired alignment.
b. Hip spica cast.
c. Buck skin traction
d. Skeletal traction.
e. Internal fixation if fractures were present.

IV. NURSING DIAGNOSES, OUTCOMES, AND INTERVENTIONS

A. See Chapter 5, Perioperative Patient Care.

B. See Table 19.2.

C. See Table 19.3.

V. PRACTICE SETTING CONSIDERATIONS

A. Office/outpatient.
1. Assist with physical exam and history of event if patient presents to this setting on injury.
2. Promote comfort.
3. Coordinate hospital admission.

B. Hospital.
1. Provide emergency, post-procedure, and postoperative care.
2. Teach hip precautions per Tables 19.2 and 19.3.
3. Assist in coordinating discharge plans.

C. Home care considerations.
1. Assess home situation for safety and functional ability of patient.
2. Teach patient/significant other home ADL management.
3. Reinforce mobility and activity restrictions.
4. Monitor/assist with and teach incision care.

HIP GIRDLESTONE PSEUDARTHROSIS (Resectional Arthroplasty)

I. OVERVIEW

A. Definition.
1. Surgical procedure in which improved joint mobility is obtained by:

a. Totally or partially excising a joint.
b. Lengthening soft tissues.
c. Developing new articulating surfaces.
2. Creation of a new false joint.

B. Etiology.
1. Prior to hip implants, was used occasionally to manage the pain of severe arthritis.
2. More frequent use of this procedure was for joint infections; pyogenic or tuberculosis.
3. Current orthopaedic techniques use this procedure for salvage of failed total hip arthroplasty or severe infection of a hip arthroplasty.

C. Pathophysiology.
1. Failed total hip arthroplasty can result from the inability to retain a prosthetic implant due to:
   a. Poor bone stock to hold a prosthesis.
   b. Fracture below a prosthesis and a resulting nonfunctional repair.
   c. Multiple hip arthroplasty revisions which remain unsuccessful with poor function and severe pain.
2. Unresolved infected total hip arthroplasty may require a Girdlestone procedure after all antibiotic possibilities are tried without success.
3. In removing the joint a fibrous pseudarthrosis is formed between the ilium and femur.
4. Results include:
   a. Pain greatly decreased.
   b. Compromised hip stability.
   c. Significant shortening of the leg.

D. Incidence.
1. Done very infrequently; only as a final option.
2. Present antibiotic combinations rarely necessitate this procedure for an infected arthroplasty.

E. Considerations across the lifespan.
1. Will greatly affect ambulation ability which may require change of occupation.
2. In the elderly, this may necessitate being wheelchair-bound or bedridden depending on ambulation/transfer ability or learning ability if confused.

F. Complications.
1. Surgical complications.
2. Complications of immobility.

II. ASSESSMENT

A. History.
1. Presenting symptoms.
   a. Severe pain.
   b. Nonfunctional hip joint.
2. Surgical history of hip arthroplasties and results.
3. Unresolved hip infection and review of treatment.

B. Physical examination.
1. Reproducible pain.
2. Inadequate hip joint range of motion.
3. Findings specific to a mechanical cause such as instability, alignment, or dislocation.

C. Diagnostic tests.
1. Radiographs.
   a. AP and lateral hip.
   b. CT/MRI for more detailed definition of the joint space and femoral shaft.
2. Laboratory and preoperative diagnostics as required for surgery.

III. COMMON THERAPEUTIC MODALITIES

A. Preoperative discussion should include review of the procedure and affect on lifestyle.

B. Surgical technique.
1. Femoral head and neck are resected which results in shortening of the femur by 2 inches or more.
2. Pseudarthrosis forms between the wing of the ilium and the proximal femur.
3. Muscle spasm is common following the procedure.
4. Skeletal traction is used postoperatively to reduce muscle spasm and provide alignment for the fibrous pseudarthrosis to form.
5. Weight bearing is restricted for about 6 months for healing.
6. May remove a prosthesis and place a spacer with antibiotic beads for a period of 4-6 weeks as treatment of infection prior to a Girdlestone procedure.
7. Many patients will require long-term use of cane or crutches.

IV. NURSING DIAGNOSES, OUTCOMES, AND INTERVENTIONS

A. See Table 19.2.

B. Physical mobility, impaired.
1. Outcome: patient will obtain highest level of function possible relative to procedure.
2. Interventions.
   a. Instruct/reinforce the ongoing permanent use of assistive device for ambulating.
   b. Assist with/refer to occupational therapy/physical therapy to obtain necessary ADL devices and home equipment.

V. PRACTICE SETTING CONSIDERATIONS

A. Office/outpatient.
1. Coordinate preoperative testing and hospital admission.
2. Assist with postoperative follow-up care and monitoring.

B. Hospital.
1. Provide postoperative care per protocol.
2. Assist in coordinating discharge plans.
3. Teach hip precautions per Tables 19.2 and 19.3.

C. Home care considerations.
1. Assess home situation for safety and functional ability of patient.
2. Reinforce mobility instruction; progress same.
3. Monitor/assist with and teach incision care.
4. Teach patient and significant other home ADL management.

HIP ARTHRODESIS

I. OVERVIEW

A. Definition.

1. Surgical fusion of a joint to relieve pain by eliminating motion.
2. Fusion of the femoral head to the acetabulum eliminating motion across the hip joint.

B. Etiology.

1. Painful, unstable joint is the broad indication.
2. Mechanical dysfunction includes:
   a. Deformities (varus/valgus).
   b. Degenerative joint disease.
   c. Rheumatoid arthritis.
   d. Malpositioned fractures.
   e. Pain.
   f. Instability or limitation in joint motion.
   g. Trauma.
   h. Neuropathic joint.
   i. Previous, unsuccessful surgery.

C. Pathophysiology.

1. Femoral head and acetabulum are fused which totally eliminates motion in the joint and relieves the pain.
2. Fused in a position of slight flexion and neutral abduction/adduction.
3. Loss of hip motion is compensated by increased motion at the lumbar spine and knee joint.
4. Increased stresses on the lumbar spine and knee of the affected extremity may result in:
   a. Osteoarthritis of the knee after many years of wear.
   b. Increasing low back pain and intermittent claudication.
   c. Contralateral hip and knee degeneration.
   d. Consideration of converting the fusion to an arthroplasty which will relieve these stresses.
5. No activity limitations once successful fusion is obtained.

D. Incidence.

1. Disadvantages of the procedure make it an infrequent choice.
2. May be the choice of younger patients (< 55) with severe osteoarthritis of the hip over arthroplasty which may limit lifestyle.

E. Considerations across the lifespan.

1. Arthrodesis allows for a more normal lifestyle for the younger adult who leads a more active life and may do heavy labor; arthroplasty would require alterations.
2. Need to monitor for effects on the lumbar spine and knee. Utilize preventive measures to minimize joint wear.
3. Elderly patient may have more difficulty adapting to the altered gait pattern.

F. Complications.

1. Wound infection/dehiscence hematoma.
2. Thromboembolism.
3. Neurovascular compromise.
4. Nonunion.
5. Malunion.
6. Pseudoarthrosis.

II. ASSESSMENT

A. History.

1. Presenting symptoms.
   a. Pain.
   b. Difficulty ambulating or awkward gait.
   c. Frustration with lack of success of prior treatment.
2. Review of prior treatment (conservative and surgical) and the results.

B. Physical examination.

1. Reproducible joint pain.
2. Instability with weight bearing, range of motion, and functional activity.
3. Severe joint trauma necessitating the procedure.

C. Diagnostic tests.

1. Radiographs.
   a. AP and lateral hip.
   b. Comparison to prior films to identify continued instability and/or malalignment.
2. Laboratory and preoperative diagnostics as required for surgery.

III. COMMON THERAPEUTIC MODALITIES

A. Desired outcome is total pain relief and joint stability.

B. Surgery.

1. Bone ends are denuded of any remaining cartilage and surfaces of the joint are smoothed.
2. Hip joint is reduced to the desired alignment.
3. Joint is fixed by means of screws, pins, plates, nails, or external fixator.
4. Bone grafts (allograft, autograft, or banked bone) often used.
5. Most important postoperative consideration is immobilizing the joint long enough for fusion to take place.
6. Spica cast or bracing may be used along with the internal fixation.
7. Resulting shortening of the extremity will likely require a shoe lift.

IV. NURSING DIAGNOSES, OUTCOMES, AND INTERVENTIONS

A. See Table 19.2.

B. See Chapter 10, Therapeutic Modalities (section on casts).

V. PRACTICE SETTING CONSIDERATIONS

A. Office/outpatient.

1. Coordinate preoperative testing and hospital admission.
2. Teach patient/significant other regarding care/management of spica cast if appropriate.
3. Refer to orthotics/prosthetics if appropriate.
4. Assist with postoperative care and monitoring.

B. Hospital.

1. Provide postoperative care per protocol.

2. Assist in coordinating discharge plans.
3. Teach hip precautions per Tables 19.2 and 19.3.
4. Teach care of hip spica cast or brace if appropriate.

C. Home care considerations.
1. Assess home situation for safety and functional ability of patient.
2. Reinforce mobility instruction; progress same.
3. Monitor/assist with and teach incision care.
4. Teach patient and significant other home ADL management.

PROXIMAL FEMORAL OSTEOTOMY

I. OVERVIEW

A. Definition.
1. Procedure indicated in early hip arthritis if conservative measures have failed; usually caused by congenital malformation.
2. Refers to realignment of the femoral neck.

B. Etiology.
1. Indicated for younger patients to provide an alternative to immediate total hip replacement.
2. Used for patients whose activities, occupation or lifestyle make them a less than ideal candidate for joint replacement.

C. Pathophysiology.
1. Early arthritis is present but joint congruency exists.
2. Hip motion is relatively normal.
3. Procedure redistributes mechanical stress over less worn areas of the femoral head.

D. Incidence.
1. Successful in approximately 80% of patients.
2. Generally a temporary alternative for up to 10 years.
3. By 10 years post-osteotomy one-half to three-quarters of patients require further surgery including joint replacement.

E. Considerations across the lifespan.
1. Middle-age adult with hip arthritis who is trying to gain some time prior to requiring a joint replacement.
   a. Desire to remain more active.
   b. Desire to delay joint replacement and potential multiple revisions.
2. If osteotomy fails, joint replacement will likely occur requiring a potential lifestyle change for these adults.

F. Complications.
1. Non-union.
2. Thromboembolism.
3. Wound infection.
4. Under/over correction.

II. ASSESSMENT

A. History.
1. Presenting symptoms similar to those noted for hip arthroplasty, though less severe.
2. See Chapter 12, Arthritis and Connective Tissue Conditions.
3. Review pain related to location, intensity, and precipitating activities.
4. Assess affect of the hip arthritis on ADL and lifestyle.
5. Obtain information on predisposing factors.
6. Obtain general health history.

B. Physical examination.
1. See hip assessment in Chapter 3, Musculoskeletal Assessment.
2. Assess range of motion and effect on lifestyle/activities.
3. Passive range of motion can exacerbate the symptoms.

C. Diagnostic tests.
1. Laboratory and preoperative diagnostics as required for surgery.
2. Radiographs.
   a. Full hip series.
   b. Compare to any prior films to determine progression of disease.

III. COMMON THERAPEUTIC MODALITIES

A. The goal of a successful osteotomy is to relieve pain and allow more vigorous activities with fewer restrictions.

B. Surgery.
1. Wedge of bone removed from the proximal femur, usually near the lesser trochanter.
2. Angle of femoral neck relative to the femoral shaft is realigned.
3. Plate and screws used to fix the proximal femur.
4. Approximately three months of partial weight bearing is necessary for healing.

IV. NURSING DIAGNOSES, OUTCOMES, AND INTERVENTIONS

A. See Table 19.2.

B. Most common diagnoses seen with these patients are:
1. Pain.
2. Physical mobility, impaired.
3. Peripheral neurovascular dysfunction, risk for.
4. Knowledge, deficient.

V. PRACTICE SETTING CONSIDERATIONS

A. Office/outpatient.
1. Coordinate preoperative testing and hospital admission.
2. Assist with postoperative care and monitoring.

B. Hospital.
1. Provide postoperative care per protocol.
2. Teach patient per Table 19.2.

C. Home care considerations.
1. Generally not required with these patients.
2. If necessary may include reinforcing mobility and monitoring incision care.

FEMORAL FRACTURES

I. OVERVIEW

A. Definition.

1. Femoral shaft fracture occurs between subtrochanteric and supracondylar area.
2. Shaft fractures may be open or closed; comminuted or non-comminuted; displaced or non-displaced.
3. Fractures involving the head, neck, greater and lesser trochanter areas defined in hip fractures.

B. Etiology.

1. Occurs when bone is subjected to more stress then it can absorb.
2. Shaft fractures may be caused by direct or indirect force, stress, or pathologic process (see Chapter 14, Trauma).
3. Femoral shaft fractures usually result from tremendous forces such as trauma of a vehicular accident.

C. Pathophysiology.

1. Amount of force required to fracture the femur varies with biologic factors.
   a. As age increases the required force decreases, such as the more elderly patient with osteoporosis or osteoarthritis.
   b. Bone size is a determining factor related to force; the femur is the largest bone.
   c. Weakened bone from pathologic disease requires less stress.
2. Femoral fractures may cause a loss of 1-2.5 liters of blood volume.

D. Incidence.

1. Femoral shaft fractures occur most often in young or middle-aged adults.
2. High-risk activities of recreation may predispose the younger adult to a higher incidence of femur fractures.

E. Considerations across the lifespan.

1. Femur fractures can require prolonged rehabilitation and thus an altered lifestyle/occupation for the younger adult.
2. In children:
   a. Fractures through the shaft of a long bone stimulates growth, therefore to avoid limb length discrepancy due to overgrowth the fracture ends may be set in a slight overlap.
   b. If prolonged bed rest is required diversional activity will be an even larger challenge than with the adult.
3. In the elderly patient with very osteoporotic bone, internal fixation can be more difficult related to poor bone stock.

F. Complications.

1. Fat embolism.
2. Compartment syndrome.
3. Shock.
4. Pulmonary embolism.
5. Nonunion.
6. Malunion.
7. Wound infection
8. Impaired mobility.
9. Limb length discrepancy in children.

II. ASSESSMENT

A. History.

1. Mechanism of injury.
2. Presenting symptoms.
   a. Pain.
   b. Deformity of femur.
   c. Leg length discrepancy.
   d. Inability to move the extremity.
   e. Complaints of altered neurovascular status to the affected extremity.
   f. An open wound related to an open fracture.
3. Altered hemodynamic status related to extensive soft tissue damage and considerable blood loss from fracture site.

B. Physical examination.

1. Appearance of the extremity.
   a. Swelling.
   b. Bruising.
   c. Open wounds.
   d. Deformity.
2. Position of extremity.
   a. External rotation.
   b. Shortened.
   c. Malalignment compared to opposite extremity.
3. Neurovascular assessment of affected extremity.
4. Assessment of vital signs for shock due to blood loss.
5. General physical examination necessary as operative preparation.

C. Diagnostic tests.

1. Radiographs.
   a. AP and lateral radiographs of femur.
   b. Used to evaluate degree of fracture to determine management.
2. Laboratory tests appropriate to trauma work up or preoperative requirements.

III. COMMON THERAPEUTIC MODALITIES

A. Goal of treatment is adequate fracture reduction with return to full mobility.

B. Care at the accident scene.

1. Assessment of neurovascular status of extremity.
2. Splinting.
3. Covering an open fracture site with a sterile dressing and observing the wound frequently.

C. Conservative.

1. Skin traction.
2. Skeletal traction.
   a. May be used short-term for several days to medically stabilize the patient prior to surgery.
   b. If chosen as treatment choice will require 4-6 weeks of traction with associated potential complications of immobility.
3. Cast brace.
4. Hip spica cast.
5. Casting is preferred treatment for children up to approximately age 10.

D. Surgical.

1. Generally preferred choice of treatment which allows early mobilization and ambulation.
2. Internal fixation.
   a. Intermedullary rods.
   b. Percutaneous pins.
   c. Plate and screws.
3. External fixation may be chosen with an open fracture.
4. Open femur fractures.
   a. Soft tissue damage generally has priority over fracture treatment.
   b. Open femur fractures should be treated as an emergency.
   c. Antibiotic therapy is used with all open femur fractures as all are considered contaminated.
   d. Debridement of the wound is performed in OR under sterile conditions followed by fracture stabilization.
   e. Wounds may have primary closure or delayed closure depending on the extent of the wound and need for grafting.
5. Approximate healing time for an adult is 8-16 weeks; for a child 6-12 weeks.

IV. NURSING DIAGNOSES, OUTCOMES, AND INTERVENTIONS

A. See Table 19.2.

B. Most common diagnoses seen with these patients are:

1. Pain.
2. Physical mobility, impaired.
3. Peripheral neurovascular dysfunction, risk for.
4. Knowledge, deficient.

C. Depending on extent of injury and extent of surgery alteration in hemodynamics may also be a priority diagnosis.

V. PRACTICE SETTING CONSIDERATIONS

A. Office/outpatient.

1. Since these are usually trauma patients they aren't seen preoperatively in this setting unless the fracture is pathologic.
2. Assist with postoperative care, teaching, evaluation, and monitoring.

B. Hospital.

1. Provide pre and postoperative care per protocol.
2. Teach patient per Table 19.2.

C. Home care considerations.

1. Generally not required with these patients.
2. If necessary may include reinforcing mobility and monitoring incision care.

PELVIC FRACTURES

I. OVERVIEW

A. Definition.

1. Fracture occurring in the ilium, ischium, or pubic bone.
2. Acetabulum is also part of the pelvis.
3. Sacral fractures occurring with pelvic ring fractures increase the severity.

B. Etiology: severe trauma is generally the cause; includes motor vehicle accidents, falls from great heights, or crushing injuries.

C. Pathophysiology.

1. Pelvic fractures can result in a high volume of blood loss.
2. Major blood vessels in the pelvic region include:
   a. Common iliac and femoral arteries.
   b. Femoral and greater saphenous veins.
   c. Severe damage to major vessels can cause hemorrhagic shock.
3. Major nerve damage can also occur related to the location of lumbar and sacral plexus.
4. With severe fractures additional abdominal trauma is likely.
5. Pelvic fractures may be stable or unstable.
   a. The location and amount of fractures in the ring will determine the stability.
   b. Displacement of fracture fragments can lead to shifting of the pelvic ring and instability.
   c. Always suspect multiple fractures in the pelvic ring due to circular construct.

D. Incidence.

1. Not a common fracture site due to the amount of trauma required.
2. Generally seen in young and middle-age adults related to higher risk recreation activities and type of employment.

E. Considerations across the lifespan.

1. Pelvic fractures require prolonged rehabilitation and physical therapy and will alter the lifestyle of an adult related to job and recreation.
2. In an elderly patient, prolonged immobility would increase the potential of altered skin integrity.
3. In the child, prolonged immobility or altered activity will be more challenging to manage related to a lower level of understanding and the need for creativity with diversional activities.

F. Complications.

1. Hemorrhagic shock.
2. Nerve damage.
3. Thromboembolism.
4. Malunion.
5. Nonunion.
6. Complications of immobility.
7. Infection.

II. ASSESSMENT

A. History.

1. Mechanism of injury.
2. Presenting symptoms.
   a. Bruising.
   b. Deformity.
   c. Pain; severe back pain may indicate retroperitoneal blood.
   d. An open wound related to an open fracture.
   e. Signs of hemorrhagic shock.

3. Alteration in neurovascular status of the lower extremities.

B. Physical examination.
1. Appearance of the abdomen and pelvis.
   a. Swelling.
   b. Bruising.
   c. Deformity.
   d. Open wounds.
2. Assess type, location, amount of pain.
3. Note any crepitus of pelvic bones; avoid movement until radiologic assessment complete.
4. Assessment of vital signs for shock due to blood loss.
5. Neurovascular assessment of bilateral lower extremities; assess peripheral pulses as absence may indicate a major artery tear.
6. Assess for injuries of abdominal organs, intestines, bladder, or rectum.
7. General physical exam as part of trauma work-up or operative prep as necessary.

C. Diagnostic tests.
1. Radiographs.
   a. Complete pelvic series.
   b. CT scan to assess for abdominal injuries.
   c. Chest x-ray if indicated as part of trauma work-up or preoperative testing.
2. Laboratory tests appropriate to trauma workup or preoperative requirements.

III. COMMON THERAPEUTIC MODALITIES

A. Goal of treatment is adequate fracture reduction with a stable pelvis and return to full mobility with full weight bearing.

B. Care at the accident scene.
1. Assessment for signs of shock.
2. Limited movement of the patient; moving slowing with support of the pelvis if necessary.
3. Covering an open fracture site with a sterile dressing.
4. Assessment of neurovascular status of the lower extremities.

C. Choice of treatment will depend on type, location, stability versus instability of fracture(s), and surgeon preference.
1. Conservative.
   a. Bed rest, progressing to ambulation with restricted weight bearing; often used with stable fractures.
   b. Buck traction.
   c. Skeletal traction.
   d. Pelvic sling traction.
2. Surgical.
   a. Open reduction internal fixation.
   b. External fixation.
   c. In some cases open reduction internal fixation (ORIF) combined with external fixation.
   d. Primary arthroplasty or arthrodesis in some acetabular fractures.
3. Combination of conservative and surgical options may be used.
4. Approximate healing time for an adult is 6-12 weeks; for a child 6-8 weeks.

IV. NURSING DIAGNOSES, OUTCOMES, AND INTERVENTIONS

A. Pain, acute.
1. Outcome.
   a. Patient's pain is controlled as evidenced by ability to rest and participate in activities.
   b. Patient progresses from IV/IM/PCA medication to use of oral medication at time of discharge.
2. Interventions.
   a. Log roll per physician order only maintaining pelvic alignment.
   b. Apply ice to incision or areas of bruising/swelling as desired.
   c. Encourage the use of relaxation techniques.
   d. Administer IV/IM/PCA medications as ordered and needed.
   e. Assess level of pain and document same.
   f. Transition to use of oral medication as patient tolerates.
   g. Communicate level of comfort to physician and other care providers.
   h. Administer pain medication prior to activity and assess effectiveness.

B. Physical mobility, impaired.
1. Outcomes.
   a. Patient will be able to perform bed-to-chair transfer with minimal assistance.
   b. Patient will be able to ambulate a functional distance with assistive device and limited weight bearing for discharge.
2. Interventions.
   a. Assess preoperative level of mobility.
   b. Encourage bed mobility within designated limitations; provide overhead frame/trapeze to facilitate.
   c. Instruct in correct positioning based on fracture site and surgeon order.
   d. Teach log rolling with proper pelvic alignment.
   e. Reinforce exercise program as instructed by physical therapy.
   f. Instruct in use of assistive devices for ambulating and with correct limited weight bearing.
   g. Help patient/family/caregiver obtain assistive device(s) for discharge.
   h. Progress mobility from bed-chair transfers to ambulating as ordered.

C. See Table 19.2 for:
1. Peripheral neurovascular dysfunction, risk for.
2. Tissue perfusion, ineffective.
3. Fluid volume, deficient.
4. Self-care deficit syndrome.
5. Knowledge, deficient.

D. If prolonged bed rest is required, see Chapter 6, Effects of Immobility, for interventions.

V. PRACTICE SETTING CONSIDERATIONS

A. Office/outpatient: assist with postoperative care and monitoring.

B. Hospital.

1. Provide post-trauma and postoperative care per protocol.
2. Teach patient per Table 19.2.

C. Home care considerations.

1. Assess home situation for safety and functional ability for patient.
2. Reinforce mobility restrictions.
3. Monitor/assist with and teach incision care.
4. Monitor lab values or medications as indicated.
5. Teach patient/significant other home ADL management.

Bibliography

Altizer, L.L. (1998). Degenerative disorder. In A.B. Maher, S.W. Salmond, & T.A. Pellino (Eds.), *Orthopaedic nursing* (2nd ed., pp. 480-543). Philadelphia: W.B. Saunders.

Lappe, J.M. (1998). Prevention of hip fractures: A nursing imperative. *Orthopaedic Nursing, 17*(3), 15-26.

Messer, B. (1998, March/April). Total joint replacement preadmission programs. *Orthopaedic Nursing,* (Suppl.), 31-33.

Taggart, H.M. (1999). *Caring for the elderly hip fracture patient. In An introduction to orthopaedic nursing* (2nd ed., pp. 113-122). Pitman, NJ: National Association of Orthopaedic Nurses.

Schoen, D.C. (2000). Care of a patient with hip and femoral surgery. In D.C. Schoen, *Adult orthopaedic nursing* (pp. 271-314). Philadelphia: Lippincott.

Slauenwhite, C., & Simpson, P. (1998). Patient and family perspectives regarding early discharge and care of the older adult undergoing fractured hip rehabilitation. *Orthopaedic Nursing, 17*(1), 30-36.

Smith, S. (Ed.). (1999). Total hip arthoplasty. In *Orthopaedic nursing core competencies: Adult acute care* (pp. 75-81). Pitman, NJ: National Association for Orthopaedic Nurses.

Theis, L.M. (1998). Cost containment and quality: Co-existing in total joint care. *Orthopaedic Nursing, 17*(6), 70-77.

STUDY QUESTIONS

Mr. Green is an 80-year-old male who presents to the emergency room after a fall at home. He is complaining of pain and holding his right hip area. A hip fracture is suspected. (Questions 1-3)

1. Which of the following is **not** a presenting symptom for a person with a fractured hip?
   a. Leg length discrepancy.
   b. Affected leg externally rotated.
   c. Pain and discoloration in the area.
   d. Affected leg is adducted.

2. Mr. Green is diagnosed with an intertrochanteric fracture. This is located:
   a. Within the joint capsule.
   b. Between the trochanters.
   c. Below the lesser trochanter.
   d. In the femoral neck.

3. Which of the following is **not** an appropriate nursing intervention?
   a. Monitor his pain level and administer medications as need.
   b. Instruct Mr. Green on the proper gait for walker/crutches.
   c. Teaching him about weight-bearing activity restrictions.
   d. Make his discharge plans with his family to prevent stress.

Mr. Anderson, a 72-year-old man, is being admitted post-operative**ly following a hip replacement due to osteoarthritis. (Questions 4-7)**

4. The physician's operative note indicates a primary total hip arthroplasty was performed. This means:
   a. The head and neck of the femur and acetabulum were replaced.
   b. Only one component of a total joint replacement was replaced.
   c. Mr. Anderson had had a hip replacement previously.
   d. The joint was totally excised due the arthritis pathology.

5. Which finding from Mr. Anderson's history and physical examination would most likely have been the indication leading to surgery?
   a. Anterior thigh pain radiating toward the knee, increasing overtime.
   b. Decreased range of motion in the joint and increased pain.
   c. Shortening of the affected extremity.
   d. Mr. Anderson needs to take ASA after his daily walks.

6. In teaching Mr. Anderson about hip precautions, which of the following is **not** appropriate?
   a. Don't sit in a low chair.
   b. Don't sit with legs crossed.
   c. Don't flex the hip more than 90 degrees.
   d. Don't flex the hip more than 120 degrees.

7. When transferring Mr. Anderson back to bed he complains of acute groin and hip pain and says he felt something "pop." What should the nurse anticipate?
   a. Subluxation.
   b. Dislocation.
   c. Infection.
   d. Fracture.

8. Which of the following is a true statement regarding a femoral osteotomy?
   a. Late-stage arthritis present with joint congruency.
   b. Procedure realigns the acetabulum with the femur.
   c. Used for a mid-age adult as an alternative to an immediate total hip arthroplasty.
   d. It is a permanent, long-term treatment option for most patients.

9. A 30-year-old female presents to the emergency room with the following symptoms after a motor vehicle accident: severe pain to the right lower extremity and inability to move it; bruising, swelling, and deformity mid-thigh with an open wound; and leg length discrepancy. Which of the following is a likely diagnosis?
   a. Closed femur fracture.
   b. Extracapsular hip fracture.
   c. Dislocated hip.
   d. Open femur fracture.

10. Which statement is **true** regarding pelvic fractures?
    a. Pelvic fractures are always unstable.
    b. Additional abdominal trauma is unlikely with severe fractures.
    c. There are no major blood vessels of concern in the pelvic area.
    d. Pelvic fractures can result in high-volume blood loss.

Chapter 20 The Knee

John P. Davis, BS, RN, ONC
Nancy Abbate, RN, CNOR, ONC

Contents

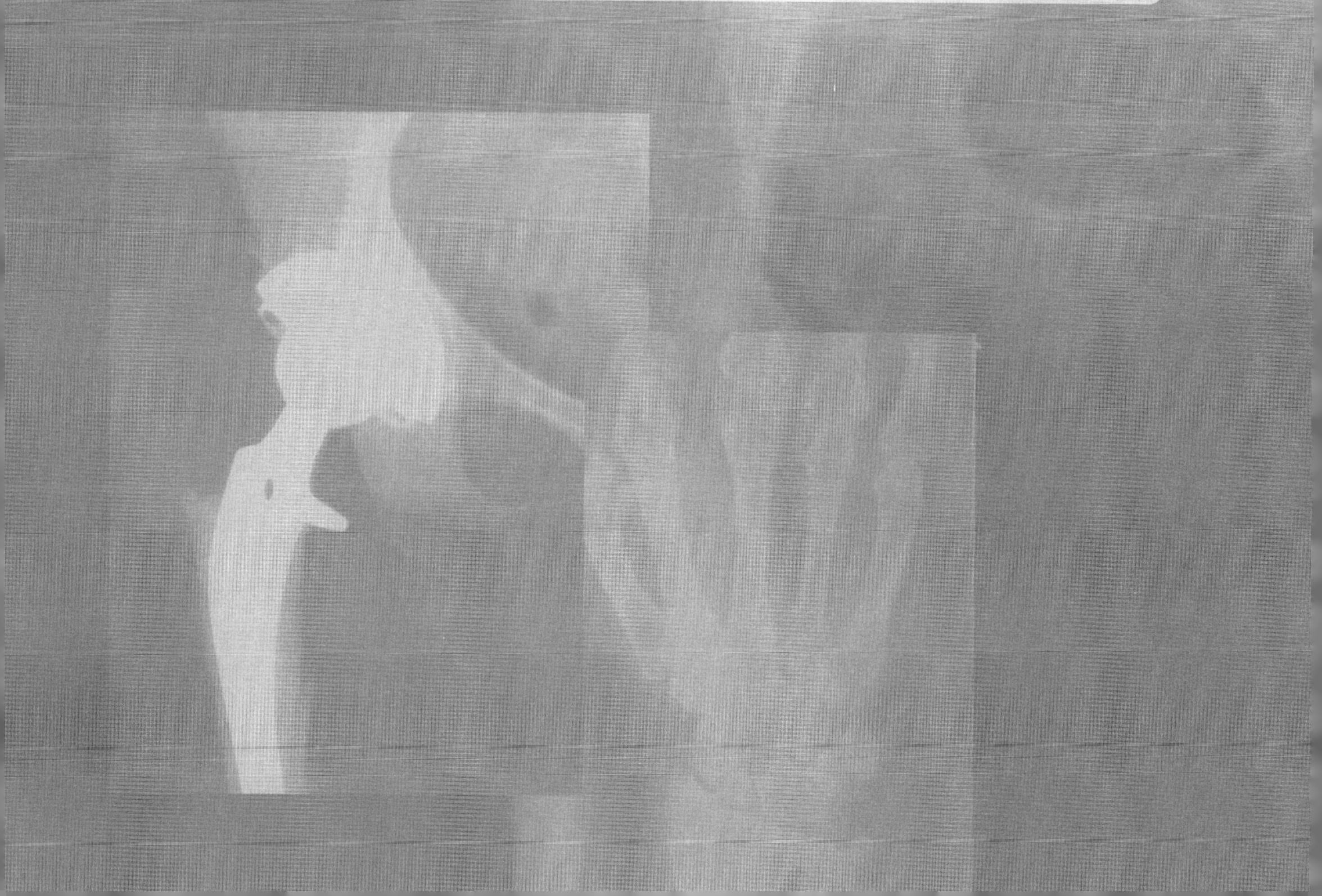

OBJECTIVES

At the completion of this chapter, the learner will be able to:

- Define the most common sports injuries to the knee.
- Discuss the surgical and nonsurgical management and treatment of the knee.
- Identify arthritic conditions to the knee.
- Identify specific conditions of the knee in pediatric patients.
- Discuss physical therapy indications.
- Identify common nursing diagnoses, outcomes, and interventions for patients with knee pathology.
- Identify home care considerations to manage patients with knee pathology.
- Identify office practice considerations.

KEY POINTS

- Assessment of the knee involves a good history and physical examination with emphasis on identifying a hierarchy of probable cause to direct one's examination.
- Knowledge of onset of symptoms and mechanism of injury can save valuable time and patient comfort during examination.
- Patient age is a significant factor when considering surgical treatment options.
- Both surgical and nonsurgical options are available for many knee pathologies.
- The use of ice, anti-inflammatory medication and compressive bracing reduces swelling.
- Many injuries to the knee require an exercise program or physical therapy to maintain/restore motion and strength.

CHAPTER 20

THE KNEE

ARTHRITIS OF THE KNEE

I. OVERVIEW

A. Definition: arthritic conditions to the knee are common with nonsurgical and surgical treatment modalities to address many symptoms and functional deficits. Arthritis, a singular and nonspecific term, refers to a variety of disease and conditions (see Chapter 12, Arthritis and Connective Tissue Disorders). These include, but are not limited to:

1. Degenerative or osteoarthritis (OA).
2. Inflammatory or rheumatoid arthritis (RA).
3. Systemic Lupus Erythematosus (SLE).
4. Psoriatic arthritis.
5. Metabolic type of arthritis or gout.
6. Post-traumatic arthritis as a result of trauma to the joint:
   a. Tibial plateau fractures.
   b. Fractures of the femoral condyles.
   c. Non-union fractures of the femoral condyles and tibial plateau.
   d. Patella fractures.

B. Etiology (see Chapter 12, Arthritis and Connective Tissue Disorders)

II. HISTORY AND PHYSICAL ASSESSMENT (See Chapter 3, Musculoskeletal Assessment)

A. Subjective information.

1. Onset of symptoms.
2. Pain severity and location.
3. Giving way and locking.
4. Assessment and disability.
   a. Walking distance.
   b. Standing ability.
   c. Climbing stairs.
5. Transferring from chair.
6. Using assistive devices and walking aids.

B. Objective information.

1. Gait analysis.
2. Effusion of the knee.
3. Tests for stability of menisci and patella.
4. Tests for determining intact ligaments.
5. Assess for crepitus.
6. Check the alignment of the knee for:
   a. Varus deformities.
   b. Valgus deformities.

C. Diagnostic tests.

1. See Chapter 4, Diagnostic Studies.
2. Radiographic examination.
   a. Standing, anterior, posterior, and lateral views.
   b. Patellofemoral or merchant/sunrise views.

III. COMMON THERAPEUTIC MODALITIES

A. Nonsurgical management.

1. Wellness promotion and disease prevention.
   a. Focus on reducing factors that cause excessive joint loading.
   b. Educate the patient regarding proper body mechanics and joint protection.
   c. Use orthotics for correction and support for pronated feet.
   d. Teach the patient to avoid excessive loading activities.
   e. Discuss ways to modify patient's workplace, if indicated.
   f. Discuss going on a weight reduction diet, if indicated.
   g. Provide gait training with the use of an assistive device.
2. Physical therapy.
   a. Reduce the impairment.
      (1) Improve joint function.
      (2) Reduce joint pain.
      (3) Decrease swelling.
   b. Increase range of motion of the knee.
      (1) Restore the strength in the muscles of the leg.
      (2) Assists in the normalization of the walking gait.
      (3) Facilitates the performance of activities of daily living (ADL).
   c. Protection of joint from damage.
      (1) Reduce stress to joint.
      (2) Improve biomechanics.
   d. Prevention of disability and poor health secondary to inactivity.
      (1) Increase the daily level of activity.
      (2) Improve physical fitness.
   e. Adjunctive treatment modalities.
      (1) Transcutaneous electrical nerve stimulation (TENS).
      (2) Cryotherapy.
      (3) Whirlpool and aquatic therapy.
3. Bracing/splinting.
   a. Joint stabilization.
   b. Compartment unloading.
4. Pharmacologic.
   a. Analgesics.
   b. Nonsteroidal anti-inflammatory drugs (NSAIDs): may be contraindicated in patients with hypertension or pitting edema.
5. Nutritional supplements and chondro-protective agents (such as glucosamine and chondroitin sulfate).
6. Joint aspiration/injection.
   a. Aspirate joint fluid.

b. Intra-articular corticosteroid treatments.
   (1) With or without local anesthetic.
   (2) Intervals of 4-6 months.
c. Viscosupplementation.
   (1) Hyalgan® (sodium hyaluronate): series of five injections at weekly intervals.
   (2) Synvisc® (hylan G-F 20): series of three injections over 15 days (day 1, 8, and 15).

B. Surgical management.

1. Synovectomy: performed as an open surgical procedure or arthroscopically to remove the inflamed synovial membrane with a rapid relief of pain and associated swelling.
   a. Indications.
      (1) Most frequently performed for rheumatoid arthritis.
      (2) After failed medical management following at least a 6-month trial.
      (3) Persistent synovitis.
      (4) Stage I or II arthropathy as defined by the American Rheumatism Association.
   b. Contraindications: if significant joint space narrowing is present in the joint.
2. Arthrodesis: usually viewed as a salvage procedure, there is a surgical femorotibial bony fusion of the joint that creates an immobile knee.
   a. Indications.
      (1) Failed arthroplasty.
      (2) Infection within the joint.
      (3) Severe ligamentous instability.
      (4) Painful ankylosis.
      (5) Painful Charcot or neuropathic arthopathy.
      (6) Malignant or highly aggressive tumors about the knee.
   b. Contraindications.
      (1) Ipsilateral hip or ankle disease.
      (2) Severe bony deficiency.
      (3) Contralateral above the knee amputation or knee fusion.
3. Arthroscopic debridement: a method of debridement within the knee, advocated for mild arthrosis with or without concurrent mechanical derangement or crystalline-induced inflammation.
   a. Indications.
      (1) Young patient with mild degenerative disease.
      (2) Early degenerative changes on radiographs.
      (3) Symptoms secondary to mechanical derangement.
      (4) Acute onset on crystalline-induced inflammation.
   b. Contraindications.
      (1) Patients with advanced arthritis.
      (2) History of long duration of symptoms.
      (3) Malalignment of knee.
4. Distal femoral osteotomy: a procedure designed to realign the proximal weight-bearing surfaces of the knee joint as a result of valgus deformity with a lateral gonarthrosis. Also used to prevent future total knee replacement.
   a. Indications.
      (1) Young patient with isolated lateral unicompartmental arthritis.
      (2) Modest activity demands.
      (3) Failed nonsurgical treatment of:
         (a) NSAID therapy.
         (b) Use of assistive device (cane).
         (c) Activity modification.
         (d) Use of unloader bracing.
   b. Contraindications.
      (1) Severe osteoporosis.
      (2) Inadequate bone stock.
      (3) Significant chondral degeneration in other compartments.
5. Proximal tibial osteotomy: a procedure designed to realign the distal articular surfaces of the knee, distribute the weight more evenly within the knee joint, and relieve pain due to varus deformities/medial compartmental osteoarthritis.
   a. Indications.
      (1) Young, healthy, highly active patient with isolated varus gonarthrosis and severe pain.
      (2) Someone who wishes to continue an active lifestyle.
      (3) Patients who demonstrate less than 10 degrees of fixed flexion and greater than 90 degrees of active flexion.
   b. Contraindications.
      (1) Significant chondral degeneration in other compartments.
      (2) Subluxation of the tibiofemoral articulation.
      (3) Anterior cruciate ligament (ACL) insufficiency, unless planning a two-stage procedure which includes ACL reconstruction.
      (4) Incompetence of the medial collateral ligament (MCL).
6. Unicompartmental knee replacement: a procedure used to treat unicompartmental femorotibial arthrosis by replacing only the arthritic affected portions of the knee joint and preserving the contralateral and patellofemoral articulations surfaces.
   a. Indications.
      (1) Elderly people who have low body weight and are sedentary.
      (2) Osteoarthritis.
      (3) Osteonecrosis.
      (4) Post-traumatic arthritis.
      (5) Adequate preoperative range of motion.
   b. Contraindications.
      (1) Young patients who have heavy body weight and are active.
      (2) Any subluxation of the tibiofemoral articulation.
      (3) ACL insufficiency.
      (4) Significant imbalance of the collateral ligament.
      (5) Inflammatory or crystalline deposition arthropathies.

7. Total knee arthroplasty (TKA): a procedure done on an injured or diseased knee to reestablish a movable functioning joint by removing the distal portions of the femur and the tibial plateau and replacing them with metal or plastic components.
    a. Indications.
        (1) Patients with severe arthritis who have failed conservative treatment including:
            (a) Medication.
            (b) Utilization of a cane.
            (c) Physical therapy.
            (d) Intra-articular injections.
            (e) Activity modification.
        (2) Disabling pain with activity.
        (3) Osteoarthritis.
        (4) Post-traumatic injury/arthritis.
        (5) Rheumatoid and other inflammatory arthritides.
        (6) Significant varus/valgus deformity.
        (7) Failed peri-articular osteotomies; rarely done prior to TKA.
    b. Contraindications.
        (1) Patients with very high demand and stress on the knee.
        (2) Young age; future need for multiple revisions.
        (3) Morbid obesity; stress wear.
        (4) Very active lifestyle; high impact activity.
        (5) Prior osteomyelitis about the knee.
        (6) Ongoing subclinical infection.
        (7) Severe peripheral vascular disease.
        (8) Any medical condition that may seriously risk the patient's ability to withstand the surgery.
    c. Strict and absolute contraindications.
        (1) Active sepsis of the knee.
        (2) Solid, painless surgical arthrodesis.
        (3) Significant genu recurvatum.
        (4) Inability to carry out and maintain active extension.

IV. NURSING DIAGNOSES, OUTCOMES, AND INTERVENTIONS

A. See Table 20.1 for specific nursing diagnoses related to the knee.
B. See Chapter 5, Perioperative Patient Care.
C. See Chapter 7, Pain, for methods of pain management.
D. See Chapter 8, Complications, on ways of combating potential complications.
E. See Chapter 9, Infections, on nursing interventions for preventing infections.
F. See Chapter 10, Therapeutic Modalities, on helping patients with assistive devices such as continuous passive motion machines, crutches, and canes.
G. See Chapter 6, Effects of Immobility.

V. HOME CARE CONSIDERATIONS (See Table 20.2)

VI. OFFICE PRACTICE CONSIDERATIONS (See Table 20.3)

MENISCAL TEARS

I. OVERVIEW

A. Definition: a tearing of the menisci within the knee joint.
1. Menisci are lunar-shaped cartilage pads between the long bones of the lower extremity.
2. They act as cushions for shock absorption between the bones, during weight-bearing activities.
3. There is a medial and a lateral meniscus.
4. The purpose of the menisci are to protect the articular cartilage that covers the ends of the tibia and femur from injury and to act as spaces to stabilize the knee.

B. Pathophysiology.
1. Menisco-capsular separation is where the meniscus is separated from its insertion at the capsule.
2. Bucket handle tear:
    a. A tear in the body of the meniscus that appears like a bucket handle.
    b. Frequently causes locked knee because handle catches in joint and prevents extension.
    c. Tear can be repaired if:
        (1) Tear is in vascular zone.
        (2) If tear is not in vascular zone, torn portion must be removed.
3. Flap tear:
    a A part of meniscus has torn and flipped up.
    b. Can cause locking
    c. Can rarely be repaired.
4. Linear tear is the most common type of tear and not repairable.
5. Cleavage tear in body of meniscus is repairable, but usually not full thickness.
6. Degenerative tears:
    a. Not related to trauma.
    b. Frequently associated with articular cartilage wear.
    c. Not repairable.

II. ASSESSMENT

A. History.
1. Mechanism of injury.
    a. Torsion injury.
    b. Squatting injury.
    c. Direct impact.
2. No trauma.
3. Congenital discoid meniscus: probable cause is lack of separation of meniscus from ligament of Wrisberg during childhood.

B. Physical examination.
1. Medial or lateral joint line pain on compression.
2. Knee locked in extension/flexion.
3. Positive Steinman test: pain with knee hanging loose when knee is sharply rotated internally and externally.

Table 20.1
Common Nursing Diagnoses, Outcomes, and Interventions for Patients with Problems of the Knee

Diagnoses	Outcomes	Interventions
A. Pain, acute	• Patient is comfortable and swelling is reduced.	• See Chapter 7, Pain. • Assess pain level. • Prevent excessive joint loading. • Encourage use of pain medication and NSAIDs. • Review potential adverse side effects of medications: narcotics – nausea, vomiting, constipation, and addiction; NSAIDs – stomach irritation and increased risk of bleeding. • Encourage cryotherapy (ice) 3-4 times a day. • Elevate as needed. (Limit time with leg in dependent position, and when elevated make sure patient does not put a pillow under the knee.) • Monitor swelling. • Brace for support and compression. • Prescribe specific exercise routine to reduce swelling and stiffness. Monitor pain relief measures for effectiveness, and modify care plan based on results.
B. Physical mobility, impaired	• Knee motion and weight bearing are restored.	• Promote range of motion activities. • Alleviate pain and swelling (see Pain, above and Chapter 7, Pain). • Instruct patient in specific exercise program as indicated by surgeon, based on type of surgery. • Provide and instruct with the use of equipment as needed (CPM machine, hinged brace, crutch walking, etc). • Discuss the potential problems of overdoing exercises.
C. Knowledge, deficient	• Patient has knowledge of the diagnosis, surgical procedure, postoperative expectations, and potential complications.	• Assess knowledge base and provide patient teaching. • Reinforce explanation of diagnosis. • Prepare patient for surgical procedure. • Prepare patient for anesthesia. • Assess and explain expectations regarding pain, function and rehabilitation. • Reinforce explanation and assessment of potential complications, such as infection, bleeding, deep vein thrombosis.
D. Infection, risk for	• Patient will remain free from infection.	• Observe for signs of infection and take preventive measures. • Assess wound for redness, swelling, drainage, odor, and increased pain. • Wash hands meticulously before and after contact.

Table 20.1 (continued)
Common Nursing Diagnoses, Outcomes, and Interventions for Patients with Problems of the Knee

Diagnoses	Outcomes	Interventions
D. Infection, risk for (continued)	• Patient will remain free from infection. (continued)	• Clean wounds and apply dressings using aseptic technique. • Administer appropriate prophylactic antibiotics. • Follow vital signs and laboratory test results. • Remove invasive lines as soon as possible (urinary catheter and intravenous). • Promote good nutrition with protein and plenty of fluids to promote healing. • Teach patient to recognize signs and symptoms and report to MD. • Instruct patient in long-term prophylaxis with dental work and other invasive procedures such as implants.
E. Tissue perfusion, ineffective	• Patient will not develop altered tissue perfusion related to deep vein thrombosis.	• Institute preventive measures. • Review ankle pumps. • Promote early ambulation. • Monitor prophylaxis-mechanical devices, compression stockings, anti-coagulants (aspirin, warfarin, and/or low molecular weight heparin). • Observe lower extremity for redness, swelling, edema, skin temperature changes, deep tenderness, positive Homan's sign. • Teach patient to recognize signs and symptoms and report to MD. • Assist with post-op monitoring of laboratory values.
F. Fluid volume, deficient	• Patient will not exhibit signs and symptoms of hemorrhage.	• Monitor for post-op hemorrhage. • Record perioperative blood loss. • Measure intake and output. • Observe amount of drainage over time. • Apply compression and ice; elevate as indicated. • Monitor blood counts and coagulation laboratory values. • Replace fluid volume with crystalloids and transfuse blood products as indicated. • Monitor vital signs. • Observe for restlessness and mental status changes.

4. Positive McMurray test: a cartilage snap or jump is appreciated along the joint line when knee is flexed and foot is rotated internally and externally.
   a. Place the patient in a supine position with legs in flat neutral position.
   b. With one hand, take hold of the affected heel and flex the leg fully.
   c. Place your other hand on the knee joint with your fingers touching the medial joint line and your thumb and thenar eminence against the lateral joint line.
   d. Rotate the leg internally and externally to loosen the joint.
   e. Push on the lateral side to apply valgus stress to the medial side of the joint, at the same time, rotating the leg externally.
   f. Maintain the valgus stress and external rotation, and extend the leg slowly as you palpate the medial joint line.
   g. If the maneuver causes a palpable or audible "click" within the joint, there is a probable tear in the medial meniscus (most likely in its posterior half).
5. Position-related joint line pain when walking/twisting knee.
6. Swelling.

C. Diagnostic tests.

1. X-rays to determine evidence of arthritis or calcific deposits, which may indicate degeneration of meniscus.
2. MRI to evaluate and describe the type and position of the tear.

III. COMMON THERAPEUTIC MODALITIES

A. Nonsurgical management

1. Reduce pain with NSAIDs and pain medications.
2. Reduce swelling with elevation and NSAIDs, as needed.
3. Reduce swelling/pain with cryotherapy (ice).
4. Restore motion and maintain quadriceps/hamstring strength with gentle physical therapy.
5. Brace for return to sport.
6. Return to sports gradually.

B. Surgical treatment.

1. Prepare patient for surgery by explaining procedure, risks, and complications.
2. Perform preadmission testing as required by hospital.
3. Repair/remove tear arthroscopically.
4. Restore motion and strength immediately with gentle exercise as indicated.
5. Brace for return to sport as indicated.
6. Return to sports gradually after 6-8 weeks.

C. Physical therapy considerations.

1. Alleviate muscle shutdown.
   a. Gentle strengthening; isometrics.
      (1) Quadriceps.
      (2) Hamstring.
      (3) Hip adductor/abductor/flexors.
   b. Gentle ROM exercises to restore normal motion.
2. Emphasize modification of activities.
   a. Avoid squatting.
   b. Avoid lunges.
   c. Reduce stair climbing.
   d. Reduce heavy lifting.
   e. No/low-impact activities.
   f. Encourage weight reduction as indicated.

IV. NURSING DIAGNOSES, OUTCOMES, AND INTERVENTIONS (See Table 20.1)

V. HOME CARE CONSIDERATIONS (See Table 20.2)

VI. OFFICE PRACTICE CONSIDERATIONS (See Table 20.3)

ANTERIOR CRUCIATE LIGAMENT INJURIES

I. OVERVIEW

A. Definition: anterior cruciate ligament (ACL) injuries are usually the result of trauma or violent injuries.

1. The ACL and posterior cruciate ligament (PCL) crisscross in the center of the knee and provide for front-to-back and rotational stability of the knee.
2. The ACL is a rope-like ligamentous structure that inserts at the tibial spine of the tibia and posterolaterally in the femur.
3. The ACL prevents excessive rotation of the knee as well as excessive anterior translation of the tibia on the femur.

B. Pathophysiology.

1. Partial ACL tear:
   a. 30%-40% of ligament is torn.
   b. Knee feels loose as compared to the opposite knee but an endpoint can be felt on examination.
2. Complete ACL tear:
   a. Most of the fibers have been torn.
   b. Knee feels grossly loose on examination.
   c. Patient feels unstable when doing pivoting or lateral motions.

C. Incidence.

1. 50% of ACL tears have meniscal tear.
2. Lateral meniscus is more frequently torn in acute tears.
3. Medial meniscus is most commonly torn in chronic ACL tears.

II. ASSESSMENT

A. History: mechanism of injury.

1. Most ACL tears occur in noncontact situations.
2. Skiing.
   a. A slow, twisting fall in which the bindings do not release.

b. Patient usually hears/feels a pop with severe pain; often associated with MCL injuries.

3. Lacrosse/soccer.
   a. A running injury when the foot gets planted or stuck on the ground and the body continues to accelerate.
   b. Patient feels/hears pop and feels pain.
   c. Often associated with meniscal injuries.
4. Football: usually a direct blow to the knee; associated MCL injury.
5. Basketball/tennis/volleyball: leaping in air then landing on one foot off balance and body falls the other way.

B. Physical examination.

1. Observe swelling: due to bleeding in joint from torn fibers.
2. Assess loss of motion.
   a. Partly due to trauma and to swelling.
   b. Patients are frequently placed in a knee immobilizer to stabilize knee until they can be evaluated by orthopaedist.
3. Examine opposite knee:
   a. Assess normal.
   b. Assess for baseline motion.
4. Examine injured knee:
   a. Perform Lachman test to assess ligament tension.
      (1) Flex the patient's knee 15-30 degrees.
      (2) Stabilize the femur.
      (3) Pull the tibia anteriorly.
      (4) A positive Lachman test is when the tibia moves forward and the infrapatellar tendon slope disappears.
   b. If possible, check for pivot shift.
      (1) Pivot shift test of Galway and MacIntosh.
         (a) Performed with the knee in full extension.
         (b) A valgus and internal stress is applied.
      (2) Reverse pivot shift test.
         (a) Performed with the knee in flexion.
         (b) An external rotation and valgus stress is applied.
   c. Perform an anterior drawer test.
      (1) Place the patient in a supine position.
      (2) Affected knee is flexed at 90 degrees and the foot flat on the table.
      (3) Sit on the patient's foot to stabilize it.
      (4) Cup your hands around the patient's knee:
         (a) Place your fingers in the area of insertion of the medial and lateral hamstrings (popliteal fossa).
         (b) Place your thumbs along the lateral and medial line of the joint.
         (c) To test the anterior cruciate ligament:
            i. Pull the head of the tibia toward you so that it glides on the femoral condyles.
            ii. If the tibia slides forward more than one centimeter, that is a positive anterior draw sign, and the ACL may be torn.
            iii. Always check the other knee for comparison.
   d. Perform a posterior drawer test as a safety check.
      (1) Position patient the same as for the anterior draw test.
      (2) Push the head of the tibia away from you.
      (3) If the tibia slides backward on the femoral condyles, that is a positive posterior draw sign, indicating that the PCL is damaged.
5. Examine for associated injuries.
   a. Menisci joint line pain: McMurray testing (see Meniscal Tears in this chapter).
   b. MCL: valgus stress test.
      (1) Position patient in a supine position on the table with one knee flexed just enough so that it unlocks from full extension.
      (2) Secure the patient's ankle with one hand.
      (3) Place the other hand around the patient's knee so that your thenar eminence is against the fibular head.
      (4) Push medially against the knee and laterally against the ankle, attempting to open the knee joint on the inside (valgus stress).
      (5) If there is a gap, the MCL is not supporting the knee properly.
      (6) When the stress is relieved you can feel the tibia and femur "clunk" together as they close.
   c. Lateral collateral ligament: varus stress test.
      (1) Position patient the same as valgus stress test.
      (2) Push laterally against the knee and medially against the ankle.
   d. Posterolateral corner injury: "spin" test.
      (1) Measures the amount of external rotation of the lower leg on the femur.
      (2) Place the patient supine with the hip flexed to 90 degrees, and knee flexed to 90 degrees.
      (3) Grasp the foot and hold the knee stable, rotate the foot laterally.
      (4) Compare with the unaffected side to assess normal function.

C. Diagnostic tests.

1. X-rays to assess any bony injury.
2. MRI to evaluate ligament and cartilage injury.
   a. Sensitivity is 90%-98% identifying ACL injury.
   b. Complete versus partial less than 50%.
3. KT-1000-Biodex mechanized test to assess degree of ligament tearing.

III. COMMON THERAPEUTIC MODALITIES

A. Initial treatment.

1. To reduce swelling:
   a. Apply ice.
   b. Elevate the extremity.
   c. Administer NSAIDs.
   d. May also need to aspirate blood from knee.
2. To reduce pain: administer mild, narcotic pain medications.

Table 20.2
Common Home Care Considerations Following Knee Surgery

A. Communication with health team.
1. Home care/extended care facility nurses for plan of care and updated report of progress.
2. Pharmacists to track and monitor medication usage.
3. Physical therapists to outline specific plan and provide updated progress report.

B. Patient and family teaching.
1. Report to MD if any of the following occur:
   a. Signs and symptoms of infection.
   b. Inability to flex or extend the knee.
   c. Excessive bleeding.
   d. Pain unrelieved by pain medication.
2. Signs and symptoms of infection.
   a. Fever.
   b. Wound drainage.
   c. Erythema.
   d. Swelling.
   e. Increased pain.
3. DVT/PE prophylaxis (see Chapter 8, Complications)
   a. Observe for signs and symptoms of:
      (1) Calf pain.
      (2) Severe lower extremity swelling.
      (3) Chest pain or shortness of breath.
   b. Medications (aspirin, Coumadin®, or lower molecular weight heparin).
   c. Laboratory monitoring.
   d. Elastic stockings.
4. Pain management (see Chapter 7, Pain)
   a. Encourage elevation and cold therapy 3 times a day to reduce swelling, bleeding, and bruising.
   b. Analgesics, opioids, and NSAIDs.
      (1) Explain dosage and frequency.
      (2) Monitor for side effects such as nausea, constipation, addiction, and potential bleeding.
      (3) Encourage taking pain medication 30 minutes before therapy.
      (4) Observe pain levels and behavioral changes.
5. Post-treatment follow-up.
   a. Schedule timely appointments.
   b. Discuss antibiotic prophylaxis following invasive procedures (such as hardware/implant) if patient is to have extensive dental work or colonoscopy.

C. Physical/occupational therapy.
1. Review muscle strengthening and range-of-motion exercises as ordered.
2. Gait training with assistive devices such as canes, walkers, crutches (see Chapter 10, Therapeutic Modalities).
3. Promote return to ADL.
4. Facilitate continuous passive motion machines as indicated (see Chapter 10, Therapeutic Modalities).

3. Bracing.
   a. For isolated ACL/meniscal tear, use a sleeve-type brace for compression and support when walking.
   b. If injuries include MCL and posterolateral corner, more significant immobilization may be required.
4. Weight bearing is usually tolerated; if not, have patient use crutches.
5. Restore motion in the joint.
   a. Physical therapy to maintain muscle tone and motion.
   b. Quadriceps exercises work in opposite direction and maybe counter-productive.
   c. Hamstring strengthening to pull tibia backward on femur with deficient cruciate ligaments.

B. Conservative management.
1. For individuals who do not plan on returning to aggressive pivoting/rotational sports.
2. Initial treatments as above.
3. ACL sports bracing for return to gentle sports.
4. Quadriceps strengthening program.

C. **Surgical treatment.**
   1. Surgical treatment is advocated for patients:
      a. Who are young adults.
      b. Who wish to return to aggressive sports.
      c. When symptoms interfere with everyday activities.
      d. When conservative measures have failed.
      e. Who have meniscal tears or posterolateral corner injuries regardless of their sport preference.
   2. Initial treatments as above.
   3. Surgical intervention:
      a. After swelling has subsided.
      b. Motion has returned to ensure good outcome with little postoperative stiffness.
   4. Graft choice.
      a. Patella tendon autograft using ipsilateral central third patella tendon.
         (1) Frequently called bone-tendon-bone (BTB) as it uses a small piece of bone from patella and tibia and tendon connected to both.
         (2) Most common choice for young adults.
         (3) Inserted into bone tunnels.
         (4) Fixed in place with interference screws.
         (5) Excellent graft incorporation due to bone with bone.
      b. Hamstring.
         (1) Uses semi-tendonosis/gracillis tendons.
         (2) Thought to be vestigial tendons that run from anterior-inferior medial tibia and insert in main hamstring behind knee.
         (3) Inserted in bone tunnels as above and fixed in place with endo-button and staple or screw in tibia-longer incorporation in tunnels.
         (4) There is no bone-to-bone contact.
      c. Patella tendon allograft (cadaver graft).
         (1) Similar to autograft BTB.
         (2) Used for patients who have had previous ACL surgery and patients over 55 years old.

D. **Physical therapy considerations.**
   1. Begin motion exercises either at home or with a physical therapist within 48 hours of surgery to help restore normal strength and motion.
   2. Communicate with physical therapist to evaluate patient's status for progression of activities, bracing, return to sports.
   3. Emphasize importance of rest during first 24-48 hours with leg elevated.

IV. NURSING DIAGNOSES, OUTCOMES, AND INTERVENTIONS (See Table 20.1)

V. HOME CARE CONSIDERATIONS (See Table 20.2)

VI. OFFICE PRACTICE CONSIDERATIONS (see Table 20.3)

MEDIAL COLLATERAL LIGAMENT INJURIES

I. OVERVIEW

A. **Definition: a medial collateral ligament (MCL) is a structure that attaches to the medial femoral condyle proximally and the medial tibia plateau distally with the major function being to resist valgus rotation of the knee.**

B. **Incidence: disruption is usually partial but ligament can be completely ruptured from the femoral insertion in violent twisting injuries.**

II. ASSESSMENT

A. **History: mechanism of injury.**
   1. Similar to those sustained with ACL tears.
   2. Frequently occur at same time.

B. **Physical examination.**
   1. Palpate along length of ligament to assess pain, most severe at site of greatest injury.
   2. Flex knee to assess pain.
   3. Apply valgus stress to assess motion (see ACL Injuries).
   4. Compare with normal knee.
   5. Examine knee for associated injuries.
      a. ACL tear – hemarthrosis.
      b. Menisci – joint line pain.
      c. Patella – apprehension when patella is moved laterally.

C. **Diagnostic tests.**
   1. X-rays to assess for bony avulsion from femur or tibia.
   2. MRI is not usually indicated unless there is an associated injury or diagnosis is in doubt.

III. COMMON THERAPEUTIC MODALITIES

A. **Initial treatment.**
   1. To reduce swelling.
      a. Apply ice.
      b. Elevate the extremity.
      c. Administer anti-inflammatory medication.
   2. Use mild narcotic pain medication, if needed.
   3. Compressive bracing.
      a. Sleeve bracing for minor injury.
      b. Hinged bracing for major injury.
   4. Physical therapy program to restore motion.

B. **Conservative management.**
   1. Appropriate for grade I and II injuries.
   2. Initial treatment as above.
   3. Refrain from sports for 6-12 weeks depending on sport and severity of injury.

C. **Surgical treatment.**
   1. Appropriate for some grade III injuries.
   2. Appropriate for injuries with associated ligamentous injuries.
   3. Initial treatment as above.
   4. Repair can be primary or may require use of graft.

D. **Physical therapy considerations. (Same as those for ACL Injuries.)**

IV. NURSING DIAGNOSES, OUTCOMES, AND INTERVENTIONS (See Table 20.1)

V. HOME CARE CONSIDERATIONS (See Table 20.2)

VI. OFFICE PRACTICE CONSIDERATIONS (See Table 20.3)

POSTERIOR CRUCIATE LIGAMENT INJURIES

I. OVERVIEW. Definition: the posterior cruciate ligament (PCL) is one of the main stabilizing ligaments of the knee. It attaches at the posterior surface of the tibia and inserts at the lateral intracondylar notch surface of the medial femoral condyle. The PCL is the primary restraint to posterior displacement of the tibia on the femur.

II. ASSESSMENT

A. History: mechanism of injury.

1. Falling directly in flexed knee where the tibia is forced backwards.
2. Direct blow to anteromedial aspect of the knee with leg extended.

B. Physical examination.

1. Observe swelling due to bleeding from torn fibers (note that swelling is less than with ACL tear).
2. Range of motion is not significantly compromised and patients frequently do not realize the extent of injury.
3. Feeling of unsteadiness when descending slopes or putting weight on bent knee.
4. Positive posterior sag sign.
   a. Can look like anterior drawer sign.
   b. Easily distinguished by observing knee from the side.
   c. Tibia sags backwards.
5. Examine uninjured knee to assess normal motion.
6. Perform posterior drawer test to assess ligamentous laxity by exerting force on the tibia with the knee flexed. Tibia will move posterior to femur (see Anterior Cruciate Ligament Injuries, physical examination, in this chapter).
7. Examine for associated injuries.
   a. Posterolateral corner injuries.
   b. Lateral collateral ligament injuries.

C. Diagnostic tests.

1. X-rays assess the alignment of tibia on femur and for any avulsion fracture.
2. MRI assesses injury to PCL and other soft tissue structure.

Table 20.3
Common Office Practice Considerations

1. Assist with patient flow and scheduling.
2. Take history and perform physical examination.
3. Provide telephone triage.
4. Support insurance certification issues.
5. Communicate effectively.
   a. Patient, family, and/or significant others.
   b. Other members of the health team.
6. Assist with patient/family education.
   a. Pre-procedure.
   b. Postoperative.
   c. Home care considerations.
7. Assist with clinical procedures.
   a. Injections/aspirations.
   b. Suture/staple removal.
8. Monitor treatment effectiveness.
9. Track medications and effects.
10. Assist with outcomes data collection and management.

III. COMMON THERAPEUTIC MODALITIES

A. Initial treatment.

1. To reduce swelling.
   a. Apply ice.
   b. Elevate the extremity.
   c. Administer anti-inflammatory medication.
2. Use mild narcotic pain medication for pain reduction.
3. Compression bracing.
   a. Support during ambulation.
   b. Help reduce swelling.
4. Crutch walking if avulsion fracture is present.
5. Restore range of motion gradually.

B. Nonsurgical management.

1. Used for tears.
2. Isolated PCL injuries without avulsion: rarely need surgical intervention as knee stability is not compromised.
3. Initial treatment as above.

C. Surgical treatment.

1. For avulsion fracture.
2. Indicated for combined ligament injury.
3. Chronic PCL injury where the tibia translates more than 15 mm.
4. Initial treatment as above.
5. Surgical intervention when motion has returned and swelling has subsided.
6. Reconstruction using patella tendon autograft or Achilles tendon allograft.

D. Physical therapy considerations.

1. Nonsurgical patient.
   a. Supervised physical therapy to restore normal motion and strength.
   b. Emphasize rest for 24-48 hours with leg elevated.

2. Surgical patients.
    a. Supervised physical therapy but no active hamstring work for 4 weeks.
    b. Communicate with physical therapist for progression of motion/bracing/return to sports.
    c. Emphasize rest for 24-48 hours with leg elevated.

IV. NURSING DIAGNOSES, OUTCOMES, AND INTERVENTIONS (See Table 20.1)

V. HOME CARE CONSIDERATIONS (See Table 20.2)

VI. OFFICE PRACTICE CONSIDERATIONS (See Table 20.3)

EXTENSOR MECHANISM DISORDERS/INJURIES

I. OVERVIEW

A. Definition: the extensor mechanism is composed of the quadriceps tendon, patella and patellar tendon.

B. Pathophysiology.

1. Patella malalignment.
2. Alteration in patella tracking in femoral trochlea causing excessive force to the under surface of the patella.
3. Quadriceps tendon rupture.
4. The tendon ruptures from its insertion on the proximal pole of the patella.
5. Rarely ruptures in the body of the tendon.
6. Frequently avulses bone.
7. Patellar tendon rupture.
8. Tendon ruptures from its insertion on the distal pole of patella can avulse bone.
9. Patella fracture.
10. Patella dislocation.

II. ASSESSMENT

A. History: mechanism of injury.

1. Patella malalignment.
2. Chronic condition that causes pain under patella during activities that high load patellofemoral joint as in:
    a. Running.
    b. Squatting.
    c. Ascending/descending stairs.
    d. Rising from sitting position, more common in females.
3. Quadriceps tendon rupture: occurs when extremely high load is exerted on the tendon with knee slightly flexed as in tripping down stairs.
4. Patellar tendon rupture:
    a. Commonly occurs when quadriceps tendon contracts violently against resistance in the extended knee as in football and soccer.
    b. Commonly occurs in patients who have a history of patellar tendinitis (jumper's knee).
5. Patella fracture:
    a. Caused by a direct blow as in a dashboard impact injury.
    b. A direct fall.
    c. Can occur when quadriceps or patella tendon ruptures.
6. Patella dislocation:
    a. May result from direct blow either medially or laterally.
    b. Frequently these patients have a history of patella malalignment.

B. Physical examination.

1. Patella malalignment.
    a. Pain on compression of patella against femur.
    b. Patella is hypermobile.
2. Poor quadriceps and vastis medialis obliques (VMO) development.
3. Quadriceps tendon rupture.
    a. Compression tenderness at site of injury.
    b. Hematoma.
    c. Inability to extend knee against gravity.
    d. Defect in tendon may be palpable.
    e. Patella may sit low (patella baja).
5. Patellar tendon rupture.
    a. Compression tenderness at site of injury.
    b. Palpable defect in tendon.
    c. Patient is unable to extend knee.
    d. Patella may sit high (patella alta).
6. Patella fracture.
    a. Severe swelling.
    b. Hemarthrosis.
    c. Severe pain on compression.
    d. May not be able to raise leg or extend knee depending upon severity of fracture.
7. Patella dislocation.
    a. Severe swelling.
    b. Hemarthrosis.
    c. Tenderness along medial/lateral retinaculum.
    d. Apprehension on examination when patella is pushed laterally or medially.

C. Diagnostic tests.

1. Patella malalignment.
    a. X-rays assess alignment of patella with trochlea.
    b. MRI rarely of any use.
2. Quadriceps tendon rupture.
    a. X-rays assess position of patella (baja) and any bony avulsion.
    b. MRI to assess extent of injury to tendon.
3. Patellar tendon rupture.
    a. X-rays assess position of patella (alta) and any bony avulsion.
    b. MRI assesses extent of injury to tendon.
4. Patella fracture.
    a. X-rays assess extent of fracture.
    b. CT and 3-D MRI assesses fracture anatomy for repair but are rarely required.
5. Patella dislocation.
    a. X-rays assess bony avulsion and position of patella.
    b. MRI assesses associated soft tissue injury.

III. COMMON THERAPEUTIC MODALITIES

A. Treatment management plan.

1. Patella malalignment.
   a. Bracing and/or taping to aid in alignment.
   b. Physical therapy to strengthen quadriceps tendon and vastis medalis obliques.
   c. Use of anti-inflammatory medication to reduce swelling and irritation.
   d. Retinacular stretching to allow centralization of patella.
2. Quadriceps tendon rupture.
   a. To reduce swelling:
      (1) Elevate the extremity.
      (2) Apply ice.
      (3) Administer anti-inflammatory medications.
   b. Reduce pain with mild narcotic pain medication, if needed.
   c. Brace leg in extension for 4 weeks (for partial tears).
   d. Surgical repair is indicated in complete rupture with/without bony avulsion.
3. Patellar tendon rupture.
   a. To reduce swelling:
      (1) Elevate the extremity.
      (2) Apply ice.
      (3) Administer anti-inflammatory medications.
   b. Reduce pain with mild narcotic pain medication, if needed.
   c. Requires early surgical repair.
4. Patella fracture.
   a. To reduce swelling:
      (1) Elevate the extremity.
      (2) Apply ice.
      (3) Administer anti-inflammatory medications.
   b. Reduce pain with mild narcotic pain medication, if needed.
   c. Brace in extension for nonsurgical patients with minimally displaced fractures.
   d. Crutch walking with partial weight bearing and knee braced in full extension.
   e. Surgical open reduction for fragmented, severe fractures.
5. Patella dislocation.
   a. Reduce pain and swelling as above.
   b. Reduce dislocation if still present at time of examination.
   c. Compressive sleeve bracing for 2-4 weeks to allow for soft tissue healing.
   d. Gentle quadriceps isometric exercises to prevent atrophy.

B. Physical therapy considerations.

1. Patella malalignment.
   a. Strengthen quadriceps/hamstring/vastis medalis obliques to aid in centralizing the patella.
   b. Avoid leg extensions.
2. Quadriceps tendon rupture: restore normal extensor mechanism function.
3. Patellar tendon rupture: restore normal extensor mechanism function.
4. Patella fracture.
   a. Strengthen quadriceps/hamstring/vastis medalis obliques to aid in centralizing the patella.
   b. Avoid leg extensions.
5. Patella dislocation:
   a. Strengthen quadriceps/hamstring/vastis medalis obliques to aid in centralizing the patella.
   b. Avoid leg extensions.

IV. NURSING DIAGNOSES, OUTCOMES, AND INTERVENTIONS (See Table 20.1)

V. HOME CARE CONSIDERATIONS (See Table 20.2)

VI. OFFICE PRACTICE CONSIDERATIONS (See Table 20.3)

CHONDROMALACIA OF PATELLA

I. OVERVIEW

A. Definition: chondromalacia of the patella is a degeneration of articular cartilage of the patella and should be described as a pathological condition of the cartilage and not a clinical syndrome. Unfortunately, it is often referred to as patellofemoral syndrome.

B. Etiology.

1. Biomechanical causes.
   a. Acute.
      (1) Dislocation of the patella with a chondral or osteochondral fracture.
      (2) Direct trauma.
      (3) Fractures of the patella, resulting in incongruous surfaces.
   b. Chronic.
      (1) Recurrent subluxation or dislocation of the patella.
      (2) Increased quadriceps angle.
      (3) Quadriceps muscle imbalance, either weakness or abnormal attachment of the vastus medialis.
      (4) Patella alta.
      (5) Post-traumatic malalignment following femoral shaft fracture.
      (6) Excessive lateral pressure syndrome.
      (7) Meniscal injury with alteration of synchronous pattern of patella movement and loss of stability.
      (8) Reflex sympathetic dystrophy.
      (9) Medial femoral condylar ridge.
2. Biochemical causes.
   a. Disease.
      (1) Rheumatoid arthritis.
      (2) Recurrent hemarthrosis.
      (3) Alkaptonuria.
      (4) Peripheral synovitis.

(5) Sepsis and adhesions.
b. Iatrogenic.
(1) Repeated intraarticular steroid injections.
(2) Prolonged immobilization.
c. Degenerative: primary osteoarthritis.

II. ASSESSMENT

A. History.
1. Trauma.
2. Pathologies.

B. Physical examination.
1. Dull, aching discomfort well localized to the anterior part of the knee that is most prominent after sitting in one position for a long time.
2. Variable crepitus.
3. Catching or giving way sensation with activity.
4. Pain and giving way especially while descending stairs.
5. Puffiness or swelling in presence of synovitis.

III. COMMON THERAPEUTIC MODALITIES

A. Nonsurgical management – preferred.
1. NSAIDs.
2. Intra-articular injections.
3. Quadriceps exercises and hamstring stretching exercises.

B. Surgical treatment – after failed conservative treatment.
1. Arthroscopic patella shaving.
2. Local excision of defects with drilling of the subchondral bone.
3. Facetectomy.
4. Mechanical decompression of the patellofemoral joint by elevating anteriorly the tibial tuberosity (Maquet procedure).
5. Patellectomy.
6. Autologous chondrocyte transplantation, a two-stage procedure.
a. Indications.
(1) Cartilaginous defects of femoral condyle, medial, lateral, or trochlear caused by repetitive motion or acute trauma.
(2) Defect size less than $10cm^2$.
(3) Patients 15-55 years old.
b. Contraindications.
(1) Patella defects.
(2) Global arthritis.
(3) Lesions greater than $10cm^2$.
(4) Kissing lesions (defects on same side of joint in both femur and tibia).
(5) More than 2 lesions.
(6) Age greater than 55 years old.
c. Two-stage procedure.
(1) First stage.
(a) Arthroscopic surgery to harvest chondrocytes.
(b) Cells are then cultured and grown in lab for approximately 6 weeks.
(2) Second stage: open procedure to transplant cultured cells back into the knee.

IV. NURSING DIAGNOSES, OUTCOMES, AND INTERVENTIONS (See Table 20.1)

V. HOME CARE CONSIDERATIONS (See Table 20.2)

VI. OFFICE PRACTICE CONSIDERATIONS

A. See Table 20.3.

B. Special planning and scheduling for two-stage autologous chondrocyte transplantation procedure.

TENDINITIS AND BURSITIS

I. OVERVIEW

A. Definition: tendinitis is the inflammation of tendons and bursitis is the inflammation of bursae.

B. Etiology.
1. Tendinitis.
a. Overuse, repetitive activity.
b. Overload, sudden increase in activity.
c. Mechanical abnormality:
(1) Leg length inequality.
(2) Leg malalignment.
(3) Foot abnormalities, excessive supination or pronation.
d. Muscle imbalance.
2. Bursitis.
a. Acute or chronic trauma.
b. Acute or chronic pyogenic infection.
c. Low-grade inflammatory conditions:
(1) Gout.
(2) Syphilis.
(3) Tuberculosis.
(4) Rheumatoid arthritis.
3. Specific bursitis conditions of the knee.
a. Prepatella bursitis.
(1) Trauma.
(a) An acute injury.
(b) Fall directly on patella.
(2) Recurrent minor injuries ("Housemaid's Knee").
(3) Pyogenic prepatella bursitis is common, especially in children.
b. Popliteal cyst (Baker cyst).
(1) Typically a distended bursa and fluid build up behind the knee with unsure etiology.
(2) Herniation of the synovial membrane through the posterior part of the capsule of the knee, or escape of fluid through the normal communication of bursa with the knee.

II. ASSESSMENT

A. History.
1. Trauma, acute or chronic.
2. Infections, acute or chronic.
3. Other inflammatory pathologies:
a. Gout.

b. Syphilis.
c. Tuberculosis.
d. Rheumatoid arthritis.
4. Occupational/recreational activities that involve repetitive motion.
5. Previous knee or foot abnormalities.

B. Physical examination.
1. Pain and tenderness.
2. Swelling.
3. Warmth.
4. Limited motion and joint stiffness.

III. COMMON THERAPEUTIC MODALITIES.

A. Conservative treatment – usually beneficial.
1. Relative rest.
2. Ice.
3. Neoprene sleeve.
4. NSAIDs.
5. Alteration in occupational/recreational habits.
6. Properly fitted orthotics to address mechanical deformities.
7. Appropriate flexibility and muscle-strengthening exercises.

B. Invasive procedures – if conservative treatment fails.
1. Aspiration and injection of an appropriate drug.
2. Incision and drainage.
3. Excision of chronically infected or thickened bursae.
4. Removal of underlying bony prominence.

C. Treatment for specific bursitis conditions.
1. Prepatella bursitis.
   a. Recurrent minor injuries ("Housemaid's Knee").
      (1) Usually responds to conservative treatment.
      (2) Excision of the bursa, if fibrosis or synovial thickening with painful nodules fail to respond with conservative treatment.
   b. Pyogenic prepatella bursitis is common, especially in children.
      (1) Often responds:
         (a) One or two daily aspirations.
         (b) Immobilization.
         (c) Antibiotic therapy.
      (2) If symptoms persist after 36-48 hours, an incision and drainage may be indicated.
2. Popliteal cyst (Baker cyst).
   a. Observation, as it may disappear on its own.
   b. Aspiration and injection of steroid.
   c. Surgical excision, if persistent recurrence.

IV. NURSING DIAGNOSES, OUTCOMES, AND INTERVENTIONS (See Table 20.1)

V. HOME CARE CONSIDERATIONS (See Table 20.2)

VI. OFFICE PRACTICE CONSIDERATIONS (See Table 20.3)

DISCOID MENISCUS IN CHILDREN

I. OVERVIEW

A. Definition: discoid meniscus is an intra-articular knee lesion in children that is characterized by round rather than crescent shaped menisci.

B. Etiology:
1. Caused by lack of anatomic attachment of the posterior horn of the lateral meniscus to the tibial plateau.
2. Results in an abnormal motion of the lateral meniscus leading to a hypertrophy into the discoid form.

II. ASSESSMENT

A. History and physical examination.
1. Pain.
2. Clicking.
3. Swelling.
4. Locking.

B. Diagnostic tests: x-ray which shows:
1. Widening of lateral joint space.
2. Flattening of lateral femoral condyle.
3. Tilt of articular surface of the lateral femoral condyle.
4. Hypoplasia of the lateral tibial spine.
5. More proximal position of the tibial head.

III. COMMON THERAPEUTIC MODALITIES

A. Nonsurgical management.
1. NSAIDs.
2. Physical therapy.

B. Surgical treatment.
1. Arthroscopic partial menisectomy, provided the remaining peripheral meniscal rim is stable.
2. Arthroscopic total menisectomy is considered due to underlying instability of the peripheral attachment of the posterior segment of the meniscus that will lead to significant osteoarthritis.

IV. NURSING DIAGNOSES, OUTCOMES, AND INTERVENTIONS

A. See Chapter 11, Pediatric/Congenital Disorders.
B. See Table 20.1.

V. HOME CARE CONSIDERATIONS

A. Modification of child's activities.
B. Parent's ability to participate in treatment plan.
C. Pain management.
D. Observation and recurrent assessment.
E. See Table 20.2.

VI. OFFICE PRACTICE CONSIDERATIONS (See Table 20.3)

OSTEOCHONDRITIS DISSECANS IN CHILDREN

I. OVERVIEW

A. Definition: osteochondritis dissecans in children is an intra-articular joint lesion.

1. Characterized by disorderly endochondral ossification of epiphyseal growth during childhood.
2. Involves medial femoral condyle block of bone from its bed.

B. Etiology: secondary to:

1. Trauma.
2. Ischemia.
3. Abnormal ossification within the epiphysis.

C. Pathophysiology.

1. In the early stage x-rays show small irregularity of medial condyle.
2. As growth proceeds, irregularity develops area of bone separated from rest of condyle by a transradiant line.
3. Articular surface overlying lesion is intact at first.
4. After skeletal maturity, fragments may become loose and separate as loose bodies within the knee.

D. Classification.

1. Category I:
   a. Involves children through early adolescence.
   b. Skeletal age 11 for girls, 13 for boys.
   c. Associated with excellent prognosis.
2. Category II:
   a. Includes the age group of skeletal age 12 for girls and 14 for boys to the age of 20 for both.
   b. The physes may continue to appear open radiographically, although their contribution to longitudinal growth is minimal.
3. Category III:
   a. Includes patients 20 years of age.
   b. Or older people with closed physes increasing risk of:
      (1) Developing significant joint deformation with possible loose fragment formation.
      (2) Extensive articular defects.

II. ASSESSMENT

A. History and physical examination.

1. Pain worse with walking and hyperextension.
2. Stiffness.
3. Swelling.
4. Locking.
5. Giving way.
6. Tenderness medial to patella ligament.

B. Diagnostic tests: x-rays.

III. COMMON THERAPEUTIC MODALITIES

A. Category I: nonsurgical.

1. Observation.
2. Activity restriction and rest.
3. Possible immobilization.

B. Category II.

1. Rest the knee joint.
2. Observation for nonprogressive lesions.
3. Arthroscopy for lesions larger than 1 cm in size or located in weight-bearing area.

C. Category III.

1. Drilling for lesions that are not separated.
2. Drilling and pin stabilization for early fragment separation.
3. Large, detached lesions are curretaged, followed by stabilization with pins and bone grafting.

IV. NURSING DIAGNOSES, OUTCOMES, AND INTERVENTIONS

A. See Chapter 11, Pediatric/Congenital Disorders.

B. See Table 20.1.

V. HOME CARE CONSIDERATIONS

A. Modification of child's activities.

B. Parent's ability to participate in treatment plan.

C. Pain management.

D. Observation and recurrent assessment.

E. See Table 20.2.

VI. OFFICE PRACTICE CONSIDERATIONS (See Table 20.3)

Bibliography

Aichroth, P., & Cannon, W.D. (1992). Patellofemoral joint disorders. In P. Aichroth & W.D. Cannon (Eds.), *Knee surgery: Current practice* (pp. 354-412). London: Martin Dunitz, Ltd.

Brandt, K. D. (1997). Management of osteoarthritis. In W.N. Kelly, S. Ridley, E.D. Harris, & C.B. Sledge (Eds.), *Textbook of rheumatology* (5th ed) (Vol. 2, pp.1394-1401). Philadelphia: W.B. Saunders.

Dee, R., Hurst, L.C., Gruber, M.A., & Kottmeier, S.A. (1997). *Principles of orthopaedic practice* (2nd ed.). New York: McGraw-Hill.

Fadale, P., & Hulstyn, M. (1997). Common athletic knee injuries. *Clinics in Sports Medicine, 16*(3), 479-497.

Fu, F.H., Harner, C.D., & Vince, K.G., (1994). *Knee surgery.* Baltimore: Williams & Wilkins.

Harris, M., Williams, C., Stanish, W.D., & Micheli, L.J. (Eds.). (1994). Acute sports injuries: The knee. In *Oxford textbook of sports medicine* (pp. 342-418). New York: Oxford Medical Publications.

Hoppenfeld, S. (Ed.). (1976). Physical examination of the knee. In *Physical examination of the spine and extremities* (pp.171-196). New York: Appleton, Centry-Crofts.

Hungerford, D.S. (1998, January-April). Treating osteoarthritis with chondroprotective agents. *Orthopaedic Special Edition, 4*(1), 1-4.

Insall, J.N. (1984). *Surgery of the knee.* New York: Churchill Livingstone.

Kotz, R., & Kolarz, G. (1999). Intra-articular hyaluronic acid: Duration of effect and results of repeated treatment cycles. *American Journal of Orthopaedics, 28*(Suppl. 11S), 5-7.

Macnicol, M.F. (1992). The conservative management of the anterior cruciate ligament deficient knee. In P.M. Aichroth, W.D. Cannon, & D.V. Poatel (Eds.) *Knee surgery: Current practice* (pp. 206-217). New York: Raven Press.

Neal, L.J. (1996). Outpatient ACL surgery: The role of the home health nurse. *Orthopaedic Nursing, 15*(4), 9-13.

Salmond, S.W., Mooney, N.E., & Verdisco, L.A. (1996). *NAON core curriculum for orthopaedic nursing* (3rd ed.). Pitman, New Jersey: National Association of Orthopaedic Nurses.

Schoen, D.C. (2000). The knee and lower leg. In D.C. Schoen, *Adult orthopaedic nursing* (pp. 317-357). Philadelphia: Lippincott.

Scuderi, G.R., Scott, W.N., & Insall, J.N. (1996). Injuries of the knee. In C.A. Rockwood, D.P.L. Green, R.W. Bucholz, & J.D. Hickman (Eds.), *Rockwood and Green's fractures in adults* (pp. 2001-2126). Philadelphia: Lippincott-Raven.

Silby, M., & Fu, F. (Eds.). (1994). Knee injuries. In *Sports injuries: Mechanisms, preventions, treatments* (pp. 949-974). Baltimore: Williams & Wilkins.

Windsor, R.E. (1994). The adult knee. In S.L. Weinstein & J.A. Buckwalter (Eds.), *Turek's orthopaedics: Principles and their application* (pp. 585-614). Philadelphia: J.B. Lippincott.

Wobig, M., Dickhut, A., Maier, R., & Vetter, G. (1998). Viscosupplementation with hylan G-F 20: A 26-week controlled trial of efficacy and safety in the osteoarthritic knee. *Clinical Therapy, 20*(3), 410-423.

STUDY QUESTIONS

Mary, a 73-year-old, retired sales clerk presents to the office with complaints of right knee pain on the medial aspect especially during weight-bearing activity. She is 54 inches, 197 pounds and describes an increasing stiffness and inability to perform activities of daily living (ADL). She reports no injury or trauma to her knee. She can ambulate two blocks without the support of a cane but she cannot do stairs at all. (Questions 1-4)

1. Which of the following are **not** necessary for determining the diagnosis?
   a. Health history and physical examination of her knee.
   b. Observation of her gait with and without the use of a cane.
   c. X-ray views to include standing AP, lateral, and patella sunrise views.
   d. The Lachman and anterior draw tests.

2. Most likely diagnosis is:
   a. Torn anterior cruciate ligament.
   b. Osteochondritis dissecans, category II.
   c. Degenerative arthritis of the knee.
   d. Fractured femur which has not calcified properly.

3. Which of the following would most likely **not** be a nonsurgical treatment for Mary's condition?
   a. Physical therapy.
   b. Course of NSAIDs.
   c. Intra-articular injection.
   d. Bed rest and/or NWB until surgery.

4. In general, which is a contraindication to total knee arthroplasty?
   a. Patients above 80 years of age.
   b. Osteonecrosis and post-traumatic arthritis.
   c. Active infection anywhere in the body.
   d. Failed previous conservative treatment.

5. Arthroscopic debridement is advocated for:
   a. Patients with advanced arthritis.
   b. Malignant tumors about the knee.
   c. Young patient with mild degenerative changes.
   d. Chronic and recurring pain in the knee.

Wally A. is a 21-year-old college student who injured his knee in a slow, twisting skiing fall. He presents in the clinic with severe swelling, loss of motion, and is wearing a knee immobilizer. (Questions 6-7)

6. The most frequent injury with this type of fall is:
   a. PCL/quad tendon rupture.
   b. ACL/MCL rupture.
   c. Patellar tendon rupture.
   d. Fractures patella.

7. Initial treatment for Wally includes:
   a. Ice, NSAIDs, pain medication, physical therapy.
   b. Immediate surgical intervention and immobilization.
   c. Continued bracing and knee aspiration to reduce swelling.
   d. Quadriceps strengthening and NWB ambulation.

8. The most common graft choice for ACL reconstruction in young adults is:
   a. Achilles tendon allograft.
   b. Hamstring tendon autograft
   c. Patellar tendon autograft.
   d. Patellar tendon allograft.

Bill C. is a plumber who accidentally tripped when walking down a flight of stairs. He presents in the clinic with swelling and pain in his thigh. He is unable to extend his knee against gravity. (Questions 9-10)

9. The most probable diagnosis of Bill's condition is:
   a. Complete patellar tendon rupture.
   b. Complete quadriceps tendon rupture.
   c. Comminuted patella fracture and dislocation.
   d. Partial rupture of the hamstring.

10. The most common treatment for Bill's condition includes:
   a. Surgical repair.
   b. Lovenox and mechanical device.
   c. Conservative treatment only.
   d. Total knee replacement.

David is a 38-year-old weekend warrior. When playing an aggressive game of singles tennis he leaped in the air for an overhead shot and landed on one foot. He felt a sharp pain on the inner aspect of his knee. He stopped playing immediately and iced his knee but noticed that when he twisted his knee the wrong way the pain returned. He presented in the clinic in no apparent distress but was concerned that he was unable to return to tennis without pain. X-rays were ordered but showed no bony abnormality. The physician felt that David most likely had a medial meniscal tear. (Questions 11-12)

11. The only definitive radiologic exam to confirm meniscal tearing is:
   a. AP weight bearing X-ray.
   b. MRI.
   c. Venogram.
   d. Myelogram.

12. When doing the physical examination, which of the following is not a sign of suspected Meniscal tearing?
   a. Joint line tenderness/pain.
   b. Knee locked in extension
   c. Pain with squatting, twisting
   d. Negative Steinman/McMurray test.

13. Chondromalacia of the patella can be the result of many things. Which of the following is **not** a causative factor?
   a. Recurrent dislocation of the patella.
   b. Direct trauma to the patella.
   c. Repeated intra-articular steroid injections.
   d. Decreased quadriceps angle.

14. Autologous chondrocyte transplantation is:
   a. A one-stage transplant procedure.
   b. Indicated for patella defects.
   c. Indicated for lesions less than $10cm^2$.
   d. Indicated for global arthritis.

15. Which of the following is not a treatment for a Baker's cyst?
   a. Observation only, since it may disappear.
   b. Aspiration and injection with steroids.
   c. Surgical excision is persistent recurrence.
   d. Whirlpool and ultrasound treatment.

Chapter 21 FOOT AND ANKLE

Maureen (Moe) Schmitt, MN, FNP, ONC

Contents

OBJECTIVES

At the completion of this chapter, the learner will be able to:

- Discuss the basic anatomy of the foot and ankle.
- List the types of injuries that occur in the foot and ankle.
- Discuss common nonsurgical treatments for foot and ankle pathologies.
- Describe surgical interventions for fractures, instabilities, and deformities.
- Identify nursing interventions for managing patients with foot and ankle problems.
- Discuss safety issues associated with foot and ankle injuries.
- Identify home care needs for the patient with foot and ankle injuries.

KEY POINTS

- The biomechanics of the foot and ankle are essential to gait.
- The swelling associated with injuries to the foot and ankle may postpone healing or surgical repair. Elevation, ice, and support are essential.
- Most fractures associated with the foot and ankle will require protected weight bearing.
- Ankle sprains are a very common musculoskeletal injury. They are best treated with early range of motion, early weight bearing if tolerated, and strengthening.
- Common foot problems are usually related to shoe wear.

CHAPTER 21

FOOT AND ANKLE

ANATOMY

I. BONES

A. Ankle (3 bones).

1. Tibia: larger bone on the medial (inner) side of the leg.
   a. Distal end flares out to make the medial malleolus.
   b. Articulates with the talus and fibula.
2. Fibula: smaller bone on the lateral side of the leg.
   a. Distal end flares out to make the lateral malleolus.
   b. Articulates with the tibia.
3. Talus: a wedged shaped bone consisting of a head, neck, and body. The wedge shape allows for little to no inversion or eversion of the ankle when it is in dorsiflexion.
   a. Also articulates with the calcaneus (subtalar joint) and the navicular bones.
   b. Has extensive articular cartilage, covering approximately 60% of its surface.
   c. Has no muscular attachments, therefore has a limited blood supply.

B. Foot (26 bones).

1. Hindfoot.
   a. Talus.
   b. Calcaneus (heelbone): largest bone of the foot.
2. Midfoot.
   a. Navicular (scaphoid).
   b. Cuboid.
   c. 3 cuneiforms.
      (1) Lateral.
      (2) Middle.
      (3) Medial.
3. Forefoot.
   a. 5 metatarsals.
   b. 5 phalanges, proximal.
   c. 4 phalanges, middle.
   d. 5 phalanges, distal.

II. JOINTS

A. Ankle.

1. Tibiofibular joint.
   a. A fibrous or syndesmosis (ligamentous) type of joint.
   b. Supported by ligaments, especially the interosseous ligament that runs the full length of the tibia and fibula.
   c. Joint movement is minimal: only 1 to 2 mm of "spread" during dorsiflexion.
2. Tibiotalar and fibulotalar joints make up the talocrural joint.
   a. As a hinged synovial joint, allows only flexion and extension.
   b. Designed for stability.
   c. Forces across the ankle joint during standing equals twice the body weight and during ambulation > 5 times the body weight.

B. Hindfoot: subtalar joint.

1. Articulation of the talus and calcaneus.
2. A gliding joint that provides most of the inversion and eversion of the foot and ankle.

C. Midfoot.

1. Talocalcaneonavicular.
2. Cuneonavicular.
3. Cuboidonavicular.
4. Intercuneiform.
5. Cuneocuboid.

D. Forefoot.

1. Tarsometatarsal: Lisfranc's.
   a. Is shaped like a stone arch with the bottom (plantar) component narrower than the top.
   b. The second metatarsal acts as the keystone.
2. Intermetatarsal.
3. Metatarsophalangeal.
4. Interphalangeal.

III. LIGAMENTS (See Table 21.1)

IV. TENDONS: all have synovial sheaths

A. Extensors.

1. Puts the foot and ankle in dorsiflexion.
2. Passes anterior to the ankle joint.

B. Flexors.

1. Puts the foot and ankle in plantar flexion.
2. Passes posterior to the ankle.

C. Peroneals.

1. Everts the foot and ankle.
2. Passes posterior to the lateral malleolus.

V. RETINACULUM

A. Thick fibrous bands that hold the tendons in place.

B. Named for the tendons they cover: extensor, flexor, peroneal.

VI. CALCANEAL FAT PAD: a layer of specialized fat and connective tissue designed to act as shock absorber.

Table 21.1
Ligaments About the Ankle

Ligament	Origin	Insertion	Purpose	Notes
Syndesmotic				
1. Anterior Tibiofibular	Anterior tibia	Anterior fibula	Supports the anterior tibiofibular joint	
2. Posterior Tibiofibular	Posterior tibia	Posterior fibula	Supports the posterior tibiofibular joint	
3. Interosseous	Tibia - entire length	Fibula - entire length	Connects the tibia and fibula throughout the entire length (knee to ankle)	
Lateral				
1. Anterior Talofibular (ATFL)	Lateral malleolus	Neck of the talus	Provides stability against excessive inversion of the talus. Most important lateral stabilizer	• Most commonly injured ligament in the ankle. • Intraarticular
2. Posterior Talobibular (PTLF)	Lateral malleolus	Posterior tubercule of the talus	Resists ankle dorsiflexion and talar adduction, medial rotation, and rotation	• Intraarticular
3. Calcaneo-Fibular (CFL)	Lateral malleolus	Calcaneus	Provides stability against maximum inversion at the ankle and subtalar joint	• Extraarticular
Medial				
Deltoid	Medial tibia	Talus	Provides stability against eversion	• Quadrangular shape • Only ligament in ankle with elastic tissue so can stretch rather than tear.

VII. ARCHES

A. Allow the foot to vary its function during weight bearing.

B. 3 main arches.

1. Medial longitudinal extends from the 1st metatarsal (MT) head to the calcaneus, and is functionally the most important.
2. Lateral longitudinal, extends from the 4th and 5th MT head to the calcaneus.
3. Transverse arch lies behind the metatarsal heads and is oriented perpendicular to the longitudinal arches.

VIII. BLOOD SUPPLY

A. Dorsalis pedis artery: supplies the anterior foot and ankle and provides branches for the plantar surface of the foot.

B. Posterior tibial artery: supplies the lateral and hind foot and provides branches for the plantar surface of the foot.

IX. NERVES

A. Motor.

1. Peripheral.
   a. Tibial: toe movement, ankle flexion and inversion.
   b. Peroneal: ankle and toe extension, ankle eversion.

2. Nerve roots.
   a. L4: anterior tibialis.
      (1) Extends and everts the ankle.
      (2) Dorsiflexes the foot.
   b. L5: extensor hallus longus, and extends (lifts) the great toe.
   c. S1: gastrocnemius.
      (1) Flexes the ankle.
      (2) Plantar flexes the foot.

B. Sensory.
1. Of all the peripheral nerves supplying the foot and ankle the most important to the nurse is the deep peroneal, which provides sensation to the 1st web space.
2. Stems from L4, L5, and S1 nerve roots.

ASSESSMENT OF THE FOOT AND ANKLE

I. HISTORY

A. Obtain description of the injury.
1. What happened.
2. Where did it happen.
3. When did it happen.
4. Whether there has been prior injuries

B. Obtain pain assessment.

C. Question patient about mobility and sensation of the ankle and foot.
1. Stability.
2. Mobility.
3. Ability to weight bear.
4. Changes in sensation.

D. Obtain a birth history in children with foot deformities.

II. PHYSICAL EXAMINATION

A. Assess the patient's gait.

B. Compare both feet and ankles.

C. Observe the area for swelling, discoloration, and deformity.

D. Palpate the area for tenderness, tenseness, swelling, and masses.

E. Assess range of motion and strength.

F. Assess stability.
1. Anterior drawer at the ankle assesses the integrity of the anterior talofibular ligament (ATFL).
2. Talar tilt test at the ankle assesses whether the ankle mortise opens medially or laterally with eversion or inversion.
3. Tests integrity of the ATFL and calcaneofibular (CFL) ligaments .

G. Do a neurovascular assessment.

H. Evaluate the shoe for wear patterns and support.
1. In normal foot, greatest wear is beneath the ball of the foot slightly to the lateral side.
2. Heel wear is centered.

III. DIAGNOSTIC TESTS (See Table 21.2)

A. X-rays (anterior-posterior, lateral, mortise views, and/or oblique views).
1. Assesses for fractures, tumors, arthritis, and joint integrity.
2. May involve stress views to assess ankle ligaments.
3. Foot films are usually done weight bearing.

B. Computed tomography (CT).
1. Helps diagnose fractures difficult to assess or evaluate with traditional x-rays.
2. Assists with assessment of soft tissue tumors or injury.

C. Magnetic Resonance Imaging (MRI).
1. Assesses high water content tissues such as ligaments, tendons, and bone marrow (osteomyelitis, tumor, etc.).
2. Able to detect avascular necrosis earlier than traditional x-rays.

D. Arthrogram.
1. Assesses joint integrity by filling the joint space with dye.
2. Is invasive and may result in hypersensitivity reactions.

ANKLE SPRAINS

I. OVERVIEW

A. Definition: injury to the ligaments.

B. Etiology.
1. Often a result of overuse or trauma.
2. Inversion forces account for 85% of all ankle sprains therefore the lateral ankle is more commonly involved.

C. Pathology.
1. As the fibers of the ligament tear they initiate an inflammatory response causing swelling and pain.
2. Bleeding may occur.
3. Depending on the extent of the tear, stability of the joint may be compromised.
4. Grading (see Table 21.3).

D. Incidence.
1. Most common ankle injury.
2. Most common athletic injury.

E. Considerations across the lifespan.
1. Aging leads to less elastic ligaments and weaker bone.
2. The same forces that would result in a low-grade sprain in a younger person may result in a more severe sprain or even a fracture in an elderly patient.

F. Complications.
1. Chronic ankle pain.
2. Instability.
3. Arthritis.

II. ASSESSMENT (See the section in this chapter on Assessment of the Foot and Ankle.)

III. COMMON THERAPEUTIC MODALITIES

A. Functional management is the most efficient way back to full activity.
1. Phase 1.
   a. Control pain and inflammation.

Table 21.2
Imaging Studies of the Foot and Ankle

Test	Technique	Purpose
X-rays Radiographs	A high electomagnetic wave that penetrates solid matter and projects it onto film. 1. Common views of the ankle are: Anterior-posterior, lateral, and mortise. 2. Common view of the foot are: Anterior-posterior, lateral, and oblique. a. Usually done weight bearing	1. Assesses for fractures, tumors, arthritis, and joint integrity. 2. May involve stress views to assess ankle ligaments.
CAT/CT Scan (Computerized Axial Tomography)	Transverse planes of tissue are swept by a pinpoint radiographic beam and then reproduced by computerized analysis	1. Helps diagnose fractures difficult to assess or evaluate with traditional x-ray. 2. Assists with assessment of soft tissue tumors or injury.
MRI (Magnetic Resonance Imaging)	A magnetic field and radio waves are used to delineate the hydrogen density of tissues in the body. The image differentiates the differing hydrogen contents among tissue.	1. Assesses high water content tissues such as ligament, tendons, and bone marrow (osteomyelitis, tumor, etc.) 2. Able to detect avascular necrosis earlier than traditional x-rays.
Arthrogram	X-ray/CT of a joint after injection of a radio-opaque dye into the joint space.	1. Assesses joint integrity by visualizing the dye-filled joint space. 2. Is invasive. 3. May result in hypersensitivity reaction.
Bone Scan	A radioisotope is injected into the blood and concentrated in areas of increased bone activity. A gamma camera picks up the emitting rays and identifies "hot spots" that may indicate abnormalities.	1. Detects osteoblastic changes only (stress fracture, infection, arthritis, certain cancers). 2. Results are usually verified by additional testing.

(1) Cryotherapy.
(2) Elevation.
(3) Anti-inflammatory medication.

b. Encourage early weight bearing, and provide protected mobilization of the ankle.
(1) Functional bracing (stirrup type brace).
(2) Assistive ambulatory devices if needed, use until the patient can walk normally.

c. Early range of motion.
(1) Full pain-free active ROM of the ankle.
(2) Heel cord flexibility – towel stretches.

2. Phase 2.
a. Cryotherapy.
b. Increasing range of motion.
c. Muscle strengthening.
(1) Ankle strength – towel slides.
(2) Heel cord flexibility.
(a) Wall stretches.
(b) Chair stretches.
(c) Heel cord board exercises.
(3) Ankle stabilizer muscles.
(a) Calf raises
(b) Inversion/eversion exercises with flexible tubing.

d. Proprioceptive training.
(1) Wobble board.
(2) Cycling.
(3) Swimming.
(4) Short sprints if tolerated.

3. Phase 3, specific exercise program designed to return the athlete back to his/her former activity level.
4. Requirements to return to sports participation.
a. Can test wearing a functional brace.
b. No pain with functional testing.
(1) Walking.

Table 21.3
Ankle Sprains

Grading	Definition	Signs & Symptoms	Treatment
One	Disruption of some ligament fibers	1. Minimal pain 2. No instability 3. Early symptom resolution	1. RICE (Rest, Ice, Compression, Elevation) 2. Use joint as normally as possible 3. Weight bearing as tolerated (WBAT)
Two	Partial ligament Rupture	1. Severe pain 2. Minimal joint instability 3. +/- ecchymosis 4. Swelling	1. RICE 2. Support/splint 3. Gentle ROM 4. WBAT. May need assistive device
Three	Complete ligament Rupture	1. Severe pain initially 2. Unstable joint 3. Swelling 4. Ecchymosis 5. Often associated with bony injury	1. RICE 2. Immobilize 3. Possible surgery 4. Protected weight bearing

(2) Running, forward and backward.
(3) Figure eights or zigzags.
(4) One-foot hops.

c. No swelling.

B. Immobilization is discouraged.

C. Surgery: indicated only for the severely unstable ankle.

IV. NURSING DIAGNOSES, OUTCOMES, AND INTERVENTIONS

A. See Table 21.4.

B. Pain, acute.

1. Outcome: patient's pain is controlled.
2. Interventions.
   a. Cryotherapy/ice.
   b. Elevation.
   c. Medications.
      (1) NSAIDS.
      (2) Analgesics.

B. Physical mobility, impaired.

1. Outcome: patient can ambulate safely within confines of splint/cast and weight-bearing restrictions.
2. Interventions.
   a. Fit or assess for appropriate fit of brace or assistive ambulatory device if prescribed.
   b. Teach or assess for correct use of assistive device.

C. Knowledge, deficient.

1. Outcome: patient understands instructions for care during acute and rehabilitative phase of injury.
2. Interventions.
   a. Reiterate use of elevation and ice for swelling throughout healing and sometimes for months after injury.
   b. Stress importance of maintaining joint mobility via exercises.
   c. Suggest planning rest periods during activity to minimize pain and swelling and to enhance safety.

V. HOME CARE CONSIDERATIONS

A. Determine patient's ability to ambulate safely with cast/splint with weight-bearing restrictions.

B. Knows when and how to control edema.

C. Demonstrates ability to exercise, knows number of times and length of time to exercise.

D. Use of pain control methods.

ACHILLES TENOSYNOVITIS

I. OVERVIEW

A. Definition: inflammation of the Achilles tendon and its lubricating sheath.

B. Etiology.

1. Usually due to overuse.
2. Repetitive microtrauma, especially of the calf muscles.

C. Incidence: commonly seen in athletes, especially runners.

D. Considerations across the lifespan: usually seen in the young to middle-aged adult because of the activities that cause it.

E. Complications.

1. Tendon thickening.
2. Chronic tendinitis.
3. Tendon rupture.

Table 21.4
Common Nursing Diagnoses, Outcomes, and Interventions for Foot and Ankle Problems

Diagnosis	Outcome	Intervention
A. Pain, acute	• Patient will remain comfortable, on a pain scale of < 3.	• RICE • NSAIDS/analgesics
B. Physical mobility, impaired	• Patient will demonstrate the ability to ambulate safely and maintain WB status with assistive devices.	• Appropriate fit and use of assistive devices. • Correct fit and use of shoes, braces, splints, etc.
C. Infection, risk for	• Patient will remain free of any infection.	• Keep dressing dry and intact. Change dressing as indicated. • Instruction on S & S of infection. • Protected WB as indicated. • Elevate foot when indicated.
D. Knowledge, deficient	• Patient/family understands plan of treatment, rationale, rehabilitation process, and their role.	• Minimum 6 weeks recovery. • Teach methods/way to minimize swelling. • Overuse/over-rehabilitation can cause re-injury. • Purpose of cast, splint, brace. Fit and purpose of assistive devices.
E. Self-care deficit syndrome	• The patient will be able to perform ADLs with minimal assistance.	• Provide appropriate devices. • Consider home assistance agencies. • Consider short-term rehabilitation programs.
F. Individual coping, ineffective	• Patient/family will be able to set realistic goals with limitations and demands.	• Instruct regarding need for limit setting. • Provide information about adaptive aids and prostheses. • Suggest alternatives to lifestyle within restriction limitations.
G. Injury, risk for	• The patient will remain safe without further injury.	• Protected WB as indicated. • Elevate foot when indicated. • Use for and care of a foot in a splint, brace care, cast. • Assessment of any potential for injury. • Correct fit and use of devices. • Assistance via family/friends/ agencies to reduce risk.

II. ASSESSMENT

A. History and physical examination.

1. Posterior ankle pain that increases with activity.
   a. Worse at the beginning of the activity.
   b. Subsides as the leg warms up.
2. Limp is common.
3. Swelling.
4. Crepitance.
5. Local tenderness.

B. Diagnostic tests (see Table 21.2).

1. Usually not indicated.
2. CT or MRI may help in some cases.

III. COMMON THERAPEUTIC MODALITIES

A. Observation.

1. Decrease the amount of running or aggravating activity by at least 50%. It is often difficult to get the patient to agree to such restrictions.
2. Avoid uneven ground or hills when running.
3. Ice the area after activity.
4. Use NSAIDs. Remember these may mask pain as well.
5. Perform stretching exercises.
6. Perform heel lifts.

7. Use of steroid injection:
    a. Provides symptomatic relief. Is not a cure.
    b. Last resort. Risk of tendon rupture if steroid is injected directly into tendon.

B. Immobilization: indicated only in severe cases.

C. Surgery: not indicated.

IV. NURSING DIAGNOSES, OUTCOMES, AND INTERVENTIONS

A. Pain, acute.
1. Outcome: patient's pain is controlled.
2. Interventions.
    a. Use ice after activity.
    b. Use NSAIDs.

B. Knowledge, deficient.
1. Outcome: patient heals with minimal complications.
2. Interventions.
    a. Explain why tendon is irritated and rest is needed.
    b. List and define complications.

C. Body image, disturbed.
1. Outcome: patient accepts limitations to running/activity.
2. Interventions.
    a. Suggest alternative methods for relaxation, exercise, and weight maintenance.
    b. Discuss future effects of present reduction in activity level.

V. HOME CARE CONSIDERATIONS

A. Follows prescribed reduction in exercise activity.

B. Discuss ways to alter behavior.

ACHILLES RUPTURE

I. OVERVIEW

A. Definition: breaking apart or disruption of the fibers of the Achilles tendon, partial or complete.

B. Etiology: overload to the tendon due to sudden forceful dorsiflexion.

C. Pathology: force applied to the tendon exceeds its strength and elasticity.

D. Considerations across the lifespan: usually seen in athletes over the age of 30.

E. Complications.
1. Impaired ankle motion.
2. Re-rupture.

II. ASSESSMENT

A. History and physical examination.
1. Sudden pain.
2. Positive/negative audible pop or click.
3. Weakness.
4. Limp.
5. Unable to rise up on toes from a standing position.
6. Positive Thompson test.
    a. With patient prone and foot hanging free or kneeling on a chair.
    b. Squeeze the calf.
    c. Foot should plantarflex.
    d. Positive, there is no response.

B. Diagnostic Tests.
1. MRI to assess extent and location.
2. Ultrasound to assess extent and location.

III. COMMON THERAPEUTIC MODALITIES

A. Observation: partial rupture.
1. Ice.
2. Taping or strapping with the ankle in plantar flexion.
3. Heel lift in shoe to relax the tendon.
4. Stretching exercises after tendon is healed.

B. Immobilization, total rupture.
1. Non-weight-bearing (NWB) cast with foot in plantar flexion (equinas).
2. The foot is gradually brought into a neutral position before final removal.
3. Stretching exercises after cast is removed.

C. Surgery.
1. Recommended in athletes, as surgery is associated with lower re-rupture rate.
2. Followed by casting (as in B. Immobilization, above).
3. Stretching exercises after cast is removed.

IV. NURSING DIAGNOSES, OUTCOMES, AND INTERVENTIONS

A. Physical mobility, impaired.
1. Outcome: patient is able to safely ambulate with assistive device maintaining NWB status.
2. Interventions.
    a. Fit or assess for appropriate fit of cane, crutches, or walker if prescribed.
    b. Teach or assess for correct use of assistive device.

B. Knowledge, deficient: cast care.
Knowledge, deficient: rehabilitation exercises.
1. Outcome: patient is able to care for and maintain the cast and performs the rehabilitative exercises as prescribed.
2. Interventions.
    a. Provide patient with written illustrated instructions for cast care and rehabilitative exercises.
    b. May need physical therapy intervention.

V. HOME CARE CONSIDERATIONS

A. Demonstrates an understanding of cast care.

B. Ambulates safely with assistive device and NWB.

C. Demonstrates correct exercises.

D. Knows appropriate exercises: how many to do and for how long.

PLANTAR FASCITIS

I. OVERVIEW

A. Definition: inflammation of the plantar fascia and periosteum at the fascial insertion site.

Table 21.5
Shoe Wear Guidelines

Suggestion	Rationale
Have both feet measured before trying on shoes. Select the shoe that fits the largest foot.	1. Foot size changes with age. 2. Most people have one foot larger than the other. 3. Sizes vary among brands and styles.
Try on shoes at the end of the day.	1. Feet are largest and widest after being on them all day.
Select a style that conforms to the shape of the foot so that the ball of the foot fits comfortably into the widest part of the shoe.	1. Prevents toe constriction. Shoes that are no more than 1/4" narrower than the foot yield the least problems. 2. Prevents pressure points. 3. Optimizes biomechanics of the foot.
When standing there should be 3/8" to 1/2" between the longest toe and the end of the shoe.	1. Prevents blisters, callus, and deformities to toes. 2. Allows air circulation.
Avoid high heels.	1. High-heeled shoes usually have triangular toe boxes causing constriction. 2. As the height of the heel rises the pressure on the forefoot increases. A 3" heel exerts 76% more pressure than a flat heel. Heel height is recommended at 1/2" to 1".
Avoid shoes with seams stitched over prominent areas of the foot.	1. Prevents blisters or calluses.
Shoe material should be breathable (leather or canvas not plastic or nylon).	1. Allows air circulation. 2. Minimizes abrasion, maceration, and microbial growth.
Do not plan to "break in" shoes.	1. This implies improper fit. The shoe should fit comfortably when it is first worn. 2. The foot conforms more often than the shoe.
Walk in the shoe before buying it.	1. Tests the comfort and fit.

B. Etiology.
1. Overuse.
2. Precipitated by trauma.
3. Risk factors.
   a. Sudden weight gain.
   b. Sudden increase in activity.
   c. Rigid pes planus or pes cavus.
   d. Poor shoe support.
   e. Training errors (inadequate stretching).

C. Pathology.
1. Plantar fascia extends from the calcaneal tuberosity to the metatarsal heads and acts as a support to the longitudinal arch.
2. Irritation and microtears at the calcaneal insertion starts the inflammatory process.

D. Incidence.
1. Most common cause of plantar heel pain.
2. High familial incidence.

E. Considerations across the lifespan: aging causes fat pads to atrophy and increases an individual's risk factor.

II. ASSESSMENT

A. History and physical examination.
1. Heel pain.
   a. Worse at beginning and end of the day.
   b. Pain especially bad when walking barefoot.
   c. Especially painful when taking first step in the morning.
   d. Pain may extend into Achilles area.
   e. Replicable with passive dorsiflexion of toes or foot.
2. Local tenderness.
3. Assess shoe wear.

B. Diagnostic tests: x-rays.
1. Usually reserved for ambiguous presentations.
2. May show bone spur at insertion site in approximately 60%.
   a. Not the cause of pain.
   b. Often present in the asymptomatic patient or foot.

III. COMMON THERAPEUTIC MODALITIES

A. Observation.

1. Time to heal and number of modalities used depends on the length of time symptoms present.
2. Stretches of the gastrocnemius, soleus, and fascia.
   a. Most effective treatment.
   b. Should be done no matter what other modalities are used.
3. Shoe change (see Table 21.5).
4. Mechanical devices.
   a. Orthotics.
   b. Heel cups.
5. Steroids.
   a. Injection.
   b. Iontophoresis (steroid gel and ultrasound).

B. Immobilization.

1. Strapping.
2. Night splints to keep foot dorsiflexed.
3. Casting.

C. Surgery.

1. Last resort.
2. Most people respond to conservative therapy.

IV. NURSING DIAGNOSES, OUTCOMES, AND INTERVENTIONS

A. See Table 21.4.

B. Knowledge, deficient.

1. Outcome: patient will understand probable etiology and treatment modalities.
2. Interventions.
   a. Help patient identify and modify risk factors.
   b. Teach stretching exercises.
      (1) Demonstrate and/or provide written material to ensure correct stretching.
      (2) May need to ice or use mild analgesic (acetaminophen, NSAIDs) before performing.
      (3) Should be gentle and not increase pain.
      (4) Need to be consistent and do at least a minimal amount each day.
   c. Provide information/handouts regarding proper shoe fit.

V. HOME CARE CONSIDERATIONS

A. Performs stretching exercises, if appropriate, and knows how often and how long to do the exercises.

B. Demonstrated and given instruction regarding the care of the foot with strapping, night splints, and/or casting.

C. Understands the importance of proper shoe wear.

VERRUCA PLANTARIS (Plantar Wart)

I. OVERVIEW

A. Definition: tumor of the skin epidermis.

B. Etiology.

1. Papillomavirus (HPV-1 and HPV-4).
2. Incubation period is from 1-20 months.
3. Variably contagious.

C. Pathology.

1. A benign, elevated area of hypertrophy of the papillae of the skin.
2. Occurs on the pressure-bearing sole of the foot.

II. ASSESSMENT: History and physical examination.

A. Pain: acts as a foreign body.

B. Rough kerototic skin nodule on sole of foot.

1. Dark red to black dots are thrombosed blood vessels.
2. Will bleed if shaved or sharp debrided.

III. COMMON THERAPEUTIC MODALITIES

A. Chemical therapy.

1. 40% salicylic acids.
   a. Soak warts
   b. Pare as much as tolerated.
   c. Apply plaster, gel, or resin as an occlusive dressing.
   d. Remove every 24 hours and abrade the macerated skin.
   e. Takes 4-6 weeks.
   f. Is 50%-60% effective.
2. Recalcitrant warts may require stronger chemicals.
   a. Vessicants (blister forms) (cantharidin).
   b. Antimetabolites (bleomycin injection).

B. Surgical.

1. Avoided to minimize scarring and chronic untreatable pain.
2. Liquid nitrogen.
3. Laser therapy.

IV. NURSING DIAGNOSES, OUTCOMES, AND INTERVENTIONS

A. See Table 21.4.

B. Knowledge, deficient.

1. Outcome: patient will understand cause and treatment modalities.
2. Interventions.
   a. Instruct patient about the following:
      (1) Treatment can be both expensive and time consuming.
      (2) There is a recurrence rate of 33%.
      (3) Treatment does not eliminate the virus.
      (4) The immune system will eventually prevent the virus from causing warts.
      (5) Plantar warts are contagious (to varying degrees).
   b. Instruct in proper treatment techniques.
      (1) Avoid sharp debridement.
      (2) Use pumice stone, emory board, or rough cloth.
      (3) Use occlusive dressing over chemical.
      (4) Minimize application of chemical to lesion to avoid damage to normal skin around lesion.
      (5) Continue treatment until skin is smooth.
      (6) Avoid sharing footwear or treatment tools with others.

V. HOME CARE CONSIDERATIONS

A. Instruct patient on how to care for surgical incision or chemical therapy area.

B. Ambulates safely.

FRACTURES

I. OVERVIEW

A. Definition: any disruption, complete or incomplete, in the continuity of a bone.

B. Etiology.

1. Trauma.
   a. Often associated with soft tissue injury.
   b. Most common cause.
2. Overuse, also known as stress fractures.
3. Systemic disease: weakens or destroys bone, making it more susceptible to fracture from minimal trauma or stress.

C. Pathology.

1. The force of the trauma or stress supersedes the strength and or elasticity of the bone.
2. Types.
   a. Distal fibula.
      (1) Distal fractures classified by location.
         (a) Weber A – below the joint line.
         (b) Weber B – at the joint line.
         (c) Weber C – above the joint line.
      (2) May be isolated or combined with a distal tibia fracture.
      (3) Proximal fibular fractures that occur with deltoid ligament tear – Maissonneuve.
   b. Distal tibia.
      (1) Usually concurrent with fibula fractures.
         (a) Bimalleolar is a fracture of the lateral malleolus (fibula) and medial malleolus (tibia).
         (b) Trimalleolar is a fracture of the lateral malleolus (fibula) and the medial and posterior malleoli of the tibia.
      (2) Fracture may extend into the joint thereby disrupting the articular surface.
         (a) Also known as pilon fracture.
         (b) Leads to joint instability and traumatic arthritis.
         (c) Often associated with severe swelling and soft tissue injury.
   c. Talus.
      (1) Associated with poor outcomes due to extensive articular cartilage and the limited blood supply.
      (2) Chondral fractures of the dome.
         (a) Consider in patients with nonhealing ankle sprain.
         (b) Leads to arthritis as the dislodged fragment becomes imbedded into the joint.
   d. Calcaneus.
      (1) Usually a result of axial loading.
      (2) Usually associated with other injuries.
         (a) Lumbar compression fractures.
         (b) Fractures of the lower extremities.
         (c) Contralateral calcaneus fracture.
   e. Metatarsals.
      (1) Lisfranc fracture dislocation.
         (a) Interrupts the arch and therefore the stability of the tarsometatarsal (TMT) joint.
         (b) May be associated with compartment syndrome.
      (2) Jones fracture.
         (a) Transverse fracture of the proximal diaphysis of the 5th metatarsal.
         (b) High incidence of nonunion.
         (c) Most often seen in industrial workers and athletes.
   f. Phalanges.
      (1) Usually of minor consequence unless open or crushed.
      (2) Treated by taping toes together and managing skin integrity and pain.

D. Considerations across the lifespan.

1. Not age related.
2. Elderly more susceptible.
   a. Increased incidence of systemic disease (osteoporosis, diabetes, etc.).
   b. Increased risk for falls.
   c. Decreased strength and soft tissue elasticity.

E. Complications.

1. Nonunion: the fracture fails to unite after an appropriate length of time.
2. Malunion: the fracture heals with an unacceptable amount of angulation, rotation, or overriding.

II. ASSESSMENT

A. History and physical examination (see Assessment of the Foot and Ankle).

B. Diagnostic tests (see Table 21.2).

III. COMMON THERAPEUTIC MODALITIES

A. Observation.

1. Rare treatment for fracture.
2. Fractures of the foot and ankle are almost always supported or immobilized in some way.

B. Immobilization.

1. Taping, used for phalangeal fractures.
2. Bracing
   a. Stirrup splint, used for chip fractures of the lateral malleolus.
   b. Rocker-bottomed or Reese shoes, used for nondisplaced metatarsal fractures.
3. Splinting, may be used initially, until the swelling subsides.
4. Casting: a nonweight bearing (NWB) short leg cast is the usual treatment for simple, nondisplaced, extraarticular fractures.

C. Surgery.

1. Operative intervention is necessary for fractures that are:
   a. Open.
   b. Displaced.

c. Complex.
d. Intraarticular.
e. Disruptive of the joint integrity.
2. Open reduction internal fixation may consist of screws, wires, pins, or plates and screws.
3. External fixation may be used alone or in addition to internal fixation.
4. Syndesmotic screw.
a. A long screw that realigns and holds the widened tibiofibular joint when the syndesmotic/interosseous ligament is torn.
b. It may be removed before total weight bearing or allowed to break.
5. Even with surgical intervention, NWB or toe-touch/touch down weight bearing (TTWB/TDWB) is required.

IV. NURSING DIAGNOSES, OUTCOMES, AND INTERVENTIONS (See Table 21.4)

V. HOME CARE CONSIDERATIONS

A. Depends on the patient's:
1. General health.
2. Social and support systems.
3. Ability to maintain weight-bearing restrictions and dressing changes (if required).

B. Home care needs may include:
1. Home health aid.
2. Visiting nurse.
3. Physical therapy in the home.

C. Short-term stay in a rehabilitation facility may be needed before returning home.

PES PLANUS

I. OVERVIEW

A. Definition: a flattening of the medial longitudinal arch of the foot. Also known as flatfoot.

B. Etiology: unknown cause of laxity of the joint capsules and ligament of the sole of the foot.

C. Pathology.
1. The head of the talus is displaced medially and plantarward from the navicular, stretching the spring ligament and tibial posterior muscle tendon.
2. Types.
a. Flexible, arch forms as if on tiptoe or when the foot is unweighted.
b. Rigid.
(1) Arch does not form even if the foot is unweighted.
(2) Usually a pathological condition.
(a) Tarsal coalition.
(b) Heel cord contracture.
(c) Trauma.
(d) Tumor.

D. Incidence: high familial incidence.

E. Considerations across the lifespan: prior to age 3, most children appear flatfooted due to a fat pad obscuring the longitudinal arch.

F. Complications: change in gait and no toe-off.

II. ASSESSMENT

A. History and physical examination.
1. Obtain family and birth history.
2. Assess type by having the patient stand on tiptoe or unweight the foot.
3. Pain.
4. Flatfoot gait does not toe-off.
5. Positive/negative callus under 1st and 2nd metatarsal heads and medial plantar calcaneus.

B. Diagnostic tests: x-rays
1. Help determine cause of rigid pes planus.
2. Help alleviate parental fears.

III. COMMON THERAPEUTIC MODALITIES

A. Observation.
1. Appropriate only in the asyptomatic flexible type.
2. Passive stretching.

B. Immobilization.
1. Orthotics or corrective shoes.
2. Not necessary in the asymptomatic child under 3 years old.

C. Surgery.
1. Reserved for the patient over 10 years old whose activities are limited due to symptoms.
2. Surgical treatment of the rigid foot depends on cause.

IV. NURSING DIAGNOSES, OUTCOMES, AND INTERVENTIONS

A. See Table 21.4.

B. Anxiety: parental.
1. Outcome: parents are reassured.
2. Interventions.
a. Instruct parents on the normal growth and development of the foot and ankle.
b. Discourage expensive corrective shoes in the child under 3 years old.

V. HOME CARE CONSIDERATIONS

A. Stretching exercises.

B. Care and application of orthotics/corrective shoes as appropriate.

C. Support for caregiver.

PES CAVUS

I. OVERVIEW

A. Definition: excessive high arch or fixed equinus deformity.

B. Etiology: usually associated with neuromuscular disorder or injury. Rarely idiopathic.

C. Pathology.
1. Muscle imbalance or isolated muscle weakness.
2. Exact cause unknown.
3. Results in a decreased plantar weight-bearing surface.

D. Incidence: high familial incidence.

E. Complications: stress fractures secondary to lowered ability to absorb shock and small weight-bearing area.

II. ASSESSMENT

A. History and physical examination.
1. Positive family history or positive neuromuscular disorder history.
2. High arch with full weight bearing.
3. Positive callus under the metatarsal heads.
4. May have stress fractures of the heel and/or foot.

B. Diagnostic tests.
1. X-rays with the patient full weight bearing.
2. May require MRI of the spine to help determine cause.

III. COMMON THERAPEUTIC MODALITIES

A. Depends on the severity of the deformity and the underlying diagnosis.

B. Observation: passive stretching.

C. Immobilization.
1. Extra depth shoe with softer sole and wide toe box.
2. Orthotics.

D. Surgical Intervention.
1. Used for severe disabling deformities.
2. Plantar release is the primary goal.

IV. NURSING DIAGNOSES, OUTCOMES, AND INTERVENTIONS

A. See Table 21.4.

B. Knowledge, deficient.
1. Outcome: patient and/or caregivers will understand and demonstrate treatment modalities.
2. Interventions.
   a. Instruct and demonstrate stretching exercises.
   b. Instruct and demonstrate use of orthotics.

V. HOME CARE CONSIDERATIONS

A. Passive stretching exercises.

B. Orthotics/special shoes.

C. Support to caregiver.

TALIPES EQUINOVARUS (Clubfoot)

I. OVERVIEW

A. Definition: a combination of bony and soft tissue abnormalities placing the ankle in plantar flexion, the forefoot in adduction and supination, and the heel in varus.

B. Etiology.
1. Unknown.
2. Intrauterine positioning verses developmental arrest in the first trimester.

C. Risk factors.
1. Family history.
2. Male: female ratio 2:1.

D. Pathology.
1. Foot is often so severely inverted and internally rotated that the sole faces up.
2. Soft tissue contractures maintain the position of the bony malalignments.

E. Incidence.
1. Occurs in 1 per 1000 births.
2. Occurs bilaterally in 50% of cases.
3. Most common congenital foot disorder.

F. Considerations across the lifespan: usually first diagnosed in the newborn or infant.

G. Complications.
1. May reoccur, regardless of treatment, up to age 7.
   a. Common, especially in girls, due to severity.
   b. More common in bilateral cases.
2. Affected foot may be smaller and stiffer and calf circumference decreased.

II. ASSESSMENT

A. History and physical examination.
1. Positive family history.
2. Positive deformity
   a. Equinus of the foot (points down).
   b. Adduction of the forefoot (turns in).
   c. Varus of the sole of the foot (turns in).
3. Decreased calf circumference on affected side related to fibrosis of the musculature.
4. Short/long leg length discrepancy.
5. Possible neurogenic component as evidenced by:
   a. Caudal dimpling.
   b. Spinal deformity.
   c. Spinal hairy patches.

B. Diagnostic tests: radiographs
1. Rarely used initially as bones are minimally ossified at birth.
2. Evaluate progress of conservative treatment.
3. Assist with perioperative planning and evaluation.

III. COMMON THERAPEUTIC MODALITIES

A. Observation.
1. Start as soon as possible, since maternal hormones keep ligamentous tissue lax for approximately 2-3 weeks.
2. Serial casting or taping every 1-2 weeks for up to 3 months.
3. Reevaluation.
4. Treatment is inconvenient and time intensive to the caregiver.

B. Immobilization
1. Casting.
2. Reverse-last shoes, worn 24-hours per day except for bathing.

C. Surgery.
1. Usually performed between 4 and 9 months of age.
2. One stage procedure with pins removed 2-6 weeks postoperatively.
3. Requires casting (2-12 weeks) then corrective shoes.

IV. NURSING DIAGNOSES, OUTCOMES, AND INTERVENTIONS

A. Growth and development, imbalanced.
1. Outcome: child will "catch up" when physical restrictions are removed.
2. Interventions.
   a. Allow normal activity within restrictions of cast.
   b. Provide diversional and substitute activities.

B. Knowledge, deficient.
1. Outcome: parents and family will be able to provide care and understand expectations of treatment.

2. Interventions.
    a. Instruct in incidence and treatment modalities.
    b. Forewarn about intensive time and inconvenience to caregiver.
3. Instruct in cast care.

V. HOME CARE CONSIDERATIONS

A. Community support for parents, as appropriate.
B. Treat the child as "normally" as possible.
C. Instructions on care for cast/reversed shoe wear.
D. Emotional support for caregivers.

CHARCOT FOOT

I. OVERVIEW

A. Definition: a neuroarthropathic foot.
B. Etiology: two controversial theories.
1. Repetitive trauma to insensate foot.
2. Increased vascularity secondary to abnormal sympathetic reflexes leading to bone resorption and ligamentous changes.

C. Pathology.
1. Marked destruction of joint surfaces often accompanied by dislocations and/or subluxation
2. Calcification or bony debris in soft tissues around the joint.

D. Incidence.
1. Affects men and women equally.
2. Approximately 30% occur bilaterally.

F. Complications.
1. Deformity.
2. Amputation.

II. ASSESSMENT

A. History and physical examination.
1. Acute.
    a. Red.
    b. Hot.
    c. Swelling of the foot and ankle.
    d. Pain is minimal or less than expected.
    e. Must distinguish from infection.
2. Chronic.
    a. Deformed foot.
        (1) Multiple bony protuberances.
        (2) May have ulcerations.
    b. Rocker bottom foot which results from collapse of longitudinal arch and midtarsal joint subluxation.

B. Diagnostic tests: acute phase (see Table 21.2).
1. X-rays may or may not show destructive changes at this point.
2. Bone scan.
3. MRI to evaluate for osteoporosis.
4. Culture and sensitivities of drainage if present.

III. COMMON THERAPEUTIC MODALITIES

A. Treatment goals.
1. Limit joint destruction.
2. Prevent further deformity.
3. Prevent soft tissue ulceration.
4. Prevent neurovascular damage.

B. Immobilization.
1. Acute phase.
    a. NWB total contact cast.
    b. Elevation.
2. Subacute phase.
    a. Orthotics.
    b. Custom-made shoes.

C. Surgery.
1. Acute phase, only for infection.
2. Chronic phase.
    a. Excision of bony prominences.
    b. Arthrodesis.
    c. May end in amputation.

IV. NURSING DIAGNOSES, OUTCOMES, AND INTERVENTIONS

A. See Table 21.4.
B. Skin integrity, impaired.
Infection, risk for.
1. Outcome: foot will remain free of infection.
2. Interventions.
    a. Inspect foot daily.
    b. Keep feet clean and dry.
    c. Moisturize skin as needed.
    d. Wear appropriate shoes and preferably white cotton socks.
    e. Treat skin breaks as soon as possible.
        (1) Relieve pressure.
        (2) Keep wound clean and dry.
        (3) Use appropriate dressing materials as directed.

FOOT DROP

I. OVERVIEW

A. Definition: inability to dorsiflex the foot.
B. Etiology: muscle weakness or damage due to:
1. Trauma.
2. Nerve injury.
    a. Local/peripheral.
    b. Central (spinal cord injury, herniated lumbar disc, stroke, etc.).
3. Systemic disease (polio, Charcot-Marie-Tooth, cerebral palsy, etc.).

C. Complications.
1. Gait changes to steppage gait.
2. Shortening of the Achilles tendon.
3. Susceptibility to pressure sores.

II. ASSESSMENT: History and Physical Examination

A. Obtain birth history if pertinent.
B. Obtain general history.
C. Assess gait.
1. Resembles high steppage gait of a horse.
2. Excessive hip and knee flexion to clear dropped foot.

3. "Slap" of forefoot as it strikes the ground. (Normally heel strikes ground first.)

D. Assess neurologic function.

E. Assess for muscle atrophy.

III. COMMON THERAPEUTIC MODALITIES

A. Immobilization.

1. Correct the cause if possible (remove the local pressure).
2. Ankle-foot-orthosis (AFO).
   a. Supports ankle in a dorsiflexed position.
   b. Must be worn in a shoe.
   c. Shoe needs to be a full size larger.

B. Surgery: Correct the cause if possible.

IV. NURSING DIAGNOSES, OUTCOMES, AND INTERVENTIONS

A. Injury, risk for.

1. Outcome: the patient will remain without skin breakdown, infection, or trauma.
2. Interventions.
   a. Wear AFO.
   b. Check skin under brace every day.
   c. Use assistive ambulatory devices as needed.
   d. Never try to ambulate without brace and shoe on.

B. Physical mobility, impaired.

1. Outcome: ambulates safely
2. Interventions:
   a. Use of ankle support
   b. AFO shoe to be worn at all times.
   c. Shoe needs to be a full size larger.

V. HOME CARE CONSIDERATIONS

A. Make sure home environment is free of clutter and safe for the patient to ambulate.

B. Instruct on how to go up and down stairs with brace and a full size larger shoe.

C. Instruct patient to wear brace and shoe even when going to the bathroom at night.

RHEUMATOID ARTHRITIS (RA)

I. OVERVIEW

A. Definition: a chronic systemic disease characterized by inflammatory changes in joints and related tissues leading to deformity.

B. Etiology: autoimmune disorder.

C. Pathology.

1. Inflammation leads to chronic synovitis and destruction of supporting structures in multiple diarthrodial joints.
2. Results in deformities.

D. Incidence.

1. 90% of RA patients have foot involvement.
2. Usually bilateral.

E. Complications.

1. Deformity.
2. Immobility.

II. ASSESSMENT

A. History and physical examination.

1. Activity of disease flare versus quiescence.
2. Medications used to treat RA interfere with wound healing.
3. Pain.
4. Deformity.
5. Callus formation, excessive or in unusual location.
6. Difficulty ambulating.
7. May have open wounds from pressure points.
8. Vascular status.

B. Diagnostic tests: x-rays.

III. COMMON THERAPEUTIC MODALITIES

A. Observation: medical management by a rheumatologist.

B. Immobilization: extra depth shoe with orthotic liners to reduce pressure.

C. Surgical.

1. Tendon repair.
2. Arthrodesis, the surgical fixation of a joint to obtain fusion.
   a. Relieve pain.
   b. Create a plantigrade foot.
   c. Stabilize the foot and ankle.
   d. Restore or improve function.
3. Arthroplasty (silicon total phalangeal replacements).

IV. NURSING DIAGNOSES, OUTCOMES, AND INTERVENTIONS

A. See Table 21.4.

B. Infection, risk for.

1. Outcome: wounds will heal without infection.
2. Interventions.
   a. Assess frequently.
   b. Nonweight bearing.
   c. Optimal disease management.

V. HOME CARE CONSIDERATIONS

A. Assistive devices as required.

B. Home help assistance to minimize ambulation.

C. Assist with ADLs.

D. Wound assessment and care.

E. Transportation assistance

F. Financial assistance if qualifies.

HALLUS VALGUS (Bunion Deformity)

I. OVERVIEW

A. Definition: lateral deviation of the great toe on the 1st metatarsal head (MTP joint).

B. Etiology.

1. Shoes.
   a. Narrow toed.
   b. High heeled.
2. Other foot pathologies.
   a. Severe flatfoot deformity.
   b. Chronic tightness of the Achilles tendon.
   c. Spasticity.
   d. Rheumatoid arthritis.

C. Pathology.

1. The 1st MTP is suspended in a sling of muscles:
   a. The tendons allow the head of the MTP to be pushed in either direction.
   b. As the proximal phalanx of the great toe deviates laterally the 1st MTP head is pushed medially resulting in a prominence medially.
   c. May range from a simple exaggeration of normal to the true bunion.
2. Bunion is the callus, thickened bursa, and excessive bone that results from hallus valgus.

D. Incidence.

1. Female to male ratio is 9:1.
2. Family history (60%).

E. Considerations across the lifespan.

1. Foot widens with age.
2. Soft tissue laxity with aging.

F. Complications.

1. Deformity.
2. Pain.
3. Gait change.

II. ASSESSMENT

A. History and physical examination.

1. Obtain history.
   a. Family.
   b. Shoe wear.
   c. Activities.
2. Deformity of the 1st toe and possibly of 2nd and/or 3rd.
3. Pain.
4. X-ray changes.

B. Diagnostic Tests: weight bearing A-P, lateral, and oblique x-rays to determine joint congruity and angle width. (Normal angle is < 15.)

III. COMMON THERAPEUTIC MODALITIES

A. Observation.

1. Shoe changes.
2. Allow sufficient space for the forefoot (see Table 21.5).

B. Immobilization.

1. Medial longitudinal arch support.
2. Toe spacers.

C. Surgery.

1. Multiple procedures are available, based on the severity and cause of the deformity (McBride, Chevon, Keller).
2. Postoperative care requires restriction of activity, special shoes, and protected weight bearing.
3. Elevation is essential to minimize edema and pain.

IV. NURSING DIAGNOSES, OUTCOMES, AND INTERVENTIONS

A. See Table 21.4.

B. Knowledge, deficient.

1. Outcome: patient will understand restrictions and postop requirements.
2. Interventions: education.
   a. Length of time out of work.
   b. Need for flat-bottomed wide-toed shoe.
   c. Dressing and incisional care.
   d. Importance of elevation.

V. HOME CARE CONSIDERATIONS

A. Due to lack of mobility and the need to keep foot elevated, patient will require assistance.

B. Minimize such potential hazards as throw rugs, clutter, etc.

C. Discuss the length of time the patient will be unable to drive a vehicle.

AMPUTATIONS

I. OVERVIEW

A. Definition: a reconstructive procedure to remove all or portions of an extremity that is injured, diseased, or no longer functional.

1. Emotional process.
2. Requires team approach.

B. Etiology.

1. Trauma
2. Systemic disease (diabetes mellitus, rheumatoid arthritis).
3. Vascular disease (peripheral vascular disease)
4. Infection.

C. Incidence: most commonly associated with diabetes mellitus.

D. Considerations across the lifespan.

1. Prosthesis for the pediatric patient need to be adapted as the child grows.
2. Energy requirements for ambulation with a prosthesis are increased.
3. Because of decreased strength and stamina, the elderly may have more problems.

E. Complications.

1. Non-healing.
2. Need for another higher level amputation.

II. ASSESSMENT

A. History and physical examination.

1. Mechanism of injury.
2. Concurrent diseases.
3. Medications.
4. Cultural or religious taboos.
5. Neurovascular assessment.
6. Skin assessment.

B. Diagnostic tests.

1. X-rays.
   a. Trauma.
   b. Osteomyelitis.
2. Vascular studies.
   a. Arteriogram.
   b. Venogram.
3. Laboratory studies consistent with pathology (serum glucose, hemoglobin A_1c, culture and sensitivity, etc.).

III. COMMON THERAPEUTIC MODALITIES

A. Surgery: requires adequate, tension free soft tissue closure to promote wound healing and provide pressure relief.

B. Types.

1. Toe.
   a. Removal of the distal and part or all of the proximal phalanx.
   b. Does not require a prosthesis.
2. Ray.
   a. Removal of the toe and all or some of the corresponding metatarsal.
   b. Narrows the foot and changes the weight-bearing surfaces.
   c. Prosthesis such as extra depth shoes with custom molded insoles.
3. Midfoot.
   a. Also known as transmetatarsal or Lisfranc.
   b. Amount of bone resected depends on soft tissue closure.
   c. Casted postoperatively.
      (1) Prevents deformity.
      (2) Controls edema.
      (3) Speeds rehabilitation.
   d. Prosthesis.
      (1) Ankle-foot orthosis (AFO) with long foot plate and toe filler.
         (a) Prevents equinas deformity.
         (b) Use for 1 year.
      (2) Stiff-soled shoe with toe filler.
      (3) Cosmetic partial foot.
4. Hindfoot.
   a. Also known as Chopart.
   b. Removes the forefoot and midfoot, leaving only the talus and calcaneus.
   c. Requires postoperative casting.
   d. Prosthesis that requires secure stabilization to prevent heel from pistoning when walking.
5. Syme's.
   a. Removal of the foot to the tibia and fibula using the heel skin and fat pad to cover the distal leg bones.
   b. Requires postoperative casting.
   c. Prosthesis required for ambulation.

IV. NURSING DIAGNOSES, OUTCOMES, AND INTERVENTIONS

A. See Table 21.4.

B. Infection, risk for.

1. Outcome: wound will heal without infection and be ready for prosthesis.
2. Interventions.
   a. Postoperative cast care.
   b. Elevation.
   c. Ice
   d. Adequate nutrition.

C. Body image, disturbed.

1. Outcome: patient and family accepts physical limitations and cosmetic change.
2. Interventions.
   a. Information regarding prosthesis types and use.
   b. Support.

D. Physical mobility, impaired.

1. Outcome: patient will be able to ambulate and perform functional activities.
2. Interventions.
   a. Appropriate prosthetic fit.
   b. Physical therapy for gait training.
   c. Support.

V. HOME CARE CONSIDERATIONS

A. Attends physical therapy sessions to gain proper gait training for ambulation.

B. Ambulates safely.

C. Works with family members and therapy to return to a "normal" life.

D. Accepts responsibility to care for self.

E. Knowledge about how to care for cast.

INTERDIGITAL NEUROMA (Morton's Neuroma)

I. OVERVIEW

A. Definition: entrapment of interdigital nerve.

B. Etiology.

1. Nerve pinched usually by mechanical means.
2. Narrow-toed, high-heeled shoes.

C. Pathology: nerve entrapped by ligaments as the toes are brought into a dorsiflexed position, leading to nerve degeneration and fibrotic reaction.

D. Incidence.

1. Most common in 2nd and 3rd web space.
2. Female:male = 10:1.

E. Considerations across the lifespan: rarely seen in children.

II. ASSESSMENT

A. History and physical examination.

1. Pain.
   a. Burning in nature.
   b. Decreased when non-weight bearing.
   c. Increases when metatarsal heads are squeezed together.
   d. May be pain free when barefoot.
2. Swelling.
3. Web space dysesthesia.
4. Palpable click when metatarsal heads squeezed together.
5. May be able to palpate neuroma.

B. Diagnostic Tests: not helpful.

III. COMMON THERAPEUTIC MODALITIES

A. Observation:

1. Shoes with wide toe box and low heel (see Table 21.5).
2. Metatarsal pads to lift adjacent MT heads.
3. Steroid injections.

B. Immobilization: not helpful.

C. Surgery: excision of the nerve.

IV. NURSING DIAGNOSES, OUTCOMES, AND INTERVENTIONS

A. Physical mobility, impaired.

1. Outcome: able to ambulate safely and without pain.

2. Interventions
   a. Wears shoes with wide toe box.
   b. Will wear only low-heeled shoes.

B. Knowledge, deficient.
1. Outcome: patient will understand relationship of problem and shoe style.
2. Interventions.
   a. Provide information/handout regarding appropriate shoe wear.
   b. Suggest pointy-toed high-heeled shoes only for special occasions and short periods.

INGROWN TOENAILS

I. OVERVIEW

A. Definition: skin along the lateral margins of the toenail becomes inflamed.

B. Etiology.
1. Most common in the great toe.
2. External factors.
   a. Tight shoes.
   b. Improper nail cutting.
   c. Toe deformities.
3. Internal factors.
   a. Masses.
   b. Nail disease.
3. Systemic factors.
   a. Circulatory.
   b. Endocrine.
   c. Metabolic.

C. Pathology.
1. 0.5-1 mm space between lateral nail fold and nail edge.
2. Space narrows secondary to above causes.
3. Nail edge penetrates the soft tissue.

D. Incidence: increased in women in the 5th and 6th decade of life.

E. Considerations across the lifespan.
1. Infections most common in those < 30 years old.
2. Toenail deformities common in the elderly secondary to chronic fungal infections.

F. Complications: infection.

II. ASSESSMENT

A. Positive medical history for nail deformities such as:
1. Fungal infection.
2. Circulatory condition.
3. Endocrine disease (fungal infection, circulatory or endocrine disease, etc).

B. Lateral margin of the nail digs into the surrounding nail fold.

C. Acute inflammation of the area often with drainage indicative of infection.

III. COMMON THERAPEUTIC MODALITIES

A. Observation.
1. Loose fitting stockings.
2. Wide-toe shoes.
3. Correctly cut nails.
4. Warm soaks (2-3 times a day).
5. Elevate corner of nail with antiseptic soaked cotton pledget.
6. Antibiotics if infected.

B. Immobilization: not helpful.

C. Surgery.
1. Required if infected.
2. Partial (lateral third) to complete excision of the nail.
3. High recurrence of ingrowth with complete excision.
4. Onychectomy.
   a. Nail edge ablation.
   b. Used for recurrent infections.
   c. Infections must be resolved.
   d. Partial or complete.
   e. Nail regrowth rate is about 10%

IV. NURSING DIAGNOSES, OUTCOMES, AND INTERVENTIONS

A. See Table 21.4.

B. Knowledge, deficient.
1. Outcome: patient will understand cause and treatment modalities.
2. Interventions.
   a. Teach proper nail cutting.
      (1) Cut straight across.
      (2) Do not trim at corners.
   b. Avoid tight-toed or high-heeled shoes (see Table 21.5).

V. HOME CARE CONSIDERATIONS

A. Instruction on wearing loose fitting stockings and wide-toe shoes.

B. Demonstrate correct procedure for cutting toenails in the future.

C. Provide instruction and demonstration of at home foot/toe care.

MALLET TOE DEFORMITY

I. OVERVIEW

A. Definition: flexion deformity of the DIP joint of the toe.

B. Etiology.
1. MTP joint is extended.
2. PIP joint is neutral
3. DIP joint is flexed.
4. The tip of the toe faces the plantar surface.

C. Pathology.
1. May be fixed or flexible.
2. Usually only involves one toe.

D. Incidence: usually involves 2nd toe because of its excessive length in relationship to the other toes.

E. Complications.
1. Ulceration at toe tip.
2. Most common in the neuropathic foot.

II. ASSESSMENT

A. History and physical examination.

1. Pain over dorsal aspect of DIP joint.
2. Pain at tip of toe from striking the ground.
3. Callus or ulceration at tip of toe.
4. Observe with patient standing.
5. Evaluate flexibility by plantar flexing the ankle.
   a. Flexible is the total straightening of DIP with plantar flexion of ankle.
   b. Fixed is where the ankle motion does not effect deformity.

B. Diagnostics tests: x-ray confirms deformity.

III. COMMON THERAPEUTIC MODALITIES

A. Observation.

1. Wide toe box shoe.
2. Extra-depth shoe depending on extent of deformity.
3. Small pad or lambs wool placed underneath the toe to prevent it from striking the ground.

B. Surgical.

1. Flexible: the release of the flexor digitorum longus tendon.
2. Fixed: the resection of the condyls of the middle phalanx (condylectomy).

IV. NURSING DIAGNOSES, OUTCOMES, AND INTERVENTIONS

A. See Table 21.4: if surgery indicated.

B. Knowledge, deficient.

1. Outcome: patient will understand cause and treatment modalities.
2. Interventions.
   a. See Table 21.5.
   b. Present rationale as well as instructions on the use of special shoes.

V. HOME CARE CONSIDERATIONS

A. Ambulates safely with special shoes.

B. If surgery was done, instruct on infection prevention.

C. Instruct regarding any correction needed in walking/standing.

HAMMER TOE DEFORMITY

I. OVERVIEW

A. Definition: plantar flexion deformity of the proximal intraphalangeal PIP joint.

B. Etiology.

1. MTP joint is extended.
2. PIP joint is flexed.
3. DIP is extended.
4. When standing, the proximal phalanx is the only part of the toe in contact with the ground.
5. The 2nd knuckle (PIP) sticks up dorsally.

C. Pathology.

1. Usually accompanied by a flexion deformity of the DIP joint as well.
2. May result from hyperextension of the MTP joint.
3. If it occurs in the 2nd toe, may be associated with hallus valgus.
4. Usually only involves one toe.

II. ASSESSMENT

A. History and physical examination.

1. Pain over the dorsal aspect of the PIP joint.
2. Deformity.
3. Callus or ulceration over dorsum of PIP joint.
4. Observe with patient standing.
5. Evaluate flexibility by plantar flexing the ankle.
   a. Flexible: the total straightening of DIP with plantar flexion of ankle.
   b. Fixed: where ankle motion does not effect deformity.

B. Diagnostic Tests: x-ray confirms deformity.

III. COMMON THERAPEUTIC MODALITIES

A. Observation.

1. Wide, soft footwear with an adequate toe box.
2. Toe slings.

B. Surgery.

1. Flexible: where flexor tendon transfers.
2. Fixed: proximal phalanx condylectomy.
3. May require treatment of hallus valgus deformity.

IV. NURSING DIAGNOSES, OUTCOMES, AND INTERVENTIONS

A. See Table 21.4 if surgery was done.

B. Knowledge, deficient.

1. Outcome: patient will understand cause and treatment modalities.
2. Interventions.
   a. See Table 21.5.
   b. Instructions regarding the importance of wearing special shoes.

V. HOME CARE CONSIDERATIONS

A. Ambulates safely with special shoes.

B. If surgery was done, instruct on infection prevention

C. Instruct regarding any correction needed in walking/standing.

CLAW TOE DEFORMITY

I. OVERVIEW

A. Definition: flexion deformity of the MTP and ITP joints.

B. Etiology.

1. MTP joint is extended
2. PIP and DIP joints are flexed.
3. Toes appear curled under like a claw.

C. Pathology.

1. Usually involves all of the lesser toes.
2. Often seen with chronic neurological problems (RA, diabetic neuropathy, degenerative disc disease, etc.)
3. May be flexible or fixed.
4. Grading is determined by evaluation of MTP and IP joints individually.

D. Complications: may affect gait.

II. ASSESSMENT

A. History and physical examination.

1. Obtain general history especially neurologic.
2. Pain over IP joints due to chafing.
3. Pain beneath MTP joints as the heads are forced into plantar flexion.
4. Deformity.
5. Observe with patient standing.
6. Evaluate flexible verses fixed.

B. Diagnostic tests: x-ray confirms deformity.

III. COMMON THERAPEUTIC MODALITIES

A. Observation.

1. Treatment of any associated problems.
2. Extra-depth shoe to decrease pressure on the lesser toes.
3. Arch supports to relieve MT head pain.

B. Surgical.

1. Depends on nature and severity of the deformity.
2. May include:
    a. Tendon transfer and/or lengthening.
    b. Condylectomy with or without fixation.

C. See Table 21.5.

IV. NURSING DIAGNOSES, OUTCOMES, AND INTERVENTIONS (See Table 21.4)

V. HOME CARE CONSIDERATIONS.

A. Ambulates safely with special shoes.

B. If surgery was done, instruct on infection prevention.

C. Instruct regarding corrections needed on walking/standing gait.

CORN

I. OVERVIEW

A. Definition: a keratotic lesion that forms over a bony prominence on the lesser toes because of excessive pressure on the skin.

B. Etiology: improperly fitted shoes.

C. Pathology.

1. Hard.
    a. Dry.
    b. Usually on the dorsal lateral aspect of the 5th toe.
2. Soft.
    a. Lesion in the web space often resulting in maceration due to moisture between the toes.
    b. Often occurs in the 4th web space.

D. Considerations across the lifespan.

1. More difficult for self care in the elderly.
2. Decreased flexibility with age to care for feet.
3. Failing eyesight with age interferes with proper foot care.

E. Complications: infection.

II. ASSESSMENT

A. History and physical examination.

1. Horny, hard, thickening of the skin.
2. May be wet or dry, depending on location.
3. Pain.
4. Assess shoe wear.

B. Diagnostic tests:

1. Not needed unless infected.
2. Culture and sensitivities.

III. COMMON THERAPEUTIC MODALITIES

A. Observation.

1. Reduce pressure on bony prominences.
    a. Corn pads/lambs wool.
    b. Shoes with wide toe box.
2. Reduce size of corn.
    a. Shaving.
    b. Chemical debrider.

B. Surgery.

1. Rare.
2. Excision of bony prominence.

IV. NURSING DIAGNOSES, OUTCOMES, AND INTERVENTIONS

A. See Table 21.4.

B. Knowledge, deficient.

1. Outcome: patient will understand cause and treatment modalities.
2. Interventions.
    a. See Table 21.5.
    b. Teach appropriate shaving techniques.
        (1) Clean, sharp tools.
        (2) Use tools designed for the job.
    c. Provide list of providers who can do shaving if required.

V. HOME CARE CONSIDERATIONS

A. Instruct on proper shoe wear.

B. Instruct on how to prevent infection.

Bibliography

The American Academy of Family Physicians. (1991). *Sports medicine: Functional management of ankle injuries.* (Syllabus). Kansas City, MO: Author.

Childs, S. (1999). Acute ankle injury. *Lippincott's Primary Care Practice, 3*(4). 428-440.

Coughlin, M.J. (1998, October). Foot problems in women. *Consultant,* 2511-2518.

Coughlin, M.J. (1998, November). Ingrown toenails: Office procedures that relieve pain, steps that prevent recurrence. *Consultant,* 2761-2774.

DiChristina, D., & Garth, W.P. (1996). Ankle sprains. In V.R. Masar (Ed.). *Primary care orthopaedics* (pp. 122-127). Philadelphia: W.B. Saunders.

Hoppenfeld, S. (1976). *Physical examination of the spine and extremities* (pp.197-236). Norwalk, CT: Appleton-Century-Crofts.

Maher, A.B., Salmond, S.W., & Pellino, T.A. (Eds.). (1998). *Orthopaedic nursing* (2nd ed.). Philadelphia: W.B. Saunders.

Magee, D.J. (1997). *Orthopedic physical assessment* (3rd ed.) (pp. 448-515). Philadelphia: W.B. Saunders Company.

Mann, R.A., & Mann, J.A. (1995). Foot and ankle. In H.B. Skinner (Ed.), *Current diagnosis & treatment in orthopedics* (pp. 385-452). Norwalk, CT: Appleton & Lange.

Quaschnick, M.S. (1996). The diagnosis and management of plantar fasciitis. *Nurse Practitioner, 21*(4), 50-63.

Rab, G.T. (1995) Pediatric orthopedic surgery. In H.B. Skinner (Ed.), *Current diagnosis & treatment in orthopedics* (pp. 512-554). Norwalk, CT: Appleton & Lange.

Richardson, J.K., & Iglarsh, Z.A. (1994). *Clinical orthopedic physical therapy* (pp. 483-562). Philadelphia: W.B. Saunders Company.

Sangeorzan, B.J. (1993). Foot and ankle joint. In S.T. Hansen, & M.F. Swiontkowski (Eds.), *Orthopaedic trauma protocols* (pp. 339-368). New York: Raven Press.

Schoen, D.C. (2000). Care of a patient with foot and ankle conditions. In D.C. Schoen, *Adult orthopaedic nursing* (pp. 357-390). Philadelphia: Lippencott.

Simon, R.R., & Koenigsknecht, S.J. (1996). *Emergency orthopedics: The extremities* (3rd ed.) (pp. 393-412). Norwalk, CT: Appleton & Lange.

Trojian, T.J., & McKeag, D.B. (1998). Ankle sprains: Expedient assessment and management. *The Physician and Sportsmedicine, 26*(10), 29-40.

STUDY QUESTIONS

John P., a 30-year-old businessman, was clearing leaves from the gutter when he fell 10 feet from a ladder, landing upright and then falling back onto the lawn. He had immediate pain in his right foot and leg but was able to limp into the house. He applied ice to his foot and laid down. Six hours later, his wife brought him to the ER. Vital signs were stable but his right foot and ankle were quite swollen with small fracture blisters forming. He was in a great deal of pain. (Questions 1-2)

1. The best nursing interventions at this point would be:
   a. Rest, ice, compression, elevation, and pain medications.
   b. Ice, elevation, pain medications, and neurovascular checks.
   c. Elevation, pain medications, and compressive dressing.
   d. Ice, neurovascular checks, and pain medications.

2. It is most likely that he will be placed in a (an):
   a. Posterior splint and soft bulky dressing.
   b. Long leg cast with the foot in dorsiflexon.
   c. Air cast splint and soft bulky dressing.
   d. Short leg cast with the foot in plantar flexion.

3. Rose G. suffers from rheumatoid arthritis. At 68, she manages quite well at home alone with assistive devices and visiting nurses check on her once a week. She is scheduled for a triple arthrodesis of her left ankle in 2 weeks. She calls your office today concerned about going home after her surgery. At this point what nursing intervention is most appropriate?
   a. Contact the local Medicare office for assistance.
   b. Reassure her that she won't need any further help at home.
   c. Contact a social worker to investigate a rehabilitation facility or help at home.
   d. Suggest that Mrs. G. stay with her sister in Canada for a few weeks.

During basketball practice today, 15-year-old Dakota sprained his left ankle. He is unable to walk on it. The trainer immediately iced it and sent him in for evaluation. Physical examination reveals a Grade 2 sprain. There are no fractures. (Questions 4-5)

4. The best treatment at this point would be:
   a. Functional brace and weight bearing as tolerated.
   b. A short leg cast and weight bearing as tolerated.
   c. A functional brace and non-weight bearing.
   d. A short leg cast and non-weight bearing.

5. Three weeks later, Dakota wants to play in the state tournament. To be eligible for full sports participation he must be able to:
   a. Cut and run without pain.
   b. Stand on his toes and heels for 30 seconds without pain.
   c. Run without a limp.
   d. Cut, run, and jump without pain.

6. Barbara, a realtor, is expected to look professional at her job. She is on her feet most of the time. Lately she has been complaining about her "bunion." It aches by the time she gets home from work and it "looks awful." She thinks it is related to her shoes and asks you for recommendations for shoe wear. You recommend:
   a. An extra depth shoe with a wide toe box.
   b. A 1-inch heel shoe with a wide toe box.
   c. A reverse-last shoe with a wide toe box.
   d. A 2-inch heel shoe with a wide toe box.

7. Ellen is pregnant with her first child, a girl. Her two brothers and her husband's father had clubfeet. She is worried that her child will be born with clubfeet. You correctly inform her that:
   a. Clubfeet are caused by intrauterine positioning and are not genetic.
   b. There is a high familial incidence and therefore a possibility her child will have clubfeet.
   c. It doesn't matter because clubfeet can be completely cured.
   d. Clubfeet only occur in males.

8. Jabar, a salesman, runs 3 miles a day on a cross-country track near his home. Recently he increased his mileage to 5 miles per day. He has noted pain in his heel when he first starts his run and again at the end. It is manageable at this time but he wants to do something about it so he can continue to train. His shoes are well worn, soft, and flexible especially around the heel. Of the following recommendations, which would not be appropriate?
   a. Buy new shoes.
   b. Perform stretching exercises.
   c. Use metatarsal pads.
   d. Use ice and NSAIDs.

Lou Phage, a 73-year-old woman with diabetes, came to the office today concerned about redness and swelling in her left foot that she first noted the day before. She denies trauma or pain. She checks her feet daily and denies any open areas. There is no evidence of infection. On examination, the skin is intact, the midfoot is red, swollen, and hot. X-rays show early destruction of the joints in the midfoot and forefoot. (Questions 9-10)

9. Based on the data related to Ms. Phage's foot, she most likely has:
   a. Chopart deformity.
   b. Rheumatoid arthritis.
   c. Charcot Foot.
   d. Reiter's Syndrome.

10. Ms. Phage gets through the acute phase without problem but the foot continues to deteriorate. She now has a rocker-bottomed foot with an infected open area under the 1st and 2nd metatarsal heads. Multiple therapies have failed. She now opts for a transmetatarsal amputation. Which of the following interventions would prepare her to ambulate after the procedure?
    a. Postoperative casting and a long AFO with toe filler.
    b. A toe filler in a stiff-soled shoe.
    c. No adaptive devices.
    d. Postoperative casting and a forefoot prosthesis.

ANSWERS TO STUDY QUESTIONS

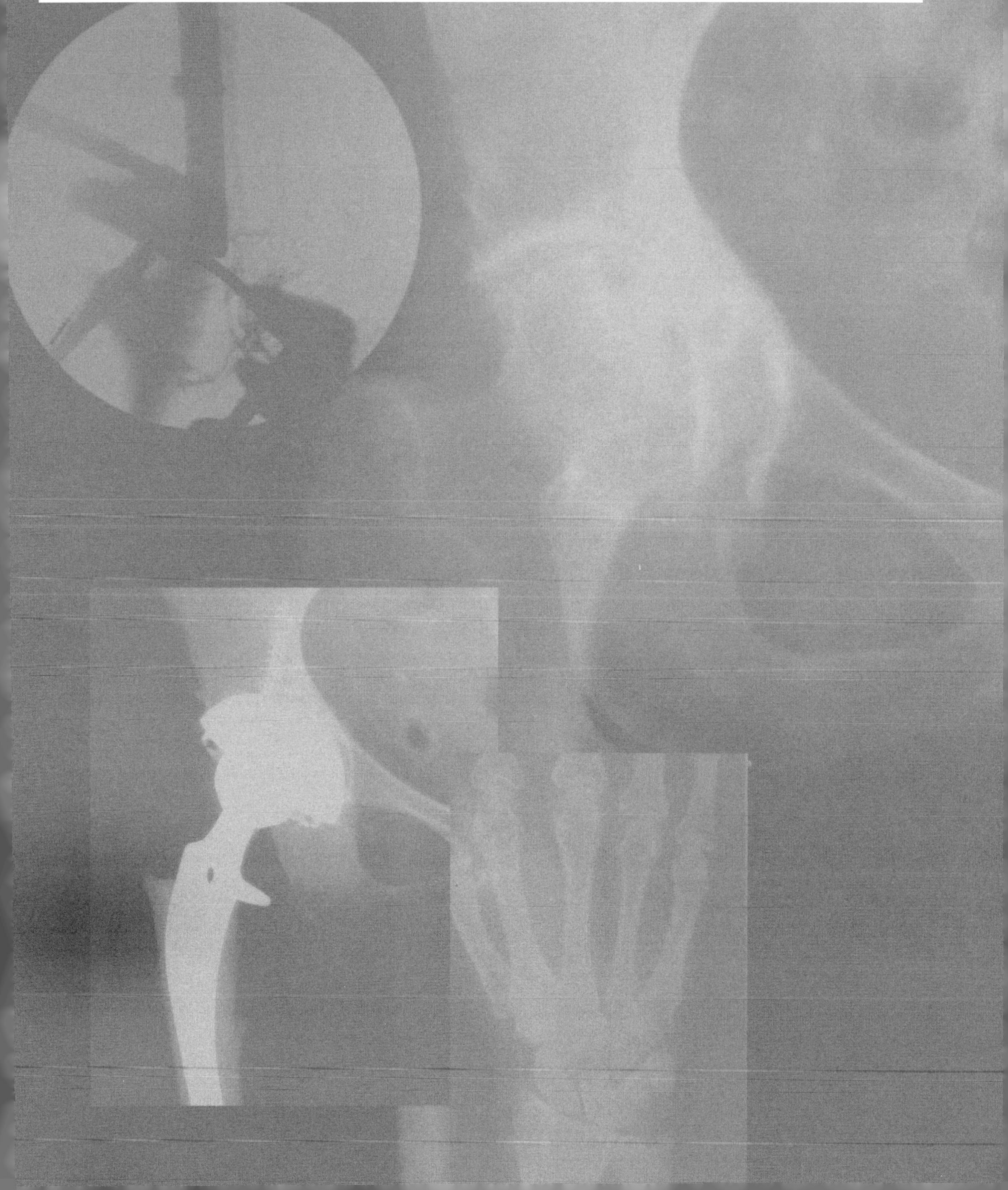

Answers to Study Questions

Chapter 1. Practice Settings for Orthopaedic Nursing

1. d
2. c
3. b
4. b
5. a
6. d
7. a
8. d
9. d
10. a

Chapter 2. Anatomy and Physiology

1. c
2. d
3. b
4. c
5. b
6. b
7. a
8. a
9. d
10. d
11. b
12. a
13. b
14. d
15. c

Chapter 3. Musculoskeletal Assessment

1. d
2. c
3. b
4. a
5. b
6. c
7. c
8. b
9. c
10. a
11. c
12. d
13. b
14. c

Chapter 4. Diagnostic Studies

1. b
2. a
3. a
4. c
5. a
6. c
7. d
8. c
9. c
10. b

Chapter 5. Perioperative Patient Care

1. b
2. d
3. c
4. a
5. c
6. b
7. a
8. b
9. b
10. a
11. c
12. d

Chapter 6. Effects of Immobility

1. b
2. d
3. c
4. b
5. d
6. b
7. b
8. c
9. c
10. a
11. b
12. a
13. b
14. a
15. d

Chapter 7. Pain

1. c
2. c
3. c
4. a
5. b
6. d
7. d
8. c
9. c
10. c
11. b
12. d
13. c
14. d
15. b
16. c
17. d
18. c
19. d

Chapter 8. Complications

1. c
2. c
3. a
4. b
5. d
6. c
7. d
8. b
9. a
10. d
11. b
12. a
13. d
14. d

Chapter 9. Infections

1. b
2. c
3. b
4. b
5. d
6. d
7. a
8. c
9. b
10. a
11. b
12. a
13. c
14. c
15. b

Chapter 10. Therapeutic Modalities

1. a
2. a
3. c
4. d
5. d
6. b
7. b
8. d
9. c
10. b
11. c
12. b

Chapter 11. Pediatric and Congenital Disorders

1. b
2. b
3. d
4. a
5. c
6. d
7. c
8. d
9. a
10. b
11. a
12. d
13. b
14. a
15. a

Chapter 12. Arthritis and Connective Tissue Disorders

1. c
2. b
3. d
4. c
5. a
6. c
7. a
8. d
9. a
10. c
11. b

Chapter 13. Metabolic Bone Conditions

1. d
2. b
3. c
4. b
5. a
6. d
7. a
8. d
9. b
10. d

Chapter 14. Trauma

1. d
2. b
3. b
4. b
5. a
6. d
7. b
8. d
9. b
10. c

Chapter 15. Tumors of the Musculoskeletal System

1. a
2. b
3. d
4. c
5. d
6. d
7. d
8. a
9. b
10. c

Chapter 16. The Shoulder

1. d
2. b
3. a
4. a
5. d
6. b
7. a
8. b
9. a
10. c

Chapter 17. Nursing Care for Hand and Wrist Problems

1. b
2. c
3. a
4. b
5. d
6. d
7. b
8. d
9. c
10. b
11. d
12. a
13. d
14. b
15. b

Chapter 18. The Spine

1. c
2. c
3. d
4. d
5. c
6. b
7. a
8. b
9. c
10. b
11. a

Chapter 19. The Hip, Femur, and Pelvis

1. d
2. b
3. d
4. a
5. b
6. d
7. b
8. c
9. d
10. d

Chapter 20. The Knee

1. d
2. d
3. d
4. c
5. c
6. b
7. a
8. c
9. b
10. a
11. b
12. d
13. d
14. c
15. d

Chapter 21. Foot and Ankle

1. b
2. a
3. c
4. a
5. d
6. b
7. b
8. c
9. c
10. a

INDEX

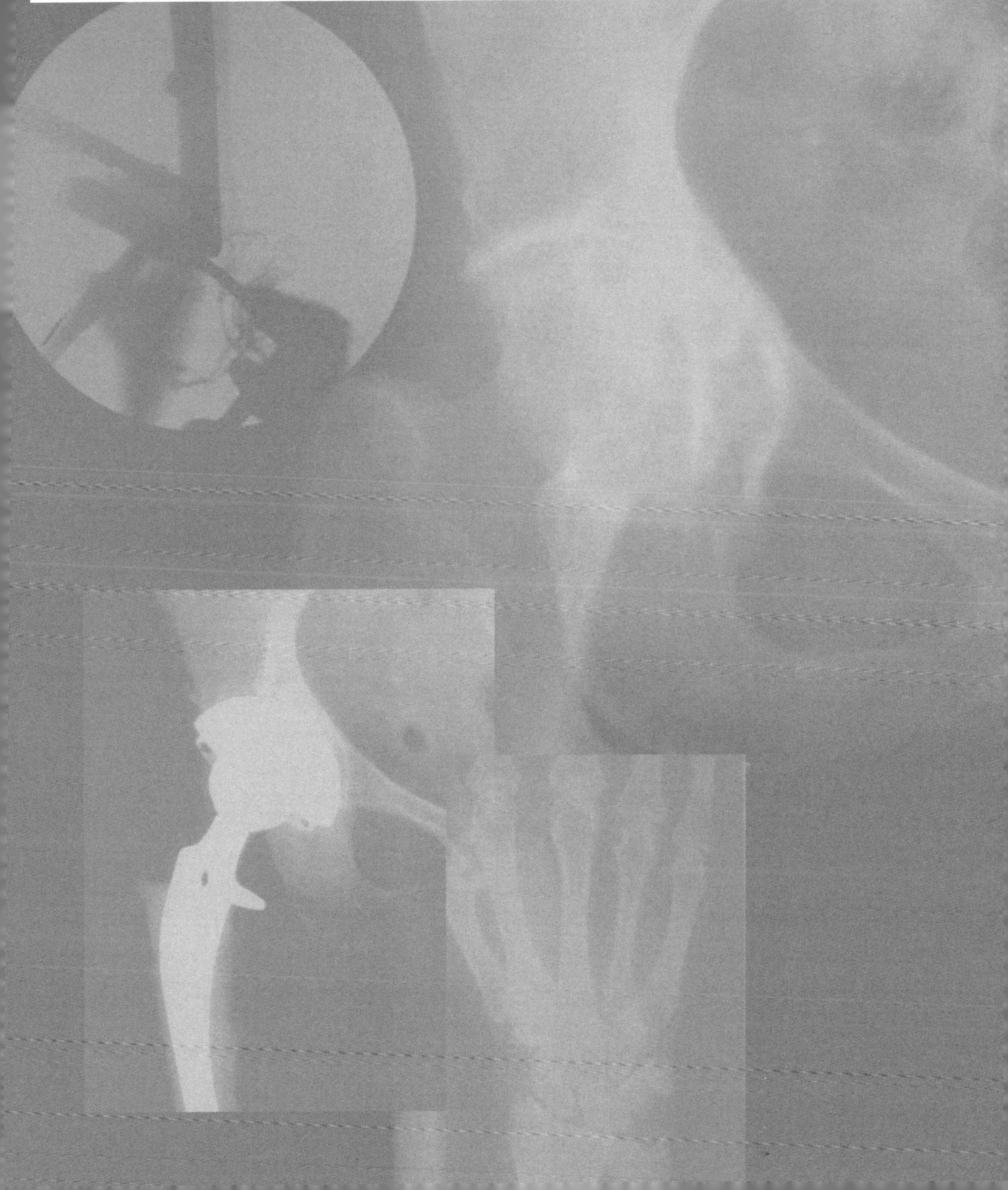

INDEX

A

B

C

D

E

F

G

H

I

J

K

L

M

N

O

P

Q

R

S

T

U

V

W

X

Y

Corporate Sponsors

The National Association of Orthopaedic Nurses thanks the following companies for their generous financial support of the Core Curriculum for Orthopaedic Nursing.

Amgen Inc.
One Amgen Center Drive
Thousand Oaks, CA 91320
Web site: www.amgen.com

Description of Company/Orthopaedic Products:
Amgen, the world's largest independent biotechnology company, was founded in Thousand Oaks, California in 1980. Amgen aspires to be the best human therapeutics company. We live the Amgen Values and use science and innovation to dramatically improve people's lives.

In-depth knowledge, developed through the utilization of state-of-the-art cellular and molecular biology, enables Amgen scientists to discover and develop both naturally occurring proteins and small molecules as potential human therapeutics.

Amgen currently markets three products: EPOGEN® (Epoetin alfa), NEUPOGEN® (Filgrastim), and INFERGEN® Interferon alfacon-1).

Imagination, technical proficiency, and dedication are the foundation for the development of innovative pipeline candidates that will be part of Amgen's future. Our search for breakthrough therapeutics remains broad and scientifically entrepreneurial.

We look for opportunities to complement our in-house research efforts by developing important synergies with academia and industry through the licensing of products, product candidates, and advances in technology. We focus our research and product development in areas such as blood cell development, neuroscience, inflammation, cancer, and endocrinology. In the future, such products may be used to treat cancer, disorders of the blood and bone marrow, infectious disease, obesity, neurodegenerative diseases such as Parkinson's, and Alzheimer's disease.

DePuy, a Johnson & Johnson Company
700 Orthopaedic Drive
PO Box 988
Warsaw, IN 46580-0988
Telephone: 800.47DEPUY
Fax: 219.268.7196
Web site: www.depuy.com

Description of Company/Orthopaedic Products:
DePuy, a Johnson & Johnson Company, is the world's oldest and largest orthopaedic company and is a leading designer, manufacturer, and distributor of orthopaedic devices and supplies. DePuy products are used in both surgical and nonsurgical therapies to treat patients with musculoskeletal conditions resulting from degenerative diseases, deformities, trauma, and sports-related injuries.

Purdue Pharma L.P.
One Stamford Forum
201 Tresser Boulevard
Stamford, CT 06901-3431
U.S. Telephone: 203.588.8000/Fax: 203.588.8850
Web site: www.purduepharma.com

Description of Company/Orthopaedic Products:
Purdue Pharma L.P. is a research-oriented pharmaceutical company which seeks to provide a benefit to patients by providing new and improved treatments for diseases and their symptoms. Purdue seeks to continually develop and sell new, high quality, innovative, pharmaceutical preparations, which together with clinical data and medical education create new value for patients and the health care system. Purdue is engaged in the research, development, marketing, sales, distribution, and licensing of prescription pharmaceuticals, over-the-counter medicines, and hospital products. Our company is dedicated to providing new and improved treatments for diseases and their symptoms. We are a world leader for delivering the best possible care for people in pain. For more information, visit the Partners Against Pain Web site, www.partnersagainstpain.com.